Neonatology Questions and Controversies
Neurology

Neonatology Questions and Controversies
Neurology
Fourth Edition

Series Editor

Richard A. Polin, MD
William T Speck Professor of Pediatrics
Executive Vice Chair Department of Pediatrics
Vagelos College of Physicians and Surgeons
Columbia University
New York, New York
United States

Other Volumes in the Neonatology Questions and Controversies Series

GASTROENTEROLOGY AND NUTRITION

HEMATOLOGY AND TRANSFUSION MEDICINE

INFECTIOUS DISEASE, IMMUNOLOGY, AND PHARMACOLOGY

NEONATAL HEMODYNAMICS

RENAL, FLUID AND ELECTROLYTE DISORDERS

THE NEWBORN LUNG

Neonatology Questions and Controversies

Neurology

Jeffrey M. Perlman, MBChB
Professor of Pediatrics
Division of Neonatology, Department of
Pediatrics
NewYork Presbyterian Hospital - Weill
Cornell Medicine
New York, New York
United States

Terrie Inder, MBChB, MD
Director
Center for Neonatal Research
Childrens Hospital of Orange County
Professor of Pediatrics
University of California
Irvine, California
United States

Consulting Editor
Richard A. Polin, MD
William T Speck Professor of Pediatrics
Executive Vice Chair Department of Pediatrics
Vagelos College of Physicians and Surgeons
Columbia University
New York, New York
United States

ELSEVIER

Elsevier
1600 John F. Kennedy Blvd.
Ste 1800
Philadelphia, PA 19103-2899

NEONATAL QUESTIONS AND CONTROVERSIES:
NEUROLOGY, FOURTH EDITION

ISBN: 978-0-3238-8077-0

Notice

Practitioners and researchers must always rely on their own experience and knowledge in evaluating and using any information, methods, compounds or experiments described herein. Because of rapid advances in the medical sciences, in particular, independent verification of diagnoses and drug dosages should be made. To the fullest extent of the law, no responsibility is assumed by Elsevier, authors, editors or contributors for any injury and/or damage to persons or property as a matter of products liability, negligence or otherwise, or from any use or operation of any methods, products, instructions, or ideas contained in the material herein.

Previous editions copyrighted 2019, 2012 and 2008.

Content Strategist: Sarah Barth
Senior Content Development Specialist: Vasowati Shome
Publishing Services Manager: Shereen Jameel
Senior Project Manager: Beula Christopher
Design Direction: Margaret M. Reid

Printed in India

Last digit is the print number: 9 8 7 6 5 4 3 2 1

Working together
to grow libraries in
developing countries

www.elsevier.com • www.bookaid.org

Contributors

Peter Anderson (John), PhD
School of Psychological Sciences
Monash University
Clayton, Victoria
Australia

Samudragupta Bora, PhD
Department of Pediatrics
University Hospitals Rainbow Babies and Children's
    Hospital
Case Western Reserve University School of Medicine
Cleveland, Ohio
United States

Dalit Cayam-Rand, MD
Staff Neurologist
Neuropediatric Unit
Shaare Zedek Medical Center
Jerusalem, Israel

Lina Chalak, MD, MSCS
Professor, Division Chief
Department of Pediatrics
UT Southwestern Dallas
Dallas, Texas
United States

Vann Chau, MD, FRCPC
Pediatric Neurologist
Department of Pediatrics (Neurology)
The Hospital for Sick Children
Associate Professor of Pediatrics
Department of Pediatrics (Neurology)
University of Toronto
Toronto, Ontario
Canada

Basil T. Darras, MD
Associate Neurologist-in-Chief
Boston Children's Hospital
Distinguished Joseph J. Volpe Chair in Neurology
Harvard Medical School
Boston, Massachusetts
United States

Jahannaz Dastgir, DO
Pediatric Neuromuscular Medicine Physician
Goryeb Children's Hospital
Morristown, New Jersey
United States

Linda S. de Vries, MD, PhD
Emeritus Professor
Department of Neonatology
University Medical Center
Utrecht
Emeritus Professor
Department of Neonatology
Leiden University Medical Center
Leiden, The Netherlands

Mohamed El-Dib, MD
Director of Neonatal Neurocritical Care
Department of Pediatrics
Brigham and Women's Hospital
Associate Professor of Pediatrics
Harvard Medical School
Boston, Massachusetts
United States

Jarred Garfinkle, MDCM, MSc, FRCPC
Assistant Professor
Department of Pediatrics
McGill University
Montréal, Québec
Canada

v

Hannah C. Glass, MDCM, MAS
Professor
Department of Neurology and Pediatrics
University of California, San Francisco
San Francisco, California
United States

Jane E. Harding, MBChB, FRACP, DPhil
Professor of Neonatology
Liggins Institute
University of Auckland
Auckland, New Zealand

Petra S. Hüppi, MD
Professor
Division of Development and Growth
Department of Pediatrics
University Childrens Hospital
University of Geneva
Geneva, Switzerland

Terrie Inder, MBChB, MD
Director
Center for Neonatal Research
Childrens Hospital of Orange County
Professor of Pediatrics
University of California
Irvine, California
United States

Nazia Kabani, MD, MSPH, BS, FAAP
Assistant Professor
Department of Pediatric Infectious Disease and
 Neonatology
University of Alabama at Birmingham
Birmingham, Alabama
United States

Ericalyn Kasdorf, MD
Associate Professor of Clinical Pediatrics
Weill Cornell Medicine
New York, New York
United States

David A. Kaufman, MD
Professor
Department of Pediatrics
University of Virginia School of Medicine
Charlottesville, Virginia
United States

Jennifer C. Keene, MD, MS, MBA
Assistant Professor
Pediatric Neurology
University of Utah
Salt Lake City, Utah
United States

David W. Kimberlin, MD
Professor of Pediatrics
Department of Pediatrics
Sergio Stagno Endowed Chair in Pediatric Infectious
 Diseases
Co-Director
Division of Pediatric Infectious Diseases
University of Alabama at Birmingham
Birmingham, Alabama
United States

Abbot R. Laptook, MD
Professor of Pediatrics
Department of Pediatrics
Warren Alpert School of Medicine at Brown
 University
Medical Director
Neonatal Intensive Care Unit
Department of Pediatrics
Women and Infants Hospital of Rhode Island
Providence, Rhode Island
United States

Gregory A. Lodygensky, MD
Associate Professor
Department of Pediatrics
CHU Sainte-Justine
Montréal, Québec
Canada

Dana McCarty, PT, DPT, PCS
Assistant Professor
Department of Health Sciences
University of North Carolina at Chapel Hill
Chapel Hill, North Carolina
United States

Caroline Menache Starobinski, MD
Department of Pediatrics
Hirslanden Group
Geneva, Switzerland

Steven Paul Miller, MDCM, MAS, FRCPC
Professor and Head
Department of Pediatrics
University of British Columbia
Chief, Pediatric Medicine
Department of Pediatrics
BC Children's Hospital
Vancouver, British Columbia
Adjunct Senior Scientist
Professor (affiliate)
Department of Paediatrics
University of Toronto
Toronto, Ontario
Canada

Shahab Noori, MD, MS, CBTI
Professor of Pediatrics
Department of Pediatrics
USC Keck School of Medicine
Fetal and Neonatal Institute
Division of Neonatology
Children's Hospital Los Angeles
Los Angeles, California
United States

Jeffrey M. Perlman, MBChB
Professor of Pediatrics
Division of Neonatology, Department of Pediatrics
NewYork Presbyterian Hospital - Weill Cornell Medicine
New York, New York
United States

Roberta Pineda, PhD, OTR/L, CNT
Assistant Professor
Chan Division of Occupational Science and Occupational Therapy
University of Southern California
Los Angeles, California
United States

Pablo J. Sánchez, MD
Professor of Pediatrics
Department of Pediatrics
Divisions of Neonatology and Pediatric Infectious Diseases
Center for Perinatal Research
Abigail Wexner Research Institute at Nationwide Children's Hospital
Nationwide Children's Hospital—The Ohio State University College of Medicine
Columbus, Ohio
United States

Mike Seed, MBBS
Division Head, Cardiology
Department of Paediatrics
The Hospital for Sick Children
Associate Professor
Department of Paediatrics
University of Toronto
Toronto, Ontario
Canada

Thiviya Selvanathan, MD, FRCPC
Neonatal Neurology Fellow
Department of Pediatrics
The Hospital for Sick Children
Toronto, Ontario
Canada

Sarbattama Sen, MD
Neonatologist
Department of Pediatric Newborn Medicine
Brigham and Women's Hospital
Assistant Professor
Department of Pediatrics
Harvard Medical School
Boston, Massachusetts
United States

Istvan Seri, MD, PhD, HonD
Professor of Pediatrics
Fetal and Neonatal Institute
Division of Neonatology
Children's Hospital Los Angeles
Department of Pediatrics
Keck School of Medicine
University of Southern California
Los Angeles, California
United States
Faculty of Medicine
First Department of Pediatrics
Semmelweis University
Budapest, Hungary

Emily W. Y. Tam, MDCM, MAS, FRCPC
Clinician Investigator
Department of Paediatrics
Hospital for Sick Children
Associate Professor
Department of Paediatrics
University of Toronto
Toronto, Ontario
Canada

Maria Luisa Tataranno, MD, PhD
Department of Neonatology
University Medical Center, Utrecht Brain Center and
    Wilhelmina Children's Hospital
Utrecht University
Utrecht, The Netherlands

Lauren C. Weeke, MD, PhD
Department of Neonatology
Radboud University Medical Center
Nijmegen, The Netherlands

Andrew Whitelaw, MD, FRCPCH
Emeritus Professor of Neonatal Medicine
Department of Translational Health Sciences
University of Bristol
Bristol, United Kingdom

Vivien L. Yap, MD
Associate Professor of Clinical Pediatrics
Division of Neonatology, Department of Pediatrics
New York Presbyterian Hospital - Weill Cornell
    Medicine
New York, New York
United States

**Crystal Jing Jing Yeo, MB BChir (Distinction), PhD,
MRCP(UK)**
Adjunct Associate Professor of Neurology
Northwestern University
Chicago, Illinois
United States

Santina A. Zanelli, MD, MSc
Professor
Department of Pediatrics
University of Virginia School of Medicine
Charlottesville, Virginia
United States

Series Foreword

Richard A. Polin, MD

"To study the phenomena of disease without books is to sail an uncharted sea, while to study books without patients is not to go to sea at all."

"Medicine is learned by the bedside and not in the classroom. Let not your conceptions of disease come from the words heard in the lecture room or read from the book. See and then reason and compare and control. But see first."

William Osler

Before the invention of the movable type by Johannes Gutenberg in the 15th century, physicians learned medicine by serving an apprenticeship with individuals considered experienced. There were no printed textbooks and medical journals were not published until the beginning of the 19th century. By apprenticing yourself to a physician over a period of years, you learned how to be a competent practitioner. Internships in the United States evolved from those apprenticeships in the 18th century. The term residency was chosen because the physicians in training had a "residence" at the hospital. Modern-day internships began at Johns Hopkins Hospital in 1904. The Johns Hopkins Hospital was founded by Osler, Halstead, Welch, and Kelly. Halstead is credited with creating the first surgical residency and coined the phrase "see one, do one, teach one" (SODOTO). That educational philosophy has been adopted by nearly every specialty in medicine including neonatology.

Modern-day trainees in neonatology still learn how to care for critically ill infants and how to perform procedures by watching, assisting, and listening to more experienced individuals at the bedside. The SODOTO approach is considered a fundamental educational tool. However, over a 3-year period, much of education occurs remote from the bedside during teaching rounds and conferences. The teaching is often more theoretical, and by design, rounds in the nursery and conferences are passive learning exercises. In those settings, trainees listen but do not take an active role in the educational process. Learning is always more effective when the recipient takes an active role in their own education. Ideally, they should be questioning what they hear, reading pertinent literature, and, when the opportunity arises, teaching others. Unfortunately, much of the information transmitted in those settings is not usually followed by an active phase of questioning and reading by the trainee.

Most graduates of fellowship programs turn out to be excellent practitioners, but once they leave the fellowship program, new information is acquired only intermittently either at conferences or from journals and textbooks. As a source of new information, journals provide access to the most up-to-date information. However, that information is unfiltered, and the conclusions of a study may not be appropriate (or perhaps risky) for a critically ill infant. Textbooks like the *Neonatology Questions and Controversies* series offer an opportunity to hear from experts in Neonatal-Perinatal Medicine who have synthesized (and filtered) the existing literature and can provide up-to-date recommendations.

The fourth edition of the *Questions and Controversies* series will also have seven volumes. Each of them has been extensively revised and we have added several new editors: Terrie Inder has joined Jeffrey Perlman for the Neurology volume; James Wynn joined William Benitz and P. Brian Smith as a coeditor for the Infectious Disease, Immunology and Pharmacology volume; and Patrick McNamara is now a coeditor with Martin Kluckow for the Neonatal Hemodynamics volume. The reader will find many completely new chapters; however, like the last edition, each of them is focused on day-to-day clinical decisions encountered by neonatologists. Nothing will replace the teaching that occurs at the bedside when confronted with a critically ill neonate and the SODOTO educational approach still has an important role in education. Procedures are best learned by simulations and guidance by experienced practitioners at the bedside. However, expertise as a practitioner can only be enhanced by reading and incorporating new information into daily practice, once proven safe and effective. Perhaps SODOTO should be changed to LQRT (listen, question, read, and teach). *Questions and Controversies* is a unique source to learn from experts in the field who have been through the LQRT process many times. Osler's quotes at the top of this preface suggest that both bedside teaching and journals/textbooks have a synergistic role in physician education, and neither alone is sufficient.

As with all prior editions, I am indebted to an exceptional group of volume editors who chose the content and authors and edited the manuscripts. I also want to thank Sarah Barth (Publisher), as well as Vasowati Shome and Vaishali Singh (Senior Content Development Specialists) at Elsevier, who have guided the development of this series.

Preface

Our understanding of the basic mechanisms contributing to perinatal brain injury continues to evolve secondary to ongoing research, which has facilitated the introduction of targeted strategies in certain instances. The fourth edition of this book again addresses some of the prominent factors/events contributing to brain injury as well as describes some of the newer treatment strategies. Three new chapters have been added. The first relates to neurological and neurobehavioral evaluation in the neonatal period (Chapter 1). In this chapter it is pointed out that early neurobehavioral assessment can define intervention targets, that is, early occupational therapy, physical therapy, and speech-language pathology services, by identifying existing problems that exist in order to build appropriate therapeutic strategies at the foundations of early development. This should optimize later outcomes. The second is a separate chapter devoted to white matter injury, the commonest form of brain injury in the preterm infant (Chapter 4). The third new chapter focuses on cerebellar hemorrhage in the premature infant (Chapter 5). It is noted that cerebellar hemorrhage has been associated with motor, visuomotor, cognitive, and behavioral problems in early childhood. In addition, hemorrhage affecting the vermis and deeper aspects of the cerebellar hemispheres is more likely to be associated with neurodevelopmental deficits than the more superficial punctate lesion. In Chapter 7, devoted to recent trials for hypoxic-ischemic encephalopathy: Extending hypothermia to infants not previously studied, it is again highlighted that there is little data to indicate benefit from therapeutic hypothermia for hypoxic-ischemic encephalopathy among infants with a mild encephalopathy, preterm infants, or infants in low- or middle-income countries. In Chapter 9, which highlights the acute management of symptomatic seizures, it is pointed out that seizures are a frequent neonatal emergency requiring the use of continuous EEG for accurate, rapid evaluation and treatment. Once identified, antiseizure medication should be promptly optimized but may be safely discontinued during the acute hospitalization, in the setting of acute provoked seizures. In Chapter 12, devoted to congenial viral meningoencephalitis, in addition to neonatal herpes simplex virus, congenital cytomegalovirus, and congenital Zika, the novel coronavirus 2019 (COVID-19) caused by severe acute respiratory syndrome coronavirus 2 (SARS-CoV-2) is discussed. It is noted that cases of vertical transmission have been described but are rare, and most infected neonates tend to have no adverse outcomes. However, given the novelty and constant changes in the virus, there is much still to be learned.

The remaining chapter updates are all outstanding in their depth and comprehensive reviews and make for compelling reading.

The primary goal of this fourth edition is to provide the reader with a clearer management strategy for common and rare neonatal neurological disorders of based on the most updated comprehension of their underlying pathophysiology. A desired secondary goal is to highlight gaps in knowledge which should serve as a strong stimulus for future research.

Contents

Chapter 1

Neurological and Neurobehavioral Evaluation

Roberta Pineda, Dana McCarty, and Terrie Inder

Chapter Outline

What Skill Sets Do Neonates Possess?

Bursts of developmental motor skills (i.e., rolling and subsequent sitting and walking) emerge around 4 months corrected age and serve as predictors for the infant's developmental trajectory.[1] This emergence of developmental skills enables fairly quick assessment of whether an infant is on target or falling behind. However, neonates also possess more subtle, spontaneous behaviors and responses that serve as the building blocks for later function. Making observations on whether developmental milestones have been achieved later in infancy may be simple, compared to the identification of early markers of alteration that are observed during the perinatal period, which often require specialized training and experience to detect.

Many early neurobehavioral assessment components evaluate the presence of reflexes that are essential to normal development and prepare the child for progressive skills.[2,3] Through the process of reflex integration, primitive (spinal and brain stem) reflexes gradually diminish in appearance as higher-order patterns of righting, equilibrium reactions, and voluntary responses manifest.[4] Early primitive reflexes do not fully disappear but instead are inhibited by the cerebral cortex.[5] Subsequently, if inhibitory control of higher centers is disrupted later in life (e.g., stroke, traumatic brain injury), these primitive reflex patterns may re-emerge.[5] When there are alterations in reflex patterns during the perinatal period, it can impact necessary sensory experiences.[6] The infant's early sensory experiences also influence later motor function, including how the infant moves their extremities (i.e., through adequate range to prevent muscle shortening and loss of joint motion) and the development of balanced flexor and extensor muscle groups necessary for postural control and fluid movement.[7-9] All of these factors can impact the achievement of developmental milestones, affect parent-infant bonding, impact reciprocal responses with others, and affect the development of healthy relationships.[10-12]

Beyond reflexes, infants demonstrate a wide range of behaviors, responses, and interactions. For example, a particular marker of infant neural maturity is the extent to which the infant reacts and habituates to environmental stimuli.[8] Other behaviors include the infant's use of the auditory and visual systems to interact with the environment. Further, how the infant responds to and interacts with caregivers is an important component of early neurobehavior. Alterations in any of these behaviors, responses, and/or interactions can indicate a departure from normal development, signaling alterations in brain development, and potentially indicating the need for therapeutic interventions.

With medical advancements in neonatal care, there has been an increased rate of survival of premature infants and other high-risk populations. However, alterations in brain structure and adverse neurodevelopmental outcomes are often observed in high-risk newborns.[13,14] This is evidenced by significant abnormalities of grey and white matter in the brain, as well as reduced overall brain size.[15-18] Subsequently, high-risk infants demonstrate neurobehavioral deficits including poorer postural control, midline behavior, exploratory behaviors, and visual motor skills as compared to their full-term counterparts.[19] High-risk infants can experience various developmental delays including motor, cognitive, or behavioral impairment(s).[20,21] Long-term motor, behavioral, and cognitive deficits may persist throughout childhood and even into adulthood.[22] Medical factors associated with prematurity, such as low birth weight, respiratory support, infection, and brain injury, may further exacerbate developmental deficits.[23-26] Consequently, there is a greater need for addressing immediate and long-term developmental outcomes. The clinician can detect alterations in the neurodevelopmental trajectory during the perinatal period, prior to discharge from the NICU, through the neurological or neurobehavioral exam.[27,28] Such exams can be done at the infant's bedside and have been shown to impose less stress on the infant than typical nursing care.[29]

Overview of the History of Neurological and Neurobehavioral Assessment

The neurological exam can be traced back to the turn of the 20th century; however, the first systemized neonatal neurological exam was reported as early as 1960, conducted by Andre Thomas.[30] Also in the 1960s, Albrecht Peiper identified an extensive portfolio of the development of reflexes and responses, which aided our understanding of neonatal behaviors, with foundational information that has been incorporated into the modern-day neurological exam. Further to his work, Lily and Victor Dubowitz developed a scale to determine gestational age of the newborn in the 1970s, which led to the pioneering development of a neurological scale for neonates in the early 1980s. Ground-breaking work by Prechtl and colleagues aided an understanding of early movement patterns during the perinatal period, including identifying a change in movement patterns that occurs in the first couple months of life (corrected) and continues through 20 weeks corrected age.[31] Refinements in the neurological exam continue to occur, as more evidence emerges and as new interventions, such as hypothermia for the infant with hypoxic-ischemic encephalopathy, are integrated into clinical care.

The difference between neurological exams and neurobehavioral assessments can be clouded, as there can be significant overlap. The purpose of the neurological exam is to test the function of the brain, spinal cord, and nerves, and the neurobehavioral exam expands upon that to the understanding of infant behavior. The use of neurobehavioral assessments can be traced back to at least 1956 when Graham and colleagues developed the Graham Scale and later the Graham-Rosenblith Scale[32,33] to better understand the behavioral differences of infants in their care. Prechtl and Beintema differentiated between behavioral states and noted that responses to the same stimulus varied based on the infant's state.[34] Beginning in the 1950s and continuing through the 1990s, several scholars developed scales to aid in quantifying early behavior including Graham and Rosenblith,[32,33] Yang,[35] Prechtl and Beintema,[36] Scanlon,[37] Parmelee,[38] and Amiel-Tison.[39] Brazelton's work, on which many of the modern-day assessments are based, recognized the complexity of newborn infants' skills and began developing formal assessments in an effort to capture this complexity as well as to chart an individual infant's development.[40] The first version of the Neonatal Behavioral Assessment Scale (NBAS), called the Cambridge Neonatal Scales, was published in 1971[41] and set the stage for a deeper understanding of neonates as social beings able to respond to and interact with their environment and their caregivers. Other pioneers, including Als, Lester, and Tronick, developed the Assessment of Preterm Infant Behavior[42] and the NICU Network Neurobehavioral Scales.[43] These tools have similarities and differences in the items and scoring represented on the original NBAS. Additional variations of the neurobehavioral exam continue to emerge, with tools that can be used in infants at very young postmenstrual ages or with infants who are on significant respiratory support, tools that can aid in the identification of behaviors that are specific to the age of the infant, and tools that target different areas of complex behavior or motoric responses.

The Neurological Exam

GENERAL FEATURES

Observation is critical in each domain of the systematic neurological examination of the newborn. Observations must be made in context of physical features, such as appearance of the skin, due to the relationships between the neurological system and ectoderm. Physical clues, such as sacral dimples, may relate to neurological integrity and can be put in the context of findings from the neurological evaluation. Head circumference can be measured with a tape measure, with a full-term infant measuring an average of 35 (+2) cm. The outward head circumference is informative, as it is reflective of underlying brain structure and development.

MENTAL STATUS

Timing of the examination is a careful consideration in the newborn so that the neurological evaluation can be captured when the infant is in a quiet and calm state. More than one assessment may be more informative than an isolated assessment at one moment in time. One of the best times to undertake the evaluation is between feedings. It is also important to ensure that the infant is not distressed in any other way, such as following a painful procedure or when affected by medications such as sedatives or analgesics. The best way to study mental state is by observation of the newborn infant's spontaneous behavior with minimal handling. Careful observation of eye opening, spontaneous movements of the face and extremities, and the extent of any response to stimulation can be informative. The state of arousal is defined by both the combination of eye opening and spontaneous movements. It is important to note that there are also developmental changes that occur from preterm birth to term equivalent. As the newborn matures toward term equivalency, there is increasing duration, frequency, and quality of alertness. After 28 weeks postmenstrual age, stimulation consistently results in the infant waking for several minutes. By 32 weeks postmenstrual age, no stimulation is needed for arousal. After 36 weeks postmenstrual age, increased alertness is readily observed, as are well-formed sleep-wake cycles. Abnormalities in mental status are recognized as alterations in the levels of arousal and alertness. These neurologic abnormalities are among the most common noted during the newborn period but often are subtle, so careful attention is needed. The general descriptions of mental status alterations include hyperalertness, lethargy, stupor, and coma. In the hyperalert state, the infant is often noted to have "wide eyes" and more frequent tremulous type movements, with reflexes that may be excessive or hyper-responsive. The hyperalert infant will often not organize to feed well and often will not easily move into a sleep state. In contrast, the lethargic infant is "sleepy" and difficult to arouse or open their eyes, even when stimulated or hungry. The lethargic infant may also be noted to have low tone and reduced movements, both spontaneously and when stimulated. Stupor and coma describe an infant who cannot be aroused to open their eyes. Lack of responsiveness often results in the infant being intubated and ventilated. In the term born infant, the distinction between stupor and coma relates specifically to the quality of the movements. In coma, all movements are reflexive withdrawal from painful stimuli, with no decrement in the withdrawal reflex response.

CRANIAL NERVES

There are 12 cranial nerves (CNs), and they can all be examined in the newborn but are often overlooked. CN I is olfaction and can be tested by introducing a smell (such as peppermint extract), which elicits a sucking arousal or withdrawal response in an infant from 30 to 32 weeks postmenstrual age. Breast milk scent has also been demonstrated to induce an olfactory response. CN II and III (optic and oculomotor nerves) can be tested by observing eye blinking in response to light, which can begin from 25 to 26 weeks postmenstrual age. These CNs can further be evaluated through consistent visual fixation on a target (e.g., human face or red object) by 34 weeks postmenstrual age and subsequently through tracking of the stimulus in a 180-degree arc by term equivalency. Random eye movements may be observed in the newborn, particularly if the infant is in a drowsy state or stressed by light in the environment. Shielding direct light from the infant may produce different results. One can detect the eyes moving conjugately in the opposite direction to head movement from 26 to 28 weeks postmenstrual age. Facial sensation

(CN V—trigeminal nerve) can be tested with pinprick and by observing facial grimace or observation of the movement with mastication and sucking. It can also be tested with the corneal reflex, which should be present starting at 26 weeks postmenstrual age. Facial motility represents the function of CN VII (facial nerve) and is best assessed by observation of the symmetry and movement of the face in both the quiet alert state and during movement with crying. Hearing (CN VIII—vestibulocochlear nerve) can be tested with any loud noise and by observing the infant's response. Such responses may be subtle and include visual blinking to the sudden, loud noise starting at 28 weeks postmenstrual age. To test CN V, VII, and XII (trigeminal, facial, and hypoglossal nerves), the newborn can be observed sucking on a pacifier to identify sucking, swallowing, and coordination with breathing. Synchronous swallowing does not occur until approximately 34 weeks postmenstrual age, and sucking is not fully coordinated with breathing until 36 to 37 weeks postmenstrual age. Cranial nerve XI (accessory nerve) controls the sternocleidomastoid muscle function, which controls flexion and rotation of the neck. This is best assessed by observation for any atrophy or fixed posture. Cranial nerve XII (hypoglossal nerve) can be examined by observing the tongue for atrophy or fasciculations.

MOTOR EXAMINATION

The major features of the motor examination of the newborn include the descriptions of muscle bulk, muscle tone, posture of the limbs, spontaneous and elicited movements, and muscle power, as well as deep tendon and primitive reflexes. Examination of the muscle bulk as well as the presence of any contractures should be identified. Tone is best evaluated by observing the resting posture and passively manipulating the limbs. It is important to avoid head turning (keep the head in midline), as it can elicit a tonic neck reflex and give false asymmetries in tone. Flexor tone tends to develop first in the lower extremities and proceed cephalad. At 28 weeks postmenstrual age, the infant lies in extended positioning with minimally flexed extremities and has minimal resistance to passive movement. By 32 weeks, distinct flexor tone begins in the lower extremities with more resistance present to passive movement. By 36 weeks, flexor tone is prominent in the lower extremities and palpable in the upper extremities with flexion at the elbows. In addition to passive tone, the nature of both the quality and the quantity of the infant's spontaneous movements matures from 28 weeks to term equivalent. For example, the more immature infant at 28 to 30 weeks postmenstrual age will have more twisting-type symmetric movements of the extremities. By term, movements may best be described as large-amplitude, slow, and asymmetric movements that are fluid and elegant and rotate around the major joints in an unpredictable (not cramped) fashion. For muscular power, one can assess the strength of lower or upper extremity withdrawal to stimulation and the infant's ability to hold their head upright when held prone in the midline.

SENSORY EXAMINATION

While use of pinprick to elicit sensory responses has been used for many decades, the response to touch can provide much information without noxious stimuli. Many early reflexes are elicited through a touch stimulus, such as palmar and plantar grasp, galant, and rooting. Eliciting these responses can tell you a lot about sensory processing. The time of greatest focus on the sensory examination is related to concerns for a spinal injury, which may produce a dermatome or spinal level where sensation is lost. This can be assessed by using a blunt end of a cotton applicator to scratch or indent the skin from the lower limbs through the truncal region and monitoring for a grimace, which indicates sensation.

REFLEXES

The deep tendon reflexes in the pectoralis, biceps, and brachioradialis as well as reflexes in the knee and ankle can be elicited in the infant from 32 to 34 weeks postmenstrual age and should be assessed, even if they are hard to elicit, which is not uncommon. Following the evolution of the reflexes can be very helpful, especially following a brain injury, as they evolve over days to weeks. Symmetric ankle clonus of 5 beats, with decrement, can be a normal finding in a healthy full-term newborn.

PRIMITIVE REFLEXES

There are five major primitive reflexes that provide useful information: the Moro reflex, palmar and plantar grasp, tonic neck responses, placing reflex, and stepping reflex. The Moro reflex is the most commonly tested primitive reflex and is elicited by dropping the infant's head in relation to the body. A full reflex consists of bilateral hand opening with upper extremity extension and abduction followed by flexion. The Moro emerges from 28 weeks postmenstrual age to 37 weeks postmenstrual age (with disappearance by 4 months corrected age). The palmar grasp reflex is tested by stimulating the palm with a finger. It is present from 28 weeks postmenstrual age and increases in strength. By 37 weeks postmenstrual age, the palmar grasp is strong enough to lift the baby off the bed. The palmar grasp integrates by 2 months corrected age. The asymmetric tonic neck reflex is elicited by rotating the head to one side, resulting in elbow extension occurring to the side the head is turned and elbow flexion on the other side. It appears after 35 weeks postmenstrual age, is well established at 1 month, and is integrated by 5 to 7 months corrected age. For the placing reflex, the infant is held under the axilla in an upright position, and the dorsal aspect of the foot is brushed against an edge, producing hip and knee flexion, with the infant appearing to take a step.

Beyond the Neuro Exam: The Neurobehavioral Assessment

The definition of neurobehavioral assessment includes evaluation of a person's neurological state by observing his or her behavior; establishing relationships between the nervous system and behavior; and connecting how the brain influences emotion, behavior, and learning.[44] Neurobehavioral assessment is an expansion of the neurological exam, which traditionally involves elicitation of a response and an observation of that response. In addition to motoric and reflexive responses, the neurobehavioral assessment further aims to identify behaviors such as capacity for self-regulation, stress reactions and responses to interactions, habituation, and an expansion of other behavioral responses and observations of orientation, posture, reflexes, and movement.

STATE REGULATION

State regulation refers to how an infant achieves and maintains an appropriate state to learn from and interact with the environment. An awake quiet state is well-understood to be the best state for learning. The infant who is unable to achieve this (their state is too low or state is too high) is unable to optimally take in and process important sensory information for appropriate behavioral outputs. The clinician can understand an infant's state regulatory capacity by identifying how well the infant transitions between states of arousal and maintains an appropriate state in the midst of environmental stimuli. How the infant copes with stressors can also provide powerful information about infant self-regulatory capacity. State regulation is an important construct influencing the neurological and neurobehavioral exam, because many items must be assessed in a particular state (e.g., awake quiet state, drowsy). For example, it is inappropriate to assess tone in a crying or sleeping infant, and orientation cannot be assessed in an infant unable to achieve an awake state. For many neurobehavioral exams, state regulation is assessed throughout the exam (or as part of a naturalistic observation during a caregiving task) as the infant shows their ability to rouse from sleep and make smooth transitions from state to state. Self-soothing or calming can also be noted when the infant becomes stressed or disorganized or demonstrates a crying response. Subsequently, whether the infant copes with the stressor on their own or needs assistance from the caregiver (and how much assistance is needed to re-achieve a stable state for interaction) can be identified.

STRESS/RESPONSES TO INTERACTIONS

Infants can demonstrate different responses to stressors within the environment. The stressor need not be a painful stimulus but may also include necessary hospital-based tasks such as increasing lighting, picking up the infant to hold, or changing the diaper. Stress responses can come in the form of autonomic/physiological (e.g., heart rate drop, color change, stooling), motor (e.g., facial grimace, back arching, finger splaying), state (e.g., going into a diffuse sleep state), or attentional (e.g., gaze aversion away from an interaction) responses. How quickly an infant demonstrates stress during the exam or caregiving interaction, what strategies they use to cope (e.g., sucking, foot bracing, or hand clasping), and if and how quickly they recover can provide important information on stress thresholds and maturity of the central nervous system.

HABITUATION

Habituation refers to the infant's ability to discriminate stimuli in the environment that are not of importance in order to tune them out. This skill is important, because a continual response to a stimulus results in increased attention to it, leading to increased energy expenditure and the infant's inability to focus on other stimuli. These continuous responses to environmental stimuli and subsequent inability to habituate can also impact infant sleep. Habituation in the newborn is usually assessed by ringing a bell or shaking a rattle for a few seconds next to the ear, observing for a motoric response, waiting for the response to stop, and then re-introducing the stimuli up to 10 times to determine if the infant habituates or stops responding to it within the sequence.

EXPANDED OBSERVATIONS OF ORIENTATION

The visual and auditory systems are important conduits for understanding the environment. Of note is that the visual system is the last to develop, with its full development not being mature until close to term equivalent age. Aside from the development of stationary visual fixating, the ability to follow a face or target continues to advance from preterm birth to term equivalent age (and beyond). Visual tracking may initially involve short periods of following a target horizontally, then the infant may lose the stimuli in its trajectory, followed by losing the target and finding it again. This will be followed by complete and smooth pursuit across midline and when the target moves vertically and then in an arc. However, during the perinatal period, visual attention and pursuit are best when close to and in line with the infant's visual field, within 12 and 18 inches of the infant's eyes. The auditory system is largely functional by 34 weeks postmenstrual age, and auditory perception and orientation advances from preterm birth to term equivalent age. The preterm infant initially may demonstrate perception (with "brightening") of an auditory stimulus to the side (and responses may be heightened with familiar voice of the parent). This is followed by visual gaze toward that side, followed by head turn. By term equivalent age, the infant can perceive an auditory stimulus, turn the head, and visually localize to the stimulus at the side.

EXPANDED OBSERVATIONS OF TONAL PATTERNS/POSTURAL REACTIONS

Tone, posture, and reflexes all provide important information for the neurobehavioral exam. Tone refers to how responsive the muscles react to movement. The full-term normal newborn assumes a position of physiological flexion with the arms and legs flexed close to the body. If an extremity is pulled into extension and then released, the response is a swift movement back into flexion. The flexed positioning enables the infant to bring the hands to midline and hands to mouth for self-soothing. Further, most primitive reflexes are related to flexion responses. Spontaneous movements during this early period are described as writhing movements. Writhing movements are fluid, elegant, and smooth with joint rotation and without restriction. They are not dominated by reflexive patterns, and there is not a repetitive pattern to the movement. The newborn's muscle tone can vary in the trunk as compared to the extremities; it can vary between upper and lower extremities; and it can vary from one side of the body to the other (as in asymmetry). It is possible for infants to demonstrate low tone and high tone simultaneously; therefore, it is important for the clinician to identify and distinguish where alterations in tone are observed. Moving the infant into a multitude of different positions and testing reflexes on both sides of the body can aid in appreciating these tonal differences. For example, an infant can appear to have increased tone in the trunk and extremities while lying supine in the bed, with increased elicitation of the tonic labyrinthine reflex and increased extension of both the trunk and extremities. However, the same infant, when placed in ventral suspension (infant suspended prone over the examiner's hand), can demonstrate low truncal tone with the extremities, head, and trunk falling into flexion with decreased righting responses.

The Value of the Bedside Exam

The development of imaging technologies has improved our understanding of brain structure and connectivity, but these technologies are not widely available in the clinical setting.[45] More research is needed to better understand brain structure and connectivity and their associations with the infant's functional capacity. Fortunately, examination tools exist to standardize the assessment of human performance during the neonatal period. Standardized neurobehavioral clinical examinations are low-cost, noninvasive methods with little to no risk to the infant that are utilized to identify developmental alterations. These tools can aid in early identification of neurological impairment, define the infant's functional strengths and limitations, and aid in establishing targets for therapeutic intervention. Early detection of developmental delays is important to facilitate early intervention and optimize the developmental trajectory for vulnerable or at-risk populations.[46] Most importantly, it can be used to educate parents so that activities to improve performance can be embedded in day-to-day positioning and tasks. Alterations in function should be determined as early as possible so that the opportunity to ameliorate the deficits through therapeutic interventions is not missed. However, it is important to choose the appropriate clinical evaluation tool in order to best characterize the infant's neurobehavioral function. This can vary according to the age of the infant, the infant's maturity or tolerance of handling, the resources and training that are available, and the purpose or information sought from the exam.

There is a larger repertoire of standardized tools that can be used to assess development later in infancy and into early childhood.[47,48] Such tools designed for after the neonatal period largely define skills that are appropriate at each developmental stage and assess whether the infant has achieved those skills. Other assessments require observation of posture and reflexive patterns to determine whether they exist within the typical timeframe of development.[49-51] However, tools used in later infancy and childhood often do not discriminate alterations in function during the neonatal period, nor are they sensitive to factors unique to the perinatal developmental stage.[52] Thus tools for the perinatal period are designed for use during a finite period of development, with most only used from preterm birth (or full-term birth) up to 6 to 8 weeks corrected age. The incompatibility of tools from the perinatal period to early childhood can pose challenges, which highlights the importance of using appropriate tools to capture the distinct stage of infant development occurring around the infant's due date.

Choosing the Right Neurobehavioral Assessment

Information derived from an assessment must be matched with knowledge about typical and atypical development, brain behavioral relationships, experience, brain malformation, nutrition, stress, and other causes of apparent dysfunction. However, determining which assessment tool to use is best guided by factors related to the infant and the type of information the assessor seeks. Different assessments are appropriate for infants at different postmenstrual or corrected ages and amid different medical interventions. Choosing the right tools can be guided by answering several key questions:

(1) What information about the infant is sought by the clinician?
(2) What medical interventions (i.e., respiratory support) are being conducted with the infant at the time the assessment is conducted?
(3) What is the infant's postmenstrual age or corrected age?
(4) What information is needed to aid education and goal setting with the family?

Refer to Table 1.1 for a list of assessments in the perinatal period to aid with determining what tool to use in context.

Neurobehavioral Assessment Training

Some tools require advanced training to conduct, while others can be conducted using standardized instruction manuals without formal training. Regardless of the need for formal assessment-specific training, conducting neurobehavioral assessments (especially on infants who are immature or experiencing acute medical conditions in the NICU) requires advanced handling and observational skills. Many of the more comprehensive assessments introduce stimuli that can be stressful to the developing infant. Although full term, healthy infants usually have appropriate adaptive responses to handle such exams, the premature infant (especially at low postmenstrual ages) may not.[53] It is critical that the examiner has a good understanding of determining risk versus benefit and gauging what tools are appropriate for those infants who can have detrimental effects from environmental stress. Advanced skill enables the examiner to be guided by infant behavioral cues and also to ensure that the infant does not expend an undesirable amount of energy or suffer physiological consequences during the exam. Important education/training that may be necessary to perform neurobehavioral exams includes: a foundational understanding of medical complications and interventions that may limit the scope of the exam, understanding and responding appropriately to infant behavioral cues, employing handling procedures that support the infant during position changes, and eliciting responses in a way that reduces infant stress. Although specific training on neurobehavioral exam techniques may be needed, there are some experiences that can aid in easier acquisition of skill in doing assessments.[54]

Skills necessary to complete a neurobehavioral exam are usually achieved by engaging in clinical practice (that involves frequent infant handling) as a neonatal nurse, occupational therapist, physical therapist, psychologist, or physician for a minimum of several months. Other assessors may achieve handling experience by functioning as a volunteer in the NICU, under mentoring experiences or internships/fellowships in the NICU, and/or through experience with caring for and actively engaging with young infants in other settings.

An assessor should be competent and safe in basic infant handling experiences including:

(1) Dressing and undressing an infant (e.g., onesie or shirt, pants, socks) less than 2 weeks old corrected age efficiently and without causing agitation;
(2) Changing a diaper;
(3) Picking up a baby from a flat surface and holding in arms at chest or shoulder level while maintaining alignment (i.e., neutral neck position);
(4) Safely and adequately positioning an infant prone, supine, side-lying, and sitting;
(5) Safely positioning the infant in the lap;
(6) Independently feeding a baby while responding to infant cues;
(7) Calming the infant using multiple strategies (e.g., hands, pacifier);
(8) Securely swaddling and un-swaddling an infant;
(9) Reading infant signs and cues and responding appropriately;

TABLE 1.1   Neurobehavioral Assessments for Use During the Perinatal Period

Assessment	Age	Considerations for Use	Observational or Elicited Items	Brief Description	Infant Characteristics Assessed	Formal Training Required?	Admin Time (min)
Amiel-Tison Neurological Assessment at Term (ATNAT)	Term equivalent age	Predictive tool	Observational and elicited—infant must be able to tolerate handling and positional changes	Identifies "optimal" vs. "nonoptimal" status to better target infants who would benefit from early intervention services	Ten domains: cranial assessment, neurosensory function, passive muscle tone, axial motor activity, primitive reflexes, palate and tongue, adaptedness to manipulations, feeding autonomy, medical status, unfavorable circumstances at time of exam	No	5
Assessment of Preterm Infant Behavior (APIB)	27 weeks PMA to 1 month corrected age	Extensive training and eligibility requirements; Discriminative tool	Observational and elicited—infant must be able to tolerate handling and positional changes	A comprehensive systematic assessment of the preterm and full-term newborn based on NBAS but with greater focus on self-regulation and disorganization	Autonomic, motor, state, attention, and self-regulation assessed via maneuvers that increase in vestibular and tactile demands on the infant	Yes—~2 years including preparatory competencies, on-site and independent practice, and established reliability with trainer	30–60
Neonatal Behavioral Assessment Scale (NBAS)	36 weeks PMA to 2 months corrected age	Not recommended for infants requiring intensive care; Discriminative tool	Elicited—infant must be able to tolerate handling and positional changes	Identifies full range of individual neurobehavioral functioning and identifies areas of difficulty	Autonomic, motor and reflexes, state, social/attentional	Yes—2-day workshop, and completion of three separate 2-hour reliability sessions	30
General Movement Assessment (GMA)	Preterm birth to 20 weeks corrected age	Predictive tool	Observational	Neuromotor assessment of observed spontaneous movements to identify early central nervous system dysfunction	Movement pattern identification: Writhing: poor repertoire, cramped-synchronous, or chaotic; Fidgety: present, absent, or abnormal	Yes—4–5-day training with GMs Trust	3–5

Continued

TABLE 1.1 Neurobehavioral Assessments for Use During the Perinatal Period—cont'd

Assessment	Age	Considerations for Use	Observational or Elicited Items	Brief Description	Infant Characteristics Assessed	Formal Training Required?	Admin Time (min)
Hammersmith Neonatal Neurological Exam) HNNE	Preterm (~34 weeks PMA) to term equivalent age	Predictive tool	Observational and elicited—infant must be able to tolerate handling and positional changes	A neurological assessment of reflexes, movement and positioning, and behavior	Six categories: posture, tone, reflexes, spontaneous movements, orientation, and behavior	No; courses are available but not required	10–15
Naturalistic Observation of Newborn Behavior (NONB)	28 weeks PMA to 1 month corrected age	Only for use within the setting of NIDCAP-trained nurseries. Useful for understanding infant behavioral organization and when too ill or immature to be examined interactively. Discriminative tool	Observational	Naturalistic observation of the infant in the course of a caregiving intervention as performed in the NIDCAP framework	Quantifies behaviors related to autonomic, state, motor, and attention subsystems	Yes—~2 years including preparatory competencies, on-site and independent practice, and established reliability with trainer prior to use	60–80
Neonatal Behavioral Observation (NBO)	Birth to 3 months corrected age	Can be used as an intervention tool to demonstrate infant capacity to parents and enhance the parent-infant relationship	Elicited—infant must be able to tolerate handling, interactions, and positional changes	Relationship-based tool, designed to sensitize parents to their baby's behavior and foster positive parent-infant interactions	Habituation, muscle tone, reflexes, visual skills, orientation, state regulation, activity, and environmental responses	3-day training	Variable–infant led
NICU Network Neurobehavioral Scale (NNNS)	~32–34 weeks PMA to 6–8 weeks corrected age	For use with preterm, full-term, and/or substance-exposed infants. Predictive tool	Observational and elicited—infant must be able to tolerate handling and positional changes	Assesses at-risk infants, documenting neurological integrity, and broad range of behavioral functioning	Arousal, self-regulation, orientation, hypertonia, hypotonia, stress, excitability, lethargy, tolerance of handling, suboptimal reflexes, and quality of movement	Yes—3-5-day training	20–25

Premie-Neuro	23–37 weeks PMA	The abbreviated form may be used while infant is still intubated or <28 weeks; full form for infants >28 weeks and extubated. Predictive tool	Elicited—reflex testing and motor responses as well as observational	A neurological examination with scoring that indicates performance expected at each week PMA	Three categories: neurological, movement, and responsiveness. Scores can be categorized into normal, questionable, or abnormal	No	3–5 (full) 1–3 (abbreviated)
Test of Infant Motor Performance (TIMP)	34 weeks PMA to 4 months corrected age	Predictive tool	Observational and elicited—infant must be able to tolerate handling and positional changes	Evaluates motor control and organization of posture and movement for functional activities	Orientation head in space, response to auditory and visual stimuli, body alignment, spontaneous limb movements	No—but training is available	30

(10) Identifying signs of infant compromise; and

(11) Demonstrating adequate communication with parents of young infants.

A comprehensive neurobehavioral assessment generally requires the examiner to complete more advanced handling activities in rapid succession while monitoring the infant's signs of tolerance.

These may include:

(1) Unswaddling;

(2) Moving extremities in a particular sequence;

(3) Picking up infant off the surface and holding suspended in a supine position over the bedspace;

(4) Pulling the infant up into a sitting position by holding the arms or shoulders;

(5) Picking the infant up under arms, holding vertically, and allowing the lower extremities to bear weight on the support surface;

(6) Suspending the infant prone over your hand and above the bed surface;

(7) Turning or rolling the infant over;

(8) Rotating the infant's head to one side and then the other.

Tools Available for the Perinatal Period

Below are tools that are available to assess neurobehavior during the perinatal period (in alphabetical order). See Fig. 1.1 for a breakdown of when (age) each assessment is appropriate to assess the infant. For each tool, we describe the information gained from the exam, how long the assessment takes to administer, training that may be required, ages it is appropriate for, and information on its validity and reliability. We have only included tools that are appropriate for the newborn, and for this reason recognize there are tools that can be used in early infancy that are not represented. Parent report measures of function are also not included.

THE AMIEL-TISON NEUROLOGICAL ASSESSMENT AT TERM

The Amiel-Tison Neurological Assessment at Term (AT-NAT) was developed by Claudine Amiel-Tison and colleagues in 1982 and updated in 2002 with the objective of creating an assessment for full-term infants and/or preterm infants at term equivalent age that was both easy to administer and well-tolerated by

the infant and parents.[55] Amiel-Tison sought to replace "at-risk" categorization with "nonoptimal neurological potential" categorization from this assessment in order to better target infants who would benefit from early intervention services.[56] The assessment is made up of 35 observational and manipulation items covering 10 domains (cranial assessment, neurosensory function, passive muscle tone, axial motor activity, primitive reflexes, palate and tongue, adaptedness to manipulations, feeding autonomy, medical status, and unfavorable circumstances at time of exam). Scores that are derived from the assessment indicate "optimal" or "nonoptimal" status, which can be further categorized into mild, moderate, and severe. The ATNAT takes approximately 5 minutes to complete. While training is not required to administer the ATNAT, the authors suggest using the manual, video instructions, and learning from someone who has experience with the assessment.[56] The ATNAT has demonstrated excellent inter-rater reliability[57] and in two small studies suggests good predictive validity with relationships to the Bayley Scales of Infant Development-II at 24 months and the Griffith Mental Scales at preschool age.[58]

ASSESSMENT OF PRETERM INFANTS' BEHAVIOR

The Assessment of Preterm Infants' Behavior (APIB) was developed by Heidelese Als with the objective of assessing infant individuality and competence through observation of behavioral subsystems.[42] The test involves 30 to 60 minutes of naturalistic observation and elicited items administered according to standardized instructions with six sections of increasingly vigorous environmental inputs. The APIB is a criterion-referenced tool that has been identified to be used from 28 weeks postmenstrual age to 1 month corrected age.[42,59] The tool may not be completed in its entirety in young, immature infants unable to tolerate extensive handling. In particular, the APIB components include determination of: (1) the infant's current, newly emerging developmental agendum and the degree of its saliency; (2) the infant's current level of subsystem balance and smoothly integrated subsystem functioning; (3) the threshold of disorganization indicated in subsystem behaviors of defense and avoidance; (4) the degree of relative modulation and regulation of the various subsystems; (5) the degree of

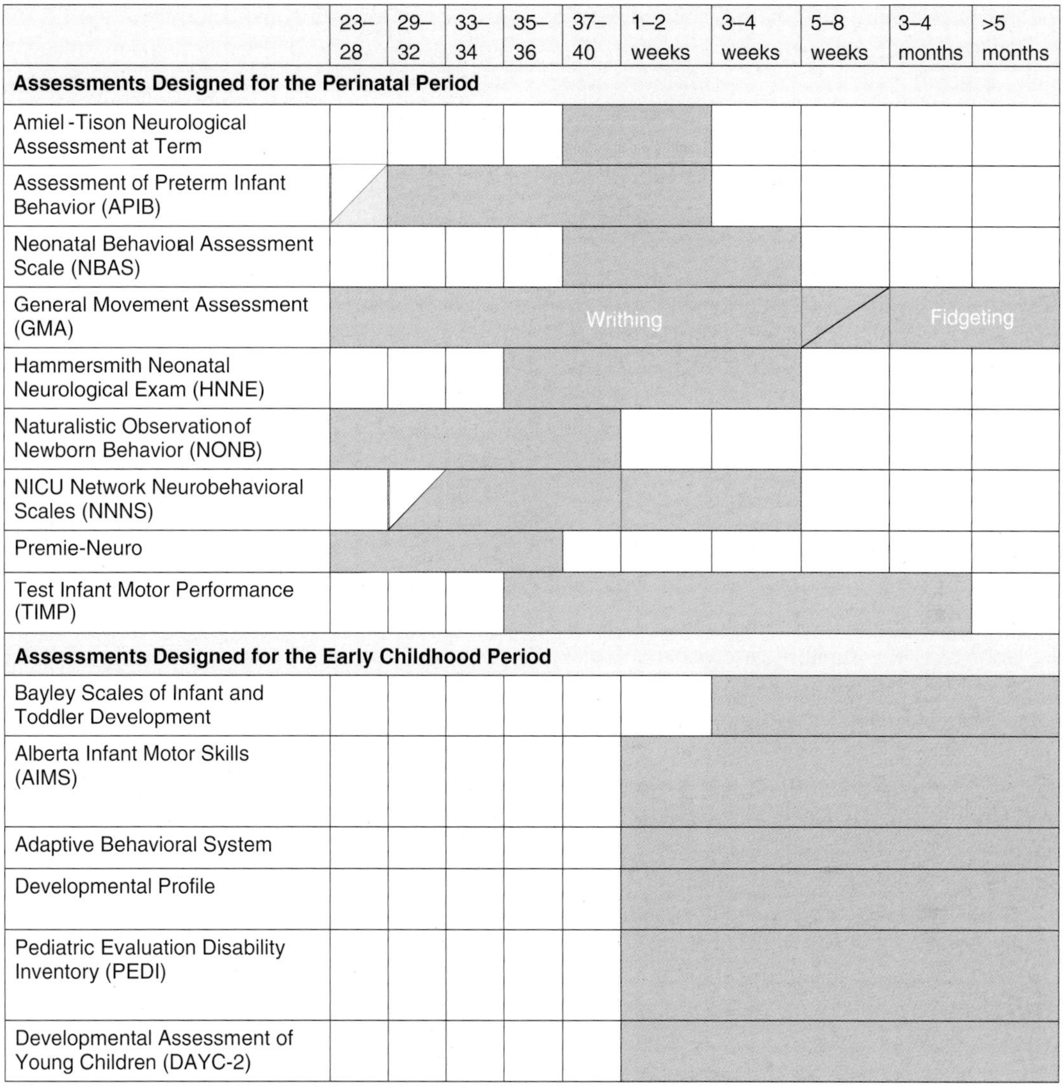

	23–28	29–32	33–34	35–36	37–40	1–2 weeks	3–4 weeks	5–8 weeks	3–4 months	>5 months
Assessments Designed for the Perinatal Period										
Amiel-Tison Neurological Assessment at Term					▓					
Assessment of Preterm Infant Behavior (APIB)	▓	▓	▓	▓	▓					
Neonatal Behavioral Assessment Scale (NBAS)					▓	▓				
General Movement Assessment (GMA)	▓	▓	▓	▓	▓ Writhing	▓	▓	▓	▓ Fidgeting	▓
Hammersmith Neonatal Neurological Exam (HNNE)	▓	▓	▓	▓	▓					
Naturalistic Observation of Newborn Behavior (NONB)	▓	▓	▓	▓	▓					
NICU Network Neurobehavioral Scales (NNNS)		▓	▓	▓	▓					
Premie-Neuro	▓	▓	▓	▓	▓					
Test Infant Motor Performance (TIMP)			▓	▓	▓	▓	▓	▓	▓	▓
Assessments Designed for the Early Childhood Period										
Bayley Scales of Infant and Toddler Development								▓	▓	▓
Alberta Infant Motor Skills (AIMS)					▓	▓	▓	▓	▓	▓
Adaptive Behavioral System					▓	▓	▓	▓	▓	▓
Developmental Profile					▓	▓	▓	▓	▓	▓
Pediatric Evaluation Disability Inventory (PEDI)					▓	▓	▓	▓	▓	▓
Developmental Assessment of Young Children (DAYC-2)					▓	▓	▓	▓	▓	▓

Fig. 1.1 Ages that each assessment are appropriate for (from weeks PMA to weeks and months corrected age).

differentiation and effectiveness in rebalancing the subsystems; (6) the degree of environmental structuring, support, and facilitation necessary to bring about optimal implementation of the new strategies; and (7) the degree of environmental structuring, support, and facilitation necessary to bring about the return to smooth, well-integrated, baseline functioning.[59] Low scores represent well-modulated and well-organized behavioral regulation, while high scores indicate that the infant is easily disorganized, demonstrates poorly modulated behavioral regulation, and has increasing levels of stress.[59,60] In 2022, the APIB required 1 to 2 years of training consisting of three separate 2½-day training sessions spread out over time with two periods of independent preparation and practice in between. The cost of training is negotiated with trainers based on their current daily salary.[61]

The APIB is well known as a tool within the Newborn Individualized and Developmental Care Program (NIDCAP). As part of research inquiry, the APIB has good test-retest reliability, interrater reliability, internal consistency, and accurate discrimination.[42] The APIB has high construct validity and concurrent validity with relationships with MRI and electroencephalography. Similar to the NBAS, it is primarily used for discriminative purposes and not as a predictive tool.

The Assessment of Behavioral Systems Organization (ABSO) scoring tool is based on the systems component (front page) of the APIB. It examines infant behavior in the following subsystems of the Synactive Theory of Development: physiologic organization, motor organization, effectiveness of self-regulatory behaviors, and need for caregiver facilitation of each infant.[62] Each subsystem is scored 1 to 9, with low scores reflecting a well-organized subsystem. The ABSO can be used after becoming reliable in the APIB.

BRAZELTON NEONATAL BEHAVIORAL ASSESSMENT SCALE

The Neonatal Behavioral Assessment Scale (NBAS), initially known as the Cambridge Neonatal Scales, was developed by Brazelton to identify a full range of individual neurobehavioral functioning and areas of difficulty.[41] It may be used with healthy preterm infants (36–37 weeks postmenstrual age and onward, up to 2 months corrected age).[63] It is not recommended for infants still requiring intensive care or recovering from illness due to the potential stress of the assessment.[63] It has a total of 53 items that are either administered or observed in the areas of behavior and neurological status, addressing four domains of neonatal functioning: autonomic regulation, organization of motor behavior, state, and infant attention/social interaction or regulation.[63] The assessment may take half an hour to administer, with additional time required for scoring.[64] The assessment is designed to give a behavioral "portrait" rather than a standard score. Training in the administration of the NBAS is required prior to reliability certification.[65] In 2022, training for the NBAS was $1600 for a 2-day workshop followed by up to three separate 2-hour reliability sessions.[65]

The NBAS has high specificity (94%–97%) and moderate to high sensitivity (50%–78% for classification of mild disability and 71%–85% for classification of severe disability).[60] The NBAS may have limitations in large multi-site studies when more than one examiner

is needed.[66] A distinguished feature of the NBAS is the ability to depict the behavioral profile of infants and to inform clinical intervention aimed at enhancing the parent-infant relationship.[63]

GENERAL MOVEMENT ASSESSMENT

The General Movement Assessment (GMA) was developed by Heinz Prechtl and his team to identify potential neurological concerns through the assessment of movement patterns.[67] At least 3 to 5 minutes of video is captured to assess the infant's movement patterns while the infant is on a flat surface. The GMA is an observational assessment, meaning that there is no elicitation of responses by the evaluator. The earliest movement pattern observed, writhing, can be seen by ultrasound during fetal development or in the NICU following preterm birth. Writhing movements are interpreted as normal, poor repertoire, chaotic, or cramped synchronized. Consistent cramped synchronized movements are related to poor neurodevelopmental outcome.[68] After 6 to 9 weeks corrected age, writhing movements are replaced by fidgety movements, which are present until 20 weeks corrected age. Fidgety movements are interpreted as present (normal), absent (abnormal), or hyperkinetic. Absent fidgety movement patterns are related to poor neurodevelopmental outcome and have higher predictive validity than the earlier writhing patterns.[69] An optimality scoring system that aids in further identification of variation in movement patterns has also been developed.[70] In 2022, training could be achieved over a 4-day course at a cost of $990.[71]

The GMA is currently considered one of the best clinical assessments for detection of early cerebral palsy in young infants.[72,73] The GMA has 98% sensitivity[74] and fair to moderate interrater reliability, with higher reliability among those with more experience.[75] GMA results used in combination with neonatal imaging are >95% accurate in diagnosing cerebral palsy when administered in routine clinical settings.[74,76,77]

HAMMERSMITH NEONATAL NEUROLOGICAL EXAMINATION

The Hammersmith Neonatal Neurological Examination (HNNE) was developed by Lilly and Victor Dubowitz.[78] The developers of the HNNE were also developers of the Ballard exam, a widely accepted scoring system for gestational age estimation focused on a number of neurological and behavioral items. The HNNE is a 34-item evaluation that takes approximately 10 to 15 minutes to administer. Although identified as a neurological examination, the HNNE includes assessment of behavior, in addition to tone, tone patterns, reflexes, spontaneous movement, and abnormal neurological signs. The HNNE Optimality Score is calculated from raw scores from each individual item (scored 0–1),[79] with Optimality Scores below 31.5 deemed "suboptimal." Subscores can also be achieved for posture and tone, tone patterns, reflexes, movements, abnormal signs/patterns, and orientation/behavior. The HNNE has some scoring differentiation for infants as young as 37 weeks postmenstrual age, but the scoring differentiation is only appropriate on a few test items.[80] Instructions on how to administer the HNNE are contained within a textbook[78] as well as on a webpage,[81] and training opportunities have recently started to be offered.

The HNNE is one of the assessment tools that is most widely documented in clinical research during the perinatal period.[82] The HNNE has been used extensively for neurobehavioral assessment of preterm and full-term infants and has been found to be valid and reliable at term equivalent age. Suboptimal HNNE scores have been associated with more brain abnormality including damage to cerebral white matter and cerebellar injury as seen on MRI when performed at term equivalent age. The HNNE also is predictive of neurodevelopmental disability at 1 year corrected age.[83,84]

NATURALISTIC OBSERVATION OF THE NEWBORN

Although not necessarily considered a neurobehavioral assessment, the Naturalistic Observation of the Newborn (NONB) includes observations of the infant for up to 20 minutes prior to a caregiving activity, during the caregiving activity, and then for at least 20 minutes after the caregiving activity.[85] The NONB is learned through the Newborn Individualized and Developmental Care Assessment Program (NIDCAP) and aims to define how robust the infant is in handling caregiving interactions and other stimuli in the environment by quantifying behaviors related to autonomic, state, motor, and attention subsystems.[85] It results in a descriptive report that identifies the infant's threshold for stimuli before becoming disorganized. Training occurs through the Newborn Individualized Developmental Care Program.[86] The NONB is not a predictive tool.

NEWBORN BEHAVIORAL OBSERVATION

The Newborn Behavioral Observation (NBO) tool encompasses 18 neurobehavioral items into a relationship-building tool that aims to provide positive reinforcement to parents and aid them in understanding their infant's language and behavior.[65] The NBO is not an examination or a test, and because it is a relationship-building tool, should only be conducted when parents are present with the infant. The tool includes items that assess the infant's ability to habituate to light and sound; motor tone and activity; self-regulation; stress responses; and visual, auditory, and social interactive capacities. The NBO gives the caregivers a behavioral profile of the infant's strengths and weaknesses to aid parents in meeting their infant's needs. It can be serially used in a variety of clinical settings during the first 3 months of life as an intervention tool focused on infants' unique capacities. The goals of the NBO are enhancement of parental confidence, parent-infant relationships, and family-provider relationships.[87,88] Research has demonstrated that families who had the NBO administered demonstrated better knowledge related to their infant's behavior.[89,90] In 2022, a 3-day training course was available at a cost of $650, a requirement before clinicians may use the tool in practice.[91]

NICU NETWORK NEUROBEHAVIORAL SCALE

The NICU Network Neurobehavioral Scales (NNNS) was developed by Barry Lester and Edward Tronick to provide a standardized, reliable, and predictable measure of infant neurobehavior that was not solely based on optimal criterion performance (such as the NBAS) but also on norm-referenced behavior.[43] The NNNS is a neurobehavioral assessment developed for infants at high risk for medical and developmental problems[92] and can be used on infants born preterm,[93,94] full-term,[95,96] and with prenatal substance exposure.[97,98] The NNNS contains 115 items, of which approximately 45 are elicited responses. It can be conducted once an infant can tolerate multiple position changes and handling over a period of 20 to 25 minutes. The NNNS has been documented to be used in infants as young as 32 and 34 weeks postmenstrual age through 6 to 8 weeks corrected age.[66,99] However, in a sample of infants at 34 weeks postmenstrual age, approximately 90% could tolerate the NNNS, with the other 10% requiring more time for maturation and resolution of medical challenges prior to tolerating the exam.[19] The NNNS assesses the infant's neurological (tone, reflexes), behavioral, and stress/abstinence responses and yields 13 summary scores: habituation, arousal, self-regulation, orientation, hypertonia, hypotonia, stress, excitability, lethargy, asymmetry, tolerance of handling, suboptimal reflexes, and quality of movement.[43]

This scale has been used extensively with preterm infants. When the NNNS is administered shortly before hospital discharge, it has demonstrated acceptable internal consistency (α = 0.87–0.90), good test-retest reliability (α = 0.30–0.44), and predictive validity with relationships to Bayley-II mental (P = .011, R^2 = 0.295) and psychomotor (P =.002, R^2 = 0.441) scores and Ages and Stages Questionnaire scores at age 3.[66,100] In 2020, the NNNS was revised, and is now referred to as the NeoNatal Neurobehavioral Scale II (NNNS-II). Major changes included removal of the asymmetry and habituation scales.[92] Extensive training is required to administer the NNNS. In 2022, this included prior study followed by 3 to 5 days of in-person training and reliability testing at a cost of $2500.[101]

There is also a variation of the NNNS, the Fetal Neurobehavior Coding System (FENS), designed to evaluate fetal neurobehavior by assessing fetal heart rate, motor activity, behavioral state, and responsiveness to extrauterine stimuli.[102] Behaviors from the NNNS are coded from videotaped ultrasound. The mother reclines in a chair, and using ultrasound, the fetus is monitored for 40 to 60 minutes followed by application of a 3-second vibroacoustic stimulus. Fetal neurobehavior using the FENS has been shown to identify infants at risk of developmental impairment.[102] FENS is only used in research at this time.

PREMIE-NEURO

The Premie-Neuro was developed by Donna Daily and Patricia Ellison to aid in detecting alterations in early function among infants who are immature or still undergoing respiratory support, with testing being able to be conducted in a short period of time.[103] The Premie-Neuro is appropriate for infants between 23 and 37 weeks postmenstrual age and intended to be

a precursor to the next in its family, the NeoNeuro[104] (from 37 weeks postmenstrual age to 1 month corrected age) followed by the Infant Neurological International Battery (INFANIB; for 1–18 months corrected age).[105] The Premie-Neuro breaks down infant behavior into three categories: neurological, movement, and responsiveness. In total, 14 out of the 24 items relate to assessment of reflexes and motor responses, with 10 of the 24 items assessing stress signs, excitability, arousal, and other behaviors. Each of the 24 items on the Premie-Neuro is scored based on expected performance for the infant's postmenstrual age. The exam takes approximately 3 to 5 minutes to administer. Raw scores can be used to categorize infant performance into abnormal, questionable, or normal. An abbreviated form is available for infants <28 weeks postmenstrual age or who are intubated. This abbreviated form includes 16 items (8 reflexes and 8 behavioral observations) from the Premie-Neuro that do not require moving the infant away from the supine position. The abbreviated form of the Premie-Neuro can be administered in 1 to 3 minutes. The Premie-Neuro can be learned by reading a manual available from the authors and checking reliability with an experienced clinician. At the time of this publication, training for the Premie-Neuro was being developed.

Validity has been established, and the Premie-Neuro has fair to moderate reliability.[53] The Premie-Neuro conducted at 30 weeks postmenstrual age has been shown to be predictive of neurobehavioral performance at term equivalent age.[28] Further, Premie-Neuro scores have been shown to be predictive of standardized outcomes at 3 months and 24 months.[53] The Premie-Neuro is unique in that it is one of the only tools that differentiate scoring based on the infant's postmenstrual age and the only tool that can be used with infants who are still on a ventilator or <28 weeks postmenstrual age.

The NeoNeuro has received little attention since an article that identified test construction and factor analysis (resulting in 32 items on the test and reported internal consistency or reliability of 0.80).[104] The NFANIB is currently available for use by clinicians and has gone through more psychometric assessment than its counterparts.[105]

TEST OF INFANT MOTOR PERFORMANCE

The Test of Infant Motor Performance (TIMP)[106] was developed by Suzann Campbell, Gay Girolami, Thubi

Kolobe, Elizabeth Osten, and Maureen Lenke.[107] It is a functional movement assessment consisting of 42 items and can be used on preterm and full-term infants as young as 34 weeks postmenstrual age up to 4 months corrected age. It takes approximately 30 minutes to administer and score. Both observation of spontaneous movements and response to elicited items from various positions are used to quantify infant delays.[108] A total score is achieved on the TIMP, with scores increasing with advancing repertoire of skills across time. There are established norms for each age group.

The TIMP is widely used for preterm infant motor developmental assessment due to its excellent reliability and predictive validity.[96,109] It has also been identified as a good tool for early detection of cerebral palsy.[73] The TIMP has good test-retest reliability (r = 0.89), strong interrater reliability (r = 0.95), and strong construct validity.[96,109] The TIMP has demonstrated sensitivity to discriminate between infants with low, medium, or high risk for developmental delays, and scores correlate with risk factors such as white matter injury, intraventricular hemorrhage, chronic lung disease, and neonatal seizures.[110-112] TIMP scores are also highly predictive of other infant and preschool motor assessment scores including the Alberta Infant Motor Scales (AIMS), the Bayley Scales of Infant Development-III (BSID-III), and the Peabody Developmental Motor Scales 2 (PDMS-2).[109,113-115] In 2022, the TIMP could be learned in 15 hours of instruction via in-person workshops or online self-instruction modules at a cost of $379.[116] A unique feature of the TIMP is that the same tool can be used in the NICU prior to discharge and at the first follow-up clinic visit, as most tools designed for the perinatal period do not extend to 4 months corrected age.

Other Assessments During the Neonatal Period

THE EINSTEIN NEONATAL NEUROBEHAVIORAL ASSESSMENT

The Einstein Neonatal Neurobehavioral Assessment was developed in 1977 by Cecilia Daum and colleagues.[117] It has 20 items that assess tone, movement, reflexes, and visual and auditory responses. It takes 30 to 45 minutes to assess. Studies have used the Einstein Neonatal Neurobehavioral Assessment and demonstrated that a normal exam during the newborn period was related to positive outcomes at ages 1 and 3 years. However, abnormal scores on the assessment during the neonatal period were not consistently associated with poor outcome.[118] Further, poorer outcome on visual and auditory responses on the Einstein Neonatal Neurobehavioral Assessment was related to poorer cognitive outcome at 1 and 6 years.[119] Despite recent publications citing the use of this tool, information on how to obtain the assessment, including at the Albert Einstein University where it was developed, could not be found.

NEONATAL NEUROBEHAVIORAL EXAMINATION

The Neonatal Neurobehavioral Examination (NNE) was developed by Andrew Morgan and colleagues due to the need for a more quantified neurological evaluation.[120] It contains 27 items in the categories of tone and motor patterns, primitive reflexes, and behavioral responses. It was developed in the late 1980s with the objective to better define the postmenstrual age that can elicit different variations of responses (modeled after the HNNE). It clusters appropriate responses for infants 37 to 42 weeks, 34 to 36 weeks, and <34 weeks.[120] Other than a publication in 1988 and online evidence that it was translated into Chinese, little more information is available on the NNE.

THE NEUROBEHAVIORAL ASSESSMENT OF THE PRETERM INFANT

The Neurobehavioral Assessment of the Preterm Infant (NAPI) is a criterion-referenced tool used to assess motor development, alertness, and orientation with infants from 32 weeks postmenstrual age until term equivalent age.[121] This tool has been used to document neurodevelopmental maturation over time, with 19 items scored on a 6-point scale along with behavioral state scores and a summary score. The NAPI has been described as having excellent clinical utility with adequate validity.[60] However, in 2022, the NAPI was no longer available on the Stanford website, which is where it was originally developed.

THE NEUROMOTOR BEHAVIORAL ASSESSMENT

The Neuromotor Behavioral Assessment was developed by Burns and O'Callaghan in 1988 to address the need for a reliable postnatal assessment that could quickly be administered with minimal handling.[122] This 10- to 15-minute assessment was designed to detect optimal subsystem functioning in infants 30 to 36 weeks postmenstrual age. The assessment is divided into four sections: neurological items, behavioral items, autonomic items, and motor functions. This tool effectively identified neonates experiencing adverse events from those who did not between 30 and 36 weeks postmenstrual age based on within-test correlations for all age groups and parameters of the assessment.[122] However, this tool has been used minimally in research and clinical practice, with no identified publications since 1988.

Developmental Assessments That Include the Birth Time Frame

There are several developmental assessments that include a timeframe of assessment from birth. Some of these include the Developmental Assessment of Young Children (birth to age 5 years), Alberta Infant Motor Scales (0–18 months), the Bayley Scales of Infant and Toddler Development (ages 16 days to 42 months), Adaptive Behavior Assessment System (birth to 21 years), Developmental Profile 3 (birth to 12 years, 11 months), and Parents' Evaluation of Developmental Status (birth to 7 years, 11 months). Because these tools assess skills over a longer developmental trajectory, with birth being the lower end, they may not discriminate early function in the same way that tools specifically designed for the perinatal age group do. However, they have great value in identifying developmental challenges after the neonatal period. While debatable, developmental assessments typically have more value at 4 months of age and beyond, when there is a burst of developmental skills to classify as present or emerging.

Opinions on timing and frequency of developmental assessment can also be variable based on organizational factors (e.g., clinic capacity) as well as individual factors (e.g., infant tolerance and family accessibility). For example, the American Academy of Cerebral Palsy and Developmental Medicine (AACPDM) have adopted "Early Detection of Cerebral Palsy" guidelines that recommend a battery of neurological exams, neurological imaging, and motor assessments from 0 to 24 months corrected age for preterm infants at risk for cerebral palsy.[74] Administration of these different assessments is suggested at term age, and then subsequently at 4 months; 6, 9, or 12 months; and 24 months corrected age. There can be great value in conducting repetitive and frequent assessment to identify alterations in developmental trajectory across infancy and early childhood due to the rapid development of skills.

Beyond the Neurobehavioral Assessment

Successful full oral feeding is often a primary goal to achieve prior to discharge from the NICU. Neuromotor, sensory, and physiologic capabilities all contribute to successful oral feeding.[123] Necessary functions and feeding behaviors include the ability to achieve and maintain an awake state, have an adequate suck in order to take fluid from the nipple, manage the bolus, protect the airway during swallowing, and coordinate the feeding process to enable intake in a reasonable amount of time.[124] Because preterm and other high-risk infants experience challenges related to many domains of function, central nervous system immaturity, and physiologic instability,[125] feeding problems are common. These can include oral-motor dysfunction, nonorganic failure to thrive, and dysphagia.[126-128] Feeding is considered a primary occupation of infancy, and problems can lead to altered feeding experiences, which can affect nutrition, developmental outcome, parent interaction, and social adaptiveness.[129-133] Preterm infants at term equivalent age and full-term infants who struggle to successfully feed as infants often continue to face feeding challenges (and other developmental concerns) throughout childhood and beyond.[134]

Research suggests a reciprocating relationship between feeding and neurodevelopment. Neurobehavioral development during infancy appears to correlate with an infant's ability to suck, swallow, and breathe in order to coordinate functionally safe feeding skills. Specifically, more arousal and visual attention have been related to more success with oral feeding in infants with congenital heart disease.[135] Feeding behaviors engage various neural mechanisms including multiple CNs, afferent and efferent neural networks, inhibitory and excitatory neurons, and central pattern generators.[123] An infant's oral feeding skills are therefore often reflective of his/her ability to organize and coordinate oral-motor functions efficiently in order to consume sufficient calories to grow and develop.[136]

Standardized Assessments of Oral Feeding During the Perinatal Period

The *Early Feeding Skills* assessment is a 36-item oral feeding assessment.[137] It is scored over a full feeding and is broken down into oral feeding readiness, oral feeding skill, and oral feeding recovery. While the middle section of the assessment provides information on four skills of oral feeding, the tool largely identifies readiness for oral feeding and the impact of the feeding on the infant.[137]

The Infant Driven Feeding Scales is not a measure of normal or abnormal feeding performance but rather a scale to aid the clinician in determining the infant's readiness to orally feed, the quality of the feeding, and the caregiver interventions provided to unsupport quality feeding behaviors.[138] The total volume consumed is not considered within this scale as the focus is on quality of feeding, not quantity. The feeding readiness scale is administered at a time when oral feeding may be attempted, and the scores inform the clinician if the infant should have an oral feeding attempt based on their arousal, medical severity, and oral motor responsiveness. If deemed appropriate to feed, the quality of nippling scale is used to observe and document the infant's feeding behaviors such as coordination, rhythm, and pacing. Finally, the caregiver techniques scale describes supports the caregiver provides to improve feeding quality, including external pacing, modified side-lying, chin support, cheek support, and oral stimulation.[138]

The Neonatal Eating Outcome Assessment assesses oral feeding skills over a 20-minute time period, and scoring is based on expected performance at each postmenstrual age.[139] It has 19 scored items and several more unscored items that provide context for the feeding. There is an abbreviated form that assesses seven nonnutritive sucking behaviors that can be administered with infants who are not yet orally feeding. It can be used from approximately 30 to 32 weeks postmenstrual age to approximately 6 to 8 weeks corrected age. It has

been demonstrated to have content, concurrent, and predictive validity as well as excellent reliability.[134,140] Training has recently started to be offered.

The Neonatal Oral Motor Assessment Scale (NOMAS) is likely the most widely used and researched assessment of feeding during the perinatal period.[141] It is a 28-item assessment of jaw and tongue movements used to assess the first 2 minutes of oral feeding. Feeding is then defined as being normal, disorganized, or dysfunctional. It can be used with breastfed or bottle-fed infants once oral feeding is initiated until the infant is approximately 6 to 8 weeks corrected age.[142,143] Validity has been well established, but there are mixed reports of reliability.[144] Formal training is required to administer the NOMAS.

The Oral Feeding Scale uses two constructs to categorize feeding ability into one of four levels with Level I being the most immature and Level IV being the most mature.[145] The two constructs assessed are proficiency (PRO), defined as a percentage (milliliters of milk consumed in 5 minutes divided by the milliliters of milk prescribed) and rate of milk transfer (RT), defined as milliliters consumed divided by the duration of the feeding. By combining these two constructs, the measure is able to define infants' actual skills prior to fatigue as well as overall skills inclusive of onset of fatigue.[145] This measure assesses feeding solely from the volume consumed.

Importance of Early Assessment

Perinatal assessments examine a wide array of infant skill sets. Some assessments define normal or abnormal movement patterns, others identify alterations in tone and posture, others focus on presence of neonatal reflexes, and others define behavioral responses. Such information can aid in early identification of developmental challenges to enable proper referral to early therapy programming. Further, early neurobehavioral assessment can define intervention targets by identifying where problems exist in order to build appropriate therapeutic strategies. Early occupational therapy, physical therapy, and speech-language pathology services can address problem areas at the foundations of early development in order to optimize later outcomes. Such interventions can begin in the NICU or

immediately after birth in the full-term infant to gar-
ner the largest impact.[46,146]

Acknowledgments

The authors wish to thank Polly Kellner, Elizabeth
Heiny Wedell, Kristen Connell, Marinthea Richter,
Carolyn Ibrahim, Bethany Gruskin, and Delaney Smith
for assisting with research, editing, and formatting.

REFERENCES

1. Yaari M, Mankuta D, Harel-Gadassi A, et al. Early developmental trajectories of preterm infants. *Res Dev Disabil.* 2018;81:12-23.
2. Salandy S, Rai R, Gutierrez S, Ishak B, Tubbs RS. Neurological examination of the infant: a comprehensive review. *Clin Anat.* 2019;32(6):770-777.
3. Chinello A, Di Gangi V, Valenza E. Persistent primary reflexes affect motor acts: potential implications for autism spectrum disorder. *Res Dev Disabil.* 2018;83:287-295.
4. Gieysztor EZ, Choinska AM, Paprocka-Borowicz M. Persistence of primitive reflexes and associated motor problems in healthy preschool children. *Arch Med Sci.* 2018;14(1):167-173.
5. Modrell AK, Tadi P. Primitive reflexes. In: *StatPearls.* Treasure Island, FL; 2022.
6. Pecuch A, Gieysztor E, Telenga M, et al. Primitive reflex activity in relation to the sensory profile in healthy preschool children. *Int J Environ Res Public Health.* 2020;17(21):8210.
7. Kobesova A, Kolar P. Developmental kinesiology: three levels of motor control in the assessment and treatment of the motor system. *J Bodyw Mov Ther.* 2014;18(1):23-33.
8. Dusing SC. Postural variability and sensorimotor development in infancy. *Dev Med Child Neurol.* 2016;58(suppl 4):17-21.
9. Righetto Greco AL, Sato NTDS, Cazotti AM, Tudella E. Is segmental trunk control related to gross motor performance in healthy preterm and full-term infants? *J Mot Behav.* 2020;52(6):666-675.
10. de Cock ESA, Henrichs J, Klimstra TA, et al. Longitudinal associations between parental bonding, parenting stress, and executive functioning in Toddlerhood. *J Child Fam Stud.* 2017;26(6):1723-1733.
11. Hofheimer JA, Smith LM, McGowan EC, et al. Psychosocial and medical adversity associated with neonatal neurobehavior in infants born before 30 weeks gestation. *Pediatr Res.* 2020;87(4):721-729.
12. White-Traut R, Norr KF, Fabiyi C, Rankin KM, Li Z, Liu L. Mother-infant interaction improves with a developmental intervention for mother-preterm infant dyads. *Infant Behav Dev.* 2013;36(4):694-706.
13. Rogers CE, Lean RE, Wheelock MD, Smyser CD. Aberrant structural and functional connectivity and neurodevelopmental impairment in preterm children. *J Neurodev Disord.* 2018;10(1):38.
14. Keunen K, Kersbergen KJ, Groenendaal F, Isgum I, de Vries LS, Benders MJ. Brain tissue volumes in preterm infants: prematurity, perinatal risk factors and neurodevelopmental outcome: a systematic review. *J Matern Fetal Neonatal Med.* 2012;25(suppl 1):89-100.
15. Alexander B, Kelly CE, Adamson C, et al. Changes in neonatal regional brain volume associated with preterm birth and perinatal factors. *Neuroimage.* 2019;185:654-663.
16. Gui L, Loukas S, Lazeyras F, Hüppi PS, Meskaldji DE, Borradori Tolsa C. Longitudinal study of neonatal brain tissue volumes in preterm infants and their ability to predict neurodevelopmental outcome. *Neuroimage.* 2019;185:728-741.
17. Pascoe MJ, Melzer TR, Horwood LJ, Woodward LJ, Darlow BA. Altered grey matter volume, perfusion and white matter integrity in very low birthweight adults. *Neuroimage Clin.* 2019;22:101780.
18. Menegaux A, Hedderich DM, Bäuml JG, et al. Reduced apparent fiber density in the white matter of premature-born adults. *Sci Rep.* 2020;10(1):17214.
19. Pineda RG, Tjoeng TH, Vavasseur C, Kidokoro H, Neil JJ, Inder T. Patterns of altered neurobehavior in preterm infants within the neonatal intensive care unit. *J Pediatr.* 2013;162(3):470-476.e1.
20. Kerstjens JM, de Winter AF, Bocca-Tjeertes IF, ten Vergert EM, Reijneveld SA, Bos AF. Developmental delay in moderately preterm-born children at school entry. *J Pediatr.* 2011;159(1):92-98.
21. Rogers EE, Hintz SR. Early neurodevelopmental outcomes of extremely preterm infants. *Semin Perinatol.* 2016;40(8):497-509.
22. Patel RM. Short- and long-term outcomes for extremely preterm infants. *Am J Perinatol.* 2016;33(3):318-328.
23. Law JB, Wood TR, Gogcu S, et al. Intracranial hemorrhage and 2-year neurodevelopmental outcomes in infants born extremely preterm. *J Pediatr.* 2021;238:124-134.e10.
24. Zonnenberg IA, van Dijk-Lokkart EM, van den Dungen FAM, Vermeulen RJ, van Weissenbruch MM. Neurodevelopmental outcome at 2 years of age in preterm infants with late-onset sepsis. *Eur J Pediatr.* 2019;178(5):673-680.
25. Zhang H, Dysart K, Kendrick DE, et al. Prolonged respiratory support of any type impacts outcomes of extremely low birth weight infants. *Pediatr Pulmonol.* 2018;53(10):1447-1455.
26. Pascal A, Govaert P, Oostra A, Naulaers G, Ortibus E, Van den Broeck C. Neurodevelopmental outcome in very preterm and very-low-birthweight infants born over the past decade: a meta-analytic review. *Dev Med Child Neurol.* 2018;60(4):342-355.
27. Pineda RG, Tjoeng TH, Vavasseur C, Kidokoro H, Neil JJ, Inder T. Patterns of altered neurobehavior in preterm infants within the neonatal intensive care unit. *J Pediatr.* 2013;162(3):470-476.e1.
28. Pineda R, Liszka L, Inder T. Early neurobehavior at 30 weeks postmenstrual age is related to outcome at term equivalent age. *Early Hum Dev.* 2020;146:105057.
29. Allinson LG, Denehy L, Doyle LW, et al. Physiological stress responses in infants at 29–32 weeks' postmenstrual age during clustered nursing cares and standardised neurobehavioural assessments. *BMJ Paediatr Open.* 2017;1(1):e000025.
30. Ashwal S. Historical aspects of the neonatal neurological examination: why child neurologists are not "little" adult neurologists. *J Hist Neurosci.* 1995;4(1):3-24.
31. Prechtl HF. State of the art of a new functional assessment of the young nervous system. An early predictor of cerebral palsy. *Early Hum Dev.* 1997;50(1):1-11.
32. Graham FK. Behavioral differences between normal and traumatized newborns: I. The test procedures. *Psychol Monogr Gen Appl.* 1956;70(20):1-16.
33. Rosenblith J. Neonatal assessment. *Psychol Rep.* 1959;5:791.
34. Prechtl HFR. The neurological examination of the full term newborn infant. In: *Clinics in Developmental Medicine.* 2nd ed. London, Philadelphia, Lippincott: Heinemann Medical for Spastics International Medical Publications; 1977.
35. Yang DC. Neurologic status of newborn infants on first and third day of life. Evaluated by a simplified neurologic examination. *Neurology.* 1962;12:72-77.

36. Prechtl HF, Beintema D. *The Neurological Examination of the Fullterm Newborn Infant*. Philadelphia: Lippincott; 1964.
37. Scanlon JW, Brown WU Jr Weiss JB, Alper MH. Neurobehavioral responses of newborn infants after maternal epidural anesthesia. *Anesthesiology*. 1974;40(2):121-128.
38. Parmelee AH, Kopp CB, Sigman M. Selection of developmental assessment techniques for infants at risk. *Merrill Palmer Q*. 1976;22(3):177-199.
39. Amiel-Tison C. Neurologic examination of the newborn infant. *Rev Prat*. 1977;27(33):2143-2151.
40. Lester BM, Tronick EZ. History and description of the Neonatal Intensive Care Unit Network Neurobehavioral Scale. *Pediatrics*. 2004;113(3 Pt 2):634-640.
41. Als H, Tronick E, Lester BM, Brazelton TB. The Brazelton neonatal behavioral assessment scale (BNBAS). *J Abnorm Child Psychol*. 1977;5(3):215-231.
42. Als H, Lester B, Tronick E, Brazelton T. Toward a research instrument for the assessment of preterm infants' behavior (APIB). *Theory Res Behav Pediatr*. 1982;1:35-132.
43. Lester BM, Tronick E. *NICU Network Neurobehavioral Scale (NNNS) Manual*. Baltimore: Paul H. Brookes Pub. Co.; 2004.
44. Brown N, Spittle A. Neurobehavioral evaluation in the preterm and term infant. *Curr Pediatr Rev*. 2014;10(1):65-72.
45. Inder TE, de Vries LS, Ferriero DM, et al. Neuroimaging of the preterm brain: review and recommendations. *J Pediatr*. 2021;237:276-287.e4.
46. Spittle A, Treyvaud K. The role of early developmental intervention to influence neurobehavioral outcomes of children born preterm. *Semin Perinatol*. 2016;40(8):542-548.
47. Cairney DG, Kazmi A, Delahunty L, Marryat L, Wood R. The predictive value of universal preschool developmental assessment in identifying children with later educational difficulties: a systematic review. *PLoS One*. 2021;16(3):e0247299.
48. Griffiths A, Toovey R, Morgan PE, Spittle AJ. Psychometric properties of gross motor assessment tools for children: a systematic review. *BMJ Open*. 2018;8(10):e021734.
49. Bayley N, Aylward GP. Technical manual. In: Pearson N, ed. *Bayley Scales of Infant and Toddler Development*. 4th ed. Bloomington: NCS Pearson; 2019.
50. Folio MR. *PDMS-2: Peabody Developmental Motor Scales*. 2nd ed. Austin: Pro-Ed. 1 case; 2000.
51. Piper M, Darrah J. *Motor Assessment of the Developing Infant*. 2nd ed. Philadelphia: Elsevier, Inc.; 2021:pages cm.
52. Spittle AJ, Doyle LW, Boyd RN. A systematic review of the clinimetric properties of neuromotor assessments for preterm infants during the first year of life. *Dev Med Child Neurol*. 2008;50(4):254-266.
53. Gagnon K, Cannon S, Weatherstone KB. The premie-neuro: opportunities and challenges for standardized neurologic assessment of the preterm infant. *Adv Neonatal Care*. 2012;12(5):310-317.
54. Pineda R. *General Competencies to Initiate NNNS-II Training with Infants*. Available at: https://www.brown.edu/research/projects/children-at-risk/sites/brown.edu.research.projects.children-at-risk/files/uploads/General%20Competencies%20to%20Initiate%20NNNS-II%20Training%20with%20Infants_0.pdf.
55. Amiel-Tison C. Update of the Amiel-Tison neurologic assessment for the term neonate or at 40 weeks corrected age. *Pediatr Neurol*. 2002;27(3):196-212.
56. Gosselin J, Gahagan S, Amiel-Tison C. The Amiel-Tison neurological assessment at term: conceptual and methodological continuity in the course of follow-up. *Ment Retard Dev Disabil Res Rev*. 2005;11(1):34-51.
57. Simard MN, Lambert J, Lachance C, Audibert F, Gosselin J. Interexaminer reliability of Amiel-Tison neurological assessments. *Pediatr Neurol*. 2009;41(5):347-352.
58. Simard MN, Lambert J, Lachance C, Audibert F, Gosselin J. Prediction of developmental performance in preterm infants at two years of corrected age: contribution of the neurological assessment at term age. *Early Hum Dev*. 2011;87(12):799-804.
59. Als H, Butler S, Kosta S, McAnulty G. The Assessment of Preterm Infants' Behavior (APIB): furthering the understanding and measurement of neurodevelopmental competence in preterm and full-term infants. *Ment Retard Dev Disabil Res Rev*. 2005;11(1):94-102.
60. Noble Y, Boyd R. Neonatal assessments for the preterm infant up to 4 months corrected age: a systematic review. *Dev Med Child Neurol*. 2012;54(2):129-139.
61. NFI Quality Assurance Training Policy. 2022. Available at: https://nidcap.org/wp-content/uploads/2014/08/QAT002-updated-logo-May2014.pdf.
62. Assessment of Behavioral Systems Organization Following Observation (ABSO). Available at: https://nidcap.org/wp-content/uploads/2013/12/ABSO-Manual.pdf.
63. Brazelton TB, Nugent JK. The neonatal behavioral assessment scale: background and conceptual basis. In: *Neonatal Behavioral Assessment Scale*. London: Mac Keith Press; 2011:4.
64. Brazelton TB. Assessment of the infant at risk. *Clin Obstet Gynecol*. 1973;16(1):361-375.
65. Newborn Behavioral Observations (NBO) and Neonatal Behavioral Assessment Scale (NBAS). https://learn.brazeltontouchpoints.org/learning-type/newborn-behavior-trainings/.
66. Tronick E, Lester BM. Grandchild of the NBAS: the NICU network neurobehavioral scale (NNNS): a review of the research using the NNNS. *J Child Adolesc Psychiatr Nurs*. 2013;26(3):193-203.
67. Einspieler C, Prechtl HFR. Prechtl's method on the qualitative assessment of general movements in preterm, term and young infants. In: *Clinics in Developmental Medicine*. London: Mac Keith Press; 2004:xi, 91.
68. Zuk L. Fetal and infant spontaneous general movements as predictors of developmental disabilities. *Dev Disabil Res Rev*. 2011;17(2):93-101.
69. Kwong AKL, Fitzgerald TL, Doyle LW, Cheong JLY, Spittle AJ. Predictive validity of spontaneous early infant movement for later cerebral palsy: a systematic review. *Dev Med Child Neurol*. 2018;60(5):480-489.
70. Einspieler C, Marschik PB, Pansy J, et al. The general movement optimality score: a detailed assessment of general movements during preterm and term age. *Dev Med Child Neurol*. 2016;58(4):361-368.
71. International Training Courses on the Prechtl General Movement Assessment. Available at: https://general-movements-trust.info/.
72. Goyen TA, Morgan C, Crowle C, et al. Sensitivity and specificity of general movements assessment for detecting cerebral palsy in an Australian context: 2-year outcomes. *J Paediatr Child Health*. 2020;56(9):1414-1418.
73. Early Detection of Cerebral Palsy Section 1: Evidence Summary. 2022. Available at: https://www.aacpdm.org/publications/care-pathways/early-detection-of-cerebral-palsy.
74. Novak I, Morgan C, Adde L, et al. Early, accurate diagnosis and early intervention in cerebral palsy: advances in diagnosis and treatment. *JAMA Pediatr*. 2017;171(9):897-907.
75. Peyton C, Pascal A, Boswell L, et al. Inter-observer reliability using the General Movement Assessment is influenced by rater experience. *Early Hum Dev*. 2021;161:105436.

76. Craciunoiu O, Holsti L. A systematic review of the predictive validity of neurobehavioral assessments during the preterm period. *Phys Occup Ther Pediatr.* 2017;37(3):292-307.

77. Støen R, Boswell L, de Regnier RA, et al. The predictive accuracy of the general movement assessment for cerebral palsy: a prospective, observational study of high-risk infants in a clinical follow-up setting. *J Clin Med.* 2019;8(11):1790.

78. Dubowitz L, Dubowitz V, Mercuri E. *The Neurological Assessment of the Preterm and Full-Term Newborn Infant.* 2nd ed. London: Mac Keith Press; 1999.

79. Spittle AJ, Walsh J, Olsen JE, et al. Neurobehaviour and neurological development in the first month after birth for infants born between 32–42 weeks' gestation. *Early Hum Dev.* 2016;96:7-14.

80. Dubowitz L, Mercuri E, Dubowitz V. An optimality score for the neurologic examination of the term newborn. *J Pediatr.* 1998; 133(3):406-416.

81. Hammersmith Neurological Examinations. Available at: http://hammersmith-neuro-exam.com/.

82. Romeo DM, Ricci M, Picilli M, Foti B, Cordaro G, Mercuri E. Early neurological assessment and long-term neuromotor outcomes in late preterm infants: a critical review. *Medicina (Kaunas).* 2020;56(9):475.

83. Eeles AL, Walsh JM, Olsen JE, et al. Continuum of neurobehaviour and its associations with brain MRI in infants born preterm. *BMJ Paediatr Open.* 2017;1(1):e000136.

84. Venkata SKRG, Pournami F, Prabhakar J, Nandakumar A, Jain N. Disability prediction by early hammersmith neonatal neurological examination: a diagnostic study. *J Child Neurol.* 2020; 35(11):731-736.

85. Als H. Manual for the naturalistic observation of newborn behavior. In: *Newborn Individualized Developmental Care and Assessment Program* (NIDCAP), NIDCAP, ed. NIDCAP Federation International; 2006.

86. Learning Center. Available at: https://nidcap.org/learning-center/.

87. McManus BM. A review of "Understanding newborn behavior & early relationships: the newborn behavioral observations (NBO) system handbook by J. K. Nugent, C. Keefer, S. Minear, L. C. Johnson, & Y. Blanchard." *Phys Occup Ther Pediatr.* 2008; 28(3):283-285.

88. Barlow J, Herath NI, Bartram Torrance C, Bennett C, Wei Y. The Neonatal Behavioral Assessment Scale (NBAS) and Newborn Behavioral Observations (NBO) system for supporting caregivers and improving outcomes in caregivers and their infants. *Cochrane Database Syst Rev.* 2018;3:CD011754.

89. Guimaraes MAP, Alves CRL, Cardoso AA, Penido MG, Magalhães LC. Clinical application of the Newborn Behavioral Observation (NBO) system to characterize the behavioral pattern of newborns at biological and social risk. *J Pediatr (Rio J).* 2018;94(3):300-307.

90. Hoifodt RS, Nordahl D, Landsem IP, et al. Newborn behavioral observation, maternal stress, depressive symptoms and the mother-infant relationship: results from the Northern Babies Longitudinal Study (NorBaby). *BMC Psychiatry.* 2020;20(1):300.

91. NBAS and NBO Trainings Around the World. Available at: https://www.newbornbehaviorinternational.org/nbas-and-nbo-trainings.

92. Brown University. *Neonatal Neurobehavioral Scale (NNNS-II).* 2022 [cited 2020 March 12]. Available at: https://www.brown.edu/research/projects/children-at-risk/about.

93. El-Dib M, Massaro AN, Glass P, Aly H. Neurobehavioral assessment as a predictor of neurodevelopmental outcome in preterm infants. *J Perinatol.* 2012;32(4):299-303.

94. Dorner RA, Allen MC, Robinson S, et al. Early neurodevelopmental outcome in preterm posthemorrhagic ventricular dilatation and hydrocephalus: Neonatal ICU Network Neurobehavioral Scale and imaging predict 3–6-month motor quotients and Capute Scales. *J Neurosurg Pediatr.* 2019:1-11.

95. Hogan WJ, Winter S, Pinto NM, et al. Neurobehavioral evaluation of neonates with congenital heart disease: a cohort study. *Dev Med Child Neurol.* 2018;60(12):1225-1231.

96. Byrne R, Noritz G, Maitre NL, NCH Early Developmental Group. Implementation of early diagnosis and intervention guidelines for cerebral palsy in a high-risk infant follow-up clinic. *Pediatr Neurol.* 2017;76:66-71.

97. Velez ML, Jansson LM, Schroeder J, Williams E. Prenatal methadone exposure and neonatal neurobehavioral functioning. *Pediatr Res.* 2009;66(6):704-709.

98. Jones HE, O'Grady KE, Johnson RE, Velez M, Jansson LM. Infant neurobehavior following prenatal exposure to methadone or buprenorphine: results from the neonatal intensive care unit network neurobehavioral scale. *Subst Use Misuse.* 2010;45(13):2244-2257.

99. de Souza Perrella VV, Marina Carvalho de Moraes B, Sañudo A, Guinsburg R. Neurobehavior of preterm infants from 32 to 48 weeks post-menstrual age. *J Perinatol.* 2019;39(6): 800-807.

100. Pineda R, Smith J, Roussin J, Wallendorf M, Kellner P, Colditz G. Randomized clinical trial investigating the effect of consistent, developmentally-appropriate, and evidence-based multisensory exposures in the NICU. *J Perinatol.* 2021;41(10):2449-2462.

101. NNNS-II Training and Certification Program. 2022. Available at: https://www.brown.edu/research/projects/children-at-risk/about/nnns-training-and-certification-program-0.

102. Salisbury AL, Fallone MD, Lester B. Neurobehavioral assessment from fetus to infant: the NICU Network Neurobehavioral Scale and the Fetal Neurobehavior Coding Scale. *Ment Retard Dev Disabil Res Rev.* 2005;11(1):14-20.

103. Daily DK, Ellison PH. The Premie-Neuro: a clinical neurologic examination of premature infants. *Neonatal Netw.* 2005;24(1): 15-22.

104. Sheridan-Pereira M, Ellison PH, Helgeson V. The construction of a scored neonatal neurological examination for assessment of neurological integrity in full-term neonates. *J Dev Behav Pediatr.* 1991;12(1):25-30.

105. Infant Neurological International Battery (INFANIB). 2022. Available at: https://www.physio-pedia.com/Infant_Neurological_International_Battery_(INFANIB).

106. Campbell SK. *The Test of Infant Motor Performance: Test User's Manual.* 3rd ed. Chicago: Infant Motor Performance Scales, LLC; 2012.

107. Campbell S, Osten ET, Kolobe THA, Fisher AG. Development of the test of infant motor performance. *Phys Med Rehabil Clin N Am.* 1993;4(3):541-550.

108. Campbell SK. Functional movement assessment with the Test of Infant Motor Performance. *J Perinatol.* 2021;41(10):2385-2394.

109. Kim SA, Lee YJ, Lee YG. Predictive value of Test of Infant Motor Performance for infants based on correlation between TIMP and Bayley scales of infant development. *Ann Rehabil Med.* 2011;35(6):860-866.

110. Lee EJ, Han JT, Lee JH. Risk factors affecting Tests of Infant Motor Performance (TIMP) in pre-term infants at post-conceptional age of 40 weeks. *Dev Neurorehabil.* 2012;15(2):79-83.

111. Peyton C, Yang E, Kochergisnky M, et al. Relationship between white matter pathology and performance on the General

Movement Assessment and the Test of Infant Motor Performance in very preterm infants. *Early Hum Dev.* 2016;95:23-27.

112. Campbell SK, Hedeker D. Validity of the Test of Infant Motor Performance for discriminating among infants with varying risk for poor motor outcome. *J Pediatr.* 2001;139(4):546-551.
113. Peyton C, Schreiber MD, Msall ME. The Test of Infant Motor Performance at 3 months predicts language, cognitive, and motor outcomes in infants born preterm at 2 years of age. *Dev Med Child Neurol.* 2018;60(12):1239-1243.
114. Campbell SK, Kolobe TH, Wright BD, Linacre JM. Validity of the test of infant motor performance for prediction of 6-, 9- and 12-month scores on the Alberta Infant Motor Scale. *Dev Med Child Neurol.* 2002;44(4):263-272.
115. Kolobe TH, Bulanda M, Susman L. Predicting motor outcome at preschool age for infants tested at 7, 30, 60, and 90 days after term age using the Test of Infant Motor Performance. *Phys Ther.* 2004;84(12):1144-1156.
116. Learn the Tests. 2022. Available at: https://www.thetimp.com/learn-the-tests.
117. Daum CKD, Grellong B, Albin S, Vaughan H, Garnter L. Neurobehavioral assessment of high-risk neonates. *Pediatr Res.* 1977;11:376.
118. Majnemer A, Rosenblatt B, Riley P. Predicting outcome in high-risk newborns with a neonatal neurobehavioral assessment. *Am J Occup Ther.* 1994;48(8):723-732.
119. Wallace IF, Rose SA, McCarton CM, Kurtzberg D, Vaughan HG Jr. Relations between infant neurobehavioral performance and cognitive outcome in very low birth weight preterm infants. *J Dev Behav Pediatr.* 1995;16(5):309-317.
120. Morgan AM, Koch V, Lee V, Aldag J. Neonatal neurobehavioral examination. A new instrument for quantitative analysis of neonatal neurological status. *Phys Ther.* 1988;68(9):1352-1358.
121. Korner A, Thom V. *Neurobehavioral Assessment of the Preterm Infant.* New York: The Psychological Corporation; 1990.
122. Carmichael K, Burns Y, Gray P, O'Callaghan M. Neuromotor behavioural assessment of preterm infants at risk for impaired development. *Aust J Physiother.* 1997;43(2):101-107.
123. Jadcherla S. Dysphagia in the high-risk infant: potential factors and mechanisms. *Am J Clin Nutr.* 2016;103(2):622S-628S.
124. Barlow SM. Oral and respiratory control for preterm feeding. *Curr Opin Otolaryngol Head Neck Surg.* 2009;17(3):179-186.
125. Moore TA, Pickler RH. Feeding intolerance, inflammation, and neurobehaviors in preterm infants. *J Neonatal Nurs.* 2017;23(3):134-141.
126. Medoff-Cooper B, Shults J, Kaplan J. Sucking behavior of preterm neonates as a predictor of developmental outcomes. *J Dev Behav Pediatr.* 2009;30(1):16-22.
127. Lefton-Greif MA. Pediatric dysphagia. *Phys Med Rehabil Clin N Am.* 2008;19(4):837-851, ix.
128. Hawdon JM, Beauregard N, Slattery J, Kennedy G. Identification of neonates at risk of developing feeding problems in infancy. *Dev Med Child Neurol.* 2000;42(4):235-239.
129. Samara M, Johnson S, Lamberts K, Marlow N, Wolke D. Eating problems at age 6 years in a whole population sample of extremely preterm children. *Dev Med Child Neurol.* 2010;52(2):e16-e22.
130. Hawdon JM, Beauregard N, Slattery J, Kennedy G. Identification of neonates at risk of developing feeding problems in infancy. *Dev Med Child Neurol.* 2000;42(4):235-239.
131. Bier JA, Ferguson A, Cho C, Oh W, Vohr BR. The oral motor development of low-birth-weight infants who underwent orotracheal intubation during the neonatal period. *Am J Dis Child.* 1993;147(8):858-862.
132. Dodrill P, McMahon S, Ward E, Weir K, Donovan T, Riddle B. Long-term oral sensitivity and feeding skills of low-risk preterm infants. *Early Hum Dev.* 2004;76(1):23-37.
133. Burklow KA, McGrath AM, Valerius KS, Rudolph C. Relationship between feeding difficulties, medical complexity, and gestational age. *Nutr Clin Pract.* 2002;17(6):373-378.
134. Kwon J, Kellner P, Wallendorf M, Smith J, Pineda R. Neonatal feeding performance is related to feeding outcomes in childhood. *Early Hum Dev.* 2020;151:105202.
135. Gakenheimer-Smith L, Glotzbach K, Ou Z, et al. The impact of neurobehavior on feeding outcomes in neonates with congenital heart disease. *J Pediatr.* 2019;214:71-78.e2.
136. Osman A. Oral feeding readiness and premature infant outcomes. *J Neonatal Nurs.* 2019;25(3):111-115.
137. Thoyre SM, Shaker CS, Pridham KF. The early feeding skills assessment for preterm infants. *Neonatal Netw.* 2005;24(3):7-16.
138. Ludwig SM, Waitzman KA. Changing feeding documentation to reflect infant-driven feeding practice. *Newborn Infant Nurs Rev.* 2007;7(3):155-160.
139. Pineda R. *Neonatal Eating Outcome Assessment.* 2016. Available at: https://chan.usc.edu/nicu/neonatal-eating-outcome-assessment.
140. Pineda R, Harris R, Foci F, Roussin J, Wallendorf M. Neonatal eating outcome assessment: tool development and inter-rater reliability. *Acta Paediatr.* 2018;107(3):414-424.
141. Bickell M, Barton C, Dow K, Fucile S. A systematic review of clinical and psychometric properties of infant oral motor feeding assessments. *Dev Neurorehabil.* 2018;21(6):351-361.
142. Zarem C, Kidokoro H, Neil J, Wallendorf M, Inder T, Pineda R. Psychometrics of the neonatal oral motor assessment scale. *Dev Med Child Neurol.* 2013;55(12):1115-1120.
143. Palmer MM, Crawley K, Blanco IA. Neonatal oral-motor assessment scale: a reliability study. *J Perinatol.* 1993;13(1):28-35.
144. Longoni L, Provenzi L, Cavallini A, Sacchi D, Scotto di Minico G, Borgatti R. Predictors and outcomes of the neonatal oral motor assessment scale (NOMAS) performance: a systematic review. *Eur J Pediatr.* 2018;177(5):665-673.
145. Lau C, Smith EO. A novel approach to assess oral feeding skills of preterm infants. *Neonatology.* 2011;100(1):64-70.
146. Khurana S, Kane AE, Brown SE, Tarver T, Dusing SC. Effect of neonatal therapy on the motor, cognitive, and behavioral development of infants born preterm: a systematic review. *Dev Med Child Neurol.* 2020;62(6):684-692.

Chapter 2

Cerebral Circulation and Hypotension in the Premature Infant: Diagnosis and Treatment

Shahab Noori and Istvan Seri

Chapter Outline

Key Points

- Although there is no consensus on the definition of hypotension in preterm infants, up to 50% of very low birth weight (VLBW) infants are diagnosed with hypotension, and about one-third of extremely preterm infants receive at least one vasopressor/inotrope medication during the first postnatal week.
- There is an association between hypotension and brain injury and poor neurodevelopmental outcome. However, it remains unclear whether hypotension, its treatment, or both play a causative role.
- Alteration in cerebral blood flow is implicated in the pathogenesis of brain injury, including peri/intraventricular hemorrhage (P/IVH). Studies using Doppler and near-infrared spectroscopy have demonstrated a period of hypoperfusion-reperfusion prior to the development of P/IVH.
- The use of advanced technologies capable of diagnosing altered systemic and cerebral blood flow and the associated changes in brain function in the VLBW population in the first hours to days after delivery has increased in the last decade but still remains largely in the experimental arena.
- Due to the limited available data from randomized control trials and the challenges associated with conducting such studies, hypotension and circulatory compromise management remain controversial. The best strategy involves identifying the underlying pathophysiology of the hypotension and circulatory compromise, selecting the supportive and pharmacological treatment with an appropriate profile for the

pathophysiology, and titrating the therapy based on the response by close monitoring.

Introduction

With the evolution of neonatology over the last few decades, improved methods of monitoring and more effective interventions have been developed to identify and manage the respiratory, fluid and electrolyte, and nutritional abnormalities frequently encountered in very low birthweight (VLBW) infants. However, the ability to continuously and effectively monitor the *hemodynamic changes* at the level of systemic and organ blood flow and tissue perfusion in the clinical setting is still limited. Yet, the advances achieved with the use of targeted neonatal echocardiography and other bedside, noninvasive continuous systemic, organ and tissue perfusion, and cerebral function monitoring modalities have ushered in a new era in developmental hemodynamics. The novel monitoring modalities include but are not restricted to electrical impedance velocimetry, continuous wave Doppler ultrasonography, near-infrared spectroscopy (NIRS), visible light spectroscopy, laser Doppler technology, and amplitude-integrated EEG (aEEG). Yet, with the improvements in hemodynamic monitoring and a better understanding of the principles of developmental cardiovascular physiology have come the realization that little is known about circulatory compromise and its effects on organ, especially brain blood flow, blood flow–metabolism coupling, and long-term outcomes. Although we can continuously and reliably monitor systemic blood pressure in absolute numbers and there are a great number of proposed interventions for "normalizing" it, blood pressure is only the dependent component among the three hemodynamic parameters regulating systemic perfusion. Accordingly, blood pressure is determined by changes in the two independent variables, cardiac output and systemic vascular resistance (SVR). Therefore, in addition to monitoring and maintaining perfusion pressure (blood pressure), the obvious goal is to preserve normal systemic and organ blood flow and thus tissue oxygenation especially in the vital organs, that is, the brain, heart, and adrenal glands. In this regard, especially for the brain, medicine is at an even greater disadvantage. For instance, measuring cerebral blood flow (CBF) is

more complex than continuously measuring systemic blood flow (left ventricular output), which itself has remained a significant challenge. Assessment of systemic blood flow becomes even more complicated when shunting through the fetal channels (ductus arteriosus and foramen ovale) occurs during the first few postnatal days in the preterm neonate. Unfortunately, in the neonate, it is more complicated to detect clinical evidence of ischemia in the brain in a timely manner and as readily as in other organs, such as the heart, liver, and kidneys. In addition, distinct regions of the brain have different sensitivity to decreased oxygen delivery. Accordingly, injury to the normally less well-perfused white matter might occur before other regions suffer damage. Alterations in normal brain activity and seizures are clear signs of a pathologic process, but they can be difficult to recognize, especially in the VLBW neonate; although the use of aEEG might be helpful in this regard. As for seizures, by the time they are present, irreversible injury may have already occurred. Most importantly, the clinician faces the formidable task of effectively supporting and protecting the enormously complex developmental processes that take place in the brain of the preterm infant during the transitional period and beyond. In addition, the understanding of how to manage hemodynamic disturbances that affect CBF, flow-metabolism coupling, brain function and structure, and, ultimately, neurodevelopmental outcome, is limited.

The intent of this chapter is to review the information available on the definition of systemic hypotension and the pathogenesis, diagnosis, and treatment of early cerebral perfusion abnormalities that have been shown to precede intracranial hemorrhage and periventricular white matter injury (PWMI) in the VLBW infant. Because CBF, flow-metabolism coupling, and cerebral oxygenation in this population are such a complex topic, we focus our discussion on the first postnatal days, during which the cardiorespiratory transition from fetal to extrauterine life occurs and most early pathological processes take place. We discuss some of the bedside modalities potentially useful for identifying changes in CBF and cerebral oxygenation. Once a pathological process is identified, provision of coherent, safe, and effective means of treating it is crucial. We present a paradigm for the treatment of the pathological processes underlying clinically evident brain injury in the VLBW infant based on the most up-to-date monitoring and clinical evidence available. Unfortunately, only little evidence exists about the appropriateness and effectiveness of the current approaches to treatment of neonatal hypotension and cardiovascular compromise. In an area as controversial and complex as this one, it is important to always highlight the vast unknown as well as the little-known pieces of the puzzle. Our goal is to provide the practitioner with recommendations for establishing the diagnosis and treatment. However, the recommendations should only be considered guidelines. Finally, although the understanding of both the normal and pathological processes in the developing preterm brain is improving, the definitive, safe, and effective clinical approach remains elusive.

Definition of Hypotension

Hypotension, defined by *population-based normative data*, is present in up to 50% of VLBW infants admitted to the neonatal intensive care unit. About one-third of extremely preterm infants receive at least one vasopressor/inotrope medication during the first postnatal week.[1] Hypotension in the immediate postnatal period has historically been thought to be one of the major factors contributing to central nervous system injury and eventual cerebral palsy and poor long-term neurologic outcome in VLBW neonates. Indeed, an *association* between hypotension and brain injury and poor neurodevelopmental outcome is well documented[2-12] and forms the basis of therapeutic efforts to normalize blood pressure. However, *causation* has not been demonstrated between hypotension and poor neurodevelopment and thus one cannot infer that long-term neurodevelopmental outcomes will improve if hypotension is rigorously avoided.[13] Therein lies the conundrum often faced by the neonatologist: when to treat early cardiovascular compromise in the VLBW neonate, what medication to use and how quickly to normalize blood pressure and CBF?

On the other hand, a prospective observational study of over one thousand infants less than 28 weeks' gestation showed that early postnatal hypotension was not associated with poor outcomes.[14] Retrospective studies have also raised additional concerns by finding an association between "treated hypotension" and poor neurodevelopmental outcomes.[15-17] Of note is that the use of the definition "treated hypotension" in these studies has introduced an additional bias by implying that, in addition to or independent of hypotension, the treatment might be a factor contributing to the described association. Although the implication of the potential negative effects of treatment of hypotension is plausible and thus needs to be prospectively studied, at present no conclusion can be drawn especially since other investigators have reported essentially the opposite finding.[18,19] Unfortunately, all of the studies to date were uncontrolled, either retrospective or observational in nature, and hypotension was treated in one way or another. There are only two randomized controlled trials (RCT) published to date that had a no-treatment arm.[20,21] The first study found that, due to difficulties in obtaining informed consent in a timely fashion or refusal of enrollment by the attending neonatologist, these trials are not feasible to perform.[20] The second trial randomized hypotensive preterm infants to dopamine or placebo for 2 hours.[21] Thereafter, if mean blood pressure in mm Hg was less than the gestational age in weeks by more than five points and/or a combination of hypotension and criteria for poor perfusion were met, the addition of another vasopressor/inotrope or inotrope was allowed. The need for other pressors/inotropes for treatment of hypotension was significantly higher in the placebo arm (66% vs. 38%). However, like the previous study, this trial was terminated early due to difficulty in enrollment with only 7% of the target sample recruited. Hence, the study remained severely underpowered for the primary outcome of survival without significant brain injury.

Therefore it remains unclear whether hypotension, its treatment, or both are implicated (either negatively or positively) in the association with neurodevelopmental outcome. Interestingly, the follow-up study[18] to a randomized prospective trial[22] comparing the effectiveness of dopamine and epinephrine in increasing blood pressure and CBF in hypotensive VLBW neonates during the first postnatal day found that neonates who responded to dopamine or epinephrine had long-term neurodevelopment outcomes comparable to those of age-matched normotensive controls, and that patients who did not respond to vasopressor-inotrope treatment had worse long-term outcome. It's important to note that, contrary to the RCT discussed earlier,[21] this study required titrating the medications to achieve the target blood pressure range. These findings suggest that careful treatment of neonatal hypotension may not be harmful and may actually be effective. However, as the primary outcome measure of the original study[18] was not long-term neurodevelopmental outcome, the follow-up study[18] was not appropriately powered to put this concern to rest. Similarly, a retrospective study of dopamine-treated preterm infants of <28 weeks' gestation found the failure to respond to dopamine treatment to be associated with almost a sixfold greater likelihood of developing peri-intraventricular hemorrhage (P/IVH), while a positive response was associated with a reduction in the risk of P/IVH.[23] In contrast, the secondary analysis of a recent RCT of peripheral perfusion- versus blood pressure-based approach to circulatory management of preterm infants during the transitional period found a higher incidence of P/IVH in a subset of the blood pressure-based management group that had responded to the treatment (volume, pressors and/or inotropes).[24] Although the reason for this discrepancy is unclear, differences in the choice and titration of vasopressor/inotropes and avoidance of the extremes in blood pressure may, at least in part, provide an explanation.[25,26]

During the last decade, the trend toward less aggressive treatment of hypotension[1] has provided a glimpse into the potential effects of the presence of sustained hypotension without clinical evidence of poor perfusion ("isolated hypotension"). For example, the analysis of the French national prospective population-based cohort study allowed for the matching of 119 extremely preterm infants with untreated isolated hypotension to 119 neonates who received treatment despite having no clinical evidence of poor perfusion.[11] Thus in this study none of the patients included had any sign of inadequacy of cardiovascular function other than hypotension. Hypotension was defined as a mean blood pressure less than gestational age in weeks during the first three postnatal days. The findings revealed that the group treated for the "isolated hypotension" had a higher rate of survival without severe morbidity and a lower rate of severe P/IVH and cerebral injury. Interestingly, the association between treatment and better outcome was even stronger when hypotension was defined as a mean blood

pressure in mm Hg less than gestational age in weeks by more than five points. Although this dose-effect relationship strengthens the possibility of causality, further studies are clearly needed to verify the impact of hypotension on long-term outcome.

Accordingly, we do not have evidence indicating that, in a given VLBW neonate, what blood pressure is associated with decreased oxygen delivery to the tissues including the brain and thus harm to the patient. In addition, there is no solid evidence that increasing blood pressure to the "normal" range will normalize oxygen delivery. A school of thought exists that because mean arterial pressure (MAP) is a dependent variable of the equation describing tissue perfusion (and thereby oxygen delivery), MAP is less important than other indirect clinical indicators of decreased perfusion such as capillary refill time (CRT), urine output, and lactic acidosis. This approach ignores the physiologic principle that a pressure gradient is necessary to drive flow (Poiseuille's law). Simplistically, in order to provide blood flow to the brain, the systemic arterial pressure has to be higher than the intracranial pressure. In other words, if blood pressure drops below the intracranial pressure, there would not be any gradient to drive blood to the brain. Obviously, the dependent variables of systemic hemodynamics (cardiac output and SVR) determine blood pressure and thus tissue oxygen delivery. However, ignoring MAP itself, as sometimes implied in the literature, may not be prudent and even feasible.[20] Furthermore, ignoring it will not refine perfusion and oxygenation of the developing brain to its essence. Instead, it will further limit our current ability to monitor the patients. Therefore in our opinion, *blood pressure should be considered as one of the markers* of adequacy of circulatory function but *not the only or primary marker*. Indeed, low blood pressure implies impairment of vasomotor tone, low cardiac output, or both. On the other hand, normal blood pressure indicates either normal cardiac output and vasomotor tone or a compensated state, in which either cardiac output is increased to compensate for the low vasomotor tone or the vasomotor tone is elevated to compensate for the low cardiac output (Fig. 2.1).[27] In older children and adults, vital organs are relatively protected in the compensated phase of shock. Unfortunately, this does not seem to be the case in the preterm, especially the very preterm infant as

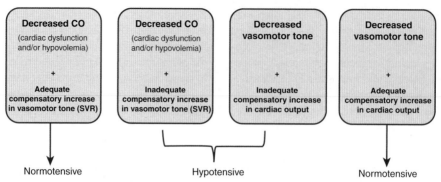

Fig. 2.1 Pathophysiology of neonatal cardiovascular compromise in primary myocardial dysfunction and primary abnormal vascular tone regulation with or without compensation by the unaffected other variable. This figure illustrates why blood pressure can be considered "normal" when there is appropriate compensatory increase in either vasomotor tone or Cardiac output. In the hypotensive scenarios, there is inadequate compensatory increase in these variables. *CO*, cardiac output. (From Wu T, Noori S, Seri I. Neonatal hypotension. In: *Polin R, Yoder M, eds. Workbook in Practical Neonatology*, 5th ed. Elsevier; 2014.)

their forebrain may not have reached "vital organ" assignment immediately after delivery (see below). Hence the limitation of primarily relying on blood pressure monitoring in an effort to assess the adequacy of circulation.

In clinical practice, hypotension is usually defined as the blood pressure value below the 5th or 10th percentile for the gestational and postnatal age–dependent normative blood pressure values (Fig. 2.2).[28,29] Interestingly, findings of a recent study suggest that the normative values may actually be low, i.e., physiologically normal blood pressure in VLBW infants may actually be higher than has been commonly accepted.[30] Moreover, due to the compensatory mechanisms, a certain blood pressure value in a given patient might be associated with normal oxygen delivery at one point in time while the same value may indicate true hypotension (abnormal tissue oxygen delivery) at another time.[27] Accordingly, there is no consensus among neonatologists about the acceptable lower limit of systemic mean or systolic arterial blood pressure, and most units have different guidelines for the initiation of treatment of hypotension. From a pathophysiological standpoint, three levels of functional alterations of increasing severity can be used to guide the definition of hypotension (Fig. 2.3). Findings of a small study[31] underscore this point. However, it is important to keep in mind that no prospectively collected information is available on mortality and morbidity associated with the different proposed blood pressure thresholds.

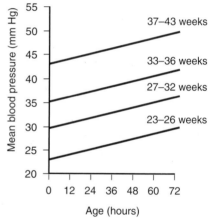

Fig. 2.2 Gestational age– and postnatal age–dependent nomogram for mean blood pressure values in preterm and term neonates during the first three postnatal days. The nomogram is derived from continuous arterial blood pressure measurements obtained from 103 neonates with gestational ages between 23 and 43 weeks. As each line represents the lower limit of 80% confidence interval of mean blood pressure for each gestational age group, 90% of infants for each gestational age group will have a mean blood pressure equal or greater than the value indicated by the corresponding line (the lower limit of confidence interval). (From Nuntnarumit P, Yang W, Bada-Ellzey HS. Blood pressure measurements in the newborn. *Clin Perinatol*. 1999;26:981–96, with permission.)

First, the mean blood pressure associated with the loss of CBF autoregulation is the generally accepted definition of hypotension (*autoregulatory blood pressure threshold*).[32] Indeed, there is considerable information in the literature indicating that CBF autoregulation is functional, albeit with a narrow range, in normotensive

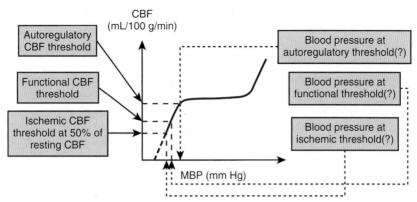

Fig. 2.3 Definition of hypotension by three pathophysiologic phenomena of increasing severity: autoregulatory, functional, and ischemic thresholds of hypotension. *CBF*, Cerebral blood flow; *MBP*, mean blood pressure.

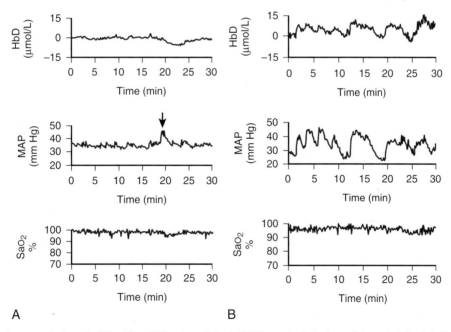

Fig. 2.4 Intact and compromised cerebral blood flow (CBF) autoregulation in VLBW neonates in the immediate postnatal period. Changes in cerebral intravascular oxygenation (HbD = HbO₂ – Hb) correlate with changes in CBF (5). A, Changes in HbD (i.e., CBF), mean arterial pressure (MAP), and oxygen saturation (SaO₂) in a 1-day-old 28-week gestation preterm infant whose subsequent head ultrasound remained normal. No change occurs in CBF in relation to the sudden increase in MAP associated with endotracheal tube suctioning (*arrow*). B, Changes in HbD (CBF), MAP, and SaO₂ in a 1-day-old 27-week GA preterm infant whose subsequent head ultrasound revealed the presence of PWMI. Changes in blood pressure are clearly associated with changes in CBF. (From Tsuji M, Saul PJ, duPlessis A, et al. Cerebral intravascular oxygenation correlates with mean arterial pressure in critically ill premature infants. *Pediatrics.* 2000;106:625, with permission.)

but not in hypotensive VLBW neonates in the immediate postnatal period (Fig. 2.4).[6,33,34] Also of interest is that CBF velocity increases in a pressure-passive fashion as systolic blood pressure is increased with dopamine during the first postnatal day.[35] A study found that cerebral pressure passivity in the VLBW neonatal population was associated with an increased risk for periventricular/intraventricular hemorrhage (P/IVH).[36] These findings implicate blood pressure and pressure passivity as risk factors for intracranial pathology.

Autoregulation is the ability of the arteries to constrict or dilate in response to an increase or decrease, respectively, in the transmural pressure to maintain blood flow relatively constant within a range of arterial blood pressure changes (see Fig. 2.4). However, in the neonate, the vascular response has a limited capacity. In addition, and as mentioned above, the autoregulatory blood pressure range is narrow in the neonatal patient population with the 50th percentile of the mean blood pressure being relatively close to the lower autoregulatory blood pressure threshold. In other words, small decreases in blood pressure may result in loss of CBF autoregulation, especially in the VLBW infant.[33] Available data suggest that the autoregulatory blood pressure threshold is around 28–29 mm Hg even in the extremely LBW (ELBW) neonate during the first postnatal day (Fig. 2.5).[33,34] At and just below this blood pressure, However, cellular function and

structural integrity are unlikely to be affected, because increased cerebral fractional oxygen extraction (CFOE), microvascular vasodilation, and a shift in the hemoglobin-oxygen dissociation curve to the left can maintain tissue oxygen delivery at levels appropriate to sustain cellular function and integrity.[25,37]

If blood pressure continues to fall, it reaches a value at which cerebral function becomes compromised (*functional blood pressure threshold*). Data suggest that the functional blood pressure threshold may be around 22 to 24 mm Hg in the VLBW neonate during the first postnatal days (Fig. 2.6).[38,39] However, caution is needed when interpreting these findings obtained in a small number of preterm infants, as their clinical relevance is unclear. Furthermore, the relationship between cerebral electrical activity, neurodevelopmental outcome, and the threshold of CBF associated with impaired brain activity is not known.

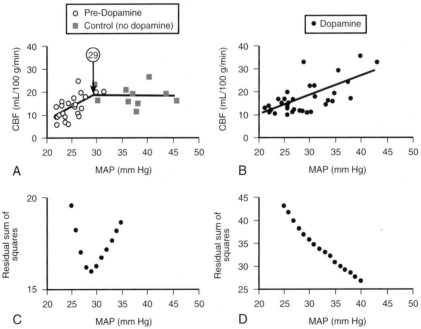

Fig. 2.5 Relationship between cerebral blood flow (CBF) and mean arterial pressure (MAP) in hypotensive and normotensive ELBW neonates during the first postnatal day and the effect of dopamine on this relationship. A, B, MAP (mm Hg) and CBF (mL/100 g/min) assessed by NIRS in normotensive ELBW neonates not requiring dopamine ("Control," closed squares; n = 5) and hypotensive ELBW neonates before dopamine administration ("Pre-dopamine," open circles; n = 12). The lower threshold of the CBF autoregulatory blood pressure limit (29 mm Hg; A) is identified as the minimum of residual sum of squares of the bilinear regression analysis (B). (C, D) MAP (mm Hg) and CBF (mL/100 g/min) in previously hypotensive ELBW neonates after dopamine treatment (filled circles). No breakpoint is evident in the CBF–MAP curve in ELBW neonates on dopamine (C), because there is no minimum identified by the bilinear regression analysis (D). (From Munro MJ, Walker AM, Barfield CP. Hypotensive extremely low birth weight infants have reduced cerebral blood flow. *Pediatrics*. 2004;114:1591, with permission.)

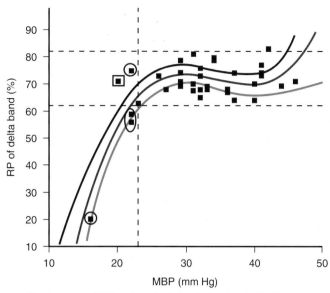

Fig. 2.6 Relationship between mean blood pressure (MBP) and cerebral electrical activity in VLBW neonates during the first 4 postnatal days. Relationship between MBP and the relative power (RP) of the delta band of the EEG, showing line of best fit with 95% confidence interval (n = 35; $R^2 = 0.627$; $p < 0.001$). Horizontal dotted lines represent the normal range of the relative power of the delta band (10th–90th percentile), while the vertical dotted line identifies the point of intercept. The open square identifies the infant with abnormal CFOE and the abnormal EEG records are circled. (From Victor S, Marson AG, Appleton RE, et al. Relationship between blood pressure, cerebral electrical activity, cerebral fractional oxygen extraction and peripheral blood flow in very low birth weight newborn infants. *Pediatr Res.* 2006;59:314–319, with permission.)

Finally, if blood pressure decreases even further, it reaches a value at which brain tissue structural integrity becomes compromised (*ischemic blood pressure threshold*). On the basis of findings in immature animals, it is assumed that the ischemic CBF threshold is around 50% of resting CBF.[33] Although it is unclear what blood pressure value represents the ischemic CBF threshold in the VLBW neonate during the first postnatal day, it may be at or below 20 mm Hg (see Fig. 2.3).[38,39] It is important to emphasize that the situation is further complicated by the fact that these numbers represent moving targets for the individual patient influenced by their ability to compensate for decreases in blood pressure and oxygen delivery. In addition, other factors, such as the different sensitivity of brain structures to perfusion changes, $PaCO_2$ levels, the presence of acidosis, preexisting insults (asphyxia), and underlying pathophysiology (sepsis, anemia) all have an impact on the critical blood pressure value at which perfusion pressure and cerebral oxygen delivery cannot satisfy cellular oxygen demand to sustain autoregulation, then cellular function, and finally structural integrity.

In addition to using the three thresholds described above, two other approaches have been proposed to define the physiologically important blood pressure threshold. These are based on identifying the cerebrovascular critical closing pressure and monitoring cerebrovascular reactivity. Cerebrovascular critical closing pressure is defined as the arterial blood pressure at which CBF ceases.[40] This blood pressure value can be estimated by analyzing simultaneously obtained systemic blood pressure and Doppler-derived CBF velocity (e.g., in the middle cerebral artery) waveforms and using an equation of impedance to flow velocity.[40,41] As the critical closing pressure is affected by the intracranial pressure and vascular properties, it could theoretically define the hypoperfusion blood pressure threshold for a specific patient at a particular time. A recent study used the diastolic closing margin defined as diastolic blood pressure minus critical closing pressure to investigate the development of early severe P/IVH.[42] Interestingly, a higher diastolic closing margin was associated with severe P/IVH, which the authors considered as evidence for a hyperperfusion injury. Therefore, this study could not demonstrate a utility for using the critical closing pressure to identify the presence of cerebral hypoperfusion that often precedes developing P/IVH. However, as the concept of critical closing pressure is physiologically relevant, it merits further investigation.

To define the optimal MAP by using cerebrovascular reactivity, the tissue oxygenation-heart rate reactivity index needs to be first calculated.[43] This index represents the correlation between the slow waves of the NIRS-defined cerebral tissue oxygenation index (TOI) and the slow fluctuations in the heart rate. As heart rate is one of the determinants of cardiac output, a positive correlation with the TOI is thought to indicate changes in cerebral circulation in response to changes in cardiac output. Therefore its positive correlation with the TOI suggests impaired cerebrovascular reactivity (regulation). Conversely, a zero or negative correlation is suggestive of intact cerebrovascular reactivity (regulation). Accordingly, the optimal MAP can be defined as the MAP associated with the lowest tissue oxygenation heart rate reactivity index in an individual for a given period. Recently, the optimal MAP averaged over the first 24 postnatal hours was calculated in 44 extremely preterm infants.[43] The mean deviation below the optimal MAP was higher in infants who developed P/IVH and those who died. In contrast, the same investigators earlier reported that an MAP greater than optimal MAP by at least 4 mm Hg to be associated with severe P/IVH.[44] As hypoperfusion-reperfusion precedes the occurrence of P/IVH,[45] the observed deviations below and above the optimal MAP leading to P/IVH may be indicative of exposure to episodes of hypoperfusion and reperfusion, respectively. Further studies are needed to validate the concept of "optimal MAP."

In most units, continuous monitoring of blood pressure and assessment of indirect signs of tissue perfusion (urine output, CRT, and lactic acidosis) still form the basis for identifying the presence of cardiovascular compromise. As discussed earlier though, "adequate" blood pressure may not always guarantee adequate organ perfusion in VLBW neonates especially during the first postnatal day.[46] Indeed, blood pressure only weakly correlates with superior vena cava (SVC) flow in VLBW neonates during the period of immediate postnatal adaptation.[47] Of note is that SVC flow has increasingly been used in the clinical practice as a surrogate for systemic blood flow in the VLBW neonate during the immediate postnatal period, when shunting through the fetal channels prohibits the use of left ventricular output to assess systemic blood flow.[48] The finding that adequate blood pressure may not always guarantee adequate systemic blood flow in these patients may be explained, at least in part, by the notion that the cerebral vascular bed, especially of the 1-day-old ELBW neonate, may not be of high priority assignment yet and thus it will constrict, as do the vessels do in the nonvital organs, rather than dilate in response to a decrease in the perfusion pressure (see below).[37,49]

Pathogenesis and Diagnosis of Pathologic Cerebral Blood Flow

Fluctuations in CBF are implicated in the pathogenesis of P/IVH and PWMI in the VLBW infant.[2,6,36,49] Both systemic and local (intracerebral) factors play a role in the pathogenesis of these central nervous system injuries and therefore are important to establish the underlying pathogenesis. In addition, the level of maturity, postnatal age, and intercurrent clinical factors (e.g., infection/inflammation, vasopressor-resistant hypotension) need to be also considered.[50] In this section, we briefly discuss the monitoring parameters that are currently in widespread clinical use (systemic arterial pressure and arterial blood gas sampling) and then delve into the emerging field of bedside monitoring of systemic and organ blood flow, especially CBF and brain activity. We review most of the existing technologies, including echocardiography and Doppler ultrasound, impedance electrical cardiometry (IEC), NIRS, and aEEG, and discuss the applicability and limitations of these modalities. We do not discuss the use of magnetic resonance imaging (MRI) for assessing CBF in the neonatal patient population, because this topic is beyond the scope of this chapter.

A logical place to begin the discussion on monitoring CBF in the VLBW infant is to ask, "What is the normal CBF in the VLBW infant?" Several investigators have addressed this issue. It is clear from these studies that CBF is lower in preterm infants than in adults, corresponding to the lower metabolic rate of the preterm brain. A study using xenon-133 clearance[51] found that, in 42 preterm infants with a mean gestational age of 31 weeks, CBF was 15.5 $\pm$ 7.2 mL/100 g/min during the first postnatal week, a value three to four times lower than that in adults. Interestingly, patients enrolled in this study who were receiving mechanical ventilation had lower CBF than their nonventilated counterparts and those supported on CPAP (11.8 ±3.2 vs. 19.8 ±5.3 and 21.3 ±12 mL/100 g/min, respectively). CBF in this study was not consistently affected by postnatal age, gestational age, birth weight, mode of delivery, $PaCO_2$, hemoglobin concentration, mean blood pressure, or phenobarbital therapy. In contrast, subsequent publications by the same group of authors investigating CBF reactivity in preterm infants during the first three postnatal days showed that, as expected, $PaCO_2$ and hemoglobin concentration significantly affect CBF in this patient population.[52–54] However, the relationship between $PaCO_2$ and CBF appears to be also affected by postnatal age during the immediate postnatal period (see below). Using positron emission tomography (PET) to measure CBF, a study found[55] lower values for CBF in preterm and term neonates compared to those obtained by the use of xenon-133 clearance. More importantly, the authors reported that, in one term and five preterm infants with CBF between 4.9 and 10 mL/100 g/min, the term neonate and three of the preterm infants had normal neurodevelopmental outcome at 24 months.[55] These data suggest but do not prove that the "neurodevelopmentally safe" lower limit of CBF in the neonate may be between 5 and 10 mL/100/min. Finally, and as also mentioned earlier, because CBF is affected by many factors other than blood pressure, it is not possible to define the blood pressure value consistently associated with a decrease of CBF below the "safe" limit that results in ischemic brain injury.

Kluckow and Evans, using SVC flow as a surrogate for CBF, established normal values of SVC flow during the first 48 postnatal hours in well preterm neonates younger than 30 weeks of gestation who were receiving minimal ventilatory support.[48] However, it must be stated that the extent to which SVC flow is representative of systemic or CBF in preterm neonates during the first postnatal days is not understood. In a subsequent study that included sick preterm infants younger than 30 weeks of gestation, the same group found that 38% of infants had a period of low SVC in the first 24 postnatal hours.[46] The incidence of low SVC flow was significantly related to the level of immaturity, and more

than 70% of low SVC flow occurred in very preterm neonates (less than 27 weeks' gestation). The sudden increase in the peripheral vascular resistance caused by the loss of the low-resistance placental circulation when the cord is clamped immediately after delivery, the complex process of cardiorespiratory transition to the postnatal circulatory pattern, and myocardial and autonomic central nervous system immaturity have all been proposed to contribute to these findings. Indeed, these factors may explain why many of these very preterm neonates struggle to maintain normal systemic blood flow during the first 12 to 24 postnatal hours. Of note is that using "physiologic" (delayed, for at least 30–60 seconds) rather than immediate cord clamping, immediate postnatal hemodynamic transition and the incidence of associated cerebral pathologies have changed.[56,57] Although physiologic cord clamping and other strategies to enhance placental transfusion do not alter the rate of severe P/IVH (grade III and IV), they do decrease the overall rate of P/IVH. The lower incidence of P/IVH with physiologic cord clamping may be due to improved postnatal cardiovascular adaptation. In addition, the higher intravascular volume may mitigate or attenuate cerebral hypoperfusion prevalent in the extremely preterm infants during the immediate transitional period, thereby decreasing the risk of P/IVH.[58] An intriguing and potentially important finding of the SVC studies was that a proportion of the very preterm babies with extremely low SVC flow was found to have systemic blood pressures in the "normal" range (i.e., equal to or greater than their gestational age in weeks), a finding supported by subsequent studies of this group of researchers.[37,47,49] Because normal blood pressure and decreased organ blood flow to nonvital organs are the hallmarks of the compensated phase of shock and because a portion of SVC flow represents blood returning from the brain, a vital organ, it is conceivable that that the proposed low-priority vessel ("nonvital organ") assignment of the vascular beds of the forebrain (cerebral cortex and white matter) in the very preterm neonate during the immediate postnatal period explain these findings. This hypothesis, which is supported by studies in different animal models[59,60] and also, indirectly, in the human neonate[37,49,61] may explain, at least in part, why SVC blood flow may be decreased in some very preterm neonates who have normal systemic blood pressure. Most preterm neonates with documented low SVC flow in the first 24 to 48 hours that do not go on to have P/IVH or PWMI are more mature (28 weeks and beyond vs. 25–26 weeks' gestation). Thus for preterm infants of less than 30 weeks' gestation, preexisting low systemic blood flow (and CBF) may be necessary but not sufficient to cause intracranial pathology. Importantly, all patients studied had an increase in SVC flow by 24 to 36 hours, and all P/IVHs occurred after the SVC flow had increased. Findings of a later prospective observational study by our group using echocardiography and NIRS confirm and expand these observations.[45] In this study, very preterm neonates who presented with lower systemic blood flow and higher cerebral vascular resistance during the first 12 postnatal hours were at a higher risk for the development of P/IVH. Importantly, the bleeding occurred only after cardiac output and brain blood flow had increased. In addition, lower cerebral tissue oxygenation levels detected by NIRS during the first 12 postnatal hours might identify the patients who will subsequently develop P/IVH.[45] Taken together, these findings implicate an ischemia-reperfusion cycle in the pathogenesis of P/IVH in very preterm neonates during the immediate transitional period.

It is important to note that the methods used to assess systemic and CBF in VLBW neonates in the immediate transitional period have significant limitations. When SVC flow is used to assess systemic and CBF, the measurements are operator dependent owing to the uncertainties associated with the accurate measurement of vessel diameter and flow velocity. The fluctuations in vessel size during the cardiac cycle and the flow velocity pattern in the SVC are important factors contributing to these technical difficulties. In addition, the shape of the SVC, the lack of data on the magnitude of the contribution of CBF to SVC flow in the human neonate, and the lack of a documented association between $PaCO_2$ and SVC flow in this patient population call for caution in the interpretation of these findings.

Yet, an association has been found between SVC flow and aEEG indices of oxygen utilization (continuity and amplitude) in the first 48 postnatal hours.[62] Finding of this study also demonstrated that hypotension, either treated or untreated, was associated with decreased levels of brain activity as assessed by aEEG. This finding supports the previously referenced

data[22,25,31] indicating that blood pressure and brain oxygen utilization are inextricably linked.

In another study, CBF was measured in both the internal carotid and vertebral arteries and the sum of the flow in the four arteries supplying the brain was used to assess the changes in CBF volume in preterm infants of 28 to 35 weeks of gestation over the first 2 postnatal weeks.[63] Although the technique, again, has significant limitations, the findings suggest that a steep rise in CBF occurs from the first to the second postnatal day and that this pattern is independent of gestational age. Thereafter, CBF continues to rise gradually (Fig. 2.7). Because brain weight does not significantly increase during the first 48 postnatal hours, the investigators inferred that the observed increase in CBF during that period was secondary to increased cerebral perfusion per unit weight of tissue. On the other hand, the more gradual increase over the ensuing 2 weeks is likely due to a combination of increased brain weight, increased cerebral metabolic rate, and increased perfusion.[55,63] This study enrolled only "healthy" preterm infants with normal brains, whereas investigations in other studies[46,47,64,65] included a group of preterm infants who were sicker and had a higher incidence of significant intracranial pathology. Nevertheless, the results in the two groups of patients are complementary as they provide evidence for a decreased CBF in the first postnatal day, followed by a significant increase by the second postnatal day. Although low CBF in the first postnatal day and the ensuing "reperfusion" appears to be a physiologic phenomenon likely occurring in all very preterm neonates, CBF is even lower in those who later develop P/IVH.[45] Therefore, the phenomenon of low CBF is also a necessary but not sufficient cause of intracranial pathology (P/IVH or PWMI) in this patient population. Interestingly, the difference in CBF may be present as early as the first few minutes after birth. A case-control study showed lower cerebral oxygen saturation in the "P/IVH group" from 7 minutes after birth compared to the "no-P/IVH control group" despite having similar arterial oxygen saturation.[66] This difference may be related to a lower CBF or hemoglobin in the P/IVH group. Similarly, a prospective study showed lower cerebral oxygen saturation in the delivery room among the four patients who later developed severe P/IVH or died in the first 72 postnatal hours.[67]

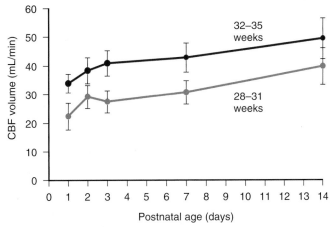

Fig. 2.7 Changes in CBF volume in preterm neonates during the first 14 days after delivery. Development of CBF volume with increasing postnatal age in two different gestational age groups (28–31 and 32–35 weeks' gestation). Mean and 95% confidence interval are shown (ANOVA; n = 29, $p < 0.0001$). (From Kehrer M, Blumenstock G, Ehehalt S, et al. Development of cerebral blood flow volume in preterm neonates during the first two weeks of life. *Pediatr Res.* 2005;58:927–30, with permission.)

However, these four patients also had higher mean airway pressure and lower arterial oxygen saturation, and as such, the lower cerebral oxygen saturation may simply reflect the poor respiratory status of these patients. Finally, although the vast majority of studies found low CBF on the first exam performed during the first few hours after birth, some have described a decrease in CBF at 12 hours compared to 3 to 6 hours after delivery.[68,69] The reason for the discrepancy in the findings is unclear at present.

The ultimate goal is to improve neurodevelopmental outcome in preterm infants. In addition to the association between low SVC flow in the early postnatal period and P/IVH, low SVC flow in the early postnatal period is also independently associated with impaired neurologic outcome at 3 years of age.[7] Therefore, infants most at risk must be identified in the immediate postnatal period. In addition to ultrasonography, NIRS and other monitoring modalities may be helpful in this regard. Indeed and as mentioned earlier, preterm infants who develop P/IVH have a pattern of changes in cerebral regional tissue oxygen saturation and oxygen extraction that is different from those without at risk for P/IVH.[45] Thus combining different systemic and organ blood flow and tissue oxygenation monitoring technologies may be helpful in the early identification of infants at greater risk for the development of intracerebral pathologies.[70]

It is clear from the large number of epidemiologic and hemodynamic studies that the level of immaturity is one of the most important predisposing factors for the occurrence of more abrupt changes in CBF and the increased vulnerability during postnatal adaptation and for poor neurologic outcome. Therefore, assessment of CBF during the first 24 to 48 postnatal hours in the most immature and vulnerable patients is important. However, owing to the technical difficulties associated with reliable and continuous assessment of CBF, clinical practice currently relies on indirect measures for diagnosis of changes in cerebral perfusion especially since the sole reliance on blood pressure in the indirect assessment of CBF in this patient population during the first postnatal day is not appropriate.

In addition to blood pressure, monitoring of the indirect clinical indicators of tissue perfusion such as urine output, CRT, and acid-base status in routine clinical practice remains important. Although these indirect clinical indicators by themselves are fairly nonspecific for evaluating systemic flow, using CRT and blood pressure together results in greater sensitivity. Indeed, when blood pressure and CRT are less than 30 mm Hg and 3 seconds or higher, respectively, the sensitivity for identifying low systemic blood flow is 86%.[71] In addition, avoidance of both hypocapnia and hypercapnia is of utmost importance because of their effect on CBF. However, and as mentioned earlier, the manifestation of the effect of $PaCO_2$ on CBF appears to be dependent on postnatal age. A study reported a gradual change in the relationship between $PaCO_2$ and middle cerebral artery mean velocity, a surrogate for CBF, from none on the first day to the expected positive linear pattern by the third postnatal day.[72] Others have also described an attenuated relationship on the first postnatal day with an increase in the reactivity of CBF to CO_2 during the following days.[73,74] Finally, inappropriately high intrathoracic pressure and elevated right heart pressure may also increase the risk of the development of P/IVH by impeding cerebral venous drainage. A recent study showed that altered internal cerebral venous flow pattern is associated with an increased rate of P/IVH.[75] In addition to the increased intrathoracic and right atrial pressures, high blood pressure and PDA have also been associated with altered internal cerebral venous flow.[76] However, the underlying mechanisms of this association are unclear.

Monitoring of Blood Pressure, Systemic and Organ Blood Flow, and Cerebral Function

Blood pressure is invasively and continuously monitored in most critically ill neonates using an indwelling arterial catheter and a calibrated pressure transducer. Available techniques are more likely to be used for systemic blood flow and CBF monitoring are ultrasound (echocardiography and Doppler ultrasound), electrical impedance, and NIRS. As for continuous monitoring of cerebral function in neonates, aEEG has also been increasingly used at the bedside. We briefly discuss these modalities used for systemic and organ blood flow monitoring in the following sections with a primary focus on those that can be performed non-invasively at the bedside.

DOPPLER ULTRASOUND

Velocity of blood flow can be measured through the use of the Doppler principle, which states that the change in frequency of reflected sound is proportional to the velocity of the passing object (in this case, blood). The calculated velocity needs to be corrected for the angle between the vessel and the emitted sound beam (angle of insonation), and the straightforward idea is complicated by the fact that arterial blood is pulsatile, and its

speed varies within the vessel (i.e., it is faster in the center of the vessel). It is important to recognize that speed of blood (distance traveled per unit time) in a vessel means little by itself; we are interested in the absolute blood flow (volume per unit time). Thus volumetric measurements are crucial and can be obtained by the product of velocity time integral (VTI) and cross-sectional area of the vessel that the blood travels in. Investigators have used several different volumetric indices, including SVC, internal carotid artery, and vertebral artery flow, as previously discussed.[48,63] The limitations of SVC flow measurements were discussed earlier. In general, major technical problems with volumetric measurements include but are not restricted to the small size of the vessels, the motion of vessel wall, and whether or not an angle of insonation of less than 20 degrees can be achieved. In addition to volumetric measurements of vessel blood flow, right ventricular and left ventricular outflow measurements have excessively been studied. However, both are fraught with pitfalls in the very preterm neonate in the immediate postnatal period, because the patent foramen ovale (PFO) and patent ductus arteriosus (PDA) represent shunts that confound measurements of the right ventricular and left ventricular flows, respectively. It is believed that right ventricular output may be a more reliable indicator of systemic blood flow during the immediate postnatal period with the fetal channels open, because shunting through the PFO is less significant than PDA shunting during the first 24 postnatal hours.[77] Indeed, right ventricular output and systemic blood pressure have been correlated with EEG parameters (brain function) in VLBW infants in the immediate postnatal period.[61] Ultrasound techniques are noninvasive and widely accessible in the intensive care setting and can be done at the bedside. The procedure itself minimally affects hemodynamic and physiological variables of the infant.[78] However, all ultrasound measurements are noncontinuous, operator dependent, and have their significant limitations. As for the issues related to operator skills, centers utilizing these methods to diagnose pathologic CBF in neonates must have a rigorous quality control system in place with neonatologists trained in functional echocardiography and available at the bedside at any time.[79]

With regard to the limitations to the use of vascular Doppler ultrasonography in assessing organ blood flow, the most important limitation is the small size of the artery of interest (e.g., middle or anterior cerebral artery), which precludes accurate measurement of its diameter. As previously mentioned, the estimation of blood flow (Q) depends on assessment of mean velocity of the blood (V) and the vessel diameter (D) $(Q = V(\pi D^2/4) \times 60)$; any small error in measuring the diameter will translate into a significant error in estimating the actual blood flow. Therefore, instead of directly measuring blood flow, investigators often use changes in various Doppler-derived indices, such as mean blood flow velocity or the pulsatility or resistance index, as surrogates for changes in blood flow. This approach is based on the premise that the vessel diameter remains constant despite the changes in blood flow. However, this concept in not universally accepted.[79] Nevertheless, both animal and human studies have shown an acceptable correlation between these indices and other measures of blood flow.[80–83]

Finally, although normative data for the Doppler ultrasonography–derived indices for various vessels are available, the previously described limitations require caution in the interpretation of a single measurement. Rather, repeated measurements and the use of trends over time are thought to be more informative of the hemodynamic status and the changes in organ blood flow.

IMPEDANCE ELECTRICAL CARDIOMETRY

IEC is a noninvasive and continuous bedside method of measuring beat-to-beat left ventricular output on the basis of detection of changes in thoracic electrical bioimpedance (Aesculon, Cardiotronic; La Jolla, CA) caused by the changes in the orientation of the red blood cells in the ascending aorta during systole and diastole normalized for the body mass of the patient.[68] The method has been validated against thermodilution and other direct methods of cardiac output measurement and has shown good correlation in adults and children.[84,85] Although the clinical utility of the bioimpedance technology in neonates is still untested, data from our group and others show clinically acceptable precision and comparable quantitation of left ventricular output to echocardiography in term neonates.[86,87] However, a recent study comparing MR and IEC in adults found poor agreement between the two methods in estimating left ventricular output.[88] In

addition to the inherent limitations of MR, in this study, the IEC measurements were done before and after MR imaging and not simultaneously. Another recent study by our group, however, also found poorer correlation with MRI-derived values of cardiac output and its changes with those obtained by simultaneous IEC monitoring in adults during rest and exercise.[89] These findings suggest that the absolute values obtained using IEC may not appropriately represent cardiac output. Yet, due to its reproducibility, continuous, beat-to-beat cardiac output measurements, and ease of application, IEC appears to possess clinical applicability when the measurements are trended over time. Finally, and to highlight the complexity of the studies comparing the utility of the different technologies in measuring systemic blood flow in the neonate, a recent study using bioreactance technology (NICOM Reliant; Cheetah Medical, MA, USA) found a poor concordance rate and wide limits of agreement with echocardiography in estimating changes in cardiac output in preterm infants.[90]

The recent publications of reference values for cardiac output measured by IEC and bioreactance in premature infants of different gestational age[91,92] may be helpful if one considers them as a screening tool for the detection of infants at risk for low cardiac output and thus cerebral injury. Further validation of these techniques is needed, especially in the premature infant population, before the routine use of IEC or bioreactance can be recommended in the neonatal patient population. As for IEC, it remains an interesting approach with the ability to obtain continuous, beat-to-beat, and noninvasively collected data in absolute numbers on stroke volume and cardiac output at the bedside in neonates, especially when trending changes in cardiac output and assessing the efficacy of therapeutic interventions.

NEAR-INFRARED SPECTROSCOPY

NIRS has received much attention since its first use in newborns in 1985[93] and numerous papers have been published describing its use and clinical relevance in neonatology. As absorption of light in the near-infrared range (600–900 nanometers) depends on the oxygenation status of "chromophores" such as hemoglobin and cytochrome aa3, the absorption during passage through brain tissue can be measured, and oxygenation indices calculated. Different wavelengths of light can be used to assess different parameters, such as oxyhemoglobin, deoxyhemoglobin, and cytochrome aa3 oxidase. Through induction of a small but rapid change in arterial oxygen saturation in the subject, CBF can even be calculated using the Fick's principle. This method assumes that during the measurement period, cerebral blood volume (CBV) and cerebral oxygen extraction remain constant. However, the technique may not be feasible in babies with severe lung disease, in whom no or very little change in oxygen saturation occurs with an increased FiO_2, and in infants with normal lungs in whom oxygen saturation is 100% when they breathe room air. To get around this problem, an injected tracer dye such as indocyanine green has been used instead of oxygen, with comparable results.[94] Some instruments use the TOI, which is the weighted average of arterial, capillary, and venous oxygenation and theoretically allows the measurement of regional cerebral hemoglobin oxygen saturation ($rScO_2$) without manipulation of FiO_2 or use of dye. However, this index also has a significant problem with reproducibility when the sensor is changed. In one study, the 95% limit of agreement was as large as -17% to $+17\%$.[95] Indeed, reproducibility of NIRS measurements in general has been an ongoing issue for investigators, especially in the detection of focal changes in cerebral hemodynamics. This is a significant problem, because focal hemodynamic changes are at least as likely as global changes to contribute to neuropathology. Despite these limitations, NIRS has been validated through comparison with xenon-133 clearance in human newborns.[96] In addition, by averaging several measurements, the precision of TOI improves and becomes clinically acceptable.[97] As the penetration depth of NIRS is around 2.5 cm, unless the patient is a very preterm neonate, TOI is primarily assessed in the frontal lobes (both gray and white matter) when the optodes are placed on the forehead.

For clinical use, an algorithm allowing for continuous monitoring of regional tissue oxygen saturation (rSO_2) in absolute numbers has been developed for adult, pediatric, and neonatal use.[98] Reference values of cerebral rSO_2 and oxygen extraction in preterm neonates during the first 3 postnatal days have been established.[99] Cerebral rSO_2 is higher in more mature preterm infants with an increase of 1% per week of gestation.

More recently, newly developed MR techniques not requiring respiratory calibration have allowed comparison of cerebral oxygen saturation measurements by NIRS and MRI in neonates. The agreement is reasonable with strong linear relation between the two methods.[100,101] Although NIRS represents a practical solution and information on its use in neonates has been encouraging,[102] accumulation of more data and prospective studies looking at both short- and long-term outcomes are needed to provide an evidence-based utilization of NIRS in neonatal medicine. A multicenter randomized clinical trial (SafeBoosC II) proposes a treatment guideline to reduce burden of cerebral hypoxia or hyperoxia of extremely preterm infants by targeting a hypothesized "acceptable" $rScO_2$ range of 55% to 85% by use of NIRS monitoring during the first 3 postnatal days.[103] Short-term outcomes have shown an overall 58% (95% CI: 35%–73%) reduction of hypoxia or hyperoxia burden in the "NIRS group" versus the control group (36.1% vs. 81.3% hours) using a preset treatment guideline.[104] However, despite the decrease in cerebral hypoxia/hyperoxia burden, no significant differences in the incidence of severe brain injury as detected by cranial ultrasound and MRI,[105] EEG (burst rates), or certain biomarkers of brain injury[85] were found between the NIRS and control groups. Similarly, the higher burden of hypoxia had no significant effect on 2-year neurodevelopmental outcomes.[106] However, there was a trend toward a better survival rate and reduction in severe brain injury at discharge in the NIRS group.[104] In addition, a statistically insignificant higher rate of cerebral palsy and severe developmental impairment was found in the high hypoxia burden group.[106] Currently, a multinational, randomized, pragmatic phase III clinical trial (SafeBoosC III) is underway.[107] This trial tests the hypothesis that intervention based on cerebral rSO_2 during the first 3 postnatal days reduces the composite outcome of either death or severe brain injury. Finally, limited animal data suggest that cerebral rSO_2 of 45% to 55% may be an important threshold below which ischemic brain injury likely occurs.[108,109] However, as the list of commercially available NIRS devices continues to expand,[110] it is important to keep in mind that different NIRS devices and even various sensors have systematic differences with up to 12 percentage points difference in measured tissue oxygen saturation.[107,111]

A case-control study comparing hypotensive preterm infants on moderate-high dose dopamine to normotensive control found no difference in percentage time spent with cerebral saturation less than 50% in the first 3 postnatal days. However, patients who spent more than 10% of the time with saturation less than 50% had worse neurodevelopmental outcome.[88] In addition to the interest in absolute $rScO_2$ values, assessment of cerebral autoregulation in premature infants using NIRS has also become a focus of active research. Assuming a constant SaO_2, hematocrit, metabolic rate, CBV, and arterial and venous blood distribution in the tissue, alteration in cerebral rSO_2 reflects changes in CBF. When coupled with mean arterial blood pressure measurement, cerebral autoregulation can be characterized. However, this is a challenging approach since maintaining a constant oxygen saturation in extremely premature infants is difficult in the clinical setting.[112,113] Another potential application of NIRS is recognition of shock in the compensated stage to avoid decompensation and the development of hypotension in the first place. A recent RCT used cerebral and peripheral NIRS to guide the management of circulatory compromise among preterm infants during the transitional period.[114] If there was a more than 5% increase in cerebral-to-peripheral saturation ratio, it was considered as evidence for peripheral vasoconstriction to aid in the preferential perfusion of the brain and therefore was regarded as an early sign of developing shock. This, in turn, prompted further evaluation of the circulatory status with echocardiography and led to predefined interventions. Unfortunately, the study population was restricted to recruiting only moderate-to-late preterm neonates with relatively stable hemodynamic status with no patient requiring catecholamine therapy. Although the burden of hypotension was not statistically different between the NIRS and control groups (33% vs. 45% hypotensive), the authors speculated there could be a value in such monitoring in more immature and unstable neonates. In summary, the clinical application of NIRS has significantly increased over the past decade. There is some evidence to support its utility in the care of hemodynamically at-risk neonates; however, before NIRS monitoring can be recommended to guide routine clinical care, well-designed, large, multicenter RCTs need to be completed.

AMPLITUDE-INTEGRATED EEG (CEREBRAL FUNCTION MONITORING)

Although video EEG is the gold standard, amplitude-integrated EEG is an acceptable bedside method to establish a neurologic prognosis in asphyxiated infants during the first several hours after birth.[115–117] Accordingly, aEEG has been used to select candidates for enrollment in head-cooling neuroprotection trials. This technology uses either a single-channel EEG recording with biparietal electrodes or duo-channel EEG with four electrodes. Frequencies lower than 2 Hz and higher than 15 Hz are selectively filtered out, and the amplitude of the signal is integrated. The signal is then recorded semilogarithmically with slow speed, effectively compressing hours of EEG recording into shorter segments that reflect global background activity and major deviations from baseline (e.g., seizures). Studies have shown that aEEG correlates with conventional EEG,[118] although recent studies have shown lower sensitivity and specificity for seizure detection.[116,119] However, aEEG has the distinct advantage of being easily applied and interpreted by nonneurologists. In an earlier study, normal aEEG findings in the first 72 postnatal hours in asphyxiated term neonates have been found to be prognostic of normal neurologic outcome at 2 years of age.[120] Coupled with early neurologic examination, simultaneous aEEG improved specificity and positive predictive value of abnormal results for abnormal neurologic outcome at 18 months of age.[121] A growing interest for the utilization of aEEG in the preterm population has enabled gathering of normative data. Typical patterns of background activity for preterm infants have been established, and a number of studies exist that point to its applicability in this group.[122] West and colleagues[123] examined the relationships among echocardiographic blood flow findings, mean arterial blood pressure, and aEEG findings in preterm infants (<30 weeks of gestation) during the first 48 hours after birth. They found that low right ventricular output, used as a surrogate for systemic blood flow due to the shunting across the fetal channels at 12 hours of postnatal age, correlated with low aEEG amplitude, whereas low mean blood pressure (<31 mm Hg) correlated with low EEG continuity. Indeed, recent studies showed a coupling between mean blood pressure and EEG and demonstrated an inverse relationship between mean blood pressure and EEG discontinuity.[124,125] Furthermore, abnormal aEEG (increased discontinuity and low voltage) has been shown to be predictive of severe P/IVH in preterm infants.[122] Taken together with evidence that early aEEG in preterm infants can be helpful in predicting long-term neurodevelopmental outcome,[126] it is reasonable to suggest that aEEG merits further study in the VLBW population, especially along with the use of NIRS, as a means of identifying infants at risk for low CBF and oxygen delivery and/or for pathologic fluctuations in CBF.

SUMMARY OF THE MONITORING METHODS DISCUSSED

Methods capable of diagnosing altered CBF and the associated changes in brain function in the VLBW population in the first hours to days after delivery are still largely in the experimental arena. It is extremely unlikely that one monitoring parameter will be sufficient to encapsulate the status of CBF and oxygen delivery. Instead, and in addition to clinical assessment, a combination of a variety of technologies will likely prove helpful, ranging from conventional (heart rate, blood pressure, oxygen saturation, transcutaneous CO_2) to advanced (Doppler ultrasonography, IEC, NIRS, aEEG) methods. Both systemic and CBF, as well as cerebral oxygen delivery and extraction have to be evaluated simultaneously and continuously to enable the collection of in-depth information allowing for more informed, minute-to-minute decisions about how, when, and what to treat. This goal has not been achieved, but it is likely that a number of these modalities will be incorporated into routine clinical use in the not-too-distant future.[127]

Fig. 2.8 illustrates an example of a comprehensive, real-time, hemodynamic bedside monitoring and data acquisition system developed by our group.[128]

Treatment Strategies

In the previous section, we discussed the available noninvasive bedside techniques with the potential to monitor CBF in the VLBW neonate. Although these techniques have been more widely used in the past few years and may aid in the management of circulatory compromise in a subset of neonates, they are not yet quite ready for widespread routine clinical use for CBF monitoring, as their application and interpretation require specialized technology and further confirmation. By extension, application of these methods in clinical practice must eventually be shown to improve long-term neurologic outcome. However, results of studies using these experimental strategies can at least be useful for tailoring routine care because they give a glimpse of how MAP and systemic blood flow interact and affect CBF. This section focuses on how routinely monitored indices such as arterial blood pressure (hypotension), acid-base status, and arterial oxygenation, the commonly used medications, presence of a PDA, and intercurrent infection may affect CBF. We discuss management options, including evidence for when and how to treat systemic hypotension and clinical signs of systemic and organ hypoperfusion. Ultimately, we propose a treatment strategy for maintaining brain perfusion and oxygenation in the VLBW infant during the first few postnatal days.

SYSTEMIC HYPOTENSION

There are several clinical approaches to the diagnosis and treatment of neonatal hypotension. First, and as mentioned earlier, two groups of researchers independently identified an MAP of approximately 28 to 29 mm Hg as a "breakpoint," below which autoregulation was absent in preterm neonates.[25,31] Use of dopamine to raise the mean blood pressure resulted in a normalization of the CBF in these hypotensive infants. Thus treatment of hypotension with dopamine quickly restores normal blood pressure and CBF.[25] However, CBF autoregulation was not immediately restored. Findings of an earlier study suggest that it may take up to an hour or more for CBF autoregulation to be restored following treatment of systemic hypotension.[129] If a mean blood pressure over 28 to 29 mm Hg was considered normal in VLBW infants, many would be treated whose overall hemodynamic status does not indicate a need for treatment or may receive a treatment modality (volume, vasopressors/inotropes, or inotropes) that does not specifically address the underlying pathophysiology of their cardiovascular compromise. Instead, the most widespread approach to the definition of hypotension in the VLBW neonate

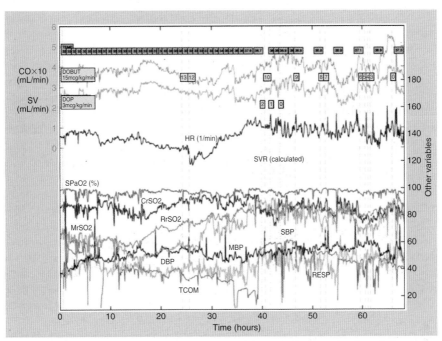

Fig. 2.8 Hemodynamic parameters continuously monitored by the hemodynamic monitoring tower in a term, 3-day-old neonate with hypoxic-ischemic encephalopathy undergoing rewarming from therapeutic whole-body hypothermia. Parameters continuously monitored included arterial oxygen saturation (SPao$_2$;%), heart rate (HR; 1/min), respiratory rate (RESP; 1/min), systolic (SBP; mm Hg), diastolic (DBP; mm Hg) and mean (MBP; mm Hg) blood pressure, beat-to-beat cardiac output (CO; mL/min) and stroke volume (SV; mL/min) using impedance electrical cardiometry, cerebral (CrSO$_2$), renal (RrSO$_2$), and muscle (MrSO$_2$) mixed venous tissue oxygen saturation using NIRS, and transcutaneous CO$_2$ (TCOM; mm Hg). These parameters are depicted on the Y-axis while age after delivery in hours is shown on the X-axis. Rewarming started at 30 hours of monitoring. Core temperature (TEMP) is shown in small boxes and dopamine (DOP) and dobutamine (DOBUT) doses are depicted over the cardiac output and stroke volume data. Automatically calculated systemic vascular resistance (SVR; mm Hg $\times$ min/mL) is also depicted. See text for details.

during the immediate transitional period is use of a mean blood pressure value that equals the gestational age in numerals. There are two major concerns with this approach. First, if the autoregulatory blood pressure breakpoint is indeed at 28 to 29 mm Hg for this patient population, blood pressure at the level of the gestational age in more immature and thus vulnerable preterm neonates will be out of the autoregulatory range. Second, as discussed earlier, some of these immature neonates even with "normal" blood pressure have low systemic and presumably CBFs,[37] especially since their cerebral vasculature may constrict rather than dilate in the first, compensated phase of shock.[37,49,59,60,130] Because low SVC flow (used as a surrogate of CBF) in the first postnatal day is a risk factor for P/IVH and poor neurodevelopmental outcome,[7] it is important to identify the babies at risk, and this identification cannot be accomplished with blood pressure monitoring alone. As discussed earlier, the combined use of blood pressure and indirect clinical signs of tissue hypoperfusion might help to identify patients with low systemic and thus low CBF. If functional echocardiography is available, VLBW neonates who are "normotensive" (their blood pressure is equal to or higher than their gestational age in numerals) but have low systemic blood flow may be identified. As this presentation mostly occurs during the first 6 to 12 hours postnatally, targeted use of functional echocardiography to measure right ventricular output and SVC blood flow may be the best approach currently available to detect low systemic perfusion. However, even if one can diagnose low systemic blood flow during the first hours after delivery, at present we do not have an effective treatment modality to improve systemic blood flow in this patient population. Further, hypotension defined by the gestational age-based criterion in VLBW neonates appears to be a risk factor for poor neurodevelopmental outcome and it is not known whether treatment with vasopressor/inotropes or inotropes does[11,18] or does not[10] ameliorate the risk. One could speculate that some of the hypotensive babies may have been treated too late to make a difference, or that the current treatment approach is ineffective in other neonates to ameliorate the hypotension-and/or the low CBF-associated brain injury. Finally, because of the uncertainties surrounding the definition of hypotension and the unexpected relationship between blood pressure and CBF in the VLBW neonate in the immediate postnatal period, as well as the potential side effects of vasopressors and or their use along with the lack of evidence that treatment of hypotension improves neurodevelopmental outcome, some authors advocate that hypotension in the VLBW neonate during the first postnatal day(s) be treated only if there is clear evidence of organ hypoperfusion (i.e., lactic acidosis). We would caution though that by the time lactic acidosis can be detected, cerebral ischemia is likely to have already occurred. Therefore, this approach carries the theoretical risk of allowing significant cerebral hypoperfusion to occur. On the other hand, unnecessary treatment may indeed be harmful. Therefore an individualized approach based on early (direct or indirect) evidence of decreases in systemic and/or brain blood flow in hypotensive preterm neonates is the only remaining choice at present.

There is general consensus that once the fetal channels are closed and the blood pressure–CBF relationship is restored after the first few days following delivery, blood pressure becomes a more reliable indicator of cerebral perfusion even in the most immature neonates. In this scenario, it can be more stringently advocated that hypotension should be treated promptly with cautious volume administration and careful titration of the most appropriate vasoactive medication (vasopressor/inotrope or inotrope) to avoid sustained changes in systemic blood pressure and blood flow.

TREATMENT OF HYPOTENSION ASSOCIATED WITH PDA

PDA, a common presentation in VLBW infants in the immediate postnatal period, with significant left-to-right shunting often manifests as hypotension.[77,131,132] It has been demonstrated that the direction of shunting through a nonrestrictive PDA is already primarily left to right in the first 6 hours after delivery and is highly associated with a low SVC flow state.[48,133] Ductal size of >2.0 mm and left atrium-to-aortic root ratio of >1.4 (especially when simultaneously present) are associated with a high risk of abnormal organ blood flow.[134] A large PDA with and without hypotension during early transition has also been associated with P/IVH.[46,132,135] Treatment of the PDA before 6 hours of postnatal life with indomethacin induces ductal constriction within 2 hours, but this effect is not associated with simultaneous improvements in systemic blood flow.[136] Indomethacin decreases CBF via a direct cerebrovascular vasoconstrictive effect that is independent of the drug's inhibitory action on prostaglandin synthesis.[137] It is possible that the documented decrease in severe P/IVH with early indomethacin use is due to this selective cerebral vasoconstrictive effect during the first 2 to 3 days after delivery when reperfusion occurs[136] and has less to do with improving systemic blood flow by constricting the ductus arteriosus.

Although treatment of a hemodynamically insignificant PDA has become more controversial in last few years, most authors agree that a symptomatic, hemodynamically significant PDA should be treated. Cardiovascular management of the hemodynamically unstable, hypotensive VLBW neonate with a large PDA should focus on measures that induce stepwise and reversible increases in pulmonary vascular resistance until pharmacologic or, if this fails, surgical or device closure of the PDA takes place. Such measures may include the avoidance of hyperventilation and respiratory (and/or metabolic) alkalosis and maintenance of oxygen saturation value at the lower end of the acceptable range. It is not known how vasopressors affect ductal shunting. Limited data suggest that dopamine may not worsen ductal shunting and might actually improve systemic blood flow along with increases in blood pressure in preterm infants.[138] However, the hemodynamic effects of dopamine or epinephrine need to be closely monitored in these patients with the use of functional echocardiography or EIC.

TREATMENT OF HYPOTENSION ASSOCIATED WITH OTHER CAUSES SUCH AS SEPSIS, ADRENAL INSUFFICIENCY, AND HYPOVOLEMIA

In the treatment of hypotension in preterm infants with sepsis, adrenal insufficiency, and hypovolemia, every effort should be made to specifically treat the underlying primary cause to the cardiovascular status. Although there is very little experimental data regarding the response of CBF to vasopressor/inotropes or inotropes in the hypotensive VLBW infant, some evidence is accumulating.

Dopamine is the first-line medication for many neonatologists because of its cardiovascular and renal effects thought to be beneficial.[139] A study of hypotensive neonates in 43 pediatric hospitals in the United States shows dopamine to be by far the most commonly used medication.[140] A more recent study reported a similar finding among extremely preterm infants.[1] Dopamine effectively increases blood pressure in the preterm infant, but its effect on organ blood flow is less well described. Evidence indicates that despite its effect on increasing blood pressure and renal perfusion, dopamine does not have a selective vasoactive action on the cerebral circulation in normotensive VLBW neonates.[141,142] However, in hypotensive VLBW infants, the dopamine-induced increase in blood pressure is associated with an increase in CBF.[25,35,129] This finding suggests strongly that cerebrovascular autoregulation is impaired in hypotensive preterm infants and that effective treatment of hypotension is associated with an increase in CBF but with a delay in the restoration of CBF autoregulation (see earlier text).

Are other vasopressors more effective in restoring "normal" CBF in this population than dopamine? An RCT compared the cerebrovascular, hemodynamic, and metabolic effects of dopamine and epinephrine using careful, stepwise titration of the two medications to achieve optimum blood pressure in VLBW neonates in the first 24 postnatal hours.[18] Both medications were effective in increasing cerebral perfusion in the medium dose range, with epinephrine being slightly more effective in infants of less than 28 weeks' gestation and dopamine being more effective in those of greater than 28 weeks' gestation. A recent double-blinded RCT compared escalating doses of dopamine and epinephrine in preterm and term infants with septic shock.[143] The study showed no difference in shock reversal or mortality between groups treated by the two medications.[143,144] Similarly, a metaanalysis of three RCTs comparing dopamine and epinephrine in pediatric septic shock found no difference in reversal of shock

and mortality between the two medications.[145] Therefore, the available data indicate that dopamine and epinephrine are comparable in increasing blood pressure and CBF and reversing septic shock. Despite the above findings, given the limited data available, the surviving sepsis campaign international guidelines suggest using epinephrine, rather than dopamine, in children with septic shock (weak recommendation, low quality of evidence).[146] It is possible that in the subset of infants with septic shock and poor contractility, having a more potent direct inotropic than dopamine, epinephrine has a theoretical advantage. Even fewer data are available on norepinephrine. A retrospective study on the use of norepinephrine in septic shock after the failure of standard therapy, which included dopamine, epinephrine, and hydrocortisone, found improvement in blood pressure and urine output after adding norepinephrine.[147] Another retrospective study showed improvement in blood pressure but no change in acidosis or urine output after adding norepinephrine in preterm infants with cardiovascular compromise due to sepsis or pulmonary hypertension.[148] Vasopressin has also been proposed for the treatment of hypotension in preterm infants during the transitional period and was found to be a viable candidate in a small pilot study.[149] However, more data are needed before vasopressin can be considered as one of the first-line medications for the treatment of hypotension. As for the inotropes and lusitropes, there has been growing interest in the potential use of milrinone, a selective phosphodiesterase III inhibitor, in neonates and infants who have undergone cardiac surgery and in VLBW neonates with low systemic blood flow during the first postnatal day. Indeed, milrinone effectively decreases the incidence of low cardiac output in infants following cardiac surgery.[150,151] Because the low-flow state in preterm infants immediately after birth is in many ways similar to the low cardiac output syndrome in postoperative cardiac patients, this drug has the potential both as treatment for and prophylaxis of low systemic blood flow (and presumably low CBF) in the VLBW patient population. A pilot study examined the safety, efficacy, and optimal dosing of milrinone in infants of less than 29 weeks' gestation during the first hours of postnatal life.[152] At the applied dose, milrinone appeared to be relatively safe in the 1-day-old VLBW neonate. However, findings of a likely somewhat underpowered RCT by the same group of researchers indicate that milrinone is likely *ineffective to prevent* the occurrence of low SVC flow (a surrogate of systemic blood flow) in the 1-day-old VLBW neonate.[153] Therefore, at present, routine use of milrinone in this population cannot be recommended. Dobutamine, another sympathomimetic amine with direct positive inotropic and mild vasodilatory effects, effectively increases cardiac output and blood pressure in the VLBW neonate, especially when the cardiovascular compromise is caused by myocardial dysfunction.[154] However, dobutamine may not improve hemodynamics if the primary underlying pathophysiology is not poor myocardial contractility. Indeed, a placebo-controlled pilot trial showed dobutamine to have no effect on SVC flow.[155] Beyond the presentation of different forms of neonatal shock treated with vasopressors/inotropes, inotropes, and lusitropes, there has been increasing recognition that "vasopressor-resistant" hypotension frequently develops in the VLBW population. This presentation is thought to be due to cardiovascular adrenergic receptor downregulation and the higher incidence of relative adrenal insufficiency in the VLBW neonate.[156–160] A prospective observational study examining the hemodynamic effects of low-dose hydrocortisone administration in preterm neonates with vasopressor resistance and borderline hypotension found no independent effect of this treatment modality on CBF.[159]

THE IMPACT OF PROVISION OF INTENSIVE CARE ON SYSTEMIC AND CEREBRAL HEMODYNAMICS

In addition to the impact of the hemodynamic changes on CBF during postnatal transition, the effects of all interventions must always be considered. They include ventilatory maneuvers, the use of medications other than vasopressors/inotropes or inotropes, and invasive procedures. Premature infants with a median gestational age of 31 weeks have been reported to have a decrease in CBF velocity (and presumably in CBF) in response to *transient hyperoxia*.[161] This occurs without a decrease in $PaCO_2$, implicating hyperoxia directly in the decrease in CBF. Indeed, brief exposure to 100% oxygen has been shown to decrease CBF by 15%.[162] In contrast, a more recent study reported a gestational age–dependent differential response of CBF velocity to hyperoxia between 24 and .48 hours after birth.[163] Keeping the increased P/IVH risk in mind and therefore

using 32 weeks' gestation as the cutoff to divide the study population into two groups, they found increased and decreased CBF velocity in the patients <32 and ≥32 weeks' gestation, respectively.

Hypocapnia is a well-described cause of cerebral vasoconstriction, and a direct association between $PaCO_2$ and CBF, and an inverse association between $PaCO_2$ and cerebral oxygen extraction have been demonstrated in VLBW infants during the first postnatal days.[37,164,165] Lower levels of $PaCO_2$ are also associated with slowing of the EEG, likely induced by decreased cerebral oxygen delivery.[165] Interestingly, the effects on aEEG are most significant in the first 24 hours, less evident on the second day, and gone by the third postnatal day. These findings support the notion that the first hours of postnatal life represent a period of heightened vulnerability to CBF fluctuations. Not surprisingly, severe hypocapnia in VLBW neonates during the immediate transition period is associated with PWMI and cerebral palsy.[166] *Hypercapnia* impacts cerebral hemodynamics by increasing CBF and attenuating CBF autoregulation. The preterm brain is fairly sensitive to acute changes in CO_2. A recent study found that a >5 mm Hg increase or decrease in end-tidal CO_2 results in a significant increase or decrease in cerebral regional oxygen saturation, respectively.[167] The increase in CBF appears to be more prominent after the first postnatal day[72,73] and with a $PaCO_2$ greater than 51–53 mm Hg.[72] $PaCO_2$ values higher than 45 mm Hg during the first two postnatal days have been shown to progressively attenuate CBF autoregulation (Fig. 2.9).[168] It is tempting to speculate that these effects may explain the findings of retrospective studies, revealing a strong independent association between hypercapnia and P/IVH in very preterm neonates.[169–171] Interestingly, a recent RCT comparing the impact of mild versus high permissive hypercapnia on the rate of bronchopulmonary dysplasia found no pulmonary benefits of high CO_2 strategy and there was also no difference in the incidence of severe P/IVH between the mild and high permissive hypercapnia groups.[172] The follow-up study of this trial also found no independent effects (positive or negative) of high CO_2 strategy on neurodevelopment.[173] However, secondary exploratory data analysis of another RCT on the subject found that higher CO_2 is an independent risk factor for severe P/IVH or death, neurodevelopmental

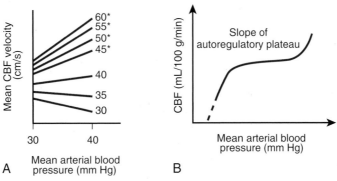

Fig. 2.9 Effect of hypercapnia on CBF autoregulation in 43 ventilated VLBW neonates during the first two postnatal days. A, Lines represent the estimated mean slopes of the autoregulatory plateau from 30 to 60 mm Hg $Paco_2$ with mean blood pressure values between 30 and 40 mm Hg. Horizontal line at slope zero indicates intact autoregulation with lines at 30, 35, and 40 mm Hg being not significantly different from zero. The estimated means of the slope of the autoregulatory plateau (cm/s/mm Hg) increased as $Paco_2$ increased from 40 mm Hg ($p = 0.004$).

impairment or death, and bronchopulmonary dysplasia or death[126] supporting the findings of the earlier retrospective studies.[168–170] Accordingly, the use of permissive hypercapnia during the immediate postnatal period may put the VLBW neonate at higher risk for cerebral injury.[174] Finally, high mean airway pressures in the immediate postnatal period have also been implicated in low systemic and CBF and a predilection for P/IVH.[47] Beyond ventilatory maneuvers and interventions, commonly used medications such as midazolam and morphine have also been associated with potentially harmful changes in CBF,[175] and even umbilical arterial blood sampling could have an effect on cerebral hemodynamics in these tiny infants.[176] The clinical relevance of the latter finding is unclear.

Summary and Recommendations

As discussed in this chapter, the management of hypotension and low systemic and CBF in the VLBW infant during the first postnatal days presents a significant challenge because immaturity, the physiologic changes during transition, and the underlying pathology all affect the hemodynamic response to pathologic processes and interventions.

Because of these factors and the lack of evidence on how treatment affects mortality and short- and long-term morbidity, straightforward recommendations on the treatment of cardiovascular compromise in the VLBW neonate during the period of transition to postnatal life cannot be given. Therefore, the following approach to diagnosis and treatment represents our view and should be considered only as such, especially because evidence on the effectiveness and impact of treatment of shock, especially on long-term neurodevelopmental outcomes, in the VLBW neonate during the first postnatal days is not available.

DIAGNOSIS OF HYPOTENSION

1. We use the 5th or 10th percentile of the gestational and postnatal age–dependent population-based blood pressure values as the crude definition of hypotension. However, we only initiate treatment at this point if signs of tissue hypoperfusion or echocardiographic evidence of decreased systemic perfusion and/or poor myocardial contractility are present. However, we attempt to maintain mean blood pressure at 23 to 24 mm Hg even if signs of tissue hypoperfusion are not present in the most immature ELBW neonates during the first postnatal day, because cerebral electrical activity appears to be depressed at blood pressure values below this level and there is some low-quality level evidence of improved outcome with treatment. However, it is important to keep in mind that cerebral metabolism is the main driver of CBF under physiologic state and when the flow-metabolism coupling is intact.

2. Irrespective of the blood pressure value, whenever there is indirect or direct evidence of poor tissue perfusion, we monitor both systemic

blood flow and blood pressure closely and attempt to maintain appropriate systemic blood flow without much fluctuation in the blood pressure. Because a blood pressure breakpoint of the CBF autoregulatory curve may exist at 28 to 29 mm Hg and because more than 90% of even ELBW neonates not receiving vasopressor support maintain their mean blood pressure at 30 mm Hg or higher by the third postnatal day, we carefully attempt to slowly increase mean blood pressure during the first 3 postnatal days and maintain it in the 28 to 30 mm Hg range by the third postnatal day. However, it must be kept in mind that an increase in blood pressure during this period does not necessarily ensure normalization of systemic and CBF and that there are no data that this approach improves long-term neurodevelopmental outcomes. Finally, the presence of a hemodynamically significant PDA affects our approach to maintaining and focusing on mean arterial blood pressure primarily and, in these cases, we carefully consider diastolic blood pressure and interrogate the cardiovascular system for evidence of systemic steal during diastole.

3. Although many neonatologists would agree with the approach described here, there is another, less frequently practiced approach that is worthy of discussion. Neonatologists using this approach initiate cardiovascular support only if there is clear evidence of poor systemic perfusion as long as mean blood pressure is at or higher than 20 mm Hg or so in the ELBW neonate during the first postnatal day. Because within the first 24 hours, it is hard to define poor perfusion, especially without the use of functional echocardiography, and because lactic acidosis heralds the presence of (ongoing or previously present) tissue ischemia, we do not practice this diagnostic and treatment philosophy and do not allow mean arterial blood pressure to stay around 20 mm Hg during the first postnatal day. Although there is no direct evidence at present that the use of "permissive hypotension" as an approach to diagnosis and management of cardiovascular compromise in VLBW neonates during the immediate postnatal

period affects outcomes, data from the EPIPAGE-II study question the wisdom of using this clinical approach.[11]

TREATMENT OF HYPOTENSION

With regard to the kind of treatment utilized, the most appropriate strategy requires identification of the underlying pathogenesis of hypotension. The most common etiologic factors are inappropriate peripheral vasoregulation and dysfunction of the myocardium complicated by the presence of a large PDA in VLBW neonates during the first postnatal days. However, recent data on physiologic ("delayed") cord clamping also implicate a certain level of hypovolemia if the cord clamped immediately after delivery.[56,57] Again, we emphasize that there is only little evidence that treatment of hypotension in this patient population improves mortality, morbidity, or long-term neurodevelopmental outcome:

1. In the case of hypotension, because low to moderate doses of dopamine (or epinephrine) improve both blood pressure and CBF, we carefully titrate dopamine in a stepwise manner using 3- to 5-minute cycles and make every effort to avoid inducing significant rapid changes in blood pressure. If there is evidence of or reasonable suspicion for hypovolemia, we carefully administer volume (usually isotonic saline unless otherwise indicated).[177] If low systemic blood flow is detected with low-normal to normal blood pressure during the first postnatal day, we use dobutamine (with or without low-dose dopamine) and monitor for indirect (CRT, urine output, base deficit) and direct (functional echocardiography) signs of improvement in systemic perfusion.

2. In the presence of a hemodynamically significant PDA, we attempt to close the ductus arteriosus with a cyclooxygenase inhibitor (we use indomethacin) along with providing appropriate supportive care. If pharmacologic closure fails in the patient with a hemodynamically significant PDA, and there is evidence of ongoing or worsening systemic tissue hypoperfusion, we use device closure or surgically ligate the ductus arteriosus. During the wait for device or surgical closure to take place, our goal is to decrease the left-to-right

shunting across the ductus. As briefly described earlier, we attempt to achieve this goal by carefully increasing pulmonary resistance in a stepwise manner. Using this approach, we frequently are successful at increasing pulmonary vascular resistance, and the associated decrease in left-to-right shunting usually results in improvement of systemic blood flow and blood pressure. We also use dopamine in babies with a hemodynamically significant PDA, because it has been shown that, in patients with increased pulmonary blood flow, dopamine increases pulmonary vascular resistance and systemic perfusion.[102] Interestingly, there is no evidence that dopamine preferentially increases pulmonary vascular resistance in neonates without preexisting pulmonary overcirculation. It is tempting to speculate that the increased pulmonary blood flow–associated "protective" upregulation of vasoconstrictive mechanisms (enhanced α-adrenergic and endothelin-1 receptor expression) and downregulation of the vasodilatory mechanisms (endogenous nitric oxide and vasodilatory prostaglandin production) in the pulmonary arteries are responsible for this observation. We add dobutamine only in the presence of impaired myocardial function, because most VLBW neonates with hemodynamically significant PDA after the first postnatal day usually have normal or hyperdynamic cardiac function. Indeed, the indiscriminate use of dobutamine in these patients may compromise diastolic function and thus cardiac filling. Finally, administration of fluids to increase blood volume must be restricted because excessive (or even liberal) use of volume is associated with greater mortality and morbidity (pulmonary hemorrhage) in this patient population.

3. Finally, because $PaCO_2$ is a more potent mediator of cerebral vascular tone than blood pressure,

we make every effort to keep $PaCO_2$ around 45 to 50 mm Hg during the first 3 postnatal days. We hope that by keeping $PaCO_2$ relatively constant, we minimize the risk for the hypocapnia-associated white matter injury and cerebral palsy and the hypercapnia-associated increased risk of P/IVH. In addition, in the presence of constant $PaCO_2$ levels, the integrity of CBF autoregulation is likely to be optimized.

Fig. 2.10 illustrates our postmenstrual age–dependent approach to the diagnosis and treatment of hypotension in preterm and term neonates. It is important to note that our definition of hypotension (*dotted line*) and the target and weaning ranges have all been arbitrarily defined with the use of epidemiologic data, extrapolation of hemodynamic findings, and the data on the association between blood pressure and systemic and CBF. As this approach, just like any other approach to manage cardiovascular compromise in the neonatal patient population, is not evidenced based, therefore it cannot be recommended for routine use and only illustrates one of the many approaches to the diagnosis and treatment of neonatal hypotension.

Finally, we use these numbers only as guidance, carefully assess the indirect clinical signs of tissue perfusion, and perform targeted echocardiographic evaluations when more information is needed. In the future and after completion of the ongoing investigations, we plan to utilize the real-time information provided by our comprehensive cardiovascular monitoring and data acquisition system.

Acknowledgment

The authors acknowledge the contributions of Claire McLean and Tai Wei-Wu to the chapter in the previous editions.

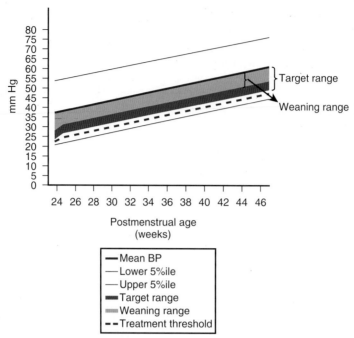

Fig. 2.10 Postmenstrual age–dependent definition of hypotension and the target and weaning blood pressure ranges. Hypotension is defined as the treatment threshold, which is 1–3 points above the 5th percentile for postmenstrual age [14-16]. Below the treatment threshold, the authors usually initiate treatment for hypotension. The target range is defined where mean blood pressure is intended to be kept. The target range is between 2 and 3 mm Hg above the treatment threshold and the 50th percentile of the mean blood pressure [14-16]. Finally, the weaning range is defined as the mean blood pressure range where careful weaning of vasopressor/inotropes and/or inotropes is commenced. This range is between 5 mm Hg above the lower limits of target range and the 50th percentile of the mean blood pressure. Note that the upper limit of the target range does not exceed the 50th percentile of the mean blood pressure in order to decrease the risk of achieving an increase in blood pressure by causing significant increases in systemic vascular resistance and thus potentially decreases in cardiac output when vasopressor/inotropes are being administered. This graph was developed in collaboration with the "Under Pressure" hemodynamic group created as part of a Vermont-Oxford Network (VON) initiative for 2004–2006. One of the authors (IS) served as the "VON expert on hemodynamics" for this initiative.

REFERENCES

1. Miller LE, Laughon MM, Clark RH, et al. Vasoactive medications in extremely low gestational age neonates during the first postnatal week. *J Perinatol*. 2021;41(9):2330-2336. doi:10.1038/s41372-021-01031-8.
2. Perlman JM, McMenamin JB, Volpe JJ. Fluctuating cerebral blood-flow velocity in respiratory-distress syndrome. Relation to the development of intraventricular hemorrhage. *N Engl J Med*. 1983;309(4):204-209. doi:10.1056/NEJM198307283090402.
3. Van Bel F, Van de Bor M, Stijnen T, Baan J, Ruys JH. Aetiological rôle of cerebral blood-flow alterations in development and extension of peri-intraventricular haemorrhage. *Dev Med Child Neurol*. 1987;29(5):601-614. doi:10.1111/j.1469-8749.1987.tb08502.x.
4. Miall-Allen VM, de Vries LS, Whitelaw AG. Mean arterial blood pressure and neonatal cerebral lesions. *Arch Dis Child*. 1987; 62(10):1068-1069.
5. Bada HS, Korones SB, Perry EH, et al. Mean arterial blood pressure changes in premature infants and those at risk for intraventricular hemorrhage. *J Pediatr*. 1990;117(4):607-614.
6. Tsuji M, Saul JP, du Plessis A, et al. Cerebral intravascular oxygenation correlates with mean arterial pressure in critically ill premature infants. *Pediatrics*. 2000;106(4):625-632. doi:10.1542/peds.106.4.625.
7. Hunt RW, Evans N, Rieger I, Kluckow M. Low superior vena cava flow and neurodevelopment at 3 years in very preterm infants. *J Pediatr*. 2004;145(5):588-592. doi:10.1016/j.jpeds.2004.06.056.
8. Goldstein RF, Thompson Jr RJ, Oehler JM, Brazy JE. Influence of acidosis, hypoxemia, and hypotension on neurodevelopmental outcome in very low birth weight infants. *Pediatrics*. 1995;95(2):238-243.
9. Dammann O, Allred EN, Kuban KCK, et al. Systemic hypotension and white-matter damage in preterm infants. *Dev Med Child Neurol*. 2002;44(2):82-90. doi:10.1017/s0012162201001724.
10. Fanaroff JM, Wilson-Costello DE, Newman NS, Montpetite MM, Fanaroff AA. Treated hypotension is associated with neonatal morbidity and hearing loss in extremely low birth weight infants. *Pediatrics*. 2006;117(4):1131-1135. doi:10.1542/peds.2005-1230.

11. Durrmeyer X, Marchand-Martin L, Porcher R, et al. Abstention or intervention for isolated hypotension in the first 3 days of life in extremely preterm infants: association with short-term outcomes in the EPIPAGE 2 cohort study. *Arch Dis Child Fetal Neonatal Ed.* 2017;102(6):490-496. doi:10.1136/archdischild-2016-312104.

12. Thewissen L, Naulaers G, Hendrikx D, et al. Cerebral oxygen saturation and autoregulation during hypotension in extremely preterm infants. *Pediatr Res.* Published online April 20, 2021. doi:10.1038/s41390-021-01483-w.

13. Dempsey E, Seri I. Definition of normal blood pressure range: the elusive target. In: Seri I, Kluckow M, eds. *Neonatology Questions and Controversies: Hemodynamics and Cardiology.* 3rd ed. Philadelphia: Elsevier; 2019:47-66.

14. Logan JW, O'Shea TM, Allred EN, et al. Early postnatal hypotension is not associated with indicators of white matter damage or cerebral palsy in extremely low gestational age newborns. *J Perinatol.* 2011;31(8):524-534. doi:10.1038/jp.2010.201.

15. Batton B, Li L, Newman NS, et al. Early blood pressure, antihypotensive therapy and outcomes at 18–22 months' corrected age in extremely preterm infants. *Arch Dis Child Fetal Neonatal Ed.* 2016;101(3):F201-F206. doi:10.1136/archdischild-2015-308899.

16. Batton B, Li L, Newman NS, et al. Use of antihypotensive therapies in extremely preterm infants. *Pediatrics.* 2013;131(6):e1865-e1873. doi:10.1542/peds.2012-2779.

17. Dempsey EM, Al Hazzani F, Barrington KJ. Permissive hypotension in the extremely low birthweight infant with signs of good perfusion. *Arch Dis Child Fetal Neonatal Ed.* 2009;94(4):F241-F244. doi:10.1136/adc.2007.124263.

18. Pellicer A, Bravo M del C, Madero R, Salas S, Quero J, Cabañas F. Early systemic hypotension and vasopressor support in low birth weight infants: impact on neurodevelopment. *Pediatrics.* 2009;123(5):1369-1376. doi:10.1542/peds.2008-0673.

19. Faust K, Härtel C, Preuß M, et al. Short-term outcome of very-low-birthweight infants with arterial hypotension in the first 24 h of life. *Arch Dis Child Fetal Neonatal Ed.* 2015;100(5):F388-F392. doi:10.1136/archdischild-2014-306483.

20. Batton BJ, Li L, Newman NS, et al. Feasibility study of early blood pressure management in extremely preterm infants. *J Pediatr.* 2012;161(1):65-69.e1. doi:10.1016/j.jpeds.2012.01.014.

21. Dempsey EM, Barrington KJ, Marlow N, et al. Hypotension in Preterm Infants (HIP) randomised trial. *Arch Dis Child Fetal Neonatal Ed.* 2021;106(4):398-403. doi:10.1136/archdischild-2020-320241.

22. Pellicer A, Valverde E, Elorza MD, et al. Cardiovascular support for low birth weight infants and cerebral hemodynamics: a randomized, blinded, clinical trial. *Pediatrics.* 2005;115(6):1501-1512. doi:10.1542/peds.2004-1396.

23. Vesoulis ZA, Ters NE, Foster A, Trivedi SB, Liao SM, Mathur AM. Response to dopamine in prematurity: a biomarker for brain injury? *J Perinatol.* 2016;36(6):453-458. doi:10.1038/jp.2016.5.

24. Ishiguro A, Sasaki A, Motojima Y, et al. Randomized trial of perfusion-based circulatory management in infants of very low birth weight. *J Pediatr.* 2022;243:27-32.e2. doi:10.1016/j.jpeds.2021.12.020.

25. Munro MJ, Walker AM, Barfield CP. Hypotensive extremely low birth weight infants have reduced cerebral blood flow. *Pediatrics.* 2004;114(6):1591-1596. doi:10.1542/peds.2004-1073.

26. Vesoulis ZA, Flower AA, Zanelli S, et al. Blood pressure extremes and severe IVH in preterm infants. *Pediatr Res.* 2020;87(1):69-73. doi:10.1038/s41390-019-0585-3.

27. Wu TW, Noori S, Seri I. Neonatal hypotension. In: Polin RA, Yoder MC, eds. *Workbook in Practical Neonatology.* 6th ed. Philadelphia: Elsevier; 2020:226-236.

28. Nuntnarumit P, Yang W, Bada-Ellzey HS. Blood pressure measurements in the newborn. *Clin Perinatol.* 1999;26(4):981-996, x.

29. Development of audit measures and guidelines for good practice in the management of neonatal respiratory distress syndrome. Report of a Joint Working Group of the British Association of Perinatal Medicine and the Research Unit of the Royal College of Physicians. *Arch Dis Child.* 1992;67(10 Spec No):1221-1227. doi:10.1136/adc.67.10_spec_no.1221.

30. Vesoulis ZA, El Ters NM, Wallendorf M, Mathur AM. Empirical estimation of the normative blood pressure in infants ,28 weeks gestation using a massive data approach. *J Perinatol.* 2016;36(4):291-295. doi:10.1038/jp.2015.185.

31. Børch K, Lou HC, Greisen G. Cerebral white matter blood flow and arterial blood pressure in preterm infants. *Acta Paediatr.* 2010;99(10):1489-1492. doi:10.1111/j.1651-2227.2010.01856.x.

32. Seri I. Circulatory support of the sick preterm infant. *Semin Neonatol.* 2001;6(1):85-95. doi:10.1053/siny.2000.0034.

33. Greisen G. Autoregulation of cerebral blood flow in newborn babies. *Early Hum Dev.* 2005;81(5):423-428. doi:10.1016/j.earlhumdev.2005.03.005.

34. Milligan DW. Failure of autoregulation and intraventricular haemorrhage in preterm infants. *Lancet.* 1980;1(8174):896-898. doi:10.1016/s0140-6736(80)90836-3.

35. Lightburn MH, Gauss CH, Williams DK, Kaiser JR. Observational study of cerebral hemodynamics during dopamine treatment in hypotensive ELBW infants on the first day of life. *J Perinatol.* 2013;33(9):698-702. doi:10.1038/jp.2013.44.

36. O'Leary H, Gregas MC, Limperopoulos C, et al. Elevated cerebral pressure passivity is associated with prematurity-related intracranial hemorrhage. *Pediatrics.* 2009;124(1):302-309. doi:10.1542/peds.2008-2004.

37. Kissack CM, Garr R, Wardle SP, Weindling AM. Cerebral fractional oxygen extraction in very low birth weight infants is high when there is low left ventricular output and hypocarbia but is unaffected by hypotension. *Pediatr Res.* 2004;55(3):400-405. doi:10.1203/01.PDR.0000111288.87002.3A.

38. Victor S, Marson AG, Appleton RE, Beirne M, Weindling AM. Relationship between blood pressure, cerebral electrical activity, cerebral fractional oxygen extraction, and peripheral blood flow in very low birth weight newborn infants. *Pediatr Res.* 2006;59(2):314-319. doi:10.1203/01.pdr.0000199525.08615.1f.

39. Victor S, Appleton RE, Beirne M, Marson AG, Weindling AM. The relationship between cardiac output, cerebral electrical activity, cerebral fractional oxygen extraction and peripheral blood flow in premature newborn infants. *Pediatr Res.* 2006;60(4):456-460. doi:10.1203/01.pdr.0000238379.67720.19.

40. Rhee CJ, Fraser CD, Kibler K, et al. Ontogeny of cerebrovascular critical closing pressure. *Pediatr Res.* 2015;78(1):71-75. doi:10.1038/pr.2015.67.

41. Elizondo LI, Rios DR, Vu E, et al. Observed and calculated cerebral critical closing pressure are highly correlated in preterm infants. *Pediatr Res.* 2019;86(2):242-246. doi:10.1038/s41390-019-0403-y.

42. Rhee CJ, Kaiser JR, Rios DR, et al. Elevated diastolic closing margin is associated with intraventricular hemorrhage in premature infants. *J Pediatr.* 2016;174:52-56. doi:10.1016/j.jpeds.2016.03.066.

43. da Costa CS, Czosnyka M, Smielewski P, Austin T. Optimal mean arterial blood pressure in extremely preterm infants within the first 24 hours of life. *J Pediatr.* 2018;203:242-248. doi:10.1016/j.jpeds.2018.07.096.

44. da Costa CS, Czosnyka M, Smielewski P, Mitra S, Stevenson GN, Austin T. Monitoring of cerebrovascular reactivity for determination of optimal blood pressure in preterm infants. *J Pediatr.* 2015;167(1):86-91. doi:10.1016/j.jpeds.2015.03.041.

45. Noori S, McCoy M, Anderson MP, Ramji F, Seri I. Changes in cardiac function and cerebral blood flow in relation to peri/intraventricular hemorrhage in extremely preterm infants. *J Pediatr.* 2014;164(2):264-270.e1-3. doi:10.1016/j.jpeds.2013.09.045.

46. Kluckow M, Evans N. Low superior vena cava flow and intraventricular haemorrhage in preterm infants. *Arch Dis Child Fetal Neonatal Ed.* 2000;82(3):F188-F194.

47. Kluckow M, Evans N. Relationship between blood pressure and cardiac output in preterm infants requiring mechanical ventilation. *J Pediatr.* 1996;129(4):506-512. doi:10.1016/s0022-3476(96)70114-2.

48. Kluckow M, Evans N. Superior vena cava flow in newborn infants: a novel marker of systemic blood flow. *Arch Dis Child Fetal Neonatal Ed.* 2000;82(3):F182-F187.

49. Seri I. Low superior vena cava flow during the first postnatal day and neurodevelopment in preterm neonates. *J Pediatr.* 2004;145(5):573-575. doi:10.1016/j.jpeds.2004.08.064.

50. Strunk T, Inder T, Wang X, Burgner D, Mallard C, Levy O. Infection-induced inflammation and cerebral injury in preterm infants. *Lancet Infect Dis.* 2014;14(8):751-762. doi:10.1016/S1473-3099(14)70710-8.

51. Greisen G. Cerebral blood flow in preterm infants during the first week of life. *Acta Paediatr Scand.* 1986;75(1):43-51. doi:10.1111/j.1651-2227.1986.tb10155.x.

52. Pryds O, Andersen GE, Friis-Hansen B. Cerebral blood flow reactivity in spontaneously breathing, preterm infants shortly after birth. *Acta Paediatr Scand.* 1990;79(4):391-396. doi:10.1111/j.1651-2227.1990.tb11482.x.

53. Pryds O, Greisen G. Effect of PaCO₂ and haemoglobin concentration on day to day variation of CBF in preterm neonates. *Acta Paediatr Scand Suppl.* 1989;360:33-36.

54. Greisen G, Trojaborg W. Cerebral blood flow, PaCO₂ changes, and visual evoked potentials in mechanically ventilated, preterm infants. *Acta Paediatr Scand.* 1987;76(3):394-400.

55. Altman DI, Powers WJ, Perlman JM, Herscovitch P, Volpe SL, Volpe JJ. Cerebral blood flow requirement for brain viability in newborn infants is lower than in adults. *Ann Neurol.* 1988;24(2):218-226. doi:10.1002/ana.410240208.

56. Backes CH, Rivera BK, Haque U, et al. Placental transfusion strategies in very preterm neonates: a systematic review and meta-analysis. *Obstet Gynecol.* 2014;124(1):47-56. doi:10.1097/AOG.0000000000000324.

57. Katheria AC, Lakshminrusimha S, Rabe H, McAdams R, Mercer JS. Placental transfusion: a review. *J Perinatol.* 2017;37(2):105-111. doi:10.1038/jp.2016.151.

58. Dekom S, Vachhani A, Patel K, Barton L, Ramanathan R, Noori S. Initial hematocrit values after birth and peri/intraventricular hemorrhage in extremely low birth weight infants. *J Perinatol.* 2018;38(11):1471-1475. doi:10.1038/s41372-018-0224-6.

59. Hernandez M, Hawkins R, Brennan R. Sympathetic control of regional cerebral blood flow in the asphyxiated newborn dog. In: Heistad D, Marcus M, eds. *Cerebral Blood Flow, Effects of Nerves and Neurotransmitters.* North Holland: Elsevier; 1982:359-366.

60. Ashwal S, Dale PS, Longo LD. Regional cerebral blood flow: studies in the fetal lamb during hypoxia, hypercapnia, acidosis, and hypotension. *Pediatr Res.* 1984;18(12):1309-1316.

61. Lightburn MH, Gauss CH, Williams DK, Kaiser JR. Cerebral blood flow velocities in extremely low birth weight infants with

62. Shah D, Paradisis M, Bowen JR. Relationship between systemic blood flow, blood pressure, inotropes, and aEEG in the first 48 h of life in extremely preterm infants. *Pediatr Res.* 2013;74(3):314-320. doi:10.1038/pr.2013.104.

63. Kehrer M, Blumenstock G, Ehehalt S, Goelz R, Poets C, Schöning M. Development of cerebral blood flow volume in preterm neonates during the first two weeks of life. *Pediatr Res.* 2005;58(5):927-930. doi:10.1203/01.PDR.0000182579.52820.C3.

64. Kluckow M, Evans N. Low systemic blood flow and hyperkalemia in preterm infants. *J Pediatr.* 2001;139(2):227-232. doi:10.1067/mpd.2001.115315.

65. Osborn D, Evans N, Kluckow M. Randomized trial of dobutamine versus dopamine in preterm infants with low systemic blood flow. *J Pediatr.* 2002;140(2):183-191. doi:10.1067/mpd.2002.120834.

66. Baik N, Urlesberger B, Schwaberger B, Schmölzer GM, Avian A, Pichler G. Cerebral haemorrhage in preterm neonates: does cerebral regional oxygen saturation during the immediate transition matter? *Arch Dis Child Fetal Neonatal Ed.* 2015;100(5):F422-F427. doi:10.1136/archdischild-2014-307590.

67. Katheria AC, Harbert MJ, Nagaraj SB, et al. The Neu-Prem trial: neuromonitoring of brains of infants born preterm during resuscitation-a prospective observational cohort study. *J Pediatr.* 2018;198:209-213.e3. doi:10.1016/j.jpeds.2018.02.065.

68. Takami T, Sunohara D, Kondo A, et al. Changes in cerebral perfusion in extremely LBW infants during the first 72 h after birth. *Pediatr Res.* 2010;68(5):435-439. doi:10.1203/00006450-201011001-00867.

69. Sortica da Costa C, Cardim D, Molnar Z, et al. Changes in hemodynamics, cerebral oxygenation and cerebrovascular reactivity during the early transitional circulation in preterm infants. *Pediatr Res.* 2019;86(2):247-253. doi:10.1038/s41390-019-0410-z.

70. Seri I, Noori S. Fetal and neonatal hemodynamics. *Semin Fetal Neonatal Med.* 2015;20(4):209. doi:10.1016/j.siny.2015.04.002.

71. Osborn DA, Evans N, Kluckow M. Clinical detection of low upper body blood flow in very premature infants using blood pressure, capillary refill time, and central-peripheral temperature difference. *Arch Dis Child Fetal Neonatal Ed.* 2004;89(2):F168-F173.

72. Noori S, Anderson M, Soleymani S, Seri I. Effect of carbon dioxide on cerebral blood flow velocity in preterm infants during postnatal transition. *Acta Paediatr.* 2014;103(8):e334-e339. doi:10.1111/apa.12646.

73. Pryds O, Greisen G, Lou H, Friis-Hansen B. Heterogeneity of cerebral vasoreactivity in preterm infants supported by mechanical ventilation. *J Pediatr.* 1989;115(4):638-645.

74. Levene MI, Shortland D, Gibson N, Evans DH. Carbon dioxide reactivity of the cerebral circulation in extremely premature infants: effects of postnatal age and indomethacin. *Pediatr Res.* 1988;24(2):175-179. doi:10.1203/00006450-198808000-00007.

75. Ikeda T, Amizuka T, Ito Y, et al. Changes in the perfusion waveform of the internal cerebral vein and intraventricular hemorrhage in the acute management of extremely low-birth-weight infants. *Eur J Pediatr.* 2015;174(3):331-338. doi:10.1007/s00431-014-2396-1.

76. Ikeda T, Ito Y, Mikami R, Matsuo K, Kawamura N, Yamoto A. Hemodynamics of infants with strong fluctuations of internal cerebral vein. *Pediatr Int.* 2019;61(5):475-481. doi:10.1111/ped.13828.

77. Evans N, Iyer P. Longitudinal changes in the diameter of the ductus arteriosus in ventilated preterm infants: correlation with

respiratory outcomes. *Arch Dis Child Fetal Neonatal Ed.* 1995;72(3):F156-F161. doi:10.1136/fn.72.3.f156.

78. Noori S, Seri I. Does targeted neonatal echocardiography affect hemodynamics and cerebral oxygenation in extremely preterm infants? *J Perinatol.* 2014;34(11):847-849. doi:10.1038/jp.2014.127.

79. Kluckow M, Seri I, Evans N. Functional echocardiography: an emerging clinical tool for the neonatologist. *J Pediatr.* 2007; 150(2):125-130. doi:10.1016/j.jpeds.2006.10.056.

80. Gilbert RD, Pearce WJ, Ashwal S, Longo LD. Effects of hypoxia on contractility of isolated fetal lamb cerebral arteries. *J Dev Physiol.* 1990;13(4):199-203.

81. Hansen NB, Stonestreet BS, Rosenkrantz TS, Oh W. Validity of Doppler measurements of anterior cerebral artery blood flow velocity: correlation with brain blood flow in piglets. *Pediatrics.* 1983;72(4):526-531.

82. Greisen G, Johansen K, Ellison PH, Fredriksen PS, Mali J, Friis-Hansen B. Cerebral blood flow in the newborn infant: comparison of Doppler ultrasound and ^{133}xenon clearance. *J Pediatr.* 1984;104(3):411-418.

83. Raju TN. Cerebral Doppler studies in the fetus and newborn infant. *J Pediatr.* 1991;119(2):165-174.

84. Suttner S, Schöllhorn T, Boldt J, et al. Noninvasive assessment of cardiac output using thoracic electrical bioimpedance in hemodynamically stable and unstable patients after cardiac surgery: a comparison with pulmonary artery thermodilution. *Intensive Care Med.* 2006;32(12):2053-2058. doi:10.1007/s00134-006-0409-x.

85. Norozi K, Beck C, Osthaus WA, Wille I, Wessel A, Bertram H. Electrical velocimetry for measuring cardiac output in children with congenital heart disease. *Br J Anaesth.* 2008;100(1):88-94. doi:10.1093/bja/aem320.

86. Noori S, Drabu B, Soleymani S, Seri I. Continuous non-invasive cardiac output measurements in the neonate by electrical velocimetry: a comparison with echocardiography. *Arch Dis Child Fetal Neonatal Ed.* 2012;97(5):F340-F343. doi:10.1136/fetalneonatal-2011-301090.

87. Wu W, Lin S, Xie C, Li J, Lie J, Qiu S. Consistency between impedance technique and echocardiogram hemodynamic measurements in neonates. *Am J Perinatol.* 2021;38(12):1259-1262. doi:10.1055/s-0040-1710030.

88. Trinkmann F, Berger M, Doesch C, et al. Comparison of electrical velocimetry and cardiac magnetic resonance imaging for the non-invasive determination of cardiac output. *J Clin Monit Comput.* 2016;30(4):399-408. doi:10.1007/s10877-015-9731-6.

89. Borzage M, Heidari K, Chavez T, Seri I, Wood JC, Blüml S. Measuring stroke volume: impedance cardiography vs phase-contrast magnetic resonance imaging. *Am J Crit Care.* 2017; 26(5):408-415. doi:10.4037/ajcc2017488.

90. Van Wyk L, Smith J, Lawrenson J, Lombard CJ, de Boode WP. Bioreactance cardiac output trending ability in preterm infants: a single centre, longitudinal study. *Neonatology.* 2021;118(5): 600-608. doi:10.1159/000518656.

91. Hsu KH, Wu TW, Wang YC, Lim WH, Lee CC, Lien R. Hemodynamic reference for neonates of different age and weight: a pilot study with electrical cardiometry. *J Perinatol.* 2016;36(6): 481-485. doi:10.1038/jp.2016.2.

92. Van Wyk L, Smith J, Lawrenson J, Lombard CJ, de Boode WP. Bioreactance-derived haemodynamic parameters in the transitional phase in preterm neonates: a longitudinal study. *J Clin Monit Comput.* Published online May 13, 2021. doi:10.1007/s10877-021-00718-9.

93. Brazy JE, Lewis DV, Mitnick MH, Jöbsis vander Vliet FF. Noninvasive monitoring of cerebral oxygenation in preterm infants: preliminary observations. *Pediatrics.* 1985;75(2):217-225.

94. Patel J, Marks K, Roberts I, Azzopardi D, Edwards AD. Measurement of cerebral blood flow in newborn infants using near infrared spectroscopy with indocyanine green. *Pediatr Res.* 1998;43(1):34-39. doi:10.1203/00006450-199801000-00006.

95. Dullenkopf A, Kolarova A, Schulz G, Frey B, Baenziger O, Weiss M. Reproducibility of cerebral oxygenation measurement in neonates and infants in the clinical setting using the NIRO 300 oximeter. *Pediatr Crit Care Med.* 2005;6(3):344-347. doi:10.1097/01.PCC.0000161282.69283.75.

96. Bucher HU, Edwards AD, Lipp AE, Duc G. Comparison between near infrared spectroscopy and ^{133}Xenon clearance for estimation of cerebral blood flow in critically ill preterm infants. *Pediatr Res.* 1993;33(1):56-60. doi:10.1203/00006450-199301000-00012.

97. Sorensen LC, Greisen G. Precision of measurement of cerebral tissue oxygenation index using near-infrared spectroscopy in preterm neonates. *J Biomed Opt.* 2006;11(5):054005. doi:10.1117/1.2357730.

98. Dujovny M, Ausman JI, Stoddart H, Slavin KV, Lewis GD, Widman R. Somanetics INVOS 3100 cerebral oximeter. *Neurosurgery.* 1995;37(1):160. doi:10.1227/00006123-199507000-00036.

99. Alderliesten T, Dix L, Baerts W, et al. Reference values of regional cerebral oxygen saturation during the first 3 days of life in preterm neonates. *Pediatr Res.* 2016;79(1):55-64.

100. Alderliesten T, De Vis JB, Lemmers PM, et al. Brain oxygen saturation assessment in neonates using T_2-prepared blood imaging of oxygen saturation and near-infrared spectroscopy. *J Cereb Blood Flow Metab.* 2017;37(3):902-913. doi:10.1177/0271678X16647737.

101. Alderliesten T, De Vis JB, Lemmers PMA, et al. T_2-prepared velocity selective labelling: a novel idea for full-brain mapping of oxygen saturation. *NeuroImage.* 2016;139:65-73. doi:10.1016/j.neuroimage.2016.06.012.

102. Toet MC, Lemmers PMA, van Schelven LJ, van Bel F. Cerebral oxygenation and electrical activity after birth asphyxia: their relation to outcome. *Pediatrics.* 2006;117(2):333-339. doi:10.1542/peds.2005-0987.

103. Pellicer A, Greisen G, Benders M, et al. The SafeBoosC phase II randomised clinical trial: a treatment guideline for targeted near-infrared-derived cerebral tissue oxygenation versus standard treatment in extremely preterm infants. *Neonatology.* 2013;104(3):171-178. doi:10.1159/000351346.

104. Hyttel-Sorensen S, Pellicer A, Alderliesten T, et al. Cerebral near infrared spectroscopy oximetry in extremely preterm infants: phase II randomised clinical trial. *BMJ.* 2015;350:g7635. doi:10.1136/bmj.g7635.

105. Plomgaard AM, Hagmann C, Alderliesten T, et al. Brain injury in the international multicenter randomized SafeBoosC phase II feasibility trial: cranial ultrasound and magnetic resonance imaging assessments. *Pediatr Res.* 2016;79(3):466-472. doi:10.1038/pr.2015.239.

106. Plomgaard AM, Schwarz CE, Claris O, et al. Early cerebral hypoxia in extremely preterm infants and neurodevelopmental impairment at 2 year of age: a post hoc analysis of the SafeBoosC II trial. *PLoS One.* 2022;17(1):e0262640. doi:10.1371/journal.pone.0262640.

107. Hansen ML, Pellicer A, Gluud C, et al. Cerebral near-infrared spectroscopy monitoring versus treatment as usual for extremely preterm infants: a protocol for the SafeBoosC randomised clinical phase III trial. *Trials.* 2019;20(1):811. doi:10.1186/s13063-019-3955-6.

108. Kurth CD, McCann JC, Wu J, Miles L, Loepke AW. Cerebral oxygen saturation-time threshold for hypoxic-ischemic injury in piglets. *Anesth Analg.* 2009;108(4):1268-1277. doi:10.1213/ane.0b013e318196ac8e.

109. Hagino I, Anttila V, Zurakowski D, Duebener LF, Lidov HGW, Jonas RA. Tissue oxygenation index is a useful monitor of histologic and neurologic outcome after cardiopulmonary bypass in piglets. *J Thorac Cardiovasc Surg.* 2005;130(2):384-392. doi:10.1016/j.jtcvs.2005.02.058.

110. Vesoulis ZA, Mintzer JP, Chock VY. Neonatal NIRS monitoring: recommendations for data capture and review of analytics. *J Perinatol.* 2021;41(4):675-688. doi:10.1038/s41372-021-00946-6.

111. Kleiser S, Ostojic D, Andresen B, et al. Comparison of tissue oximeters on a liquid phantom with adjustable optical properties: an extension. *Biomed Opt Express.* 2018;9(1):86-101. doi:10.1364/BOE.9.000086.

112. Eriksen VR, Hahn GH, Greisen G. Cerebral autoregulation in the preterm newborn using near-infrared spectroscopy: a comparison of time-domain and frequency-domain analyses. *J Biomed Opt.* 2015;20(3):037009. doi:10.1117/1.JBO.20.3.037009.

113. Greisen G. Cerebral autoregulation in preterm infants. How to measure it—and why care? *J Pediatr.* 2014;165(5):885-886. doi:10.1016/j.jpeds.2014.07.031.

114. Pichler G, Höller N, Baik-Schneditz N, et al. Avoiding arterial hypotension in preterm neonates (AHIP)—a single center randomised controlled study investigating simultaneous near infrared spectroscopy measurements of cerebral and peripheral regional tissue oxygenation and dedicated interventions. *Front Pediatr.* 2018;6:15. doi:10.3389/fped.2018.00015.

115. Toet MC, Hellström-Westas L, Groenendaal F, Eken P, de Vries LS. Amplitude integrated EEG 3 and 6 hours after birth in full term neonates with hypoxic-ischaemic encephalopathy. *Arch Dis Child Fetal Neonatal Ed.* 1999;81(1):F19-F23. doi:10.1136/fn.81.1.f19.

116. Dilena R, Raviglione F, Cantalupo G, et al. Consensus protocol for EEG and amplitude-integrated EEG assessment and monitoring in neonates. *Clin Neurophysiol.* 2021;132(4):886-903. doi:10.1016/j.clinph.2021.01.012.

117. Chandrasekaran M, Chaban B, Montaldo P, Thayyil S. Predictive value of amplitude-integrated EEG (aEEG) after rescue hypothermic neuroprotection for hypoxic ischemic encephalopathy: a meta-analysis. *J Perinatol.* 2017;37(6):684-689. doi:10.1038/jp.2017.14.

118. Toet MC, van der Meij W, de Vries LS, Uiterwaal CSPM, van Huffelen KC. Comparison between simultaneously recorded amplitude integrated electroencephalogram (cerebral function monitor) and standard electroencephalogram in neonates. *Pediatrics.* 2002;109(5):772-779. doi:10.1542/peds.109.5.772.

119. Buttle SG, Lemyre B, Sell E, et al. Combined conventional and amplitude-integrated EEG monitoring in neonates: a prospective study. *J Child Neurol.* 2019;34(6):313-320. doi:10.1177/0883073819829256.

120. ter Horst HJ, Sommer C, Bergman KA, Fock JM, van Weerden TW, Bos AF. Prognostic significance of amplitude-integrated EEG during the first 72 hours after birth in severely asphyxiated neonates. *Pediatr Res.* 2004;55(6):1026-1033. doi:10.1203/01.pdr.0000127019.52562.8c.

121. Shalak LF, Laptook AR, Velaphi SC, Perlman JM. Amplitude-integrated electroencephalography coupled with an early neurologic examination enhances prediction of term infants at risk for persistent encephalopathy. *Pediatrics.* 2003;111(2):351-357. doi:10.1542/peds.111.2.351.

122. Magalhães LV da S, Winckler MIB, Bragatti JA, Procianoy R, Silveira R de CS. The role of amplitude integrated electroencephalogram in very low-birth-weight preterm infants: a literature review. *Neuropediatrics.* 2017;48(6):413-419. doi:10.1055/s-0037-1604403.

123. West CR, Groves AM, Williams CE, et al. Early low cardiac output is associated with compromised electroencephalographic activity in very preterm infants. *Pediatr Res.* 2006;59(4 Pt 1):610-615. doi:10.1203/01.pdr.0000203095.06442.ad.

124. Semenova O, Lightbody G, O'Toole JM, Boylan G, Dempsey E, Temko A. Coupling between mean blood pressure and EEG in preterm neonates is associated with reduced illness severity scores. *PLoS One.* 2018;13(6):e0199587. doi:10.1371/journal.pone.0199587.

125. Pereira SS, Kempley ST, Wertheim DF, Sinha AK, Morris JK, Shah DK. Investigation of EEG activity compared with mean arterial blood pressure in extremely preterm infants. *Front Neurol.* 2018;9:87. doi:10.3389/fneur.2018.00087.

126. Fogtmann EP, Plomgaard AM, Greisen G, Gluud C. Prognostic accuracy of electroencephalograms in preterm infants: a systematic review. *Pediatrics.* 2017;139(2):e20161951. doi:10.1542/peds.2016-1951.

127. Elsayed YN, Amer R, Seshia MM. The impact of integrated evaluation of hemodynamics using targeted neonatal echocardiography with indices of tissue oxygenation: a new approach. *J Perinatol.* 2017;37(5):527-535. doi:10.1038/jp.2016.257.

128. Azhibekov T, Soleymani S, Lee BH, Noori S, Seri I. Hemodynamic monitoring of the critically ill neonate: an eye on the future. *Semin Fetal Neonatal Med.* 2015;20(4):246-254. doi:10.1016/j.siny.2015.03.003.

129. Seri I, Rudas G, Bors Z, Kanyicska B, Tulassay T. Effects of low-dose dopamine infusion on cardiovascular and renal functions, cerebral blood flow, and plasma catecholamine levels in sick preterm neonates. *Pediatr Res.* 1993;34(6):742-749. doi:10.1203/00006450-199312000-00009.

130. Noori S, Stavroudis TA, Seri I. Systemic and cerebral hemodynamics during the transitional period after premature birth. *Clin Perinatol.* 2009;36(4):723-736, v. doi:10.1016/j.clp.2009.07.015.

131. Evans N, Moorcraft J. Effect of patency of the ductus arteriosus on blood pressure in very preterm infants. *Arch Dis Child.* 1992;67(10 Spec No):1169-1173.

132. Aldana-Aguirre JC, Deshpande P, Jain A, Weisz DE. Physiology of low blood pressure during the first day after birth among extremely preterm neonates. *J Pediatr.* 2021;236:40-46.e3. doi:10.1016/j.jpeds.2021.05.026.

133. Kluckow M, Evans N. Early echocardiographic prediction of symptomatic patent ductus arteriosus in preterm infants undergoing mechanical ventilation. *J Pediatr.* 1995;127(5):774-779.

134. Hsu KH, Nguyen J, Dekom S, Ramanathan R, Noori S. Effects of patent ductus arteriosus on organ blood flow in infants born very preterm: a prospective study with serial echocardiography. *J Pediatr.* 2020;216:95-100.e2. doi:10.1016/j.jpeds.2019.08.057.

135. Noori S, Seri I. Hypotension and significant patent ductus arteriosus in infants born extremely preterm during the postnatal transitional period: normal adaptation? *J Pediatr.* 2022;240:314-315. doi:10.1016/j.jpeds.2021.09.023.

136. Osborn DA, Evans N, Kluckow M. Effect of early targeted indomethacin on the ductus arteriosus and blood flow to the

upper body and brain in the preterm infant. *Arch Dis Child Fetal Neonatal Ed.* 2003;88(6):F477-F482. doi:10.1136/fn. 88.6.f477.

137. Yanowitz TD, Yao AC, Werner JC, Pettigrew KD, Oh W, Stonestreet BS. Effects of prophylactic low-dose indomethacin on hemodynamics in very low birth weight infants. *J Pediatr.* 1998;132(1): 28-34. doi:10.1016/s0022-3476(98)70480-9.

138. Bouissou A, Rakza T, Klosowski S, Tourneux P, Vanderborght M, Storme L. Hypotension in preterm infants with significant patent ductus arteriosus: effects of dopamine. *J Pediatr.* 2008; 153(6):790-794. doi:10.1016/j.jpeds.2008.06.014.

139. Seri I. Cardiovascular, renal, and endocrine actions of dopamine in neonates and children. *J Pediatr.* 1995;126(3):333-344. doi:10.1016/s0022-3476(95)70445-0.

140. Rios DR, Moffett BS, Kaiser JR. Trends in pharmacotherapy for neonatal hypotension. *J Pediatr.* 2014;165(4):697-701.e1. doi:10.1016/j.jpeds.2014.06.009.

141. Seri I, Abbasi S, Wood DC, Gerdes JS. Regional hemodynamic effects of dopamine in the sick preterm neonate. *J Pediatr.* 1998;133(6):728-734. doi:10.1016/s0022-3476(98)70141-6.

142. Lundstrøm K, Pryds O, Greisen G. The haemodynamic effects of dopamine and volume expansion in sick preterm infants. *Early Hum Dev.* 2000;57(2):157-163. doi:10.1016/s0378-3782(00)00048-7.

143. Baske K, Saini SS, Dutta S, Sundaram V. Epinephrine versus dopamine in neonatal septic shock: a double-blind randomized controlled trial. *Eur J Pediatr.* 2018;177(9):1335-1342. doi:10.1007/s00431-018-3195-x.

144. Sasidharan R, Gupta N, Chawla D. Dopamine versus epinephrine for fluid-refractory septic shock in neonates. *Eur J Pediatr.* 2019;178(1):113-114. doi:10.1007/s00431-018-3252-5.

145. Wen L, Xu L. The efficacy of dopamine versus epinephrine for pediatric or neonatal septic shock: a meta-analysis of randomized controlled studies. *Ital J Pediatr.* 2020;46(1):6. doi:10.1186/s13052-019-0768-x.

146. Weiss SL, Peters MJ, Alhazzani W, et al. Surviving sepsis campaign international guidelines for the management of septic shock and sepsis-associated organ dysfunction in children. *Intensive Care Med.* 2020;46(suppl 1):10-67. doi:10.1007/s00134-019-05878-6.

147. Rizk MY, Lapointe A, Lefebvre F, Barrington KJ. Norepinephrine infusion improves haemodynamics in the preterm infants during septic shock. *Acta Paediatr.* 2018;107(3):408-413. doi:10.1111/apa.14112.

148. Rowcliff K, de Waal K, Mohamed AL, Chaudhari T. Noradrenaline in preterm infants with cardiovascular compromise. *Eur J Pediatr.* 2016;175(12):1967-1973. doi:10.1007/s00431-016-2794-7.

149. Rios DR, Kaiser JR. Vasopressin versus dopamine for treatment of hypotension in extremely low birth weight infants: a randomized, blinded pilot study. *J Pediatr.* 2015;166(4): 850-855. doi:10.1016/j.jpeds.2014.12.027.

150. Chang AC, Atz AM, Wernovsky G, Burke RP, Wessel DL. Milrinone: systemic and pulmonary hemodynamic effects in neonates after cardiac surgery. *Crit Care Med.* 1995;23(11): 1907-1914. doi:10.1097/00003246-199511000-00018.

151. Hoffman TM, Wernovsky G, Atz AM, et al. Efficacy and safety of milrinone in preventing low cardiac output syndrome in infants and children after corrective surgery for congenital heart disease. *Circulation.* 2003;107(7):996-1002. doi:10.1161/01.cir.0000051365.81920.28.

152. Paradisis M, Evans N, Kluckow M, Osborn D, McLachlan AJ. Pilot study of milrinone for low systemic blood flow in very

preterm infants. *J Pediatr.* 2006;148(3):306-313. doi:10.1016/j.jpeds.2005.11.030.

153. Paradisis M, Evans N, Kluckow M, Osborn D. Randomized trial of milrinone versus placebo for prevention of low systemic blood flow in very preterm infants. *J Pediatr.* 2009; 154(2):189-195. doi:10.1016/j.jpeds.2008.07.059.

154. Noori S, Friedlich P, Seri I. The use of dobutamine in the treatment of neonatal cardiovascular compromise. *Neo Reviews.* 2004;5(1):E22-E26.

155. Bravo MC, López-Ortego P, Sánchez L, et al. Randomized, placebo-controlled trial of dobutamine for low superior vena cava flow in infants. *J Pediatr.* 2015;167(3):572-578.e1-2. doi:10.1016/j.jpeds.2015.05.037.

156. Ng PC, Lee CH, Lam CWK, et al. Transient adrenocortical insufficiency of prematurity and systemic hypotension in very low birthweight infants. *Arch Dis Child Fetal Neonatal Ed.* 2004;89(2):F119-F126. doi:10.1136/adc.2002.021972.

157. Fernandez E, Schrader R, Watterberg K. Prevalence of low cortisol values in term and near-term infants with vasopressor-resistant hypotension. *J Perinatol.* 2005;25(2):114-118. doi:10.1038/sj.jp.7211211.

158. Seri I, Tan R, Evans J. Cardiovascular effects of hydrocortisone in preterm infants with pressor-resistant hypotension. *Pediatrics.* 2001;107(5):1070-1074.

159. Noori S, Friedlich P, Wong P, Ebrahimi M, Siassi B, Seri I. Hemodynamic changes after low-dosage hydrocortisone administration in vasopressor-treated preterm and term neonates. *Pediatrics.* 2006;118(4):1456-1466. doi:10.1542/peds.2006-0661.

160. Kumbhat N, Noori S. Corticosteroids for neonatal hypotension. *Clin Perinatol.* 2020;47(3):549-562. doi:10.1016/j.clp.2020.05.015.

161. Niijima S, Shortland DB, Levene MI, Evans DH. Transient hyperoxia and cerebral blood flow velocity in infants born prematurely and at full term. *Arch Dis Child.* 1988;63(10 Spec No):1126-1130. doi:10.1136/adc.63.10_spec_no.1126.

162. Leahy FA, Cates D, MacCallum M, Rigatto H. Effect of CO2 and 100% O2 on cerebral blood flow in preterm infants. *J Appl Physiol.* 1980;48(3):468-472.

163. Basu S, Barman S, Shukla V, Kumar A. Effect of oxygen inhalation on cerebral blood flow velocity in premature neonates. *Pediatr Res.* 2014;75(2):328-335. doi:10.1038/pr.2013.219.

164. Tyszczuk L, Meek J, Elwell C, Wyatt JS. Cerebral blood flow is independent of mean arterial blood pressure in preterm infants undergoing intensive care. *Pediatrics.* 1998;102(2 Pt 1):337-341.

165. Victor S, Appleton RE, Beirne M, Marson AG, Weindling AM. Effect of carbon dioxide on background cerebral electrical activity and fractional oxygen extraction in very low birth weight infants just after birth. *Pediatr Res.* 2005;58(3): 579-585. doi:10.1203/01.pdr.0000169402.13435.09.

166. Murase M, Ishida A. Early hypocarbia of preterm infants: its relationship to periventricular leukomalacia and cerebral palsy, and its perinatal risk factors. *Acta Paediatr.* 2005; 94(1):85-91.

167. Dix LML, Weeke LC, de Vries LS, et al. Carbon dioxide fluctuations are associated with changes in cerebral oxygenation and electrical activity in infants born preterm. *J Pediatr.* 2017;187:66-72.e1. doi:10.1016/j.jpeds.2017.04.043.

168. Kaiser JR, Gauss CH, Williams DK. The effects of hypercapnia on cerebral autoregulation in ventilated very low birth weight infants. *Pediatr Res.* 2005;58(5):931-935. doi:10.1203/01.pdr.0000182180.80645.0c.

169. Kaiser JR, Gauss CH, Pont MM, Williams DK. Hypercapnia during the first 3 days of life is associated with severe intraventricular hemorrhage in very low birth weight infants. *J Perinatol.* 2006;26(5):279-285. doi:10.1038/sj.jp.7211492.

170. Kaiser JR. Both extremes of arterial carbon dioxide pressure and the magnitude of fluctuations in arterial carbon dioxide pressure are associated with severe intraventricular hemorrhage in preterm infants. *Pediatrics.* 2007;119(5):1039; author reply 1039-1040. doi:10.1542/peds.2007-0353.

171. Vela-Huerta MM, Amador-Licona M, Medina-Ovando N, Aldana-Valenzuela C. Factors associated with early severe intraventricular haemorrhage in very low birth weight infants. *Neuropediatrics.* 2009;40(5):224-227. doi:10.1055/s-0030-1248249.

172. Thome UH, Genzel-Boroviczeny O, Bohnhorst B, et al. Permissive hypercapnia in extremely low birthweight infants (PHELBI): a randomised controlled multicentre trial. *Lancet Respir Med.* 2015;3(7):534-543. doi:10.1016/S2213-2600(15)00204-0.

173. Thome UH, Genzel-Boroviczeny O, Bohnhorst B, et al. Neurodevelopmental outcomes of extremely low birthweight infants randomised to different PCO_2 targets: the PHELBI follow-up study. *Arch Dis Child Fetal Neonatal Ed.* 2017;102(5):F376-F382. doi:10.1136/archdischild-2016-311581.

174. McKee LA, Fabres J, Howard G, Peralta-Carcelen M, Carlo WA, Ambalavanan N. $PaCO_2$ and neurodevelopment in extremely low birth weight infants. *J Pediatr.* 2009;155(2):217-221.e1. doi:10.1016/j.jpeds.2009.02.024.

175. van Alfen-van der Velden AA, Hopman JC, Klaessens JH, Feuth T, Sengers RC, Liem KD. Effects of midazolam and morphine on cerebral oxygenation and hemodynamics in ventilated premature infants. *Biol Neonate.* 2006;90(3):197-202. doi:10.1159/000093489.

176. Roll C, Hüning B, Käunicke M, Krug J, Horsch S. Umbilical artery catheter blood sampling volume and velocity: impact on cerebral blood volume and oxygenation in very-low-birthweight infants. *Acta Paediatr.* 2006;95(1):68-73. doi:10.1080/08035250500369577.

177. Wu TW, Noori S. Recognition and management of neonatal hemodynamic compromise. *Pediatr Neonatol.* 2021;62(suppl 1):S22-S29. doi:10.1016/j.pedneo.2020.12.007.

Chapter 3

Intraventricular Hemorrhage in the Premature Infant

Vivien L. Yap, and Jeffrey M. Perlman

Chapter Outline

Background

Case History

HW was a 500 g, 23-week premature twin B male infant born to a 34-year-old G1P0 (gravida 1, para 0) mother whose pregnancy was complicated by the onset of premature labor. The mother received a dose of betamethasone approximately 6 hours before a vaginal delivery. She also received antibiotics and was given magnesium sulfate. The infant was delivered with minimal respiratory effort and a heart rate of 70 beats/min. Resuscitation included bag-mask ventilation with room air and intubation, with a rapid improvement in heart rate. The infant was admitted to the intensive care unit and was given one dose of a surfactant for respiratory distress syndrome (RDS). The early course was complicated by a pneumothorax as well as a pulmonary hemorrhage, with associated hypoxic respiratory failure and significant metabolic acidosis. A head ultrasound scan showed a grade III intraventricular hemorrhage on the left with dilation of the ventricle and an associated ipsilateral intraparenchymal echodensity involving frontoparietal white matter. In addition, the infant developed a hemodynamically significant patent ductus arteriosus (PDA) that was initially treated with indomethacin. The infant was weaned to continuous positive airway pressure by day of life (DOL) 14 and was briefly reintubated for the surgical ligation of the PDA and, on another occasion, for a late-onset sepsis. Other issues included recurrent apnea, bradycardia, and desaturation episodes. He required supplemental oxygen through the 35th week of postmenstrual age. He required parenteral nutrition for 3 weeks and subsequently received enteral breast milk. Serial head ultrasound scans on DOLs 7, 14, 28, 42, and 56 revealed progressive communicating hydrocephalus involving the lateral third and fourth ventricles that peaked in dilation by DOL 28 and then gradually decreased in size by DOL 56. The parenchymal lesion evolved into a small left porencephalic cyst. The infant underwent a magnetic resonance imaging (MRI) evaluation on DOL 92 that revealed mild ventriculomegaly and the left cystic lesion and some periventricular white matter loss. The infant was discharged on DOL 100. He was seen and evaluated at 18 months. At that time, the clinical findings indicated mild right hemiparesis. He recently started walking, was very active, and had minimal speech. Evaluation using the Bayley Scales of Infant and Toddler Development (BSID) found that he had a cognitive score of 75 and a motor score of 82.

This case illustrates the course of an extremely premature infant who is at greatest risk for severe periventricular-intraventricular hemorrhage (PV-IVH) even when managed in the current era of neonatology. Although the overall incidence of PV-IVH in the premature infant decreased throughout the 1980s–1990s, it has been relatively static over the last two decades.[1] High-grade intraventricular hemorrhage remains a particularly common morbidity in the extremely preterm infant, particularly in cases of rapid delivery when the potential for full dosing of glucocorticoids around the time of delivery is not possible.[2,3] This chapter focuses on a brief review of the pathogenesis of germinal matrix hemorrhage (GMH) and PV-IVH. Various approaches or strategies for the prevention, diagnosis, and treatment as well as outcomes are discussed, with gaps in knowledge highlighted.

The overall incidence of GMH and PV-IVH declined during the era of the 1970s–1990s with the evolution of modern obstetric and neonatal intensive care practices, although severe intraventricular hemorrhage remains a significant clinical problem in the extremely preterm population.[1,4,5] For those born at or before 28 weeks' gestation, 15% continue to have the most severe forms of hemorrhage, occurring more frequently at younger gestational ages.[1,5] This observation continues to be highly relevant because the survival of the infants born at the limits of viability continues to increase, with mortality and long-term neuromotor deficits among survivors more likely with severe hemorrhage.[6–8] However, evidence also points to neurodevelopmental deficits even with lower grades of hemorrhage and even when the cranial sonogram is interpreted as being normal (see later discussion).[7,9–11] These observations are important because they point to the limitations of cranial sonography in identifying more subtle injury to the cortex, deep gray matter, or cerebellum. These additional findings may not be clearly evident in infancy or may be more readily identified by MRI studies performed closer to term.[12,13]

Neuropathology: Relevance to Clinical Findings

The primary lesion in PV-IVH is bleeding from small vessels in the subependymal germinal matrix (GM), a transitional gelatinous region that provides limited support for the luxurious but very immature capillary bed that courses through it.[14] With maturation, this matrix region becomes less prominent and is essentially absent by term gestation. The hemorrhage, when it evolves, may be confined to the GM region (grade I IVH), or it may extend and rupture into the adjacent ventricular system (grade II or III IVH, depending on the extent of hemorrhage), or extend into the white matter (termed a grade IV or intraparenchymal echogenicity [IPE], more appropriately termed periventricular hemorrhagic infarction [PVHI]) (Fig. 3.1A).[2,15,16] PVHI, which is invariably unilateral, represents an area of hemorrhagic necrosis of varying size within periventricular white matter, dorsal and lateral to the external angle of the lateral ventricle (Fig. 3.1B).[2,17,18]

Pathogenesis

The genesis of bleeding from capillaries within the GM is complex and includes a combination of intravascular, vascular, and extravascular influences.

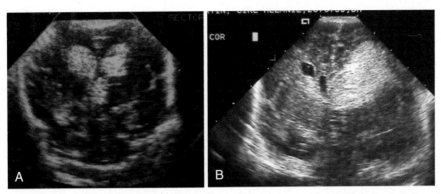

Fig. 3.1 Coronal ultrasound scans. A, Note a bilateral germinal matrix and intraventricular hemorrhage (grade III). B, Note the large left-sided germinal matrix and intraventricular hemorrhage. There is a large ipsilateral intraparenchymal echodensity involving periventricular white matter.

Intravascular factors, especially those that involve perturbations in cerebral blood flow (CBF), have a critical role in capillary rupture and hemorrhage. It has been shown, through the use of different methods to assess CBF, including Doppler ultrasonography, near-infrared spectroscopy, and xenon-enhanced computed tomography (CT), that the cerebral circulation of the sick infant is pressure passive; that is, CBF varies directly with changes in systemic blood pressure.[19–21] This state would be expected to increase the vulnerability of the GM capillaries to periods of both hypotension and hypertension, and this is supported in experimental studies and clinical observations. In a beagle puppy model GM hemorrhage can be produced by systemic hypertension with or without prior hypotension.[22,23] In addition, clinical temporal associations have been demonstrated between fluctuations in systemic blood pressure and simultaneous fluctuations in CBF velocity as may occur in the ventilated premature infant with RDS, increases in CBF as may occur with rapid volume expansion or a pneumothorax, and the subsequent development of PV-IVH.[24–27] Conversely, decreases in CBF secondary to systemic hypotension, which may occur in utero or postnatally, may also play a prominent role in the genesis of PV-IVH in certain infants.[28] Hypercarbia, producing potential modulation of autoregulation and of CBF, increases the risk for severe IVH.[29,30] A presumed mechanism in this context is that of rupture upon reperfusion.[3,20] Finally, elevations in venous pressure may be an important additional intravascular mechanism of hemorrhage and may reflect the peculiarity of the anatomy of the venous drainage of GM and the white matter.[2] Thus at the level of the head of the caudate nucleus and the foramen of Monro, the terminal, choroidal, and thalamostriate veins course anteriorly to a point of confluence to form the internal cerebral vein. The blood flow then makes a U-turn at the usual site of hemorrhage, raising the possibility that an elevation in venous pressure increases the potential for venous distention with obstruction of the terminal and medullary veins and hemorrhagic infarction. Indeed, simultaneous increases in venous pressure have been observed in infants who exhibit variability in arterial blood pressure, such as when it occurs with RDS and associated complications, such as pneumothorax and pulmonary interstitial emphysema, or with mechanical or high-frequency ventilation.[31] In addition, certain anatomic patterns of subependymal veins are more predisposed to hemorrhage, as seen in susceptibility-weighted imaging venography.[32] To summarize, it is likely that both arterial and venous perturbations contribute to the genesis of IVH. Later evidence suggests that these intravascular responses may be modulated by inflammation or the administration of medications to the mother, such as glucocorticoids (see later discussion).[33–35]

In addition to the intravascular factors, vascular and extravascular influences—the poorly supported blood vessels, excessive fibrinolytic activity noted within the matrix region, and a prominent postnatal decrease in extravascular tissue pressure—may all contribute to hemorrhage.[2,36,37]

Periventricular White Matter Injury Associated With IVH

The pathogenesis of white matter injury associated with hemorrhage remains unclear but appears to be closely linked to the adjacent bleed. Two potential pathways have been proposed to explain this intricate relationship. The first suggests a direct relationship to the PV-IVH, on the basis of several clinical observations, as follows: (1) the white matter lesion is always noted concurrent with or following a large GM and/or IVH and is rarely, if ever, observed before the hemorrhage; and (2) the white matter injury is always observed ipsilateral to the side of the larger hemorrhage when there is bilateral involvement of the ventricular system.[2,3,18] This consistent relationship between the GM and the white matter injury may in part be explained by the venous drainage of the deep white matter (see earlier discussion). A second explanation is a de novo evolution of white matter injury. Thus it is thought that the PV-IVH and white matter injury generally occur concurrently. Because both the GM and the periventricular white matter are border-zone regions, the risk for ischemic injury is increased during periods of systemic hypotension, particularly in the presence of a pressure-passive cerebral circulation.[2,3,20] Hemorrhage in these regions may then occur as a secondary phenomenon, or reperfusion injury. In support of this theory is the fairly consistent observation of the simultaneous detection of PV-IVH and white matter injury on cranial ultrasonography. Moreover, elevated hypoxanthine and uric acid levels (as markers of reperfusion injury) have been observed on the first postnatal day in infants in whom white matter injury subsequently developed.[38,39]

Identification of the mechanisms contributing to periventricular white matter injury is crucial to the prevention of this lesion. If the white matter injury is directly related to PV-IVH, then prevention of the latter should reduce the occurrence of the white matter injury. However, if the PV-IVH and the white matter injury occur simultaneously as a result of a primary ischemic event, with the hemorrhage occurring as a secondary phenomenon, then prevention of the secondary hemorrhage may not affect the primary ischemic lesion. Indeed, the two follow-up studies on indomethacin treatment to prevent IVH in the neonatal period are supportive of this latter concern. Thus although the incidence of severe IVH was reduced in infants treated with indomethacin in both studies, neurodevelopmental outcomes at 18-month follow-up, including cerebral palsy, were comparable in the indomethacin-treated group controls.[40,41]

Clinical Features

In most cases (up to 70% of less severe IVH cases) the diagnosis is made with a screening sonogram. In the earlier descriptions of PV-IVH the majority of cases, about 90%, evolved within the first 72 hours of postnatal life.[42] However, the time to initial diagnosis of hemorrhage has shifted to a later onset in recent years.[15,43] Thus for premature infants weighing less than 1000 g, the IVH diagnosis is made early, within the first 24 hours in approximately 80% of infants. However, some cases are now noted after the 10th postnatal day. This changing pattern may reflect the complexity of disease in the tiniest infants and the extent of supportive medical care. Infants with the more severe IVH frequently exhibit clinical signs such as a bulging fontanel, seizures, a drop in hematocrit, hyperglycemia, metabolic acidosis, and pulmonary hemorrhage.[3]

Complications

The two most significant complications of IVH are extension into adjacent white matter (see earlier discussion) and the development of posthemorrhagic hydrocephalus.

Prevention

PERINATAL STRATEGIES

Antenatal Steroids

Various perinatal and postnatal strategies have been investigated for the prevention of PV-IVH. The antenatal administration of glucocorticoids to augment pulmonary maturation has had the positive, unanticipated benefit of a significant reduction in the incidence of IVH and severe IVH.[35,44–49] An updated systematic review of 27 trials showed antenatal corticosteroid therapy to be associated with a reduction in the occurrence of PV-IVH (relative risk [RR] 0.58, 95% confidence interval [CI] 0.45–0.75; 12 studies, 8475 infants) and likely lead to a reduction in developmental delay in childhood (RR 0.51, 95% CI 0.27–0.97, 3 studies, 600 children).[35] The mechanisms whereby glucocorticoids reduce severe IVH remain unclear but may relate to less severe RDS, possibly minimizing fluctuation in CBF, and accelerated stabilization of the GM vasculature by modulating vascular growth factors.[26,37,50–52] Serial courses of antenatal corticosteroids are not recommended; a single rescue course is to be considered if preterm birth does not occur within a week to further decrease the risk of RDS but has no further impact on the rate of IVH or severe IVH.[53] There are concerns that multiple courses of antenatal corticosteroids may have adverse effects on the developing brain. Thus infants who were exposed to multiple courses (median of 4) of antenatal steroids had a higher incidence of cerebral palsy than a placebo group, although the difference was not statistically significant (6/206 vs. 1/195; $P = .12$).[54]

PREGNANCY-INDUCED HYPERTENSION

One maternal medical condition that may be associated with a lower incidence of IVH is pregnancy-induced hypertension (PIH). In one report a lower incidence of severe PV-IVH was found in infants born to mothers with PIH (8.2%) than to those without PIH (14%), with an odds ratio (OR) estimate of 0.43 (95% CI 0.30–0.61),[55] a finding consistent with other reports.[56–59] The mechanisms through which the risk of IVH may be reduced by the presence of PIH remain unclear, but accelerated brain maturation in such infants is possible.[60,61] However, there are retrospective studies that have reported an increased risk of PV-IVH in mothers with severe preeclampsia and HELLP syndrome.[62]

MAGNESIUM SULFATE

The use of magnesium sulfate in these women was initially suggested to be contributory to the reduction in IVH,[57,63] but subsequent studies have shown that it is not.[64–66] Tocolytic agents, in general, including magnesium sulfate, are associated with an increased risk for IVH.[67–69] However, a large prospective, randomized controlled trial of magnesium sulfate administered to mothers at 24 to 31 weeks' gestation demonstrated a reduced rate of cerebral palsy among infant survivors.[70] Subsequent randomized controlled trials showed similar neuroprotection. Thus a metaanalysis of antenatal magnesium sulfate therapy given to women at risk for preterm birth concluded that it substantially reduced the risk of cerebral palsy in the child (RR 0.68; 95% CI 0.54–0.87; in 5 trials involving 6145 infants).[71] The number of women who needed to be treated to benefit one infant by avoiding cerebral palsy is 63 (95% CI 43–155).[72] The American Congress of Obstetricians and Gynecologists (ACOG) recommends intrapartum magnesium for women at less than 32 weeks' gestation who are at risk for delivery within 7 days.[73]

ROUTE OF DELIVERY

There are conflicting data regarding the route of delivery and subsequent IVH.[57,74–76] Interpretation of the data is difficult because most studies are retrospective, but this does not exclude the possibility that, under certain circumstances, intrapartum events may contribute to the pathogenesis of severe IVH. Some studies show a higher risk for IVH with increasing duration of the active phase of labor, and a lower risk in infants delivered via cesarean section before active phase of labor.[57,74] Many of these studies were analyzed before the more frequent use of antenatal glucocorticoids.[77] In a study of infants born at less than 750 g whose mothers were given steroids, vaginal delivery was a predictor for severe IVH.[78] By contrast, in a retrospective cohort study of extremely low birth weight (ELBW) infants, the influence of labor on those born by cesarean delivery was examined and this analysis revealed that labor does not appear to play a significant role in the genesis of IVH.[79] Similarly, in a later retrospective analysis, severe IVH was not influenced by mode of delivery in vertex-presenting, singleton, very LBW infants after data were controlled for gestational age.[80] Any analysis that evaluates the impact of labor or route of delivery must account for an important role of placental inflammation, in particular fetal vasculitis, in the genesis of IVH, a role that may supersede the influence of the route of delivery. Thus in one study, although vaginal delivery was associated with an increased risk of IVH by univariate analysis, the risks attributable to vaginal delivery were no longer increased when adjustments were made in multivariate analysis for fetal vasculitis and other potential confounding factors.[81]

DELAYED CORD CLAMPING

Several randomized controlled trials have shown improved preterm newborn outcomes, including mortality, with delayed cord clamping.[82,83] The Cochrane metaanalysis showed a reduction of all grades of IVH (aRR 0.83, 95% CI 0.7–0.99 in 15 trials involving 2333 infants), although with little effect on Grades 3 or 4 IVH (aRR 0.94, 95% CI 0.63–1.39, comprising 10 studies involving 2058 newborns), consistent with the metaanalysis by the International Liaison Committee on Resuscitation.[83,84] Other benefits to preterm newborns include improved transitional circulation, decreased need for blood transfusions, and a lower risk for necrotizing enterocolitis.[82,83] One study in preterm infants born before 32 weeks showed that delayed cord clamping was protective against low motor scores at 18 to 22 months corrected age.[85] ACOG and the American Academy of Pediatrics (AAP) recommend a delay in cord clamping for vigorous preterm infants for at least 30 to 60 seconds.[86] Proposed mechanisms for the benefits associated with delayed cord clamping include an improved cardiovascular transition.[87,88] However, cord milking has been associated with increased rates of IVH in very preterm infants below 28 weeks' gestational age and should be avoided.[89]

NEONATAL TRANSPORT

Preterm infants who require interfacility transport are more likely to develop IVH or severe IVH.[90–93] While the etiology remains uncertain, transport may introduce CBF fluctuations with the additional movement, handling, and care. Maternal transport in cases of high-risk pregnancy is preferred but may be limited by regional obstetric and NICU infrastructures.

POSTNATAL STRATEGIES

Any approach to intervention should at the least consider the following: (1) the target population should be those infants in whom severe IVH is most likely to develop—that is, in those that are extremely preterm or extremely low birth weight[4]; and (2) the condition of the infant at delivery, which appears to be an important mediator of subsequent IVH (Box 3.1). The latter appears to be strongly influenced in part by perinatal events and, in particular, the administration of antenatal glucocorticoids[35] or the presence of fetal vasculitis.[81]

BOX 3.1 FACTORS ASSOCIATED WITH RISK FOR THE DEVELOPMENT OF SEVERE INTRAVENTRICULAR HEMORRHAGE

High Risk
  Minimal intrapartum care
  No glucocorticoid exposure
  Chorioamnionitis/funisitis
  Fetal distress
  Lower gestational age
  Lower birth weight
  Interfacility transport
  Respiratory distress syndrome
  Respiratory morbidity (i.e., pneumothorax)
  Fluctuations or rapid elevations in systemic blood pressure and/or cerebral blood flow
  Hypotension
  Sudden and repeated increases in venous pressure
Lower Risk
  Antenatal glucocorticoids (short course)
  Medical condition (e.g., pregnancy-induced hypertension)
  Intrauterine growth restriction
  Higher gestational age
  Higher birth weight
  Postnatal medications (e.g., indomethacin)

Postnatal Factors Associated With an Increased Risk

Postnatal factors associated with a higher risk for IVH include decreasing gestational age, lower birth weight (<1000 g), male sex, intubation, and RDS (see Box 3.1).[2,94,95] In contrast, the risk for severe IVH in the nonintubated infant is low (<10%).[96] For infants with RDS, the risk for IVH is even greater with associated perturbations in arterial and venous pressures as well as with hypercarbia.[24,25,29,30,97] These vascular perturbations are in part related to the infant's breathing patterns, which are usually out of synchrony with the ventilator breath.[98] The perturbations can be minimized with careful ventilator management, including the use of synchronized mechanical ventilation, assist/control ventilation, sedation, or, in more difficult cases, paralysis.[2,99] Interestingly enough, although surfactant administration improved respiratory ventilation, the improvement was not accompanied by a significant reduction in the incidence of IVH.[100]

Postnatal Administration of Medications to Reduce Severe IVH

Medications administered postnatally to reduce or prevent IVH have included phenobarbital,[101–104] vitamin E,[105] ethamsylate,[106] and indomethacin.[41,107–109] Although there was initial enthusiasm for the use of each of these medications in the prevention of IVH, there have been none thus far that have been of clear benefit. In one noteworthy study infants who received phenobarbital exhibited a higher incidence of severe IVH than controls,[104] and the systematic review of its postnatal use showed increased risk of mechanical ventilation.[102]

Indomethacin

Currently, the early postnatal administration of indomethacin is believed to be of benefit in the prevention of severe hemorrhage.[41,108,110] Two studies demonstrated a significant reduction in the incidence of severe IVH in infants who received indomethacin in comparison with control group infants. However, at long-term follow-up, the incidence of cerebral palsy was comparable in the two groups.[41,108] This observation, coupled with the known reduction in CBF that accompanies indomethacin administration, warrants cautious use of this agent.[109,111] We administer indomethacin to those infants at greatest risk, such as those delivered precipitously without the benefit of antenatal steroids.

Nursing Care Interventions

Rapid changes in cerebral blood volume are a major risk factor for developing IVH, which may be influenced by arterial blood withdrawal or the flushing of arterial or IV lines or by changes in head or body/leg position. Based on these assumptions, some NICU centers adopted a minimal handling approach following several small retrospective studies, which suggested that decreased monitoring and procedures were associated with a reduced incidence of IVH, although this benefit was not confirmed in a prospective study.[112] More recently, De Bijl-Marcus and colleagues reported on a care bundle consisting of maintaining the head in the midline, elevating the head of the incubator, and avoiding rapid arterial blood withdrawal, IV flushes, and elevation of the legs during diaper changes.[113] These measures targeted the optimization of venous drainage and avoidance of rapid changes in CBF and lowered the risk of IVH in the group receiving the nursing intervention bundles (aOR 0.42, 95% CI 0.27–0.65). The simple nature of this care bundle, which could readily be introduced in any neonatal unit with minimal cost and training, makes this data truly compelling.

Outcome

Mortality increases with severity of intraventricular hemorrhage, up to 40% for those with severe PVHI.[8,114] The surviving infant with severe IVH is at highest risk for adverse neurodevelopmental outcome in motor and cognitive domains.[115] For the extremely preterm infants (24 to 27-6/7 weeks gestational age) enrolled in the Preterm Erythropoietin Neuroprotection Trial (PENUT), cerebral palsy increased with increasing grade of hemorrhage, with 33% of those with grade III IVH, and 64% of those with PVHI, with significant reduction in BSID-III Cognitive, Motor, and Language scores for those with PVHI.[43] The risk is related in part to the extent of the white matter involvement that may be noted on cranial ultrasonography. Thus with a large IPE (>1 cm in diameter; see Fig. 3.1B), the outcome is invariably affected, with major motor and cognitive defects consistently noted at follow-up.[2,18,43,116]

However, as noted previously, even infants with lesser grades of hemorrhage or with no hemorrhage seen on ultrasound are at risk for motor and cognitive deficits.[7,9,10,115] Population studies have suggested that preterm infants with low-grade IVH are not at an increased risk of adverse neurodevelopmental outcome compared to those without IVH[11,117]; this has been contrasted by several studies showing increased risk. In one study, among extremely preterm infants without IVH, moderate to severe neurosensory impairment was seen in 12% and was higher in those with Grade I-II IVH, even without evidence of white matter injury.[7] In addition, the comparable neurodevelopmental outcomes for infants with and without IVH in the indomethacin study clearly indicate that the genesis of brain injury in the sick premature infant is more complex than can be deduced from the neonatal neurologic ultrasonographic appearance.[118]

Gaps in Knowledge

Prevention of IVH and its complications remain elusive, despite the increase in antenatal glucocorticoid administration and delayed cord clamping, both associated with reducing the risk. There are no specific treatments known to limit the extent of injury after it has occurred or effective ways to prevent sequelae such as posthemorrhagic ventricular dilation or white matter injury.

The mechanisms contributing to the motor and cognitive deficits in preterm infants with normal sonogram findings and/or lower grades of IVH remain unclear but critical to delineate. Also, although prophylactic administration of indomethacin has been shown to result in a reduction in the incidence of severe hemorrhage, it remains unclear why the incidence of cerebral palsy at 18 months in treated infants was comparable to that observed in control infants.[41] Furthermore, incidences of moderate to severe cognitive deficits were comparable in the two groups and were substantially higher than incidences of motor deficits.

Other than motor or cognitive disabilities, preterm survivors also have significant risks for language, behavioral, and neurosensory deficits; autism-spectrum disorders; and attention-deficit/hyperactivity disorder that are increasingly being recognized. The neuropathologic correlates are beginning to be identified, including the role of the cerebellar injury. For example, cerebellar hemorrhage may be more common than previously thought, especially as new MRI sequences are being added to routine imaging of preterm infants.[119,120] Severe IVH is much more common in infants without perinatal glucocorticoid exposure, identifying them as a target group for future interventions. Indomethacin at the current time remains the best intervention to use in this high-risk target population.

Conclusions

Current standards of obstetric and neonatal care have led to increased survival of the extremely preterm infant. However, GMH and intraventricular hemorrhage remain significant causes of brain injury in this population. The potential mechanisms contributing to injury are complex and involve factors related to CBF and its regulation. Antenatal glucocorticoid administration and delayed cord clamping have been shown to reduce the risk of IVH. Prophylactic indomethacin has been shown to reduce the risk of severe IVH. However, the reduction has not translated into long-term neurodevelopmental benefit. Complications of IVH include posthemorrhagic ventricular dilation and white matter injury, with no specific therapy to prevent their occurrence. Increasing severity of IVH is associated with increased mortality, as well as increased risk of morbidity for survivors.

REFERENCES

1. Stoll BJ, Hansen NI, Bell EF, et al. Trends in care practices, morbidity, and mortality of extremely preterm neonates, 1993–2012. *JAMA*. 2015;314(10):1039-1051. doi:10.1001/jama.2015.10244.
2. Volpe JJ, Volpe JJ. *Volpe's Neurology of the Newborn*. 6th ed. Philadelphia, PA: Elsevier; 2018.
3. Shalak L, Perlman JM. Hemorrhagic-ischemic cerebral injury in the preterm infant: current concepts. *Clin Perinatol*. 2002;29(4):745-763. doi:10.1016/s0095-5108(02)00048-9.
4. Stoll BJ, Hansen NI, Bell EF, et al. Neonatal outcomes of extremely preterm infants from the NICHD Neonatal Research Network. *Pediatrics*. 2010;126(3):443-456. doi:10.1542/peds.2009-2959.
5. Bell EF, Hintz SR, Hansen NI, et al. Mortality, in-hospital morbidity, care practices, and 2-year outcomes for extremely preterm infants in the US, 2013–2018. *JAMA*. 2022;327(3):248-263. doi:10.1001/jama.2021.23580.
6. O'Shea TM, Allred EN, Kuban KC, et al. Intraventricular hemorrhage and developmental outcomes at 24 months of age in extremely preterm infants. *J Child Neurol*. 2012;27(1):22-29. doi:10.1177/0883073811424462.
7. Bolisetty S, Dhawan A, Abdel-Latif M, et al. Intraventricular hemorrhage and neurodevelopmental outcomes in extreme preterm infants. *Pediatrics*. 2014;133(1):55-62. doi:10.1542/peds.2013-0372.
8. Christian EA, Jin DL, Attenello F, et al. Trends in hospitalization of preterm infants with intraventricular hemorrhage and hydrocephalus in the United States, 2000–2010. *J Neurosurg Pediatr*. 2016;17(3):260-269. doi:10.3171/2015.7.PEDS15140.
9. Laptook AR, O'Shea TM, Shankaran S, Bhaskar B, Network NN. Adverse neurodevelopmental outcomes among extremely low birth weight infants with a normal head ultrasound: prevalence and antecedents. *Pediatrics*. 2005;115(3):673-680. doi:10.1542/peds.2004-0667.
10. Patra K, Wilson-Costello D, Taylor HG, Mercuri-Minich N, Hack M. Grades I–II intraventricular hemorrhage in extremely low birth weight infants: effects on neurodevelopment. *J Pediatr*. 2006;149(2):169-173. doi:10.1016/j.jpeds.2006.04.002.

11. Ann Wy P, Rettiganti M, Li J, et al. Impact of intraventricular hemorrhage on cognitive and behavioral outcomes at 18 years of age in low birth weight preterm infants. *J Perinatol.* 2015;35(7):511-515. doi:10.1038/jp.2014.244.

12. Melbourne L, Chang T, Murnick J, Zaniletti I, Glass P, Massaro AN. Clinical impact of term-equivalent magnetic resonance imaging in extremely-low-birth-weight infants at a regional NICU. *J Perinatol.* 2016;36(11):985-989. doi:10.1038/jp.2016.116.

13. Inder TE, Anderson NJ, Spencer C, Wells S, Volpe JJ. White matter injury in the premature infant: a comparison between serial cranial sonographic and MR findings at term. *AJNR Am J Neuroradiol.* 2003;24(5):805-809. Available at: https://www.ncbi.nlm.nih.gov/pubmed/12748075.

14. Hambleton G, Wigglesworth JS. Origin of intraventricular haemorrhage in the preterm infant. *Arch Dis Child.* 1976;51(9):651-659. doi:10.1136/adc.51.9.651.

15. Perlman JM, Rollins N. Surveillance protocol for the detection of intracranial abnormalities in premature neonates. *Arch Pediatr Adolesc Med.* 2000;154(8):822-826. doi:10.1001/archpedi.154.8.822.

16. Papile LA, Burstein J, Burstein R, Koffler H. Incidence and evolution of subependymal and intraventricular hemorrhage: a study of infants with birth weights less than 1,500 gm. *J Pediatr.* 1978;92(4):529-534. doi:10.1016/s0022-3476(78)80282-0.

17. Gould SJ, Howard S, Hope PL, Reynolds EO. Periventricular intraparenchymal cerebral haemorrhage in preterm infants: the role of venous infarction. *J Pathol.* 1987;151(3):197-202. doi:10.1002/path.1711510307.

18. Guzzetta F, Shackelford GD, Volpe S, Perlman JM, Volpe JJ. Periventricular intraparenchymal echodensities in the premature newborn: critical determinant of neurologic outcome. *Pediatrics.* 1986;78(6):995-1006. Available at: https://www.ncbi.nlm.nih.gov/pubmed/3537951.

19. Lou HC, Lassen NA, Friis-Hansen B. Impaired autoregulation of cerebral blood flow in the distressed newborn infant. *J Pediatr.* 1979;94(1):118-121. doi:10.1016/s0022-3476(79)80373-x.

20. Pryds O, Greisen G, Lou H, Friis-Hansen B. Heterogeneity of cerebral vasoreactivity in preterm infants supported by mechanical ventilation. *J Pediatr.* 1989;115(4):638-645. doi:10.1016/s0022-3476(89)80301-4.

21. Tsuji M, Saul JP, du Plessis A, et al. Cerebral intravascular oxygenation correlates with mean arterial pressure in critically ill premature infants. *Pediatrics.* 2000;106(4):625-632. doi:10.1542/peds.106.4.625.

22. Goddard-Finegold J, Armstrong D, Zeller RS. Intraventricular hemorrhage, following volume expansion after hypovolemic hypotension in the newborn beagle. *J Pediatr.* 1982;100(5):796-799. doi:10.1016/s0022-3476(82)80596-9.

23. Ment LR, Stewart WB, Duncan CC, Lambrecht R. Beagle puppy model of intraventricular hemorrhage. *J Neurosurg.* 1982;57(2):219-223. doi:10.3171/jns.1982.57.2.0219.

24. Goldberg RN, Chung D, Goldman SL, Bancalari E. The association of rapid volume expansion and intraventricular hemorrhage in the preterm infant. *J Pediatr.* 1980;96(6):1060-1063. doi:10.1016/s0022-3476(80)80642-1.

25. Hill A, Perlman JM, Volpe JJ. Relationship of pneumothorax to occurrence of intraventricular hemorrhage in the premature newborn. *Pediatrics.* 1982;69(2):144-149. Available at: https://www.ncbi.nlm.nih.gov/pubmed/6799932.

26. Perlman JM, McMenamin JB, Volpe JJ. Fluctuating cerebral blood-flow velocity in respiratory-distress syndrome. relation to the development of intraventricular hemorrhage. *N Engl J Med.* 1983;309(4):204-209. doi:10.1056/NEJM198307283090402.

27. Mehrabani D, Gowen CW Jr, Kopelman AE. Association of pneumothorax and hypotension with intraventricular haemorrhage. *Arch Dis Child.* 1991;66(1 Spec No):48-51. doi:10.1136/adc.66.1_spec_no.48.

28. Bada HS, Korones SB, Perry EH, et al. Mean arterial blood pressure changes in premature infants and those at risk for intraventricular hemorrhage. *J Pediatr.* 1990;117(4):607-614. doi:10.1016/s0022-3476(05)80700-0.

29. Fabres J, Carlo WA, Phillips V, Howard G, Ambalavanan N. Both extremes of arterial carbon dioxide pressure and the magnitude of fluctuations in arterial carbon dioxide pressure are associated with severe intraventricular hemorrhage in preterm infants. *Pediatrics.* 2007;119(2):299-305. doi:10.1542/peds.2006-2434.

30. Kaiser JR, Gauss CH, Pont MM, Williams DK. Hypercapnia during the first 3 days of life is associated with severe intraventricular hemorrhage in very low birth weight infants. *J Perinatol.* 2006;26(5):279-285. doi:10.1038/sj.jp.7211492.

31. Perlman JM, Volpe JJ. Are venous circulatory abnormalities important in the pathogenesis of hemorrhagic and/or ischemic cerebral injury? *Pediatrics.* 1987;80(5):705-711. Available at: https://www.ncbi.nlm.nih.gov/pubmed/3670971.

32. Tortora D, Severino M, Malova M, et al. Differences in subependymal vein anatomy may predispose preterm infants to GMH-IVH. *Arch Dis Child Fetal Neonatal Ed.* 2018;103(1):F59-F65. doi:10.1136/archdischild-2017-312710.

33. Yanowitz TD, Potter DM, Bowen A, Baker RW, Roberts JM. Variability in cerebral oxygen delivery is reduced in premature neonates exposed to chorioamnionitis. *Pediatr Res.* 2006;59(2):299-304. doi:10.1203/01.pdr.0000196738.03171.f1.

34. Salhab WA, Wyckoff MH, Laptook AR, Perlman JM. Initial hypoglycemia and neonatal brain injury in term infants with severe fetal acidemia. *Pediatrics.* 2004;114(2):361-366. doi:10.1542/peds.114.2.361.

35. McGoldrick E, Stewart F, Parker R, Dalziel SR. Antenatal corticosteroids for accelerating fetal lung maturation for women at risk of preterm birth. *Cochrane Database Syst Rev.* 2020;12:CD004454. doi:10.1002/14651858.CD004454.pub4.

36. Takashima S, Tanaka K. Microangiography and vascular permeability of the subependymal matrix in the premature infant. *Can J Neurol Sci.* 1978;5(1):45-50. Available at: https://www.ncbi.nlm.nih.gov/pubmed/647497.

37. Georgiadis P, Xu H, Chua C, et al. Characterization of acute brain injuries and neurobehavioral profiles in a rabbit model of germinal matrix hemorrhage. *Stroke.* 2008;39(12):3378-3388. doi:10.1161/STROKEAHA.107.510883.

38. Russell GA, Jeffers G, Cooke RW. Plasma hypoxanthine: a marker for hypoxic-ischaemic induced periventricular leucomalacia? *Arch Dis Child.* 1992;67(4 Spec No):388-392. doi:10.1136/adc.67.4_spec_no.388.

39. Perlman JM, Risser R. Relationship of uric acid concentrations and severe intraventricular hemorrhage/leukomalacia in the premature infant. *J Pediatr.* 1998;132(3 Pt 1):436-439. doi:10.1016/s0022-3476(98)70016-2.

40. Allan WC, Vohr B, Makuch RW, Katz KH, Ment LR. Antecedents of cerebral palsy in a multicenter trial of indomethacin for intraventricular hemorrhage. *Arch Pediatr Adolesc Med.* 1997;151(6):580-585. doi:10.1001/archpedi.1997.02170430046010.

41. Schmidt B, Davis P, Moddemann D, et al. Long-term effects of indomethacin prophylaxis in extremely-low-birth-weight

infants. *N Engl J Med*. 2001;344(26):1966-1972. doi:10.1056/NEJM200106283442602.

42. Perlman JM, Volpe JJ. Intraventricular hemorrhage in extremely small premature infants. *Am J Dis Child*. 1986;140(11):1122-1124. doi:10.1001/archpedi.1986.02140250048034.

43. Law JB, Wood TR, Gogcu S, et al. Intracranial hemorrhage and 2-year neurodevelopmental outcomes in infants born extremely preterm. *J Pediatr*. 2021;238:124-134.e10. doi:10.1016/j.jpeds.2021.06.071.

44. Garite TJ, Rumney PJ, Briggs GG, et al. A randomized, placebo-controlled trial of betamethasone for the prevention of respiratory distress syndrome at 24 to 28 weeks' gestation. *Am J Obstet Gynecol*. 1992;166(2):646-651. doi:10.1016/0002-9378(92)91691-3.

45. Jobe AH, Mitchell BR, Gunkel JH. Beneficial effects of the combined use of prenatal corticosteroids and postnatal surfactant on preterm infants. *Am J Obstet Gynecol*. 1993;168(2):508-513. doi:10.1016/0002-9378(93)90483-y.

46. Kari MA, Hallman M, Eronen M, et al. Prenatal dexamethasone treatment in conjunction with rescue therapy of human surfactant: a randomized placebo-controlled multicenter study. *Pediatrics*. 1994;93(5):730-736. Available at: https://www.ncbi.nlm.nih.gov/pubmed/8165070.

47. Leviton A, Dammann O, Allred EN, et al. Antenatal corticosteroids and cranial ultrasonographic abnormalities. *Am J Obstet Gynecol*. 1999;181(4):1007-1017. doi:10.1016/s0002-9378(99)70344-3.

48. Maher JE, Cliver SP, Goldenberg RL, Davis RO, Copper RL. The effect of corticosteroid therapy in the very premature infant. March of Dimes Multicenter Study Group. *Am J Obstet Gynecol*. 1994;170(3):869-873. doi:10.1016/s0002-9378(94)70300-0.

49. Wright LL, Horbar JD, Gunkel H, et al. Evidence from multicenter networks on the current use and effectiveness of antenatal corticosteroids in low birth weight infants. *Am J Obstet Gynecol*. 1995;173(1):263-269. doi:10.1016/0002-9378(95)90211-2.

50. Vinukonda G, Dummula K, Malik S, et al. Effect of prenatal glucocorticoids on cerebral vasculature of the developing brain. *Stroke*. 2010;41(8):1766-1773. doi:10.1161/STROKEAHA.110.588400.

51. Demarini S, Dollberg S, Hoath SB, Ho M, Donovan EF. Effects of antenatal corticosteroids on blood pressure in very low birth weight infants during the first 24 hours of life. *J Perinatol*. 1999;19(6 Pt 1):419-425. doi:10.1038/sj.jp.7200245.

52. Garland JS, Buck R, Leviton A. Effect of maternal glucocorticoid exposure on risk of severe intraventricular hemorrhage in surfactant-treated preterm infants. *J Pediatr*. 1995;126(2):272-279. doi:10.1016/s0022-3476(95)70560-0.

53. Crowther CA, McKinlay CJ, Middleton P, Harding JE. Repeat doses of prenatal corticosteroids for women at risk of preterm birth for improving neonatal health outcomes. *Cochrane Database Syst Rev*. 2015;(7):CD003935. doi:10.1002/14651858.CD003935.pub4.

54. Wapner RJ, Sorokin Y, Mele L, et al. Long-term outcomes after repeat doses of antenatal corticosteroids. *N Engl J Med*. 2007;357(12):1190-1198. doi:10.1056/NEJMoa071453.

55. Perlman JM, Risser RC, Gee JB. Pregnancy-induced hypertension and reduced intraventricular hemorrhage in preterm infants. *Pediatr Neurol*. 1997;17(1):29-33. doi:10.1016/s0887-8994(97)00073-8.

56. Leviton A, Pagano M, Kuban KC, Krishnamoorthy KS, Sullivan KF, Allred EN. The epidemiology of germinal matrix hemorrhage

during the first half-day of life. *Dev Med Child Neurol*. 1991;33(2):138-145. doi:10.1111/j.1469-8749.1991.tb05092.x.

57. Kuban KC, Leviton A, Pagano M, Fenton T, Strassfeld R, Wolff M. Maternal toxemia is associated with reduced incidence of germinal matrix hemorrhage in premature babies. *J Child Neurol*. 1992;7(1):70-76. doi:10.1177/088307389200700113.

58. Gagliardi L, Rusconi F, Da Fre M, et al. Pregnancy disorders leading to very preterm birth influence neonatal outcomes: results of the population-based ACTION cohort study. *Pediatr Res*. 2013;73(6):794-801. doi:10.1038/pr.2013.52.

59. Ancel PY, Marret S, Larroque B, et al. Are maternal hypertension and small-for-gestational age risk factors for severe intraventricular hemorrhage and cystic periventricular leukomalacia? Results of the EPIPAGE cohort study. *Am J Obstet Gynecol*. 2005;193(1):178-184. doi:10.1016/j.ajog.2004.11.057.

60. Gould JB, Gluck L, Kulovich MV. The relationship between accelerated pulmonary maturity and accelerated neurological maturity in certain chronically stressed pregnancies. *Am J Obstet Gynecol*. 1977;127(2):181-186. doi:10.1016/s0002-9378(16)33247-1.

61. Hadi HA. Fetal cerebral maturation in hypertensive disorders of pregnancy. *Obstet Gynecol*. 1984;63(2):214-219. Available at: https://www.ncbi.nlm.nih.gov/pubmed/6694816.

62. Kim HY, Sohn YS, Lim JH, et al. Neonatal outcome after preterm delivery in HELLP syndrome. *Yonsei Med J*. 2006;47(3):393-398. doi:10.3349/ymj.2006.47.3.393.

63. van de Bor M, Verloove-Vanhorick SP, Brand R, Keirse MJ, Ruys JH. Incidence and prediction of periventricular-intraventricular hemorrhage in very preterm infants. *J Perinat Med*. 1987;15(4):333-339. doi:10.1515/jpme.1987.15.4.333.

64. Leviton A, Paneth N, Susser M, et al. Maternal receipt of magnesium sulfate does not seem to reduce the risk of neonatal white matter damage. *Pediatrics*. 1997;99(4):E2. doi:10.1542/peds.99.4.e2.

65. Nelson KB, Grether JK. Can magnesium sulfate reduce the risk of cerebral palsy in very low birthweight infants? *Pediatrics*. 1995;95(2):263-269. Available at: https://www.ncbi.nlm.nih.gov/pubmed/7838646.

66. Paneth N, Jetton J, Pinto-Martin J, Susser M. Magnesium sulfate in labor and risk of neonatal brain lesions and cerebral palsy in low birth weight infants. The Neonatal Brain Hemorrhage Study Analysis Group. *Pediatrics*. 1997;99(5):E1. doi:10.1542/peds.99.5.e1.

67. Canterino JC, Verma UL, Visintainer PF, Figueroa R, Klein SA, Tejani NA. Maternal magnesium sulfate and the development of neonatal periventricular leucomalacia and intraventricular hemorrhage. *Obstet Gynecol*. 1999;93(3):396-402. doi:10.1016/s0029-7844(98)00455-4.

68. Atkinson MW, Goldenberg RL, Gaudier FL, et al. Maternal corticosteroid and tocolytic treatment and morbidity and mortality in very low birth weight infants. *Am J Obstet Gynecol*. 1995;173(1):299-305. doi:10.1016/0002-9378(95)90218-x.

69. Groome LJ, Goldenberg RL, Cliver SP, Davis RO, Copper RL. Neonatal periventricular-intraventricular hemorrhage after maternal beta-sympathomimetic tocolysis. The March of Dimes Multicenter Study Group. *Am J Obstet Gynecol*. 1992;167(4 Pt 1):873-879. doi:10.1016/0002-9378(12)80004-4.

70. Rouse DJ, Hirtz DG, Thom E, et al. A randomized, controlled trial of magnesium sulfate for the prevention of cerebral palsy. *N Engl J Med*. 2008;359(9):895-905. doi:10.1056/NEJMoa0801187.

71. Doyle LW, Crowther CA, Middleton P, Marret S, Rouse D. Magnesium sulphate for women at risk of preterm birth for

neuroprotection of the fetus. *Cochrane Database Syst Rev.* 2009;(1):CD004661. doi:10.1002/14651858.CD004661.pub3.

72. Doyle LW, Crowther CA, Middleton P, Marret S. Antenatal magnesium sulfate and neurologic outcome in preterm infants: a systematic review. *Obstet Gynecol.* 2009;113(6):1327-1333. doi:10.1097/AOG.0b013e3181a60495.

73. Committee Opinion No 652: magnesium sulfate use in obstetrics. *Obstet Gynecol.* 2016;127(1):e52-e53. doi:10.1097/AOG.0000000000001267.

74. Anderson GD, Bada HS, Shaver DC, et al. The effect of cesarean section on intraventricular hemorrhage in the preterm infant. *Am J Obstet Gynecol.* 1992;166(4):1091-1099; discussion 1099-1101. doi:10.1016/s0002-9378(11)90594-8.

75. Low JA, Galbraith RS, Sauerbrei EE, et al. Maternal, fetal, and newborn complications associated with newborn intracranial hemorrhage. *Am J Obstet Gynecol.* 1986;154(2):345-351. doi:10.1016/0002-9378(86)90669-1.

76. Strauss A, Kirz D, Modanlou HD, Freeman RK. Perinatal events and intraventricular/subependymal hemorrhage in the very low-birth weight infant. *Am J Obstet Gynecol.* 1985;151(8):1022-1027. doi:10.1016/0002-9378(85)90373-4.

77. Ment LR, Oh W, Ehrenkranz RA, Philip AG, Duncan CC, Makuch RW. Antenatal steroids, delivery mode, and intraventricular hemorrhage in preterm infants. *Am J Obstet Gynecol.* 1995;172(3):795-800. doi:10.1016/0002-9378(95)90001-2.

78. Deulofeut R, Sola A, Lee B, Buchter S, Rahman M, Rogido M. The impact of vaginal delivery in premature infants weighing less than 1,251 grams. *Obstet Gynecol.* 2005;105(3):525-531. doi:10.1097/01.AOG.0000154156.51578.50.

79. Wadhawan R, Vohr BR, Fanaroff AA, et al. Does labor influence neonatal and neurodevelopmental outcomes of extremely-low-birth-weight infants who are born by cesarean delivery? *Am J Obstet Gynecol.* 2003;189(2):501-506. doi:10.1067/s0002-9378(03)00360-0.

80. Riskin A, Riskin-Mashiah S, Bader D, et al. Delivery mode and severe intraventricular hemorrhage in single, very low birth weight, vertex infants. *Obstet Gynecol.* 2008;112(1):21-28. doi:10.1097/AOG.0b013e31817cfdf1.

81. Hansen A, Leviton A. Labor and delivery characteristics and risks of cranial ultrasonographic abnormalities among very-low-birth-weight infants. The Developmental Epidemiology Network Investigators. *Am J Obstet Gynecol.* 1999;181(4):997-1006. doi:10.1016/s0002-9378(99)70339-x.

82. American College of Obstetricians, Gynecologists' Committee on Obstetric Practice. Delayed umbilical cord clamping after birth: ACOG Committee Opinion, Number 814. *Obstet Gynecol.* 2020;136(6):e100-e106.doi:10.1097/AOG.0000000000004167.

83. Rabe H, Gyte GM, Diaz-Rossello JL, Duley L. Effect of timing of umbilical cord clamping and other strategies to influence placental transfusion at preterm birth on maternal and infant outcomes. *Cochrane Database Syst Rev.* 2019;9:CD003248. doi:10.1002/14651858.CD003248.pub4.

84. Seidler AL, Gyte GML, Rabe H, et al. Umbilical cord management for newborns <34 weeks' gestation: a meta-analysis. *Pediatrics.* 2021;147(3). doi:10.1542/peds.2020-0576.

85. Mercer JS, Erickson-Owens DA, Vohr BR, et al. Effects of placental transfusion on neonatal and 18 month outcomes in preterm infants: a randomized controlled trial. *J Pediatr.* 2016;168:50-55.e1. doi:10.1016/j.jpeds.2015.09.068.

86. Committee Opinion No. 684: delayed umbilical cord clamping after birth. *Obstet Gynecol.* 2017;129(1):1. doi:10.1097/AOG.0000000000001860.

87. Elimian A, Goodman J, Escobedo M, Nightingale L, Knudtson E, Williams M. Immediate compared with delayed cord clamping in the preterm neonate: a randomized controlled trial. *Obstet Gynecol.* 2014;124(6):1075-1079. doi:10.1097/AOG.0000000000000556.

88. Chiruvolu A, Tolia VN, Qin H, et al. Effect of delayed cord clamping on very preterm infants. *Am J Obstet Gynecol.* 2015;213(5):676.e1-7. doi:10.1016/j.ajog.2015.07.016.

89. Katheria A, Reister F, Essers J, et al. Association of umbilical cord milking vs delayed umbilical cord clamping with death or severe intraventricular hemorrhage among preterm infants. *JAMA.* 2019;322(19):1877-1886. doi:10.1001/jama.2019.16004.

90. Mohamed MA, Aly H. Transport of premature infants is associated with increased risk for intraventricular haemorrhage. *Arch Dis Child Fetal Neonatal Ed.* 2010;95(6):F403-F407. doi:10.1136/adc.2010.183236.

91. Amer R, Moddemann D, Seshia M, et al. Neurodevelopmental outcomes of infants born at <29 weeks of gestation admitted to Canadian neonatal intensive care units based on location of birth. *J Pediatr.* 2018;196:31-37.e1. doi:10.1016/j.jpeds.2017.11.038.

92. Helenius K, Longford N, Lehtonen L, et al. Association of early postnatal transfer and birth outside a tertiary hospital with mortality and severe brain injury in extremely preterm infants: observational cohort study with propensity score matching. *BMJ.* 2019;367:l5678. doi:10.1136/bmj.l5678.

93. Hirata K, Kimura T, Hirano S, et al. Outcomes of outborn very-low-birth-weight infants in Japan. *Arch Dis Child Fetal Neonatal Ed.* 2021;106(2):131-136. doi:10.1136/archdischild-2019-318594.

94. Vohr B, Ment LR. Intraventricular hemorrhage in the preterm infant. *Early Hum Dev.* 1996;44(1):1-16. doi:10.1016/0378-3782(95)01692-9.

95. Leviton A, VanMarter L, Kuban KC. Respiratory distress syndrome and intracranial hemorrhage: cause or association? Inferences from surfactant clinical trials. *Pediatrics.* 1989;84(5):915-922. Available at: https://www.ncbi.nlm.nih.gov/pubmed/2677963.

96. Perlman JM. Intraventricular hemorrhage. *Pediatrics.* 1989;84(5):913-915. Available at: https://www.ncbi.nlm.nih.gov/pubmed/2797987.

97. Ambalavanan N, Carlo WA, Wrage LA, et al. PaCO2 in surfactant, positive pressure, and oxygenation randomised trial (SUPPORT). *Arch Dis Child Fetal Neonatal Ed.* 2015;100(2):F145-F419. doi:10.1136/archdischild-2014-306802.

98. Perlman J, Thach B. Respiratory origin of fluctuations in arterial blood pressure in premature infants with respiratory distress syndrome. *Pediatrics.* 1988;81(3):399-403. Available at: https://www.ncbi.nlm.nih.gov/pubmed/3344182.

99. Perlman JM, Goodman S, Kreusser KL, Volpe JJ. Reduction in intraventricular hemorrhage by elimination of fluctuating cerebral blood-flow velocity in preterm infants with respiratory distress syndrome. *N Engl J Med.* 1985;312(21):1353-1357. doi:10.1056/NEJM198505233122104.

100. Jobe AH. Pulmonary surfactant therapy. *N Engl J Med.* 1993;328(12):861-868. doi:10.1056/NEJM199303253281208.

101. Bedard MP, Shankaran S, Slovis TL, Pantoja A, Dayal B, Poland RL. Effect of prophylactic phenobarbital on intraventricular hemorrhage in high-risk infants. *Pediatrics.* 1984;73(4):435-439. Available at: https://www.ncbi.nlm.nih.gov/pubmed/6369238.

102. Smit E, Odd D, Whitelaw A. Postnatal phenobarbital for the prevention of intraventricular haemorrhage in preterm

infants. *Cochrane Database Syst Rev.* 2013;(8):CD001691. doi:10.1002/14651858.CD001691.pub3.

103. Donn SM, Roloff DW, Goldstein GW. Prevention of intraventricular haemorrhage in preterm infants by phenobarbitone. A controlled trial. *Lancet.* 1981;2(8240):215-217. doi:10.1016/s0140-6736(81)90470-0.

104. Kuban KC, Leviton A, Krishnamoorthy KS, et al. Neonatal intracranial hemorrhage and phenobarbital. *Pediatrics.* 1986;77(4):443-450. Available at: https://www.ncbi.nlm.nih.gov/pubmed/3515304.

105. Sinha S, Davies J, Toner N, Bogle S, Chiswick M. Vitamin E supplementation reduces frequency of periventricular haemorrhage in very preterm babies. *Lancet.* 1987;1(8531):466-471. doi:10.1016/s0140-6736(87)92087-3.

106. Morgan ME, Benson JW, Cooke RW. Ethamsylate reduces the incidence of periventricular haemorrhage in very low birthweight babies. *Lancet.* 1981;2(8251):830-831. doi:10.1016/s0140-6736(81)91103-x.

107. Bada HS, Green RS, Pourcyrous M, et al. Indomethacin reduces the risks of severe intraventricular hemorrhage. *J Pediatr.* 1989;115(4):631-637. doi:10.1016/s0022-3476(89)80300-2.

108. Ment LR, Oh W, Ehrenkranz RA, et al. Low-dose indomethacin and prevention of intraventricular hemorrhage: a multicenter randomized trial. *Pediatrics.* 1994;93(4):543-550. Available at: https://www.ncbi.nlm.nih.gov/pubmed/8134206.

109. Edwards AD, Wyatt JS, Richardson C, et al. Effects of indomethacin on cerebral haemodynamics in very preterm infants. *Lancet.* 1990;335(8704):1491-1495. doi:10.1016/0140-6736(90)93030-s.

110. Fowlie PW, Davis PG, McGuire W. Prophylactic intravenous indomethacin for preventing mortality and morbidity in preterm infants. *Cochrane Database Syst Rev.* 2010;(7):CD000174. doi:10.1002/14651858.CD000174.pub2.

111. Pryds O, Greisen G, Johansen KH. Indomethacin and cerebral blood flow in premature infants treated for patent ductus arteriosus. *Eur J Pediatr.* 1988;147(3):315-316. doi:10.1007/BF00442705.

112. Bada HS, Korones SB, Perry EH, et al. Frequent handling in the neonatal intensive care unit and intraventricular hemorrhage.

J Pediatr. 1990;117(1 Pt 1):126-131. doi:10.1016/s0022-3476(05)72460-4.

113. de Bijl-Marcus K, Brouwer AJ, De Vries LS, Groenendaal F, Wezel-Meijler GV. Neonatal care bundles are associated with a reduction in the incidence of intraventricular haemorrhage in preterm infants: a multicentre cohort study. *Arch Dis Child Fetal Neonatal Ed.* 2020;105(4):419-424. doi:10.1136/archdischild-2018-316692.

114. Cizmeci MN, de Vries LS, Ly LG, et al. Periventricular hemorrhagic infarction in very preterm infants: characteristic sonographic findings and association with neurodevelopmental outcome at age 2 years. *J Pediatr.* 2020;217:79-85.e1. doi:10.1016/j.jpeds.2019.09.081.

115. Hollebrandse NL, Spittle AJ, Burnett AC, et al. School-age outcomes following intraventricular haemorrhage in infants born extremely preterm. *Arch Dis Child Fetal Neonatal Ed.* 2021;106(1):4-8. doi:10.1136/archdischild-2020-318989.

116. Stewart AL, Reynolds EO, Hope PL, et al. Probability of neurodevelopmental disorders estimated from ultrasound appearance of brains of very preterm infants. *Dev Med Child Neurol.* 1987;29(1):3-11. doi:10.1111/j.1469-8749.1987.tb02101.x.

117. Payne AH, Hintz SR, Hibbs AM, et al. Neurodevelopmental outcomes of extremely low-gestational-age neonates with low-grade periventricular-intraventricular hemorrhage. *JAMA Pediatr.* 2013;167(5):451-459. doi:10.1001/jamapediatrics.2013.866.

118. Foglia EE, Roberts RS, Stoller JZ, et al. Effect of prophylactic indomethacin in extremely low birth weight infants based on the predicted risk of severe intraventricular hemorrhage. *Neonatology.* 2018;113(2):183-186. doi:10.1159/000485172.

119. Neubauer V, Djurdjevic T, Griesmaier E, Biermayr M, Gizewski ER, Kiechl-Kohlendorfer U. Routine magnetic resonance imaging at term-equivalent age detects brain injury in 25% of a contemporary cohort of very preterm infants. *PLoS One.* 2017;12(1):e0169442. doi:10.1371/journal.pone.0169442.

120. Gano D, Ho ML, Partridge JC, et al. Antenatal exposure to magnesium sulfate is associated with reduced cerebellar hemorrhage in preterm newborns. *J Pediatr.* 2016;178:68-74. doi:10.1016/j.jpeds.2016.06.053.

Chapter 4

White Matter Injury in the Premature Infant

Dalit Cayam-Rand and Steven Paul Miller

Chapter Outline

Case History

JD is a 30-week appropriate for gestational-age male infant born to a 26-year-old primigravida woman whose pregnancy was complicated by intermittent vaginal bleeding from 20 weeks' gestation. Partial placental abruption was diagnosed and mom was placed on bedrest, given a course of steroids and treated with magnesium sulfate. At 30 weeks, she had spontaneous rupture of membranes. Within several hours, labor progressed, and the infant was delivered vaginally with delayed cord clamping. He initially cried vigorously, followed by a series of apneas in the delivery room necessitating continuous positive airway pressure (CPAP). Apgar scores were 7 and 7 at 1 and 5 minutes, respectively and he was brought to the neonatal intensive care unit on CPAP with 40% FiO_2. He was treated empirically with antibiotics until cultures came back sterile. He was weaned off respiratory support at 12 days of life. The clinical course was complicated by recurrent apneas, for which he was treated with caffeine. Cranial ultrasound (US) on the third day of life showed bilateral periventricular echogenicities

(Fig. 4.1). Follow-up US 1 week later showed white matter cysts (Fig. 4.2) and magnetic resonance imaging (MRI) performed at 33 weeks postmenstrual age showed cystic periventricular leukomalacia (PVL) (Fig. 4.3). Repeat MRI at term-equivalent age (TEA) demonstrated white matter volume loss and ventriculomegaly. Developmentally, at 9 months of age, he was a communicative and curious infant with significant motor delays. He was diagnosed with diplegic spastic cerebral palsy (CP) for which he received occupational and physical therapies. Follow-up at 2 years old revealed language delays requiring speech therapy and at 6 years old he has an individualized education plan including physical therapy and special education services at his school.

This case illustrates the classic evolution of severe white matter injury (WMI) in the preterm infant characterized by hyperechogenicity or "flaring," the subsequent appearance of cystic changes, and eventually, enlarged lateral ventricles indicating progressive volume loss. While MRI is a more sensitive modality for visualizing WMI, cranial US is the most frequent bedside imaging modality used in the NICU. Recognition

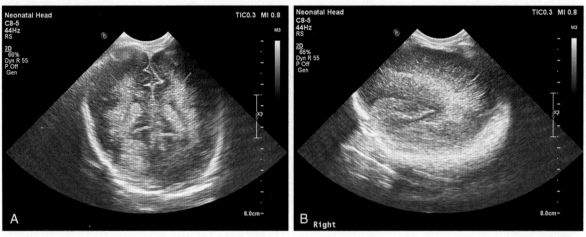

Fig. 4.1 Ultrasound images from the third day of life demonstrating periventricular echogenicities or "flaring" (*orange arrows*), on the coronal plane bilaterally (A) and the sagittal plane on the right side (B).

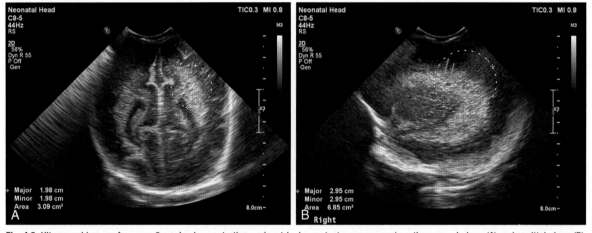

Fig. 4.2 Ultrasound images from age 2 weeks demonstrating periventricular cysts (*orange arrows*) on the coronal plane (A) and sagittal plane (B).

of the patterns of injury prior to discharge enables providers to refer to developmental follow-up and support for those at highest risk for neurodevelopmental impairments.

The Scope and Spectrum of White Matter Injury

WMI, the most common form of brain injury in preterm infants, occurs most often among infants born between 23 and 32 weeks' gestation with a peak incidence at 28 weeks' gestational age. The prevalence of WMI varies according to the gestational age of the cohort, as well as the timing and modality of imaging. A recent systematic review has described that up to 40% of preterm infants are born before 28 weeks' gestational age.[1] The spectrum of preterm WMI ranges from discrete lesions to diffuse volume loss and includes three pathologic forms: cystic necrosis, microscopic necrosis, and nonnecrotic lesions. The most severe injury consists of destructive lesions of all cellular elements with areas of cystic necrosis greater than 2 mm in diameter, known as cystic PVL. The incidence of these lesions has decreased substantially

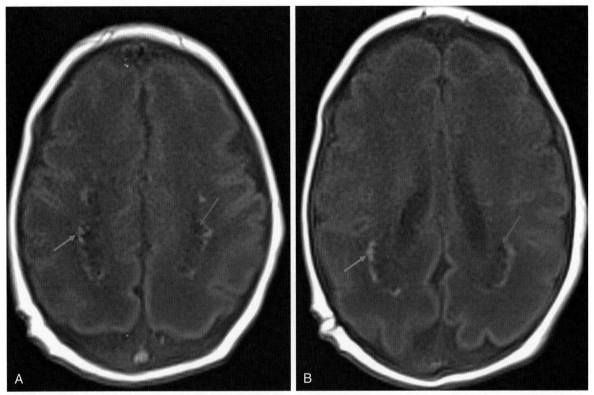

Fig. 4.3 Magnetic resonance T1 axial images from 3 weeks of age demonstrating periventricular hyperintense lesions (*orange arrows*) adjacent to cystic injury (*blue arrows*) at the level of the deep white matter directly superior to the ventricles (A) and more inferiorly and posteriorly (B).

in the last few decades and occurs in current cohorts of very low birth weight infants at a rate of less than 5%.[2,3] More commonly, microscopic foci less than 1 mm in diameter occur and evolve into areas of gliosis, commonly referred to as noncystic PVL. Interestingly, the incidence of noncystic WMI is decreasing over time in some cohorts of preterm neonates, without a clear explanation.[4] In contemporary cohorts of preterm newborns, the most common form of injury is diffuse WMI. Unlike necrotic injury, diffuse WMI is caused by selective degeneration of premyelinating oligodendrocytes (pre-OLs) that fail to mature into oligodendrocytes, leading to myelination failure and secondary axonal disturbances.[5]

Notably, the patterns of WMI associated with very preterm infants, born before 32 weeks, are increasingly being recognized in other populations. Recent studies have demonstrated WMI in a substantial number of moderate to late preterm infants, though severe lesions are less common than at lower gestational ages.[6–8] In a prospective study of neonates born between 32 and 36 weeks, WMI was the most frequent form of brain injury encountered, with MRI at TEA revealing diffuse injury in 23% and punctate lesions in 16%.[8] Term-born infants with severe congenital heart disease demonstrate similar lesions,[9,10] postulated to be a result of destructive and dysmaturational disturbances that overlap with the mechanisms in preterm infants.[11] Punctate lesions have also been reported among near-term and term-born infants associated with perinatal asphyxia and genetic diagnoses.[12] Nevertheless, as the hallmark brain lesion among very preterm infants, the imaging characteristics, pathogenesis, and outcomes of WMI are currently best understood in the context of prematurity as illustrated below.

Diagnosis and Imaging

The evolution of preterm WMI from the first few days of life until TEA has been extensively characterized by serial cranial US imaging.[13] This method has been used to diagnose cystic WMI since the 1980s due to its availability, safety, and reliability. Typically, the initial presentation of WMI on US is enhanced periventricular echogenicity. This may persist or resolve within several days; after resolution, it may then evolve into gliotic or cystic changes or, alternatively, leave no abnormality.[13] Cysts may only appear after 2 to 6 weeks and may subsequently disappear due to resorption of fluid within gliotic brain tissue and can therefore be missed without sequential imaging. At TEA, US may only demonstrate ex vacuo ventriculomegaly and enlarged extra-axial spaces. Thus the number and timing of US studies are critical to consider when evaluating the diagnostic performance of this imaging modality.

When cystic WMI persists, it is associated with significant developmental abnormalities that are primarily motor impairments, classically, spastic diplegic CP. A widely utilized grading classification for the severity of cystic PVL was developed by de Vries et al.[14] and increasing severity of PVL according to this classification is associated with increased incidence and severity of CP.[15] Prolonged duration of periventricular hyperechogenicities, even in the absence of cystic evolution, has also been associated with adverse motor outcomes.[16,17]

MRI is the preferred modality to diagnose diffuse WMI. At TEA and onward, diffuse WMI may appear on MRI as ventriculomegaly, irregularly shaped ventricles, white matter loss (enlarged cerebrospinal fluid spaces surrounding the sulci), white matter tract thinning (e.g., thin corpus callosum), diffuse signal intensity changes, and myelination disturbances.[18] Scoring systems for these white matter abnormalities have been developed that are inversely associated with neurodevelopmental outcomes at preschool age.[19–21]

Many centers also perform early MRIs, at approximately 32 weeks postmenstrual age, or as soon as infants are sufficiently stable to undergo the exam. Increased use of early MRI has demonstrated more subtle focal lesions that may not be appreciated on US imaging or follow-up TEA imaging.[22] Visualized soon after the insult, WMI lesions may appear as clusters of punctate hyperintense T1 signal abnormalities often accompanied by diffusion restriction.[18,23,24] Linear punctate lesions with a hemorrhagic component, indicated by signal loss on susceptibility-weighted imaging, may also be seen.[23,25] Clinical factors associated with punctate lesions include higher gestational age and birth weight among very preterm neonates and the presence of intraventricular hemorrhage (IVH).[26,27] These multifocal WMI lesions are most readily visualized on early-life MRI. In a significant number of infants, these early lesions fade or become challenging to detect on MRI at TEA, though they are still associated with neurodevelopmental outcomes, even if harder to detect on these later age MRI scans. The change in imaging characteristics of these lesions over time supports the destructive/necrotic nature of these early lesions and not that they are transient imaging phenomena.[22,28] Importantly for clinicians, both the volume and location of lesions on early-life MRI are predictive of outcomes, with anterior lesions being most concerning for motor and cognitive deficits.[29,30] A summary of US and MRI findings can be found in Table 4.1.

TABLE 4.1	Summary of Potential Imaging Findings According to Timing and Modality of Imaging		
Age	**US**	**MRI**	**Pathology**
<7 days	Echogenicity		Uncertain
1–4 weeks	Persistent echogenicity or resolution	Punctate T1-hyperintense ischemic lesions, hemorrhagic lesions	Microscopic necrosis, gliosis
2–6 weeks	Cysts	Cysts	Necrosis
TEA	Ex-vacuo ventriculomegaly	Diffuse volume loss, irregularly shaped ventricles, myelination disturbances	Dysmaturation of pre-OLs and neurons

MRI, magnetic resonance imaging; *pre-OLs*, premyelinating oligodendrocytes; *TEA*, term-equivalent age; *US*, ultrasound.

More sophisticated imaging modalities reveal microstructural disturbances and aberrant connectivity patterns among preterm infants with WMI. Diffusion tensor imaging (DTI) shows reduced fractional anisotropy in white matter tracts, indicating delayed maturation among preterm neonates with focal lesions,[31,32] including distal to the original site of injury[33] and even in the absence of overt injury on conventional MRI.[34] Diffuse white matter abnormalities are also associated with abnormal radial and axial diffusivities on DTI.[35,36] Functional resting state MRI has also demonstrated altered connectivity among neonates with WMI.[37–39]

WMI does not typically have a clinical correlate in the immediate neonatal period and the diagnosis is usually made by routine imaging. Guidelines from the American Academy of Pediatrics and Canadian Paediatric Society recommend performing serial cranial US in very preterm infants in the first week of life, at 4 to 6 weeks, and again prior to discharge, with minor differences between the guidelines regarding the gestational age cutoff and timing of the first US.[40,41] The first US is primarily meant for the detection of IVH and the latter for WMI, although, as discussed earlier, US may miss the more prevalent diffuse WMI, better demonstrated on MRI. Some controversy exists surrounding the routine use of MRI as a screening tool at TEA given its limited overall predictive value for long-term outcomes,[42–44] and in current guidelines, MRI is suggested for infants with abnormal imaging findings on US. Other experts offer evidence-based indications for using routine MRI in high-risk infants in conversation with the family concerning the performance of this imaging modality to predict long-term neurodevelopment.[45] It is important to note that the absence of WMI carries a particularly high negative predictive value for significant adverse outcomes,[46] allowing clinicians to be reassuring when WMI is not demonstrated. And, as noted above, multifocal WMI lesions are more readily detected on early-life MRI rather than at TEA.

Pathogenesis

The central mechanisms of WMI in preterm neonates are hypoxia-ischemia and infection-inflammation, leading to oxidative stress, glutamate-mediated excitotoxicity, and the production of proinflammatory cytokines and reactive oxygen species (ROS) that are toxic to the developing white matter. The primary cellular target of injury is oligodendrocyte precursors, called premyelinating oligodendrocytes (pre-OLs). Extensive human and experimental studies have demonstrated the vulnerability of pre-OLs, the predominant white matter cells in the preterm brain during the peak window of WMI.[47] Oligodendrocytes, primarily derived from radial glial cells, mature in four principal stages that have distinct morphology, immune markers, and functional characteristics.[48] The earliest form of oligodendrocyte progenitors can migrate and proliferate, whereas pre-OLs are proliferative but nonmigratory, and the more mature oligodendrocytes have myelinating properties. Pre-OLs are uniquely vulnerable to oxidative stress due to maturation-dependent features, including an immature antioxidant system that renders them vulnerable to ROS.[49,50] This intrinsic susceptibility is not seen in earlier and later oligodendrocyte lineage stages, or in cortical neurons,[51] and it is potentiated by both hypoxia-ischemia and inflammation, which in turn, potentiate each other.[52] The role of hypoxia-ischemia is postulated to be a result of disturbances in cerebral autoregulation, heart-rate-dependent cardiac output, and the immature vasculature precipitated by episodes of hypoxia, bradycardia, and hypotension.[53] Infection-inflammation is mediated by microglial activation via Toll-like receptors (TLRs), as a result of common inflammatory disturbances in the preterm neonate, including sepsis and necrotizing enterocolitis (NEC).[54] These mechanisms trigger a cascade of events, leading to the degeneration of pre-OLs and a subsequent increase in dysmature oligodendrocyte progenitors that are unable to fully differentiate into myelin-producing cells, causing diffuse injury characterized by impaired myelination and volume loss.[55]

HYPOXIA-ISCHEMIA

The specific factors in the preterm neonate that predispose to hypoxia-ischemia are low basal cerebral blood flow (CBF), impaired autoregulatory mechanisms, and underdeveloped vasculature.[53] These clinical issues are of particular concern given the role of repeated hypoxia-ischemia in experimental models leading to severe WMI.[56] Furthermore, the regenerated pool of pre-OLs, the vulnerable cell type, leads to an ongoing vulnerability of the white matter to repeated hypoxic-ischemic events. Repeated hypoxic-ischemic events also generate an inflammatory response culminating in

WMI, as well as related comorbidities, such as bronchopulmonary dysplasia (BPD) and retinopathy of prematurity (ROP), that predispose to WMI, further exacerbating the damage.[57,58]

Cerebral Blood Flow and Autoregulation

Basal CBF in preterm infants is low, even in the absence of disturbances.[59,60] CBF is impacted by changes in blood oxygen and carbon dioxide, acidosis, and hypoglycemia, common occurrences in sick preterm neonates. Under physiologic conditions, CBF is maintained by cerebral autoregulation, a mechanism that allows for relatively stable CBF across a range of systemic blood pressures. Above and below the limits of this range, CBF increases or decreases passively along with changes in systemic blood pressure, known as pressure-passive circulation. Preterm infants, especially those who are critically ill or mechanically ventilated, often display pressure-passive circulation, as well as impaired responses to metabolic derangements.[61–66] Cerebral autoregulation is a complex protective phenomenon involving neurogenic, myogenic, hormonal, and metabolic processes and the immature vasculature in the second and third trimesters has not developed the full capacity for autoregulation.[67] Studies in preterm sheep demonstrate development of the muscular layers of arteries, critical for vasoreactive responses, at 13 weeks' gestation, and functional autoregulation at 19 weeks' gestation, corresponding to the human equivalent of 25 and 36 weeks' gestation, respectively.[68] This is consistent with human studies showing progression of autoregulation in the third trimester.[69] Vasoreactivity is further impaired in the presence of brain injury.[70,71]

Developing Vasculature

The vascular supply of the white matter arises from the external surface of the brain via perforating branches of leptomeningeal arteries in a centripetal fashion. These penetrating vessels include shorter subcortical branches and longer medullary branches supplying the deep white matter[72] and extend in length and complexity with increasing gestational age.[73] During the second trimester of gestation, these vessels may remain short with limited anastomoses, potentially leaving the periventricular deep white matter vulnerable to ischemic injury.[74] The existence of an additional centrifugal vascular supply to the deep white matter via perforating branches of choroidal arteries, initially described by Van den Bergh,[75] remains controversial.[76] Past studies hypothesized that brain tissue at the boundary of the centripetal and centrifugal territories served as a watershed border zone that is susceptible to ischemic injury, possibly explaining the distribution and location of PVL.[77,78] More recent studies dispute this on several fronts; first, anatomic studies using histological and stereoscopic methods in the past three decades have revealed these centrifugal vessels to be early subependymal veins draining the periventricular area and do not support the existence of centrifugal arteries.[79–83] Moreover, as demonstrated by Nelson et al.,[82] in addition to the long medullary arteries originating at the gyral crests supplying the periventricular white matter, shorter medullary arteries extending from the depths of the sulci also supply these areas, giving it a rich vascular supply. Abundant arterioles from peripheral branches of medullary arteries were also found on autopsy in neonates born 20 to 41 weeks of gestation by Nakamura,[79] further challenging a hypovascular border zone hypothesis.

Physiologic evidence further refuting the end artery and border zone theory can be found in animal studies on ischemia in the immature brain. McClure et al.[84] measured CBF in various brain regions after ischemia-reperfusion caused by carotid occlusion and found no significant difference in CBF between the cortex and periventricular white matter during ischemia or reperfusion. Moreover, no differences were found in CBF between inferior, middle, and superior white matter regions, despite the predilection of the inferior areas to develop WMI. Areas of WMI, which localized to deeper white matter, were not associated with higher levels of ischemia, suggesting that the susceptibility of these areas is unrelated to blood flow.

INFECTION-INFLAMMATION

Mounting evidence in animal and human studies supports inflammatory mechanisms triggered by hypoxia-ischemia that injure the developing white matter due to its intrinsic susceptibility. Episodes of intermittent hypoxemia have been linked to local microglial activation,[85] proinflammatory cytokines,[86] and elevated levels of the products of lipid peroxidation.[87] A small study recently showed a relationship between intermittent episodes of hypoxia and plasma CRP level, a marker of systemic inflammation.[88] These inflammatory changes are associated with DTI measures and histological evidence of diffuse WMI, impaired myelination, and functional outcomes.[86,89–91] Thus it is important not to consider hypoxia-ischemia and inflammation as completely independent phenomena.

Evidence for a primary role for infectious and inflammatory processes in the pathogenesis of WMI initially came from autopsy studies showing increased WMI among neonates with bacteremia.[92] This observation led to experimentally induced infection in kittens implicating the bacterial lipopolysaccharide endotoxin,[93] later found to activate Toll-like receptor 4 (TLR4).[94–96] This receptor is highly expressed on microglia, but not on pre-OLs, the primary site of damage.[97] The final link to WMI was elucidated with studies demonstrating the unique susceptibility of pre-OL and the developing white matter to the products of activated microglia and oxidative stress, as discussed below. These experimental findings are supported by the clinical observation of higher rates of WMI in preterm neonates with multiple infections.[98]

Glutamate-Mediated Excitotoxicity

Glutamate, the primary excitatory neurotransmitter in the central nervous system, is vital to physiologic processes in the developing brain, regulating survival, proliferation, migration, and differentiation of neural progenitor cells.[99] However, when excessively accumulated in pathologic conditions, glutamate also functions as a neurotoxin.[100] Following ischemia, glutamate is released from dying cells and the buildup of extracellular glutamate is toxic to adjacent pre-OLs, as first shown by Oka et al.[101] This injury is mediated by both glutamate transporters and glutamate receptors.[102] Glutamate shares a transporter with cystine; excess extracellular glutamate inhibits the uptake of cystine which is critical for the synthesis of glutathione, a potent endogenous antioxidant. The ensuing cellular glutathione depletion renders the cells vulnerable to free radical toxicity.[101] Parallel to the transporter mechanism of injury, glutamate activates AMPA, kainate, and NMDA receptors that are expressed by developing oligodendrocytes.[103–105] The activation of

AMPA and kainate receptors causes an influx of calcium that accumulates in the mitochondria, leading to increased production of free radicals and triggering caspases, causing apoptosis.[106] Cell death then leads to additional glutamate being released, creating a feedback loop that enhances cell injury.[47] The exact mechanism of injury mediated by NMDA receptors is still unclear. Notably, the discovery of receptor-mediated damage has revealed a potential therapeutic target for WMI; rodent models of preterm WMI treated with memantine, an NMDA-receptor antagonist, and topiramate, an AMPA-receptor antagonist, have shown attenuation of oligodendrocyte degeneration.[107,108]

The excitotoxicity of glutamate may also be mediated by astrocytes via the excitatory amino acid transporter, EAAT2, a glutamine transporter encoded by the gene SLC1A2. The transient expression of this transporter in immature oligodendrocytes has been discovered at the peak time of WMI, as well as in reactive astrocytes after hypoxic-ischemic injury[109–111] and may play a role in chronic white matter dysfunction.[100]

Activated Microglia and Proinflammatory Cytokines

Microglia, the immune cells of the brain, play a key role in normal processes of brain development including apoptosis of excessive neurons, synaptic pruning, phagocytosis of cellular debris, and maintaining brain homeostasis.[112] As such, microglia are abundant in the developing white matter during the peak window of WMI,[113] including a recently discovered unique subset with myelinogenic properties.[114] Although initial activation of microglia is beneficial to the brain, prolonged activation triggers neurodegeneration.[115] Microglia are activated by TLRs, a family of receptors that recognize pathogen-associated molecular patterns, expressed by bacterial pathogens, as well as endogenous danger-associated molecular patterns, released after cellular stress or tissue injury.[116] Microglia migrate to the pathogen or site of injury and release proinflammatory cytokines, such as tumor necrosis factor-alpha, interferon-gamma, interleukin-2, and interleukin-6 that exert a toxic effect on oligodendrocytes.[117–120] Elevated levels of these cytokines and their receptors have been found in the brains of preterm infants with cystic injury[119,121,122] and with diffuse noncystic WMI.[123]

Reactive Oxygen and Nitrogen Species

Animal and human studies implicate ROS, and reactive nitrogen species, the by-products of lipid peroxidation and protein oxidation, and biomarkers of oxidative stress, in preterm WMI.[51,124–126] An increase in ascorbyl radicals was found in the brains of fetal sheep exposed to intrauterine asphyxia and reperfusion[125] and several studies have shown elevated isoprostanes, a marker of lipid peroxidation, among preterm neonates with WMI.[51] ROS are kept in check by endogenous antioxidants, such as superoxide dismutase, catalase, and glutathione peroxidase. The predilection of preterm periventricular white matter for damage due to ROS may be related to delayed expression of some of these enzymes. The expression of superoxide dismutases one and two are significantly lower in preterm oligodendrocytes at 20 to 29 weeks, rendering them susceptible to free radical damage and ill-equipped for the oxygen-rich postnatal environment.[127] This vulnerability, unique to periventricular white matter, was shown by Back et al., who found elevated levels of isoprostanes in white matter lesions, but not in the cortex.[51] This biomarker for oxidative injury has been shown to be predictive of WMI, but not predictive of 2-year outcomes, highlighting the complexity of factors relating to outcomes.[128]

Chronic Diffuse WMI

The final common pathway for these mechanisms of injury is the degeneration of pre-OLs and subsequent myelination failure. In severe focal lesions, myelination failure results from pan-cellular necrosis causing degeneration of glial cells and axons within the foci of injury, as initially described by Banker and Larroche,[129] as well as axonal injury in surrounding gliotic areas beyond the regions of necrosis.[130] The immature unmyelinated axons demonstrate a vulnerability to ischemia that is similar to pre-OLs[131] and the severity of axonopathy seems to be related to the severity of WMI necrosis.[132]

In the more prevalent chronic form of diffuse non-necrotic WMI, myelination failure is not mediated by severe axonal injury, but rather by dysmaturation. This milder form of injury is characterized by the acute degeneration of pre-OLs that is accompanied by inflammatory astrocytosis and microgliosis. Interestingly, the loss of pre-OLs also stimulates a reactive proliferation of oligodendrocyte progenitor cells, resulting in a paradoxical *increase* in the pre-OL population.[133] Human and animal studies have shown a marked increase in progenitor cells primarily within WMI lesions, with a small increase also in the subventricular zone, the transient fetal structure where they are naturally generated.[133–135] These progenitors give rise to a large pool of regenerated pre-OLs in the injured areas; however, these pre-OLs are unable to differentiate into myelinating cells.[5] The mechanisms behind their disrupted maturation are still being elucidated but seem to be related to the surrounding astrogliosis and microgliosis in the damaged extracellular matrix. Reactive astrocytes in the extracellular matrix secrete hyaluronic acid and the products of hyaluronic acid degradation by specific hyaluronidases inhibit the maturation of pre-OLs.[136–138] Increased levels of hyaluronic acid have been found in preterm sheep models of WMI and reactive astrocytes with the hyaluronic acid receptor CD44 have been found in human preterm WMI.[55,56] The accumulation of selective bioactive hyaluronic acid fragments resulting from this degradation induce signal transduction via TLRs to attenuate the transcription of myelin basic protein, thereby impeding myelination. Other proposed mechanisms for myelination failure include interactions between CD44 and hyaluronic acid that involve recognizing and producing these fragments, independent of signaling.[139]

Data from studies on adult demyelinating diseases have revealed additional potential mechanisms for dysmaturation involving signaling pathways such as Notch and Wnt-beta catenin that disrupt oligodendrocyte maturation,[140] as well as epidermal growth factor receptor (EGFR) signaling that promotes maturation.[141] The Wnt signaling pathway was subsequently found to be involved in neonatal WMI mediated by hypoxia-inducible factor alpha (HIFα), critical for angiogenesis and myelination.[142,143] More recently, HIFα was also found to regulate myelination, independent of this signaling pathway.[144] Elucidating the exact mechanisms is crucial for developing targeted treatments. In contrast to irreversible necrotic injury with resultant death of all cellular components, dysmaturation seems to be a form of regeneration and plasticity that may be potentially modifiable and reversible. Novel treatments that have been investigated include hyaluronidase blockers that have been shown to promote pre-OL maturation[145] and a selective EGFR ligand administered intranasally to mice with diffuse WMI that promotes recovery and maturation of oligodendrocytes.[146]

Clinical Risk Factors for WMI

Numerous neonatal complications, including comorbid conditions and NICU procedures and therapies, are associated with neonatal WMI. Hemorrhagic infarcts of deep white matter that accompany IVH and evolve into porencephalic cysts are discussed in the chapter on IVH. As noted above, the prevalence of WMI is higher in neonates with IVH for a given gestational age at birth. White matter dysmaturation can also occur following IVH, via the release of blood products such as iron and thrombin that induce oxidative stress, inflammation, and glutamate excitotoxicity.[147,148]

Neonatal infections are highly associated with WMI in multiple studies.[98,149–152] This association has been observed in culture-positive infections from the cerebrospinal fluid,[152] as well as from sites remote from the brain (blood and tracheal cultures),[151] and in culture-negative clinical sepsis.[153] Regarding the type of WMI, cystic PVL has been linked with neonatal sepsis,[154] while noncystic progressive WMI has been linked to recurrent infections in the neonatal period.[149] Multiple infections (≥3) have also been associated with indices of dysmaturation in white matter tracts on DTI in the absence of overt injury on conventional MRI.[98] The pathogenesis is related to proinflammatory cytokines and activated microglia via expression of TLRs as discussed above.[54,155]

NEC has also been associated with an increased risk of WMI, particularly when it requires surgical management.[156–158] The mechanism of NEC-related brain injury, long suspected to be mediated by the innate immune response and TLRs,[54,97] has only recently begun to be elucidated in mouse models, shedding new light on the gut-brain signaling axis. Nino et al.[159] discovered the release of proteins functioning as TLR ligands in the intestine that promote microglial activation and accumulation of ROS in the brain.

This group of researchers subsequently demonstrated a key role for intestinal CD4+ T-lymphocytes in inducing brain injury via release of interferon-gamma and microglial activation.[160] Importantly, inhibition of these lymphocytes and neutralization of interferon-gamma with targeted antibodies were able to prevent WMI, revealing a potential therapeutic avenue to avert brain injury in neonates with NEC.

Severe ROP is associated with altered microstructural integrity and delayed maturation of white matter tracts, predominantly in the posterior white matter.[161–163] These changes are predictive of lower motor and cognitive scores at 18 months old.[162] The pathogenesis is postulated to be linked to levels of insulin growth factor one,[164] an anabolic hormone which exerts effects on the retina and the brain, but the exact mechanisms have yet to be clarified. Other hypotheses include a role of systemic inflammation and hyperoxia, as recently reviewed by Morken et al.[165]

BPD or prolonged mechanical ventilation is associated with a spectrum of WMI and delayed maturation of white matter at TEA.[166–170] Several underlying factors seem to be related to adverse white matter development in BPD including duration of mechanical ventilation,[171,172] and precursors to BPD, such as cumulative supplemental oxygen and mean airway pressure in the first few weeks of life, which are independently associated with adverse neurodevelopmental outcomes.[173] Respiratory disturbances that are often associated with mechanical ventilation such as hypocarbia and hyperoxia are also linked to WMI.[174–176]

There is conflicting evidence to support a role for chorioamnionitis as a risk factor for WMI. Intrauterine inflammation leading to the release of proinflammatory cytokines and fetal immune response syndrome is related to neonatal morbidities, such as postnatal infection, IVH, and adverse outcomes, that are also associated with WMI,[177–179] but several studies have been unable to show an independent association between chorioamnionitis and WMI.[171,180–182]

Outcome

Given the function of myelinated white matter in the rapid transmittal of information across neural networks, it is not surprising that WMI can have a significant and broad impact on motor, cognitive, and social development. Motor-wise, white matter enables efficient and accurate communication between brain regions that include the motor cortex, basal ganglia, and cerebellum; intact myelination between these areas is vital for motor skills requiring fluency, coordination, and automatization. Accordingly, WMI is associated with a spectrum of motor deficits of varying severity, ranging from developmental coordination disorder (DCD) to CP, with more severe imaging abnormalities predicting more severe impairment.[18,46,183,184]

Although the incidence of the severe lesion of cystic WMI has decreased, when it occurs, it remains highly predictive of CP. In a recent population-based study over two decades in Canada, approximately 80% of infants with this injury were diagnosed with CP,[3] consistent with other studies.[185-187] In the absence of cystic injury, myelination disturbances in the corticospinal tract are also associated with CP.[188,189] Clinically, motor abnormalities predictive of CP may be detected early in infancy; in the first few weeks of life, abnormal general movements, including the absence of normal fidgety movements, are highly sensitive and specific for the subsequent diagnosis of CP.[190] In preterm infants, these aberrant patterns of general movements are associated with WMI on TEA-MRI, white matter microstructural abnormalities, lower regional white matter volumes, and adverse motor and cognitive outcomes.[191,192] Diffuse white matter microstructural abnormalities, in the absence of gross abnormalities on conventional MRI, are also associated with childhood DCD. Clinically, DCD manifests as difficulty learning and executing coordinated motor movements and reduced fluency in motor skills and the neuroanatomical correlates of these deficits last into childhood.[193,194]

Several studies have demonstrated increased rates of long-term cognitive impairments at school age among preterm-born children with overt WMI and, as with motor outcomes, the severity of injury is related to the severity of impairment.[21,195-199] Microstructural disturbances on DTI, even in the absence of lesions on conventional imaging, are also associated with cognitive outcomes.[200] Specifically, impairments in complex skills such as executive functions, responsible for cognitive flexibility, self-control, and working memory

are associated with white matter microstructural abnormalities among children born preterm who suffered inflammatory neonatal complications, such as BPD, NEC, and sepsis.[201] The link between executive dysfunction and inflammatory complications is bolstered by the association between elevated neonatal inflammatory markers in the first month of life and executive function deficits at age 10 years.[202] These impairments may explain the increased rates of attention deficit hyperactivity disorder seen in the preterm population.[203]

The fundamental role of white matter in these higher-order cognitive skills has been gaining recognition[204,205] and is likely related to connectivity and network efficiency.[206-208] The development of the connectome between 30 and 40 gestational weeks is heavily mediated by white matter microstructure[209] and microstructural disturbances among preterm-born children result in impaired connectivity and network efficiency.[210] These disturbances may also underlie the higher prevalence of autism spectrum disorder (ASD) and anxiety disorders that are seen among children born preterm.[211,212] Long-distance connectivity along several white matter tracts, such as the superior longitudinal fasciculus, is integral to the normal development of social cognition and theory of mind.[207] Disruptions to the integrity of these tracts are commonly found in children with ASD[213,214] and aberrant fractional anisotropy values in white matter tracts at 6 months of age can be found among infants who are subsequently diagnosed with ASD.[215] Among preterm-born children, frank WMI on conventional MRI at TEA has been associated with ASD[216] and animal models of preterm diffuse WMI provide evidence of inflammatory mechanisms mediating autistic behaviors in mice, mimicking human ASD.[217]

Cognitive outcomes are also likely mediated by grey matter changes that may accompany WMI. MRI studies have shown reduced cortical and thalamic volumes among children with WMI[218-220] and reduced caudate neuronal maturation observed experimentally with hypoxia-ischemia.[221] Furthermore, the interaction between early neonatal WMI and diminished childhood thalamic volumes has been associated with cognitive outcomes at school age.[220] Among neonates with PVL, pathology studies have demonstrated gliosis and neuronal loss in the thalamus[222] and DTI studies have demonstrated abnormal microstructure both within the thalamus and in white matter tracts that is associated with diminished thalamic volumes.[219,223,224] Animal models of diffuse WMI have attributed grey matter loss to a reduction in the complexity of the dendritic armor and reduced synaptic activity in cortical neurons and corticothalamic pathways.[221,225–227]

Cognitive outcomes are also modified by environmental and genetic influences that are not readily accessible on imaging. The substantial impact of socioeconomic status on outcomes[228] suggests potential interventions to improve outcomes, as well as important limitations for predicting outcomes with imaging alone.

Treatment

There is currently no effective treatment to prevent or to cure WMI and therefore mitigate its long-term consequences. In the neonatal period, avoiding associated risk factors for WMI, such as ventilatory complications, neonatal infection, and NEC, is key. When WMI is diagnosed on imaging, surveillance programs for early intervention are put in place to identify any neurodevelopmental impairments and start physical, occupational, and speech and language therapies. These programs have demonstrated a positive influence on outcomes at preschool age.[229]

The more prevalent chronic diffuse WMI that is seen in contemporary preterm populations opens a window for possible therapeutic strategies to mitigate or prevent the maturation and myelination failure that progressively occurs over many weeks. Potential interventions include treatments targeting inflammation and the immune response. Erythropoietin has been investigated over the last decade as a neuroprotective agent due to its antioxidant and anti-inflammatory effects and as a promotor of neurogenesis. In animal models of neonatal WMI, it prevents pre-OL death and promotes pre-OL development.[230,231] Randomized trials subsequently showed improved white matter development and better cognitive outcomes in preterm infants who received erythropoietin.[232–234] A recent randomized, double-blind trial of prophylactic erythropoietin treatment did not show differences in outcome between the placebo and erythropoietin groups.[235]

This finding is surprising given the mechanisms of WMI outlined above; as such, erythropoietin as a potential neuroprotection strategy requires further attention (e.g., longer duration of therapy). Other potentially promising interventions in preclinical trials include anti-inflammatory treatments, such as tumor necrosis factor antagonists, associated with reduced gliosis among preterm sheep exposed to inflammation,[236] and anti-interleukin-1 monoclonal antibodies, that reduce brain injury in fetal sheep exposed to ischemia.[237]

Supportive measures such as providing adequate nutrition and nutrient intake have also been shown to improve outcomes and diminish brain injury in preclinical and some clinical studies.[238] Specifically, studies on full-term infants suggest that iron may improve myelination; a recent randomized controlled trial showed greater myelin content at 1 year of age among term-born infants who underwent delayed cord clamping associated with higher ferritin levels at 4 months of age.[239] The long-term outcomes of adequate nutritional intake are still being evaluated.[238] Preventing painful procedures is also an important component of improving brain maturation and neurodevelopmental outcomes.[240] Painful procedures are associated with impaired white matter development that persists to school age and is linked with cognitive outcomes.[241–243] Optimal strategies to measure pain and provide analgesia in neonates require further investigation.

Gaps in Knowledge

1. The dysmaturation that leads to diffuse WMI develops over weeks, providing a potential window for therapeutic intervention to prevent further injury. It remains unclear how much time there is to prevent the long-term neurological complications in the chronic form of diffuse WMI and when the window for intervention closes.

2. Recent studies have demonstrated the feasibility of early intervention including inpatient NICU rehabilitation programs and home-based programs for preterm neonates at risk for adverse outcomes,[244–246] with promising results in the prevention of short-term complications, such as

duration of oxygen supplementation and hospitalization, and the incidence of BPD, ROP, and NEC.[247] The choice of therapy, optimal timing, and long-term effect on outcomes warrant further investigation.

3. Anxiety among parents of survivors of preterm birth may be heightened when brain injury is diagnosed, particularly given the wide spectrum of WMI and outcomes. How best to support parents in understanding the implications of WMI and putting it into a broader context within the confluence of factors that impact outcomes needs to be elucidated. Incorporating parental input in WMI research may be a potential avenue to enable clinicians to assist parents to optimally support their children born preterm.

REFERENCES

1. Romero-Guzman GJ, Lopez-Munoz F. [Prevalence and risk factors for periventricular leukomalacia in preterm infants. A systematic review]. *Rev Neurol.* 2017;65(2):57-62. Prevalencia y factores de riesgo de leucomalacia periventricular en recien nacidos prematuros. Revision sistematica.
2. Hamrick SE, Miller SP, Leonard C, et al. Trends in severe brain injury and neurodevelopmental outcome in premature newborn infants: the role of cystic periventricular leukomalacia. *J Pediatr.* 2004;145(5):593-599. doi:10.1016/j.jpeds.2004.05.042.
3. Ghotra S, Vincer M, Allen VM, Khan N. A population-based study of cystic white matter injury on ultrasound in very preterm infants born over two decades in Nova Scotia, Canada. *J Perinatol.* 2019;39(2):269-277. doi:10.1038/s41372-018-0294-5.
4. Gano D, Andersen SK, Partridge JC, et al. Diminished white matter injury over time in a cohort of premature newborns. *J Pediatr.* 2015;166(1):39-43. doi:10.1016/j.jpeds.2014.09.009.
5. Back SA. White matter injury in the preterm infant: pathology and mechanisms. *Acta Neuropathol.* 2017;134(3):331-349. doi:10.1007/s00401-017-1718-6.
6. Ballardini E, Tarocco A, Baldan A, Antoniazzi E, Garani G, Borgna-Pignatti C. Universal cranial ultrasound screening in preterm infants with gestational age 33–36 weeks. A retrospective analysis of 724 newborns. *Pediatr Neurol.* 2014;51(6):790-794. doi:10.1016/j.pediatrneurol.2014.08.012.
7. Fumagalli M, Ramenghi LA, De Carli A, et al. Cranial ultrasound findings in late preterm infants and correlation with perinatal risk factors. *Ital J Pediatr.* 2015;41:65. doi:10.1186/s13052-015-0172-0.
8. Boswinkel V, Kruse-Ruijter MF, Nijboer-Oosterveld J, et al. Incidence of brain lesions in moderate-late preterm infants assessed by cranial ultrasound and MRI: the BIMP-study. *Eur J Radiol.* 2021;136:109500. doi:10.1016/j.ejrad.2020.109500.
9. Peyvandi S, De Santiago V, Chakkarapani E, et al. Association of prenatal diagnosis of critical congenital heart disease with postnatal brain development and the risk of brain injury. *JAMA Pediatr.* 2016;170(4):e154450. doi:10.1001/jamapediatrics.2015.4450.
10. Guo T, Chau V, Peyvandi S, et al. White matter injury in term neonates with congenital heart diseases: topology & comparison with preterm newborns. *Neuroimage.* 2019;185:742-749. doi:10.1016/j.neuroimage.2018.06.004.
11. Volpe JJ. Encephalopathy of congenital heart disease–destructive and developmental effects intertwined. *J Pediatr.* 2014;164(5):962-965. doi:10.1016/j.jpeds.2014.01.002.
12. Hayman M, van Wezel-Meijler G, van Straaten H, Brilstra E, Groenendaal F, de Vries LS. Punctate white-matter lesions in the full-term newborn: underlying aetiology and outcome. *Eur J Paediatr Neurol.* 2019;23(2):280-287. doi:10.1016/j.ejpn.2019.01.005.
13. Agut T, Alarcon A, Cabanas F, et al. Preterm white matter injury: ultrasound diagnosis and classification. *Pediatr Res.* 2020;87(suppl 1):37-49. doi:10.1038/s41390-020-0781-1.
14. de Vries LS, Eken P, Dubowitz LM. The spectrum of leukomalacia using cranial ultrasound. *Behav Brain Res.* 1992;49(1):1-6. doi:10.1016/s0166-4328(05)80189-5.
15. Pierrat V, Duquennoy C, van Haastert IC, Ernst M, Guilley N, de Vries LS. Ultrasound diagnosis and neurodevelopmental outcome of localised and extensive cystic periventricular leucomalacia. *Arch Dis Child Fetal Neonatal Ed.* 2001;84(3):F151-F156. doi:10.1136/fn.84.3.f151.
16. Jongmans M, Henderson S, de Vries L, Dubowitz L. Duration of periventricular densities in preterm infants and neurological outcome at 6 years of age. *Arch Dis Child.* 1993;69(1 Spec No):9-13. doi:10.1136/adc.69.1_spec_no.9.
17. Ancel PY, Livinec F, Larroque B, et al. Cerebral palsy among very preterm children in relation to gestational age and neonatal ultrasound abnormalities: the EPIPAGE cohort study. *Pediatrics.* 2006;117(3):828-835. doi:10.1542/peds.2005-0091.
18. Martinez-Biarge M, Groenendaal F, Kersbergen KJ, et al. MRI based preterm white matter injury classification: the importance of sequential imaging in determining severity of injury. *PLoS One.* 2016;11(6):e0156245. doi:10.1371/journal.pone.0156245.
19. Brouwer MJ, Kersbergen KJ, van Kooij BJM, et al. Preterm brain injury on term-equivalent age MRI in relation to perinatal factors and neurodevelopmental outcome at two years. *PLoS One.* 2017;12(5):e0177128. doi:10.1371/journal.pone.0177128.
20. Kidokoro H, Neil JJ, Inder TE. New MR imaging assessment tool to define brain abnormalities in very preterm infants at term. *AJNR Am J Neuroradiol.* 2013;34(11):2208-2214. doi:10.3174/ajnr.A3521.
21. Woodward LJ, Clark CA, Bora S, Inder TE. Neonatal white matter abnormalities an important predictor of neurocognitive outcome for very preterm children. *PLoS One.* 2012;7(12):e51879. doi:10.1371/journal.pone.0051879.
22. Miller SP, Ferriero DM, Leonard C, et al. Early brain injury in premature newborns detected with magnetic resonance imaging is associated with adverse early neurodevelopmental outcome. *J Pediatr.* 2005;147(5):609-616. doi:10.1016/j.jpeds.2005.06.033.
23. Kersbergen KJ, Benders MJ, Groenendaal F, et al. Different patterns of punctate white matter lesions in serially scanned preterm infants. *PLoS One.* 2014;9(10):e108904. doi:10.1371/journal.pone.0108904.
24. Cornette LG, Tanner SF, Ramenghi LA, et al. Magnetic resonance imaging of the infant brain: anatomical characteristics and clinical significance of punctate lesions. *Arch Dis Child Fetal Neonatal Ed.* 2002;86(3):F171-F177.
25. Malova M, Morelli E, Cardiello V, et al. Nosological differences in the nature of punctate white matter lesions in preterm infants. *Front Neurol.* 2021;12:657461. doi:10.3389/fneur.2021.657461.

26. Tusor N, Benders MJ, Counsell SJ, et al. Punctate white matter lesions associated with altered brain development and adverse motor outcome in preterm infants. *Sci Rep.* 2017;7(1):13250. doi:10.1038/s41598-017-13753-x.

27. Wagenaar N, Chau V, Groenendaal F, et al. Clinical risk factors for punctate white matter lesions on early magnetic resonance imaging in preterm newborns. *J Pediatr.* 2017;182:34-40.e1. doi:10.1016/j.jpeds.2016.11.073.

28. George JM, Pannek K, Rose SE, Ware RS, Colditz PB, Boyd RN. Diagnostic accuracy of early magnetic resonance imaging to determine motor outcomes in infants born preterm: a systematic review and meta-analysis. *Dev Med Child Neurol.* 2018;60(2):134-146. doi:10.1111/dmcn.13611.

29. Guo T, Duerden EG, Adams E, et al. Quantitative assessment of white matter injury in preterm neonates: association with outcomes. *Neurology.* 2017;88(7):614-622. doi:10.1212/WNL.0000000000003606.

30. Cayam-Rand D, Guo T, Grunau RE, et al. Predicting developmental outcomes in preterm infants: a simple white matter injury imaging rule. *Neurology.* 2019;93(13):e1231-e1240. doi:10.1212/WNL.0000000000008172.

31. Bassi L, Chew A, Merchant N, et al. Diffusion tensor imaging in preterm infants with punctate white matter lesions. *Pediatr Res.* 2011;69(6):561-566. doi:10.1203/PDR.0b013e3182182836.

32. Zhang F, Liu C, Qian L, Hou H, Guo Z. Diffusion tensor imaging of white matter injury caused by prematurity-induced hypoxic-ischemic brain damage. *Med Sci Monit.* 2016;22:2167-2174. doi:10.12659/msm.896471.

33. Huppi PS, Murphy B, Maier SE, et al. Microstructural brain development after perinatal cerebral white matter injury assessed by diffusion tensor magnetic resonance imaging. *Pediatrics.* 2001;107(3):455-460. doi:10.1542/peds.107.3.455.

34. Anjari M, Srinivasan L, Allsop JM, et al. Diffusion tensor imaging with tract-based spatial statistics reveals local white matter abnormalities in preterm infants. *Neuroimage.* 2007;35(3):1021-1027. doi:10.1016/j.neuroimage.2007.01.035.

35. Counsell SJ, Allsop JM, Harrison MC, et al. Diffusion-weighted imaging of the brain in preterm infants with focal and diffuse white matter abnormality. *Pediatrics.* 2003;112(1 Pt 1):1-7. doi:10.1542/peds.112.1.1.

36. Counsell SJ, Shen Y, Boardman JP, et al. Axial and radial diffusivity in preterm infants who have diffuse white matter changes on magnetic resonance imaging at term-equivalent age. *Pediatrics.* 2006;117(2):376-386. doi:10.1542/peds.2005-0820.

37. Smyser CD, Snyder AZ, Shimony JS, Blazey TM, Inder TE, Neil JJ. Effects of white matter injury on resting state fMRI measures in prematurely born infants. *PLoS One.* 2013;8(7):e68098. doi:10.1371/journal.pone.0068098.

38. He L, Parikh NA. Aberrant executive and frontoparietal functional connectivity in very preterm infants with diffuse white matter abnormalities. *Pediatr Neurol.* 2015;53(4):330-337. doi:10.1016/j.pediatrneurol.2015.05.001.

39. Duerden EG, Halani S, Ng K, et al. White matter injury predicts disrupted functional connectivity and microstructure in very preterm born neonates. *Neuroimage Clin.* 2019;21:101596. doi:10.1016/j.nicl.2018.11.006.

40. Hand IL, Shellhaas RA, Milla SS, Committee on Fetus and Newborn, Section on Neurology, Section on Radiology. Routine neuroimaging of the preterm brain. *Pediatrics.* 2020;146(5):e2020029082. doi:10.1542/peds.2020-029082.

41. Guillot M, Chau V, Lemyre B. Routine imaging of the preterm neonatal brain. *Paediatr Child Health.* 2020;25(4):249-262. doi:10.1093/pch/pxaa033.

42. Janvier A, Barrington K. Trying to predict the future of ex-preterm infants: who benefits from a brain MRI at term? *Acta Paediatr.* 2012;101(10):1016-1017. doi:10.1111/j.1651-2227.2012.02788.x.

43. Ho T, Dukhovny D, Zupancic JA, Goldmann DA, Horbar JD, Pursley DM. Choosing wisely in newborn medicine: five opportunities to increase value. *Pediatrics.* 2015;136(2):e482-e489. doi:10.1542/peds.2015-0737.

44. Edwards AD, Redshaw ME, Kennea N, et al. Effect of MRI on preterm infants and their families: a randomised trial with nested diagnostic and economic evaluation. *Arch Dis Child Fetal Neonatal Ed.* 2018;103(1):F15-F21. doi:10.1136/archdischild-2017-313102.

45. Inder TE, de Vries LS, Ferriero DM, et al. Neuroimaging of the preterm brain: review and recommendations. *J Pediatr.* 2021;237:276-287.e4. doi:10.1016/j.jpeds.2021.06.014.

46. Van't Hooft J, van der Lee JH, Opmeer BC, et al. Predicting developmental outcomes in premature infants by term equivalent MRI: systematic review and meta-analysis. *Syst Rev.* 2015;4:71. doi:10.1186/s13643-015-0058-7.

47. Volpe JJ, Kinney HC, Jensen FE, Rosenberg PA. The developing oligodendrocyte: key cellular target in brain injury in the premature infant. *Int J Dev Neurosci.* 2011;29(4):423-440. doi:10.1016/j.ijdevneu.2011.02.012.

48. Back SA. Perinatal white matter injury: the changing spectrum of pathology and emerging insights into pathogenetic mechanisms. *Ment Retard Dev Disabil Res Rev.* 2006;12(2):129-140. doi:10.1002/mrdd.20107.

49. Back SA, Gan X, Li Y, Rosenberg PA, Volpe JJ. Maturation-dependent vulnerability of oligodendrocytes to oxidative stress-induced death caused by glutathione depletion. *J Neurosci.* 1998;18(16):6241-6253.

50. Back SA, Han BH, Luo NL, et al. Selective vulnerability of late oligodendrocyte progenitors to hypoxia-ischemia. *J Neurosci.* 2002;22(2):455-463.

51. Back SA, Luo NL, Mallinson RA, et al. Selective vulnerability of preterm white matter to oxidative damage defined by F2-isoprostanes. *Ann Neurol.* 2005;58(1):108-120. doi:10.1002/ana.20530.

52. Galinsky R, Lear CA, Dean JM, et al. Complex interactions between hypoxia-ischemia and inflammation in preterm brain injury. *Dev Med Child Neurol.* 2018;60(2):126-133. doi:10.1111/dmcn.13629.

53. Vesoulis ZA, Mathur AM. Cerebral autoregulation, brain injury, and the transitioning premature infant. *Front Pediatr.* 2017;5:64. doi:10.3389/fped.2017.00064.

54. Volpe JJ. Postnatal sepsis, necrotizing enterocolitis, and the critical role of systemic inflammation in white matter injury in premature infants. *J Pediatr.* 2008;153(2):160-163. doi:10.1016/j.jpeds.2008.04.057.

55. Buser JR, Maire J, Riddle A, et al. Arrested preoligodendrocyte maturation contributes to myelination failure in premature infants. *Ann Neurol.* 2012;71(1):93-109. doi:10.1002/ana.22627.

56. Hagen MW, Riddle A, McClendon E, et al. Role of recurrent hypoxia-ischemia in preterm white matter injury severity. *PLoS One.* 2014;9(11):e112800. doi:10.1371/journal.pone.0112800.

57. Di Fiore JM, Vento M. Intermittent hypoxia and oxidative stress in preterm infants. *Respir Physiol Neurobiol.* 2019;266:121-129. doi:10.1016/j.resp.2019.05.006.

58. Di Fiore JM, Raffay TM. The relationship between intermittent hypoxemia events and neural outcomes in neonates. *Exp Neurol.* 2021;342:113753. doi:10.1016/j.expneurol.2021.113753.

59. Greisen G. Cerebral blood flow in preterm infants during the first week of life. *Acta Paediatr Scand.* 1986;75(1):43-51. doi:10.1111/j.1651-2227.1986.tb10155.x.

60. Kehrer M, Blumenstock G, Ehehalt S, Goelz R, Poets C, Schoning M. Development of cerebral blood flow volume in preterm neonates during the first two weeks of life. *Pediatr Res.* 2005;58(5):927-930. doi:10.1203/01.PDR.0000182579.52820.C3.

61. Lou HC, Lassen NA, Friis-Hansen B. Impaired autoregulation of cerebral blood flow in the distressed newborn infant. *J Pediatr.* 1979;94(1):118-121. doi:10.1016/s0022-3476(79)80373-x.

62. Boylan GB, Young K, Panerai RB, Rennie JM, Evans DH. Dynamic cerebral autoregulation in sick newborn infants. *Pediatr Res.* 2000;48(1):12-17. doi:10.1203/00006450-200007000-00005.

63. Jayasinghe D, Gill AB, Levene MI. CBF reactivity in hypotensive and normotensive preterm infants. *Pediatr Res.* 2003;54(6):848-853. doi:10.1203/01.PDR.0000088071.30873.DA.

64. Soul JS, Hammer PE, Tsuji M, et al. Fluctuating pressure-passivity is common in the cerebral circulation of sick premature infants. *Pediatr Res.* 2007;61(4):467-473. doi:10.1203/pdr.0b013e31803237f6.

65. Wong FY, Leung TS, Austin T, et al. Impaired autoregulation in preterm infants identified by using spatially resolved spectroscopy. *Pediatrics.* 2008;121(3):e604-e611. doi:10.1542/peds.2007-1487.

66. Wong FY, Silas R, Hew S, Samarasinghe T, Walker AM. Cerebral oxygenation is highly sensitive to blood pressure variability in sick preterm infants. *PLoS One.* 2012;7(8):e43165. doi:10.1371/journal.pone.0043165.

67. Rhee CJ, da Costa CS, Austin T, Brady KM, Czosnyka M, Lee JK. Neonatal cerebrovascular autoregulation. *Pediatr Res.* 2018;84(5):602-610. doi:10.1038/s41390-018-0141-6.

68. Helou S, Koehler RC, Gleason CA, Jones MD, Jr., Traystman RJ. Cerebrovascular autoregulation during fetal development in sheep. *Am J Physiol.* 1994;266(3 Pt 2):H1069-H1074. doi:10.1152/ajpheart.1994.266.3.H1069.

69. Rhee CJ, Fraser CD, 3rd, Kibler K, et al. The ontogeny of cerebrovascular pressure autoregulation in premature infants. *J Perinatol.* 2014;34(12):926-931. doi:10.1038/jp.2014.122.

70. Ment LR, Duncan CC, Ehrenkranz RA, et al. Intraventricular hemorrhage in the preterm neonate: timing and cerebral blood flow changes. *J Pediatr.* 1984;104(3):419-425. doi:10.1016/s0022-3476(84)81109-9.

71. Vesoulis ZA, Liao SM, Trivedi SB, Ters NE, Mathur AM. A novel method for assessing cerebral autoregulation in preterm infants using transfer function analysis. *Pediatr Res.* 2016;79(3):453-459. doi:10.1038/pr.2015.238.

72. Nonaka H, Akima M, Hatori T, Nagayama T, Zhang Z, Ihara F. Microvasculature of the human cerebral white matter: arteries of the deep white matter. *Neuropathology.* 2003;23(2):111-118. doi:10.1046/j.1440-1789.2003.00486.x.

73. Raybaud C. Normal and abnormal embryology and development of the intracranial vascular system. *Neurosurg Clin N Am.* 2010;21(3):399-426. doi:10.1016/j.nec.2010.03.011.

74. Takashima S, Itoh M, Oka A. A history of our understanding of cerebral vascular development and pathogenesis of perinatal brain damage over the past 30 years. *Semin Pediatr Neurol.* 2009;16(4):226-236. doi:10.1016/j.spen.2009.09.004.

75. Van den Bergh R. Centrifugal elements in the vascular pattern of the deep intracerebral blood supply. *Angiology.* 1969;20(2):88-94. doi:10.1177/000331976902000205.

76. Smirnov M, Destrieux C, Maldonado IL. Cerebral white matter vasculature: still uncharted? *Brain.* 2021;144(12):3561-3575. doi:10.1093/brain/awab273.

77. DeReuck J, Chattha AS, Richardson EP Jr. Pathogenesis and evolution of periventricular leukomalacia in infancy. *Arch Neurol.* 1972;27(3):229-236. doi:10.1001/archneur.1972.00490150037007.

78. Takashima S, Tanaka K. Development of cerebrovascular architecture and its relationship to periventricular leukomalacia. *Arch Neurol.* 1978;35(1):11-16. doi:10.1001/archneur.1978.00500250015003.

79. Nakamura Y, Okudera T, Hashimoto T. Vascular architecture in white matter of neonates: its relationship to periventricular leukomalacia. *J Neuropathol Exp Neurol.* 1994;53(6):582-589. doi:10.1097/00005072-199411000-00005.

80. Kuban KC, Gilles FH. Human telencephalic angiogenesis. *Ann Neurol.* 1985;17(6):539-548. doi:10.1002/ana.410170603.

81. Moody DM, Bell MA, Challa VR. Features of the cerebral vascular pattern that predict vulnerability to perfusion or oxygenation deficiency: an anatomic study. *AJNR Am J Neuroradiol.* 1990;11(3):431-439.

82. Nelson MD Jr, Gonzalez-Gomez I, Gilles FH. Dyke Award. The search for human telencephalic ventriculofugal arteries. *AJNR Am J Neuroradiol.* 1991;12(2):215-222.

83. Mayer PL, Kier EL. The controversy of the periventricular white matter circulation: a review of the anatomic literature. *AJNR Am J Neuroradiol.* 1991;12(2):223-228.

84. McClure MM, Riddle A, Manese M, et al. Cerebral blood flow heterogeneity in preterm sheep: lack of physiologic support for vascular boundary zones in fetal cerebral white matter. *J Cereb Blood Flow Metab.* 2008;28(5):995-1008. doi:10.1038/sj.jcbfm.9600597.

85. Nagata N, Saji M, Ito T, Ikeno S, Takahashi H, Terakawa N. Repetitive intermittent hypoxia-ischemia and brain damage in neonatal rats. *Brain Dev.* 2000;22(5):315-320. doi:10.1016/s0387-7604(00)00123-6.

86. Darnall RA, Chen X, Nemani KV, et al. Early postnatal exposure to intermittent hypoxia in rodents is proinflammatory, impairs white matter integrity, and alters brain metabolism. *Pediatr Res.* 2017;82(1):164-172. doi:10.1038/pr.2017.102.

87. Shah VP, Raffay TM, Martin RJ, et al. The relationship between oxidative stress, intermittent hypoxemia, and hospital duration in moderate preterm infants. *Neonatology.* 2020;117(5):577-583. doi:10.1159/000509038.

88. Abu Jawdeh EG, Huang H, Westgate PM, et al. Intermittent hypoxemia in preterm infants: a potential proinflammatory process. *Am J Perinatol.* 2021;38(12):1313-1319. doi:10.1055/s-0040-1712951.

89. Goussakov I, Synowiec S, Yarnykh V, Drobyshevsky A. Immediate and delayed decrease of long term potentiation and memory deficits after neonatal intermittent hypoxia. *Int J Dev Neurosci.* 2019;74:27-37. doi:10.1016/j.ijdevneu.2019.03.001.

90. Cai J, Tuong CM, Zhang Y, et al. Mouse intermittent hypoxia mimicking apnoea of prematurity: effects on myelinogenesis and axonal maturation. *J Pathol.* 2012;226(3):495-508. doi:10.1002/path.2980.

91. Juliano C, Sosunov S, Niatsetskaya Z, et al. Mild intermittent hypoxemia in neonatal mice causes permanent neurofunctional deficit and white matter hypomyelination. *Exp Neurol.* 2015;264:33-42. doi:10.1016/j.expneurol.2014.11.010.

92. Leviton A, Gilles FH. An epidemiologic study of perinatal telencephalic leucoencephalopathy in an autopsy population. *J Neurol Sci.* 1973;18(1):53-66. doi:10.1016/0022-510x(73)90020-8.

93. Gilles FH, Leviton A, Kerr CS. Endotoxin leucoencephalopathy in the telencephalon of the newborn kitten. *J Neurol Sci.* 1976;27(2):183-191. doi:10.1016/0022-510x(76)90060-5.

94. Poltorak A, He X, Smirnova I, et al. Defective LPS signaling in C3H/HeJ and C57BL/10ScCr mice: mutations in Tlr4 gene. *Science*. 1998;282(5396):2085-2088. doi:10.1126/science.282.5396.2085.

95. Hoshino K, Takeuchi O, Kawai T, et al. Cutting edge: Toll-like receptor 4 (TLR4)-deficient mice are hyporesponsive to lipopolysaccharide: evidence for TLR4 as the Lps gene product. *J Immunol*. 1999;162(7):3749-3752.

96. Qureshi ST, Lariviere L, Leveque G, et al. Endotoxin-tolerant mice have mutations in Toll-like receptor 4 (Tlr4). *J Exp Med*. 1999;189(4):615-625. doi:10.1084/jem.189.4.615.

97. Lehnardt S, Lachance C, Patrizi S, et al. The toll-like receptor TLR4 is necessary for lipopolysaccharide-induced oligodendrocyte injury in the CNS. *J Neurosci*. 2002;22(7):2478-2486. doi:10.1523/JNEUROSCI.22-07-02478.2002.

98. Glass TJA, Chau V, Grunau RE, et al. Multiple postnatal infections in newborns born preterm predict delayed maturation of motor pathways at term-equivalent age with poorer motor outcomes at 3 years. *J Pediatr*. 2018;196:91-97.e1. doi:10.1016/j.jpeds.2017.12.041.

99. Jansson LC, Akerman KE. The role of glutamate and its receptors in the proliferation, migration, differentiation and survival of neural progenitor cells. *J Neural Transm (Vienna)*. 2014;121(8):819-836. doi:10.1007/s00702-014-1174-6.

100. Pregnolato S, Chakkarapani E, Isles AR, Luyt K. Glutamate transport and preterm brain injury. *Front Physiol*. 2019;10:417. doi:10.3389/fphys.2019.00417.

101. Oka A, Belliveau MJ, Rosenberg PA, Volpe JJ. Vulnerability of oligodendroglia to glutamate: pharmacology, mechanisms, and prevention. *J Neurosci*. 1993;13(4):1441-1453.

102. Matute C, Domercq M, Sanchez-Gomez MV. Glutamate-mediated glial injury: mechanisms and clinical importance. *Glia*. 2006;53(2):212-224. doi:10.1002/glia.20275.

103. Karadottir R, Cavelier P, Bergersen LH, Attwell D. NMDA receptors are expressed in oligodendrocytes and activated in ischaemia. *Nature*. 2005;438(7071):1162-1166. doi:10.1038/nature04302.

104. Talos DM, Follett PL, Folkerth RD, et al. Developmental regulation of alpha-amino-3-hydroxy-5-methyl-4-isoxazole-propionic acid receptor subunit expression in forebrain and relationship to regional susceptibility to hypoxic/ischemic injury. II. Human cerebral white matter and cortex. *J Comp Neurol*. 2006;497(1):61-77. doi:10.1002/cne.20978.

105. Salter MG, Fern R. NMDA receptors are expressed in developing oligodendrocyte processes and mediate injury. *Nature*. 2005;438(7071):1167-1171. doi:10.1038/nature04301.

106. Sanchez-Gomez MV, Alberdi E, Ibarretxe G, Torre I, Matute C. Caspase-dependent and caspase-independent oligodendrocyte death mediated by AMPA and kainate receptors. *J Neurosci*. 2003;23(29):9519-9528.

107. Follett PL, Deng W, Dai W, et al. Glutamate receptor-mediated oligodendrocyte toxicity in periventricular leukomalacia: a protective role for topiramate. *J Neurosci*. 2004;24(18):4412-4420. doi:10.1523/JNEUROSCI.0477-04.2004.

108. Manning SM, Talos DM, Zhou C, et al. NMDA receptor blockade with memantine attenuates white matter injury in a rat model of periventricular leukomalacia. *J Neurosci*. 2008;28(26):6670-6678. doi:10.1523/JNEUROSCI.1702-08.2008.

109. DeSilva TM, Borenstein NS, Volpe JJ, Kinney HC, Rosenberg PA. Expression of EAAT2 in neurons and protoplasmic astrocytes during human cortical development. *J Comp Neurol*. 2012;520(17):3912-3932. doi:10.1002/cne.23130.

110. Desilva TM, Kinney HC, Borenstein NS, et al. The glutamate transporter EAAT2 is transiently expressed in developing human cerebral white matter. *J Comp Neurol*. 2007;501(6):879-890. doi:10.1002/cne.21289.

111. Desilva TM, Billiards SS, Borenstein NS, et al. Glutamate transporter EAAT2 expression is up-regulated in reactive astrocytes in human periventricular leukomalacia. *J Comp Neurol*. 2008;508(2):238-248. doi:10.1002/cne.21667.

112. Tremblay ME, Stevens B, Sierra A, Wake H, Bessis A, Nimmerjahn A. The role of microglia in the healthy brain. *J Neurosci*. 2011;31(45):16064-16069. doi:10.1523/JNEUROSCI.4158-11.2011.

113. Billiards SS, Haynes RL, Folkerth RD, et al. Development of microglia in the cerebral white matter of the human fetus and infant. *J Comp Neurol*. 2006;497(2):199-208. doi:10.1002/cne.20991.

114. Wlodarczyk A, Holtman IR, Krueger M, et al. A novel microglial subset plays a key role in myelinogenesis in developing brain. *EMBO J*. 2017;36(22):3292-3308. doi:10.15252/embj.201696056.

115. Lehnardt S. Innate immunity and neuroinflammation in the CNS: the role of microglia in Toll-like receptor-mediated neuronal injury. *Glia*. 2010;58(3):253-263. doi:10.1002/glia.20928.

116. Hagberg H, Mallard C, Ferriero DM, et al. The role of inflammation in perinatal brain injury. *Nat Rev Neurol*. 2015;11(4):192-208. doi:10.1038/nrneurol.2015.13.

117. Yoon BH, Romero R, Yang SH, et al. Interleukin-6 concentrations in umbilical cord plasma are elevated in neonates with white matter lesions associated with periventricular leukomalacia. *Am J Obstet Gynecol*. 1996;174(5):1433-1440. doi:10.1016/s0002-9378(96)70585-9.

118. Deguchi K, Mizuguchi M, Takashima S. Immunohistochemical expression of tumor necrosis factor alpha in neonatal leukomalacia. *Pediatr Neurol*. 1996;14(1):13-16. doi:10.1016/0887-8994(95)00223-5.

119. Kadhim H, Tabarki B, De Prez C, Rona AM, Sebire G. Interleukin-2 in the pathogenesis of perinatal white matter damage. *Neurology*. 2002;58(7):1125-1128. doi:10.1212/wnl.58.7.1125.

120. Folkerth RD, Keefe RJ, Haynes RL, Trachtenberg FL, Volpe JJ, Kinney HC. Interferon-gamma expression in periventricular leukomalacia in the human brain. *Brain Pathol*. 2004;14(3):265-274. doi:10.1111/j.1750-3639.2004.tb00063.x.

121. Yoon BH, Romero R, Kim CJ, et al. High expression of tumor necrosis factor-alpha and interleukin-6 in periventricular leukomalacia. *Am J Obstet Gynecol*. 1997;177(2):406-411. doi:10.1016/s0002-9378(97)70206-0.

122. Kadhim H, Tabarki B, Verellen G, De Prez C, Rona AM, Sebire G. Inflammatory cytokines in the pathogenesis of periventricular leukomalacia. *Neurology*. 2001;56(10):1278-1284. doi:10.1212/wnl.56.10.1278.

123. Verney C, Pogledic I, Biran V, Adle-Biassette H, Fallet-Bianco C, Gressens P. Microglial reaction in axonal crossroads is a hallmark of noncystic periventricular white matter injury in very preterm infants. *J Neuropathol Exp Neurol*. 2012;71(3):251-264. doi:10.1097/NEN.0b013e3182496429.

124. Haynes RL, Folkerth RD, Keefe RJ, et al. Nitrosative and oxidative injury to premyelinating oligodendrocytes in periventricular leukomalacia. *J Neuropathol Exp Neurol*. 2003;62(5):441-450. doi:10.1093/jnen/62.5.441.

125. Welin AK, Sandberg M, Lindblom A, et al. White matter injury following prolonged free radical formation in the 0.65 gestation fetal sheep brain. *Pediatr Res*. 2005;58(1):100-105. doi:10.1203/01.PDR.0000163388.04017.26.

126. Ahola T, Fellman V, Kjellmer I, Raivio KO, Lapatto R. Plasma 8-isoprostane is increased in preterm infants who develop bronchopulmonary dysplasia or periventricular leukomalacia. *Pediatr Res.* 2004;56(1):88-93. doi:10.1203/01.PDR. 0000130478.05324.9D.

127. Folkerth RD, Haynes RL, Borenstein NS, et al. Developmental lag in superoxide dismutases relative to other antioxidant enzymes in premyelinated human telencephalic white matter. *J Neuropathol Exp Neurol.* 2004;63(9):990-999. doi:10.1093/jnen/63.9.990.

128. Coviello C, Perrone S, Buonocore G, et al. Isoprostanes as biomarker for white matter injury in extremely preterm infants. *Front Pediatr.* 2020;8:618622. doi:10.3389/fped.2020.618622.

129. Banker BQ, Larroche JC. Periventricular leukomalacia of infancy. A form of neonatal anoxic encephalopathy. *Arch Neurol.* 1962;7:386-410. doi:10.1001/archneur.1962.04210050022004.

130. Haynes RL, Billiards SS, Borenstein NS, Volpe JJ, Kinney HC. Diffuse axonal injury in periventricular leukomalacia as determined by apoptotic marker fractin. *Pediatr Res.* 2008;63(6): 656-661. doi:10.1203/PDR.0b013e31816c825c.

131. Alix JJ, Zammit C, Riddle A, et al. Central axons preparing to myelinate are highly sensitive [corrected] to ischemic injury. *Ann Neurol.* 2012;72(6):936-951. doi:10.1002/ana.23690.

132. Riddle A, Maire J, Gong X, et al. Differential susceptibility to axonopathy in necrotic and non-necrotic perinatal white matter injury. *Stroke.* 2012;43(1):178-184. doi:10.1161/STROKEAHA. 111.632265.

133. Segovia KN, McClure M, Moravec M, et al. Arrested oligodendrocyte lineage maturation in chronic perinatal white matter injury. *Ann Neurol.* 2008;63(4):520-530. doi:10.1002/ana. 21359.

134. Billiards SS, Haynes RL, Folkerth RD, et al. Myelin abnormalities without oligodendrocyte loss in periventricular leukomalacia. *Brain Pathol.* 2008;18(2):153-163. doi:10.1111/j.1750-3639.2007.00107.x.

135. Zaidi AU, Bessert DA, Ong JE, et al. New oligodendrocytes are generated after neonatal hypoxic-ischemic brain injury in rodents. *Glia.* 2004;46(4):380-390. doi:10.1002/glia.20013.

136. Back SA, Tuohy TM, Chen H, et al. Hyaluronan accumulates in demyelinated lesions and inhibits oligodendrocyte progenitor maturation. *Nat Med.* 2005;11(9):966-972. doi:10. 1038/nm1279.

137. Srivastava T, Diba P, Dean JM, et al. A TLR/AKT/FoxO3 immune tolerance-like pathway disrupts the repair capacity of oligodendrocyte progenitors. *J Clin Invest.* 2018;128(5): 2025-2041. doi:10.1172/JCI94158.

138. Srivastava T, Sherman LS, Back SA. Dysregulation of hyaluronan homeostasis during white matter injury. *Neurochem Res.* 2020;45(3):672-683. doi:10.1007/s11064-019-02879-1.

139. Diao S, Xiao M, Chen C. The role of hyaluronan in myelination and remyelination after white matter injury. *Brain Res.* 2021;1766:147522. doi:10.1016/j.brainres.2021.147522.

140. Fancy SP, Baranzini SE, Zhao C, et al. Dysregulation of the Wnt pathway inhibits timely myelination and remyelination in the mammalian CNS. *Genes Dev.* 2009;23(13):1571-1585. doi:10.1101/gad.1806309.

141. Aguirre A, Dupree JL, Mangin JM, Gallo V. A functional role for EGFR signaling in myelination and remyelination. *Nat Neurosci.* 2007;10(8):990-1002. doi:10.1038/nn1938.

142. Yuen TJ, Silbereis JC, Griveau A, et al. Oligodendrocyte-encoded HIF function couples postnatal myelination and white matter angiogenesis. *Cell.* 2014;158(2):383-396. doi:10.1016/j.cell. 2014.04.052.

143. Chavali M, Ulloa-Navas MJ, Perez-Borreda P, et al. Wnt-dependent oligodendroglial-endothelial interactions regulate white matter vascularization and attenuate injury. *Neuron.* 2020;108(6): 1130-1145.e5. doi:10.1016/j.neuron.2020.09.033.

144. Zhang S, Wang Y, Xu J, Kim B, Deng W, Guo F. HIFalpha regulates developmental myelination independent of autocrine Wnt signaling. *J Neurosci.* 2021;41(2):251-268. doi:10. 1523/JNEUROSCI.0731-20.2020.

145. Preston M, Gong X, Su W, et al. Digestion products of the PH20 hyaluronidase inhibit remyelination. *Ann Neurol.* 2013;73(2):266-280. doi:10.1002/ana.23788.

146. Scafidi J, Hammond TR, Scafidi S, et al. Intranasal epidermal growth factor treatment rescues neonatal brain injury. *Nature.* 2014;506(7487):230-234. doi:10.1038/nature12880.

147. Ballabh P, de Vries LS. White matter injury in infants with intraventricular haemorrhage: mechanisms and therapies. *Nat Rev Neurol.* 2021;17(4):199-214. doi:10.1038/s41582-020-00447-8.

148. Ou X, Glasier CM, Ramakrishnaiah RH, et al. Impaired white matter development in extremely low-birth-weight infants with previous brain hemorrhage. *AJNR Am J Neuroradiol.* 2014;35(10):1983-1989. doi:10.3174/ajnr.A3988.

149. Glass HC, Bonifacio SL, Chau V, et al. Recurrent postnatal infections are associated with progressive white matter injury in premature infants. *Pediatrics.* 2008;122(2):299-305. doi:10. 1542/peds.2007-2184.

150. Shah DK, Doyle LW, Anderson PJ, et al. Adverse neurodevelopment in preterm infants with postnatal sepsis or necrotizing enterocolitis is mediated by white matter abnormalities on magnetic resonance imaging at term. *J Pediatr.* 2008;153(2):170-175, 175.e1. doi:10.1016/j.jpeds.2008.02.033.

151. Graham EM, Holcroft CJ, Rai KK, Donohue PK, Allen MC. Neonatal cerebral white matter injury in preterm infants is associated with culture positive infections and only rarely with metabolic acidosis. *Am J Obstet Gynecol.* 2004;191(4): 1305-1310. doi:10.1016/j.ajog.2004.06.058.

152. Tsimis ME, Johnson CT, Raghunathan RS, Northington FJ, Burd I, Graham EM. Risk factors for periventricular white matter injury in very low birthweight neonates. *Am J Obstet Gynecol.* 2016;214(3):380.e1-e6. doi:10.1016/j.ajog.2015. 09.108.

153. Chau V, Brant R, Poskitt KJ, Tam EW, Synnes A, Miller SP. Postnatal infection is associated with widespread abnormalities of brain development in premature newborns. *Pediatr Res.* 2012;71(3):274-279. doi:10.1038/pr.2011.40.

154. Wang LW, Lin YC, Tu YF, Wang ST, Huang CC, Taiwan Premature Infant Developmental Collaborative Study G. Isolated cystic periventricular leukomalacia differs from cystic periventricular leukomalacia with intraventricular hemorrhage in prevalence, risk factors and outcomes in preterm infants. *Neonatology.* 2017;111(1):86-92. doi:10.1159/000448615.

155. Strunk T, Inder T, Wang X, Burgner D, Mallard C, Levy O. Infection-induced inflammation and cerebral injury in preterm infants. *Lancet Infect Dis.* 2014;14(8):751-762. doi:10.1016/S1473-3099(14)70710-8.

156. Hintz SR, Kendrick DE, Stoll BJ, et al. Neurodevelopmental and growth outcomes of extremely low birth weight infants after necrotizing enterocolitis. *Pediatrics.* 2005;115(3):696-703. doi:10.1542/peds.2004-0569.

157. Merhar SL, Ramos Y, Meinzen-Derr J, Kline-Fath BM. Brain magnetic resonance imaging in infants with surgical necrotizing enterocolitis or spontaneous intestinal perforation versus medical necrotizing enterocolitis. *J Pediatr.* 2014;164(2): 410-412.e1. doi:10.1016/j.jpeds.2013.09.055.

158. Shin SH, Kim EK, Yoo H, et al. Surgical necrotizing enterocolitis versus spontaneous intestinal perforation in white matter injury on brain magnetic resonance imaging. *Neonatology.* 2016;110(2):148-154. doi:10.1159/000444387.

159. Nino DF, Zhou Q, Yamaguchi Y, et al. Cognitive impairments induced by necrotizing enterocolitis can be prevented by inhibiting microglial activation in mouse brain. *Sci Transl Med.* 2018;10(471):eaan0237. doi:10.1126/scitranslmed.aan0237.

160. Zhou Q, Nino DF, Yamaguchi Y, et al. Necrotizing enterocolitis induces T lymphocyte-mediated injury in the developing mammalian brain. *Sci Transl Med.* 2021;13(575):eaay6621. doi:10.1126/scitranslmed.aay6621.

161. Thompson DK, Thai D, Kelly CE, et al. Alterations in the optic radiations of very preterm children-Perinatal predictors and relationships with visual outcomes. *Neuroimage Clin.* 2014;4:145-153. doi:10.1016/j.nicl.2013.11.007.

162. Glass TJA, Chau V, Gardiner J, et al. Severe retinopathy of prematurity predicts delayed white matter maturation and poorer neurodevelopment. *Arch Dis Child Fetal Neonatal Ed.* 2017;102(6):F532-F537. doi:10.1136/archdischild-2016-312533.

163. Ahn SJ, Park HK, Lee BR, Lee HJ. Diffusion tensor imaging analysis of white matter microstructural integrity in infants with retinopathy of prematurity. *Invest Ophthalmol Vis Sci.* 2019;60(8):3024-3033. doi:10.1167/iovs.18-25849.

164. Lofqvist C, Engstrom E, Sigurdsson J, et al. Postnatal head growth deficit among premature infants parallels retinopathy of prematurity and insulin-like growth factor-1 deficit. *Pediatrics.* 2006;117(6):1930-1938. doi:10.1542/peds.2005-1926.

165. Morken TS, Dammann O, Skranes J, Austeng D. Retinopathy of prematurity, visual and neurodevelopmental outcome, and imaging of the central nervous system. *Semin Perinatol.* 2019;43(6):381-389. doi:10.1053/j.semperi.2019.05.012.

166. Gagliardi L, Bellu R, Zanini R, Dammann O, Network Neonatale Lombardo Study Group. Bronchopulmonary dysplasia and brain white matter damage in the preterm infant: a complex relationship. *Paediatr Perinat Epidemiol.* 2009;23(6):582-590. doi:10.1111/j.1365-3016.2009.01069.x.

167. Ball G, Counsell SJ, Anjari M, et al. An optimised tract-based spatial statistics protocol for neonates: applications to prematurity and chronic lung disease. *Neuroimage.* 2010;53(1):94-102. doi:10.1016/j.neuroimage.2010.05.055.

168. Neubauer V, Junker D, Griesmaier E, Schocke M, Kiechl-Kohlendorfer U. Bronchopulmonary dysplasia is associated with delayed structural brain maturation in preterm infants. *Neonatology.* 2015;107(3):179-184. doi:10.1159/000369199.

169. Parikh NA, Sharma P, He L, et al. Perinatal risk and protective factors in the development of diffuse white matter abnormality on term-equivalent age magnetic resonance imaging in infants born very preterm. *J Pediatr.* 2021;233:58-65.e3. doi:10.1016/j.jpeds.2020.11.058.

170. Anjari M, Counsell SJ, Srinivasan L, et al. The association of lung disease with cerebral white matter abnormalities in preterm infants. *Pediatrics.* 2009;124(1):268-276. doi:10.1542/peds.2008-1294.

171. Barnett ML, Tusor N, Ball G, et al. Exploring the multiple-hit hypothesis of preterm white matter damage using diffusion MRI. *Neuroimage Clin.* 2018;17:596-606. doi:10.1016/j.nicl.2017.11.017.

172. Guillot M, Guo T, Ufkes S, et al. Mechanical ventilation duration, brainstem development, and neurodevelopment in children born preterm: a prospective cohort study. *J Pediatr.* 2020;226:87-95.e3. doi:10.1016/j.jpeds.2020.05.039.

173. Grelli KN, Keller RL, Rogers EE, et al. Bronchopulmonary dysplasia precursors influence risk of white matter injury and adverse neurodevelopmental outcome in preterm infants. *Pediatr Res.* 2021;90(2):359-365. doi:10.1038/s41390-020-01162-2.

174. Resch B, Neubauer K, Hofer N, et al. Episodes of hypocarbia and early-onset sepsis are risk factors for cystic periventricular leukomalacia in the preterm infant. *Early Hum Dev.* 2012;88(1):27-31. doi:10.1016/j.earlhumdev.2011.06.011.

175. Shankaran S, Langer JC, Kazzi SN, et al. Cumulative index of exposure to hypocarbia and hyperoxia as risk factors for periventricular leukomalacia in low birth weight infants. *Pediatrics.* 2006;118(4):1654-1659. doi:10.1542/peds.2005-2463.

176. Giannakopoulou C, Korakaki E, Manoura A, et al. Significance of hypocarbia in the development of periventricular leukomalacia in preterm infants. *Pediatr Int.* 2004;46(3):268-273. doi:10.1111/j.1442-200x.2004.01886.x.

177. Yoon BH, Jun JK, Romero R, et al. Amniotic fluid inflammatory cytokines (interleukin-6, interleukin-1beta, and tumor necrosis factor-alpha), neonatal brain white matter lesions, and cerebral palsy. *Am J Obstet Gynecol.* 1997;177(1):19-26. doi:10.1016/s0002-9378(97)70432-0.

178. Pappas A, Kendrick DE, Shankaran S, et al. Chorioamnionitis and early childhood outcomes among extremely low-gestational-age neonates. *JAMA Pediatr.* 2014;168(2):137-147. doi:10.1001/jamapediatrics.2013.4248.

179. Strunk T, Campbell C, Burgner D, et al. Histological chorioamnionitis and developmental outcomes in very preterm infants. *J Perinatol.* 2019;39(2):321-330. doi:10.1038/s41372-018-0288-3.

180. Chau V, Poskitt KJ, McFadden DE, et al. Effect of chorioamnionitis on brain development and injury in premature newborns. *Ann Neurol.* 2009;66(2):155-164. doi:10.1002/ana.21713.

181. Bierstone D, Wagenaar N, Gano DL, et al. Association of histologic chorioamnionitis with perinatal brain injury and early childhood neurodevelopmental outcomes among preterm neonates. *JAMA Pediatr.* 2018;172(6):534-541. doi:10.1001/jamapediatrics.2018.0102.

182. Granger C, Spittle AJ, Walsh J, et al. Histologic chorioamnionitis in preterm infants: correlation with brain magnetic resonance imaging at term equivalent age. *BMC Pediatr.* 2018;18(1):63. doi:10.1186/s12887-018-1001-6.

183. Woodward LJ, Anderson PJ, Austin NC, Howard K, Inder TE. Neonatal MRI to predict neurodevelopmental outcomes in preterm infants. *N Engl J Med.* 2006;355(7):685-694. doi:10.1056/NEJMoa053792.

184. Spittle AJ, Cheong J, Doyle LW, et al. Neonatal white matter abnormality predicts childhood motor impairment in very preterm children. *Dev Med Child Neurol.* 2011;53(11):1000-1006. doi:10.1111/j.1469-8749.2011.04095.x.

185. De Vries LS, Van Haastert IL, Rademaker KJ, Koopman C, Groenendaal F. Ultrasound abnormalities preceding cerebral palsy in high-risk preterm infants. *J Pediatr.* 2004;144(6):815-820. doi:10.1016/j.jpeds.2004.03.034.

186. Beaino G, Khoshnood B, Kaminski M, et al. Predictors of cerebral palsy in very preterm infants: the EPIPAGE prospective population-based cohort study. *Dev Med Child Neurol.* 2010;52(6):e119-e125. doi:10.1111/j.1469-8749.2010.03612.x.

187. Martinez-Biarge M, Groenendaal F, Kersbergen KJ, et al. Neurodevelopmental outcomes in preterm infants with white matter injury using a new MRI classification. *Neonatology.* 2019;116(3):227-235. doi:10.1159/000499346.

188. De Bruine FT, Van Wezel-Meijler G, Leijser LM, et al. Tractography of white-matter tracts in very preterm infants: a 2-year

follow-up study. *Dev Med Child Neurol.* 2013;55(5):427-433. doi:10.1111/dmcn.12099.

189. Kelly CE, Chan L, Burnett AC, et al. Brain structural and microstructural alterations associated with cerebral palsy and motor impairments in adolescents born extremely preterm and/or extremely low birthweight. *Dev Med Child Neurol.* 2015;57(12):1168-1175. doi:10.1111/dmcn.12854.

190. Bosanquet M, Copeland L, Ware R, Boyd R. A systematic review of tests to predict cerebral palsy in young children. *Dev Med Child Neurol.* 2013;55(5):418-426. doi:10.1111/dmcn.12140.

191. Spittle AJ, Boyd RN, Inder TE, Doyle LW. Predicting motor development in very preterm infants at 12 months' corrected age: the role of qualitative magnetic resonance imaging and general movements assessments. *Pediatrics.* 2009;123(2):512-517. doi:10.1542/peds.2008-0590.

192. Peyton C, Yang E, Msall ME, et al. White matter injury and general movements in high-risk preterm infants. *AJNR Am J Neuroradiol.* 2017;38(1):162-169. doi:10.3174/ajnr.A4955.

193. Dewey D, Thompson DK, Kelly CE, et al. Very preterm children at risk for developmental coordination disorder have brain alterations in motor areas. *Acta Paediatr.* 2019;108(9):1649-1660. doi:10.1111/apa.14786.

194. Brown-Lum M, Izadi-Najafabadi S, Oberlander TF, Rauscher A, Zwicker JG. Differences in white matter microstructure among children with developmental coordination disorder. *JAMA Netw Open.* 2020;3(3):e201184. doi:10.1001/jamanetworkopen.2020.1184.

195. Woodward LJ, Clark CA, Pritchard VE, Anderson PJ, Inder TE. Neonatal white matter abnormalities predict global executive function impairment in children born very preterm. *Dev Neuropsychol.* 2011;36(1):22-41. doi:10.1080/87565641.2011.540530.

196. Iwata S, Nakamura T, Hizume E, et al. Qualitative brain MRI at term and cognitive outcomes at 9 years after very preterm birth. *Pediatrics.* 2012;129(5):e1138-e1147. doi:10.1542/peds.2011-1735.

197. Hintz SR, Vohr BR, Bann CM, et al. Preterm neuroimaging and school-age cognitive outcomes. *Pediatrics.* 2018;142(1):e20174058. doi:10.1542/peds.2017–4058.

198. Kostovic Srzentic M, Raguz M, Ozretic D. Specific cognitive deficits in preschool age correlated with qualitative and quantitative MRI parameters in prematurely born children. *Pediatr Neonatol.* 2020;61(2):160-167. doi:10.1016/j.pedneo.2019.09.003.

199. Campbell H, Check J, Kuban KCK, et al. Neonatal cranial ultrasound findings among infants born extremely preterm: associations with neurodevelopmental outcomes at 10 years of age. *J Pediatr.* 2021;237:197-205.e4. doi:10.1016/j.jpeds.2021.05.059.

200. Keunen K, Benders MJ, Leemans A, et al. White matter maturation in the neonatal brain is predictive of school age cognitive capacities in children born very preterm. *Dev Med Child Neurol.* 2017;59(9):939-946. doi:10.1111/dmcn.13487.

201. Dubner SE, Dodson CK, Marchman VA, Ben-Shachar M, Feldman HM, Travis KE. White matter microstructure and cognitive outcomes in relation to neonatal inflammation in 6-year-old children born preterm. *Neuroimage Clin.* 2019;23:101832. doi:10.1016/j.nicl.2019.101832.

202. Leviton A, Joseph RM, Fichorova RN, et al. Executive dysfunction early postnatal biomarkers among children born extremely preterm. *J Neuroimmune Pharmacol.* 2019;14(2):188-199. doi:10.1007/s11481-018-9804-7.

203. Franz AP, Bolat GU, Bolat H, et al. Attention-deficit/hyperactivity disorder and very preterm/very low birth weight: a meta-analysis. *Pediatrics.* 2018;141(1):e20171645. doi:10.1542/peds.2017-1645.

204. Filley CM, Fields RD. White matter and cognition: making the connection. *J Neurophysiol.* 2016;116(5):2093-2104. doi:10.1152/jn.00221.2016.

205. Filley CM. Prematurity, white matter, and cognition: support for leukocentrism. *Dev Med Child Neurol.* 2017;59(9):888. doi:10.1111/dmcn.13503.

206. Goddings AL, Roalf D, Lebel C, Tamnes CK. Development of white matter microstructure and executive functions during childhood and adolescence: a review of diffusion MRI studies. *Dev Cogn Neurosci.* 2021;51:101008. doi:10.1016/j.dcn.2021.101008.

207. Wang Y, Metoki A, Alm KH, Olson IR. White matter pathways and social cognition. *Neurosci Biobehav Rev.* 2018;90:350-370. doi:10.1016/j.neubiorev.2018.04.015.

208. Moeller K, Willmes K, Klein E. A review on functional and structural brain connectivity in numerical cognition. *Front Hum Neurosci.* 2015;9:227. doi:10.3389/fnhum.2015.00227.

209. van den Heuvel MP, Kersbergen KJ, de Reus MA, et al. The neonatal connectome during preterm brain development. *Cereb Cortex.* 2015;25(9):3000-3013. doi:10.1093/cercor/bhu095.

210. Kline JE, Illapani VSP, Li H, He L, Yuan W, Parikh NA. Diffuse white matter abnormality in very preterm infants at term reflects reduced brain network efficiency. *Neuroimage Clin.* 2021;31:102739. doi:10.1016/j.nicl.2021.102739.

211. Agrawal S, Rao SC, Bulsara MK, Patole SK. Prevalence of autism spectrum disorder in preterm infants: a meta-analysis. *Pediatrics.* 2018;142(3):e20180134. doi:10.1542/peds.2018-0134.

212. Fitzallen GC, Sagar YK, Taylor HG, Bora S. Anxiety and depressive disorders in children born preterm: a meta-analysis. *J Dev Behav Pediatr.* 2021;42(2):154-162. doi:10.1097/DBP.0000000000000898.

213. Billeci L, Calderoni S, Tosetti M, Catani M, Muratori F. White matter connectivity in children with autism spectrum disorders: a tract-based spatial statistics study. *BMC Neurol.* 2012;12:148. doi:10.1186/1471-2377-12-148.

214. Libero LE, Burge WK, Deshpande HD, Pestilli F, Kana RK. White matter diffusion of major fiber tracts implicated in autism spectrum disorder. *Brain Connect.* 2016;6(9):691-699. doi:10.1089/brain.2016.0442.

215. Wolff JJ, Gu H, Gerig G, et al. Differences in white matter fiber tract development present from 6 to 24 months in infants with autism. *Am J Psychiatry.* 2012;169(6):589-600. doi:10.1176/appi.ajp.2011.11091447.

216. Ure AM, Treyvaud K, Thompson DK, et al. Neonatal brain abnormalities associated with autism spectrum disorder in children born very preterm. *Autism Res.* 2016;9(5):543-552. doi:10.1002/aur.1558.

217. van Tilborg E, Achterberg EJM, van Kammen CM, et al. Combined fetal inflammation and postnatal hypoxia causes myelin deficits and autism-like behavior in a rat model of diffuse white matter injury. *Glia.* 2018;66(1):78-93. doi:10.1002/glia.23216.

218. Inder TE, Huppi PS, Warfield S, et al. Periventricular white matter injury in the premature infant is followed by reduced cerebral cortical gray matter volume at term. *Ann Neurol.* 1999;46(5):755-760. doi:10.1002/1531-8249(199911)46:5<755::aid-ana11>3.0.co;2-0.

219. Kersbergen KJ, de Vries LS, Groenendaal F, et al. Corticospinal tract injury precedes thalamic volume reduction in preterm infants with cystic periventricular leukomalacia. *J Pediatr*. 2015;167(2):260-268.e3. doi:10.1016/j.jpeds.2015.05.013.

220. Cayam-Rand D, Guo T, Synnes A, et al. Interaction between preterm white matter injury and childhood thalamic growth. *Ann Neurol*. 2021;90(4):584-594. doi:10.1002/ana.26201.

221. McClendon E, Chen K, Gong X, et al. Prenatal cerebral ischemia triggers dysmaturation of caudate projection neurons. *Ann Neurol*. 2014;75(4):508-524. doi:10.1002/ana.24100.

222. Pierson CR, Folkerth RD, Billiards SS, et al. Gray matter injury associated with periventricular leukomalacia in the premature infant. *Acta Neuropathol*. 2007;114(6):619-631. doi:10.1007/s00401-007-0295-5.

223. Nagasunder AC, Kinney HC, Blüml S, et al. Abnormal microstructure of the atrophic thalamus in preterm survivors with periventricular leukomalacia. *AJNR Am J Neuroradiol*. 2011;32(1):185-191. doi:10.3174/ajnr.A2243.

224. Zubiaurre-Elorza L, Soria-Pastor S, Junqué C, et al. Thalamic changes in a preterm sample with periventricular leukomalacia: correlation with white-matter integrity and cognitive outcome at school age. *Pediatr Res*. 2012;71(4 Pt 1):354-360. doi:10.1038/pr.2011.70.

225. Dean JM, McClendon E, Hansen K, et al. Prenatal cerebral ischemia disrupts MRI-defined cortical microstructure through disturbances in neuronal arborization. *Sci Transl Med*. 2013;5(168):168ra7. doi:10.1126/scitranslmed.3004669.

226. McClendon E, Shaver DC, Degener-O'Brien K, et al. Transient hypoxemia chronically disrupts maturation of preterm fetal ovine subplate neuron arborization and activity. *J Neurosci*. 2017;37(49):11912-11929. doi:10.1523/JNEUROSCI.2396-17.2017.

227. Liu N, Tong X, Huang W, Fu J, Xue X. Synaptic injury in the thalamus accompanies white matter injury in hypoxia/ischemia-mediated brain injury in neonatal rats. *Biomed Res Int*. 2019;2019:5249675. doi:10.1155/2019/5249675.

228. Benavente-Fernández I, Synnes A, Grunau RE, et al. Association of socioeconomic status and brain injury with neurodevelopmental outcomes of very preterm children. *JAMA Netw Open*. 2019;2(5):e192914. doi:10.1001/jamanetworkopen.2019.2914.

229. Spittle A, Orton J, Anderson PJ, Boyd R, Doyle LW. Early developmental intervention programmes provided post hospital discharge to prevent motor and cognitive impairment in preterm infants. *Cochrane Database Syst Rev*. 2015;(11):CD005495. doi:10.1002/14651858.CD005495.pub4.

230. Iwai M, Stetler RA, Xing J, et al. Enhanced oligodendrogenesis and recovery of neurological function by erythropoietin after neonatal hypoxic/ischemic brain injury. *Stroke*. 2010;41(5):1032-1037. doi:10.1161/STROKEAHA.109.570325.

231. Mazur M, Miller RH, Robinson S. Postnatal erythropoietin treatment mitigates neural cell loss after systemic prenatal hypoxic-ischemic injury. *J Neurosurg Pediatr*. 2010;6(3):206-221. doi:10.3171/2010.5.PEDS1032.

232. Leuchter RH, Gui L, Poncet A, et al. Association between early administration of high-dose erythropoietin in preterm infants and brain MRI abnormality at term-equivalent age. *JAMA*. 2014;312(8):817-824. doi:10.1001/jama.2014.9645.

233. O'Gorman RL, Bucher HU, Held U, et al. Tract-based spatial statistics to assess the neuroprotective effect of early erythropoietin on white matter development in preterm infants. *Brain*. 2015;138(Pt 2):388-397. doi:10.1093/brain/awu363.

234. Fischer HS, Reibel NJ, Buhrer C, Dame C. Prophylactic early erythropoietin for neuroprotection in preterm infants: a meta-analysis. *Pediatrics*. 2017;139(5):e20164317. doi:10.1542/peds.2016-4317.

235. Juul SE, Comstock BA, Wadhawan R, et al. A Randomized trial of erythropoietin for neuroprotection in preterm infants. *N Engl J Med*. 2020;382(3):233-243. doi:10.1056/NEJMoa1907423.

236. Galinsky R, Dhillon SK, Dean JM, et al. Tumor necrosis factor inhibition attenuates white matter gliosis after systemic inflammation in preterm fetal sheep. *J Neuroinflammation*. 2020;17(1):92. doi:10.1186/s12974-020-01769-6.

237. Chen X, Hovanesian V, Naqvi S, et al. Systemic infusions of anti-interleukin-1beta neutralizing antibodies reduce short-term brain injury after cerebral ischemia in the ovine fetus. *Brain Behav Immun*. 2018;67:24-35. doi:10.1016/j.bbi.2017.08.002.

238. Hortensius LM, van Elburg RM, Nijboer CH, Benders M, de Theije CGM. Postnatal nutrition to improve brain development in the preterm infant: a systematic review from bench to bedside. *Front Physiol*. 2019;10:961. doi:10.3389/fphys.2019.00961.

239. Mercer JS, Erickson-Owens DA, Deoni SCL, et al. The effects of delayed cord clamping on 12-month brain myelin content and neurodevelopment: a randomized controlled trial. *Am J Perinatol*. 2022;39(1):37-44. doi:10.1055/s-0040-1714258.

240. McPherson C, Miller SP, El-Dib M, Massaro AN, Inder TE. The influence of pain, agitation, and their management on the immature brain. *Pediatr Res*. 2020;88(2):168-175. doi:10.1038/s41390-019-0744-6.

241. Brummelte S, Grunau RE, Chau V, et al. Procedural pain and brain development in premature newborns. *Ann Neurol*. 2012;71(3):385-396. doi:10.1002/ana.22267.

242. Zwicker JG, Grunau RE, Adams E, et al. Score for neonatal acute physiology-II and neonatal pain predict corticospinal tract development in premature newborns. *Pediatr Neurol*. 2013;48(2):123-129.e1. doi:10.1016/j.pediatrneurol.2012.10.016.

243. Vinall J, Miller SP, Bjornson BH, et al. Invasive procedures in preterm children: brain and cognitive development at school age. *Pediatrics*. 2014;133(3):412-421. doi:10.1542/peds.2013–1863.

244. Beani E, Menici V, Cecchi A, et al. Feasibility analysis of caretoy-revised early intervention in infants at high risk for cerebral palsy. *Front Neurol*. 2020;11:601137. doi:10.3389/fneur.2020.601137.

245. Menici V, Antonelli C, Beani E, et al. Feasibility of early intervention through home-based and parent-delivered infant massage in infants at high risk for cerebral palsy. *Front Pediatr*. 2021;9:673956. doi:10.3389/fped.2021.673956.

246. Letzkus L, Conaway M, Miller-Davis C, Darring J, Keim-Malpass J, Zanelli S. A feasibility randomized controlled trial of a NICU rehabilitation program for very low birth weight infants. *Sci Rep*. 2022;12(1):1729. doi:10.1038/s41598-022-05849-w.

247. Liu Y, Li ZF, Zhong YH, et al. Early combined rehabilitation intervention to improve the short-term prognosis of premature infants. *BMC Pediatr*. 2021;21(1):269. doi:10.1186/s12887-021-02727-8.

Chapter 5

Cerebellar Hemorrhage in the Preterm Newborn

Jarred Garfinkle and Emily W.Y. Tam

Chapter Outline

Key Points

- Cerebellar hemorrhages (CBH) likely originate from the external granular layer, which is a superficial germinal matrix within the immature cerebellum.
- The anterior lobe of the cerebellum is principally connected with sensorimotor cortex, while the posterior lobe is connected with association regions of the cerebral cortex.
- Cranial ultrasound is only capable of detecting relatively large CBH, while MRI can detect punctate CBH, which are typically classified as those less than 4 mm in diameter.
- CBH has been associated with motor, visuomotor, cognitive, and behavioral problems in early childhood.

- Larger CBH and those affecting the vermis and deeper aspects of the cerebellar hemispheres are more likely to be associated with neurodevelopmental deficits than superficial punctate CBH.

Case History

AM was a 600 g 24-week male neonate born to a 30-year-old mother after preterm labor. The mother received two doses of betamethasone but not magnesium sulfate. He was delivered vaginally and his umbilical cord was quickly clamped. At birth he demonstrated minimal respiratory effort and was intubated in the delivery room with a subsequent rise in heart rate. He was subsequently given surfactant for respiratory distress syndrome. On day of life 2 he developed hypotension and anemia for which he

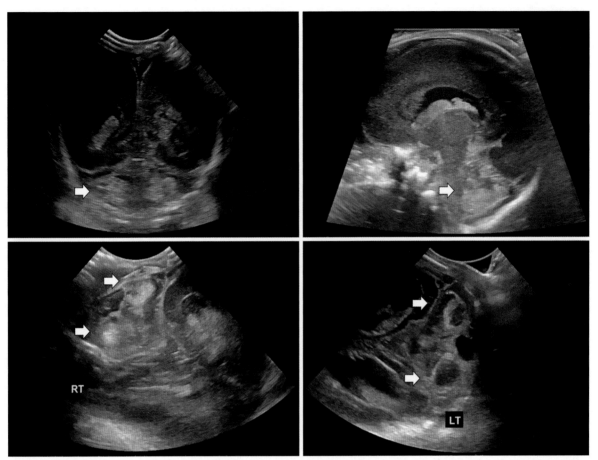

Fig. 5.1 Ultrasound images over time of the 24-week preterm male depicted in the case study. *Upper left panel:* Coronal image on day of life (DOL) 3 via the anterior fontanel demonstrating bilateral intraventricular hemorrhage within the posterior horns of the lateral ventricles with left periventricular hemorrhagic infarction and bilateral cerebellar hemisphere echogenicities suspicious for hemorrhage (*arrowhead*). *Upper right panel:* Sagittal right image on DOL 3 via the anterior fontanel demonstrating echogenicity within the inferior portion of the cerebellar hemisphere (*arrowhead*). *Bottom left panel:* Ultrasound image on DOL 6 via the left mastoid fontanel demonstrating echogenicities within both cerebellar hemispheres suggestive of cerebellar hemorrhage (*arrowheads*). Ultrasound image on DOL 19 via the left mastoid fontanel demonstrating lesions with echogenic rims in both cerebellar hemispheres, likely representing the subacute phase of the cerebellar hemorrhages (*arrowheads*).

received a packed red blood cell transfusion and inotropes. His head ultrasound on day of life 3 revealed bilateral intraventricular hemorrhage with left periventricular hemorrhagic infarction and echogenicities within both cerebellar hemispheres. A repeat head ultrasound on day of life 6 with dedicated views via the mastoid fontanel confirmed bilateral cerebellar hemorrhages (CBH) (Fig. 5.1). Subsequent head ultrasounds showed the evolution of the CBH and an MRI at 34 weeks postmenstrual age showed severe cerebellar atrophy in addition to supratentorial pathologies (Fig. 5.2).

Several questions related to CBH were asked by the bedside staff and the parents: Why did AM develop CBH? Could they have been prevented? How will the CBH impact his life?

Introduction

Cerebellar hemorrhage (CBH) is a category of preterm brain injury and typically affects newborns born at the lowest gestational ages.[1,2] Similar to the supratentorial intraventricular hemorrhages, CBH likely originate

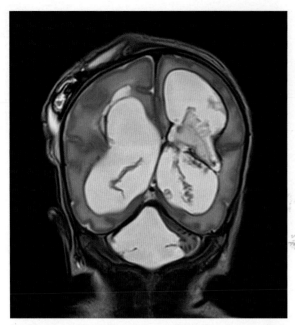

Fig. 5.2 Coronal T2 weighted MRI image of the 24-week preterm male depicted in the case study at 34 weeks postmenstrual age. The cerebellum is atrophic secondary to the early cerebellar hemorrhages. This patient also developed posthemorrhagic ventricular dilatation requiring a ventricular shunt and periventricular leukomalacia.

from the germinal matrices of the immature cerebellum, and in particular the external granular layer (EGL) which is superficially located beneath the pial layer.[3–5] The original reports of CBH in preterm neonates relied on postmortem examinations.[6] Subsequently, in the 1980s, reports of CBH detected by ultrasound (US) via the anterior fontanel were described, including by the editor of this textbook.[7] In the 1990s cranial US via the mastoid fontanel provided greater details of CBH.[2] These large hemorrhages described before the more widespread use of MRI in neonatology were associated with death and severe neurodevelopmental impairments.[2,8]

More recently, large CBH have become less common with improvements in the care of the preterm newborn. However, with the increasing use of MRI, smaller CBH referred to as punctate CBH have been increasingly reported in the preterm population.[9–13] These punctate CBH are typically defined as those only visible on MRI and measuring <4 mm in diameter on any given imaging plane.[14,15] Two recent

systematic reviews found wide variations in reported outcomes of preterm children with CBH, likely due to the heterogeneity of the hemorrhages themselves.[16,17] Thus it is important to assess the size and location of the CBH and understand the functional topography of the cerebellum.

This chapter reviews the development and function of the cerebellum and the diagnosis and implications of CBH in preterm newborns.

Cerebellar Development, Organization, Functional Topography, and Injury

In order to understand the impact of CBH on neurodevelopment, an understanding of the developmental processes that occur in the immature cerebellum and its ultimate anatomic and functional organization is essential. The cerebellum is vulnerable during the preterm period because the cerebellum is in a state of rapid development in the third trimester.[3] During the third trimester, cerebellar volume increases fivefold and the cerebellar surface area increases 20-fold.[3,18] Cerebellar proliferation continues into the second postnatal year, by which point the cerebellum contains the majority of all neurons in the central nervous system.[19] The cerebellar cortex is folded into multiple lobes and lobules to accommodate such a large number of cells.

CEREBELLAR DEVELOPMENT AND VASCULOGENESIS

There are two primary neuronal progenitor zones in the developing cerebellum: the rhombic lip, which forms in the dorsolateral part of the alar plate adjacent to the fourth ventricle, and the ventricular zone, which forms on the ventral surface of the alar plate along the lining of the fourth ventricle.[4,20,21] Progenitor cells from the rhombic lip migrate outward to beneath the pial membrane, to form the EGL.[22] The EGL, therefore constitutes a secondary germinal zone, or transit amplifying center, as it still contains progenitor cells. Neurogenesis in the ventricular zone peaks in the first trimester, whereas neurogenesis in the EGL appears at the end of the embryonic period and persists for several months to 2 years after birth (Fig. 5.3). The Purkinje cells, GABAergic projection neurons, and later the Golgi, stellate and basket interneurons and Bergmann glia arise from the ventricular zone whereas

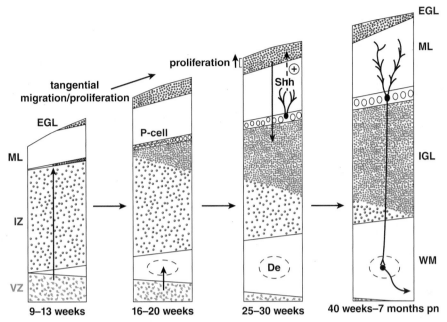

Fig. 5.3 Major events in the histogenesis of the cerebellum in four major time periods from 9 weeks of gestation to 7 months postnatal (pn). The two zones of proliferation are the ventricular zone (VZ) and the external granule cell layer (EGL). Three directions of migration are indicated by arrows, that is, radial from the VZ, tangential over the surface of the cerebellum to form the EGL, and later, inward to form the internal granular layer (IGL). Proliferation in the outer half of the EGL is under positive control by Sonic hedgehog (Shh) secreted by Purkinje cells (P-cells). Note the markedly active proliferation and migration of the granule precursor cells of the EGL during the premature period. Not shown is the marked increase in size of the molecular layer (ML) during the postnatal period. *De*, dentate; *IZ*, intermediate zone; *pn*, postnatal; *WM*, white matter. (Adapted from Rakic P, Sidman RL. Histogenesis of cortical layers in human cerebellum, particularly the lamina dissecans. *J Comp Neurol*. 1970;139(4):473–500; Sidman RL, Rakic P. Neuronal migration, with special reference to developing human brain: a review. *Brain Res*. 1973;62(1):1–35; and ten-Donkelaar HJ, Lammens M, Wesseling P, Thijssen HOM, Renier WO. Development and developmental disorders of the human cerebellum. *J Neurol*. 2003;250(9):1025–1036.)

the granule cells, glutaminergic projection neurons, and unipolar brush cells arise from the EGL.[23]

The EGL comprises two sublayers: an external proliferating zone and an inner differentiating zone, which are separated by a vascular bed.[4,21] Neuronal precursor proliferation peaks in magnitude during the third trimester in the EGL, induced by sonic hedgehog (SHH) protein secreted by differentiating Purkinje cells.[24] As a result, the EGL and its vascular bed are susceptible to myriad insults during the preterm period. Peak EGL proliferation occurs around postnatal day 7 in mice, which approximately corresponds to the first half of the third trimester in humans. The progenitor pool of the EGL persists longest in the posterior lobe.[21] As precursor neurons mature, they exit the EGL by migrating radially inward to settle beneath the Purkinje cell layer to form the internal granule layer, resulting in the final laminar arrangement of the mature cerebellum.

The development of the cerebellar vasculature may also play an important role in the topography of preterm CBH and as such is worth reviewing. Early in embryogenesis, only the superior cerebellar arteries supply the cerebellar precursor.[25] The posterior inferior cerebellar artery (PICA) is visible in the human embryo only weeks later.[26] In addition the ultimate course of the PICA is the most highly variable among the cerebellar arteries. Macchi et al. speculated that for these reasons, the PICA may represent an acquired source of vascularization via angiotrophic vasculogenesis.[26] In adults the superior cerebellar artery perfuses the anterior lobe, while the PICA perfuses the posterior.[27] It is possible that as an acquired source of vasculogenesis the PICA is more susceptible to the cardiorespiratory perturbations typical of extreme prematurity, although this hypothesis is speculative and not currently supported by experimental evidence.[28]

The posterior cerebellum not only has a distinct arterial supply, but it also has a separate venous system. The superior cortical surface of the cerebellum is drained by the superior vermian veins and the superior hemispheric veins, which empty into the great vein of Galen in the midline.[29,30] The posterior inferior cortical surface of the cerebellum is drained by the inferior hemispheric veins, which empty into the transtentorial sinuses, and the inferior vermian veins, which empty into the straight sinus directly or via the medial transtentorial sinuses. The significance of the differential venous drainage toward the topography of preterm CBH is unclear.

CEREBELLAR ORGANIZATION

The cerebellar cortex is organized into three rostro-caudally oriented compartments: the midline vermis, the paravermis, and the lateral cerebellar hemispheres. The cerebellar cortex of the cerebellar hemispheres connects to the brainstem via three paired cerebellar peduncles, via the cerebellar deep nuclei. The cerebellar deep nuclei are embedded in the white matter of

the cerebellum and include, medially to laterally, the fastigial, interpositus (globose and emboliform), and dentate nuclei. The final cerebellar output arises from these deep cerebellar nuclei and exits the cerebellum via the superior and inferior peduncles. The cerebellum projects to specific cerebral destinations and receives input back from these same regions via the middle cerebellar peduncle, and thus forms reciprocal and functional circuits, or closed loops.[31]

The primary fissure divides the cerebellar hemispheres into the anterior and posterior lobes. The cerebellar hemispheres are further folded into multiple lobules.[32] There are 10 lobules in the cerebellar cortex: lobules I–V represent the anterior lobe; lobules VI–IX the posterior lobe; and lobule X the flocculonodular lobe.[33] Lobule VII comprises almost 50% of the cerebellar cortex in humans and is subdivided into crus I, crus II, and VIIB (Fig. 5.4).[34,35]

FUNCTIONAL TOPOGRAPHY

Accumulating evidence suggests that the role of the human cerebellum extends much beyond motor

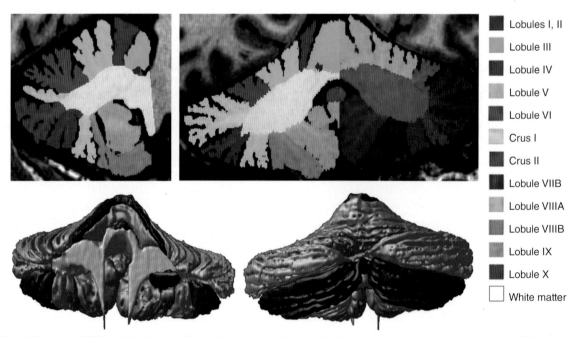

Fig. 5.4 Segmented MRI T1-weighted images of the adult cerebellum. *Top panel:* Cerebellar lobules defined according to fissures with the left and right hemispheres containing a different set of labels in a sagittal (*left*) and coronal (*right*) section. *Bottom panel:* 3D surface representation of the cerebellar lobules. (Adapted from Park MT, Pipitone J, Baer LH, et al. Derivation of high-resolution MRI atlases of the human cerebellum at 3T and segmentation using multiple automatically generated templates. *Neuroimage.* 2014;95:217–231.)

control to include nonmotor behaviors. This impression originates mainly from functional adult neuroimaging studies showing cerebellar involvement during a range of nonmotor tasks and clinical populations in whom cerebellar damage produces nonmotor deficits in cognition and behavior.[36]

The cerebellum is reciprocally connected with sensorimotor and association regions of the cerebral cortex via the feedforward cortico-ponto-cerebellar and the feedback cerebello-thalamo-cortical pathways. Sensory and motor projections to the cerebellum reveal body maps in the anterior lobe of the cerebellum. The remaining lobules of the posterior lobe of the cerebellum are linked with the parietal and prefrontal association cortices.[37] Much of our knowledge around the functional organization of the human cerebellum comes from task-based and resting-state functional MRI (fMRI) studies. In task-based fMRI studies activations related to cognitive and emotional-affective processes are usually observed in the lateral posterior lobe.[38,39]

Functional and structural imaging studies have revealed regional differences in neonatal and childhood development within the cerebellum. Recently, Herzmann et al. demonstrated via resting-state fMRI that cortico-cerebellar functional connectivity is well-established by term in even preterm newborns.[40] One important difference between functional organization of the cerebellum during the neonatal period relative to that of the adult was discovered in the somatomotor network. In the adult, the cerebellar sensorimotor network is mainly located in the anterior lobe.[39] In contrast to adult studies the study by Herzmann et al. did not find evidence for somatomotor representation in the anterior lobe of the cerebellum. The authors speculated that the somatomotor network and with it the anterior lobe of the cerebellum matures over the first years of life. This discrepancy between the neonatal and adult somatomotor representation in the cerebellum may herald discrepant deficits from similarly located injuries between the two age groups.

ADULT CEREBELLAR INFARCT

In the adult cerebellar functional topography is readily examined when the effects of cerebellar injury are studied in clinical populations. Infarcts affecting the superior cerebellar artery, which perfuses the anterior cerebellar lobe, are more likely to cause limb and gait ataxia. In contrast infarcts affecting the PICA, which perfuses most of the posterior lobe of the cerebellum, are more likely to result in the cerebellar cognitive affective syndrome (CCAS).[27,41] In adults posterior lobe infarcts occur more often than anterior lobe infarcts.[42]

The CCAS is characterized by deficits in language, visual-spatial function, executive function, and emotional-affective dysregulation following cerebellar injury. A recent voxel-based lesion symptom-mapping study reported that patients with cerebellar motor syndrome but no cognitive deficits had damage to the anterior lobe with spared posterolateral hemispheres; patients with CCAS but no motor deficits had an inverse pattern of injury.[43] These findings suggest good agreement between functional connectivity and lesion-deficit studies of the adult cerebellum.

Preterm Cerebellar Hemorrhage

EPIDEMIOLOGY AND DIAGNOSIS WITH IMAGING

CBH is one of the classic forms of preterm brain injury and ranges in size from punctate hemorrhages to larger hemispheric and vermian hemorrhages.[1] The original reports of CBH were derived from postmortem studies.[6,7] In the mid-1990s routine posterior fossa imaging through the mastoid fontanel became more commonly applied to improve the ultrasonographic visualization of the posterior fossa in neonates.[2] These CBH visualized on the US have historically been associated with adverse neurodevelopmental outcomes as only larger CBH can be visualized on cranial US (Fig. 5.1).

The reported frequency of CBH in preterm neonates in contemporary studies varies and depends on whether diagnosis was made by cranial US or brain MRI (Fig. 5.5). Cranial US is only capable of detecting relatively large CBH that are greater than 4 mm in diameter; as such, reported rates of CBH diagnosed by cranial US are lower than those reported by brain MRI. For example, one prospective cohort study scanning preterm neonates with both serial cranial US and MRI reported that 7/140 (5%) had CBH on cranial US but 28/140 (20%) had CBH on MRI with susceptibility-weighted imaging (SWI).[44] The reported rates of CBH range from 14% to 37% in recent cohort studies of very preterm neonates using MRI with different

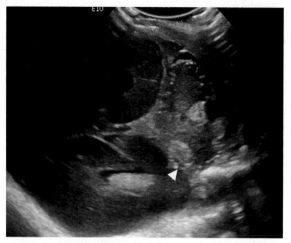

Fig. 5.5 Cranial ultrasound image via the right mastoid fontanel of a cerebellar hemorrhage in the left cerebellar hemisphere in a 25-week preterm male on day of life 8.

sequences.[9,10,12,13,44] The specific MRI imaging protocol is also important, with SWI sequences possibly identifying more hemorrhages.[2,10,12,45] SWI identifies iron deposition from degraded hemoglobin, and as such is highly sensitive for hemorrhage.

Massive CBH can be diagnosed on cranial US through the anterior fontanel, but imaging via the mastoid fontanel is more sensitive for smaller hemorrhages.[2,7,44] Different US features of large CBH can be observed according to timing. In the acute phase a globular and ill-defined area of increased echogenicity is seen within the cerebellar parenchyma; in the subacute phase, less echogenic and some echolucent lesions are observed; and in the subsequent weeks, reduced volume of the cerebellum can be appreciated.[46] Punctate hemorrhages, which are typically classified as those less than 4 mm in diameter, can by definition only be diagnosed on MRI and are imperceptible on US (Table 5.1, Fig. 5.6).[14] Studies comparing the diagnostic accuracy of US against the gold-standard of MRI for nonpunctate CBH have found that

US via the mastoid fontanel is capable of detecting the majority, but not all, of these CBH.[12,44]

The typical location of preterm CBH within the surface layers of the inferior posterior lobe has been demonstrated in two separate imaging cohorts (Fig. 5.7).[13,47] This area likely corresponds to the EGL, which is the germinal matrix for granule cells that proliferates during the third trimester and into the second postnatal year.[4] The reasons behind the predilection of the inferior posterior lobe for CBH is unknown, but may relate to the later development of the posterior lobe and its unique arterial vascularization, as discussed above.

PATHOGENESIS AND RISK FACTORS

Volpe proposed that cerebellar hemispheric hemorrhages originate in the germinal matrix of the EGL, while cerebellar vermian hemorrhages originate in the residual germinal matrix of the ventricular zone in the roof of the fourth ventricle.[3] The co-occurrence of CBH and germinal matrix-intraventricular hemorrhages further supports the hypothesis that CBH, like germinal matrix-intraventricular hemorrhages, originate in the germinal matrices.[12,45] The richly vascularized EGL germinal matrix, like the subependymal germinal matrices adjacent to the lateral ventricles, is more vulnerable to rupture in the perinatal period. The human fetal EGL achieves its maximum thickness between the 20th and 32nd gestational week and therefore requires a significant blood supply during this period.[48] Circulatory factors related to impaired cerebrovascular autoregulation and shunts via a large patent ductus arteriosus may be important in the pathogenesis, as in supratentorial germinal matrix-intraventricular hemorrhages.[49] US studies of CBH indicate detection in the first days of life, similar to germinal matrix-intraventricular hemorrhages.[12,50] In punctate CBH in which the diagnosis is made by MRI, the timing of CBH occurrence is undeterminable as the MRIs are performed weeks or months into postnatal life.

Preterm neonates born at <28 weeks' gestation are at highest risk for CBH.[10,45] Other documented risk factors

TABLE 5.1 Punctate Versus Larger Cerebellar Hemorrhages		
	Punctate Cerebellar Hemorrhage	**Larger Cerebellar Hemorrhage**
Size	<4 mm	≥4 mm
Visible on ultrasound	No	Possibly

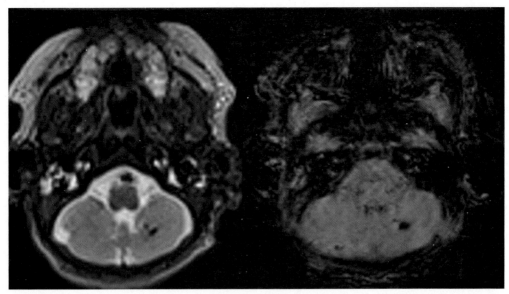

Fig. 5.6 MRI of a 25-week newborn imaged at 32 weeks postmenstrual age demonstrating a punctate left cerebellar hemorrhage with (*left panel*) low signal intensity on T2-weighted imaging and (*right panel*) blooming artifact on susceptibility-weighted imaging. Note that susceptibility-weighted imaging may exaggerate the size of the hemorrhage. Image courtesy of Drs. Steven Miller and Ting Guo.

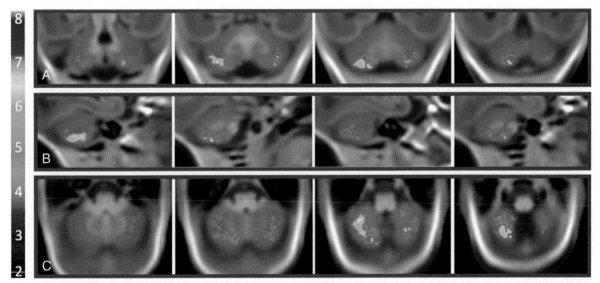

Fig. 5.7 Probabilistic cerebellar hemorrhage (CBH) map of 35 very preterm neonates overlaid on a T1-weighted early preterm brain template. CBH from preterm magnetic resonance imaging that occurred at a homologous region in two or more very preterm neonates are displayed. CBH seen only in a single neonate are omitted. The cumulative (summed) CBH map is overlaid on the neonatal brain template in (A) coronal (left to right: anterior to posterior), (B) sagittal (left to right: left to right), and (C) axial (left to right: superior to inferior) planes. The color bar on the left indicates the color coding of the CBH summation. The maximum value on the map is 8. (Adapted from Garfinkle J, Guo T, Synnes A, et al. Location and size of preterm cerebellar hemorrhage and childhood development. *Ann Neurol.* 2020;88:1095–1108.)

BOX 5.1 RISK FACTORS FOR PRETERM CEREBELLAR HEMORRHAGE

- Low gestational age
- Low birth weight
- Intubation at birth
- Mechanical ventilation
- Early hypotension
- Patent ductus arteriosus

for preterm CBH include birth weight <750 g, hypotension, inotrope exposure, intubation during resuscitation, and mechanical ventilation (Box 5.1).[10,12,13,45,49,51] There is no consistent relationship between mode of delivery and CBH with conflicting results from several studies.[17] Two cohort studies reported a reduced risk of CBH in preterm neonates exposed to antenatal magnesium sulfate for an obstetric or neuroprotective indication.[10,13]

The association between magnesium sulfate and CBH is of particular interest because it may represent the only known pharmacologic preventative intervention.[10] In the late 1990s reports of preterm neonates born to mothers given magnesium sulfate to prevent eclamptic seizures or as tocolysis showed a consistent association with reduced cerebral palsy (CP).[52] In those babies born preterm and exposed to magnesium sulfate the odds ratio (OR) for CP was 0.11 (95% CI 0.02–0.81). Since then, at least six randomized controlled trials and subsequent meta-analyses have demonstrated that magnesium sulfate administered to women at imminent risk for preterm delivery decreases the offspring's risk of CP; the relative risk in a recent meta-analysis was 0.68 (95% CI 0.54–0.85).[53,54] However, antenatal magnesium sulfate has not been associated with a reduction in brain injuries known to cause CP, such as severe germinal matrix-intraventricular hemorrhages or cystic periventricular leukomalacia, in randomized trials that used US imaging to diagnose brain injury.[55–57] It is therefore possible that the association between antenatal magnesium sulfate and reduced CP may be mediated through a reduction in CBH.[10,13]

Although the exact mechanisms of action of magnesium as a neuroprotective agent are unknown, it has several biologically plausible actions which may contribute to its neuroprotective effect on the preterm brain. For instance, magnesium has a vasodilatory effect in the cerebral microcirculation, thus playing an important role in the regulation of the cerebral circulation by maintaining normal blood flow and pressure.[58] In preterm fetal sheep exposed to asphyxia, magnesium increased systemic perfusion after umbilical cord occlusion without impairing arterial blood pressure to cerebral blood flow.[59] As such, magnesium may stabilize against rapid fluctuation in cerebral blood flow.

PATHOLOGY

One of the original descriptions of CBH involved 20 neonates born at <1500 g admitted to the NICU at The Hospital for Sick Children between 1973 and 1974.[6] They reported, "The smaller hemorrhages were often multiple and occurred in various locations: subpial in the external granular cell layer; subependymal in the germinal plate region of the fourth ventricle, in the region of the dentate nucleus, or in the superior cerebellar peduncle." Several of these cases involved the destruction of a complete cerebellar hemisphere or complete encasement of the cerebellum in blood.

A large recent autopsy cohort of 19 preterm neonates born at <37 weeks between 1999 and 2010 with CBH reported that in all cases, a destructive hematoma occupied the inferior aspect of the posterior lobe of the cerebellum in a distribution that roughly corresponded to the territory supplied by the PICA (Fig. 5.8).[28] The hematomas typically involved the superficial cortex, possibly having originated in the EGL, and the adjacent white matter. Most of the specimens demonstrated multiple hemorrhages, with satellite hemorrhages appearing near the larger ones. Other authors have speculated that larger hemorrhages could have occurred due to the coalescence of multiple smaller hemorrhages.[60] In addition, histopathology of the lesions showed acute hemorrhages admixed with subacute or chronic changes, suggesting that at least some hemorrhages may evolve over time and are due to repeated episodes of bleeding rather than a single hemorrhagic event.

In the recent autopsy cohort, there was often significant associated pathology in the inferior olivary and dentate nuclei. In addition, supratentorially, there was a high frequency of germinal matrix-intraventricular hemorrhages and white matter injury. The damage sustained

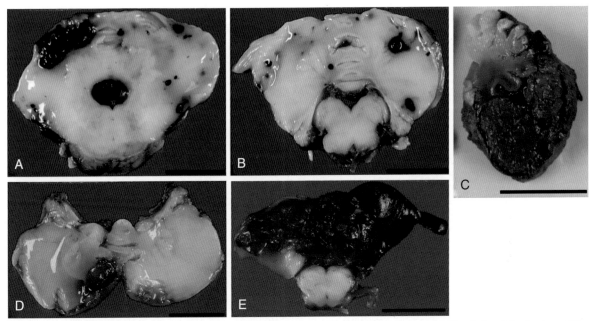

Fig. 5.8 Gross photographs of the cut surface of CBH. (A) Horizontal sections at the level of the mid pons and (B) rostral medulla showing multifocal hemorrhages and a crescentic larger superficial hemorrhage in panel (A) from a 29 weeks' gestation infant who survived 3 weeks. (C) Sagittal section through a CBH showing replacement of inferior cerebellar tissue by a hematoma that is partially covered by leptomeninges. The remaining cerebellar cortex is atrophic. (D) Unilateral CBH in an infant born at 30.5 weeks' gestation who survived 1 week. Note the dusky appearance of the hemisphere involved by the hemorrhage relative to the uninvolved contralateral hemisphere. (E) Horizontal section at the level of the rostral medulla showing near total replacement of the cerebellum by hematoma covered with leptomeninges. Bar is 1 cm in all panels. (Reproduced from Haines KM, Wang W, Pierson CR. Cerebellar hemorrhagic injury in premature infants occurs during a vulnerable developmental period and is associated with wider neuropathology. *Acta Neuropathol Commun.* 2013;1:69.)

by these adjacent and interconnected structures is important because it has the potential to exacerbate cerebellar hemispheric injury. In particular, injury to the dentate nucleus, which supplies the output from the cerebellar hemispheres to the cerebrum, may be critical. Importantly, autopsy cohorts may not be representative of the brain pathology of premature neonates with CBH who survive beyond the perinatal period.

EXPERIMENTAL MODELS

Yoo et al. developed an animal model of preterm CBH in neonatal mouse pups.[61] They used pups at postnatal day 2, which corresponds developmentally to the third trimester in humans,[4] to examine the anatomical features of CBH and the associated behavioral phenotype. They injected bacterial collagenase, which disrupts the blood vessels, into the cerebral aqueduct, which is rostral to the cerebellum. On histopathology, the area

of EGL in the CBH mice was reduced on postnatal day 7. Behaviorally, mice with CBH spent more time in the center of an open field, which is considered to be maladaptive and may be associated with increased risk-taking. In addition mice with CBH displayed deficits in motor coordination and balance on the rotarod and horizontal ladder rung walking test.

In a second experiment by the same authors, bacterial collagenase was injected directly in the cerebellar hemisphere rather than adjacent to it.[62] They found that cerebellar volume at postnatal day 15 was affected only when the CBH was inflicted in conjunction with systemic inflammation. CBH alone did not significantly affect cerebellar volume. Overall, their findings demonstrate that inflammation, which is associated with preterm birth, neonatal infections, and chronic lung disease, may amplify the consequences of CBH.

CONSEQUENCES ON THE DEVELOPING CEREBELLUM

Cerebellar hypoplasia is a relatively common finding in preterm newborns and is thought to occur from primary injury like CBH and from more remote, secondary factors, including supratentorial brain injury and exposure to glucocorticoids and morphine.[63–65] The preterm cerebellum is particularly at risk during the preterm period as it undergoes rapid growth. When assessed in the fetus by 3-dimensional volumetric US, the cerebellar volume increases fivefold from 24 to 40 weeks' gestation.[18] When assessed in the fetus by 3-dimensional volumetric MRI, cerebellar volume increases 3.5-fold from 27 to 40 weeks' gestation.[66] On fetal brain MRI, the cerebellum grows disproportionately more relative to the rest of the brain during the last 20 weeks of gestation.[67] On histologic examination the surface area of the cerebellar cortex increases more than 30-fold from 24 weeks of gestation to term.[3,48]

Kim et al. reported that CBH was associated with slower growth in the inferior aspect posterior lobe of the cerebellum. The authors speculated that CBH, which was mainly distributed along the inferior aspect of the posterior lobe, disrupted neurogenesis within the active EGL and thus resulted in locally reduced cerebellar volume.[47] In another contemporary cohort in which subjects underwent a preterm MRI around 32 weeks' gestation followed by an MRI around term-equivalent age, CBH was associated with reduced cerebellar growth after adjusting for confounders. In addition the cerebellar hemisphere with a greater volume of CBH grew less than the contralateral hemisphere.[47]

Outcomes Following Preterm Cerebellar Hemorrhage

The large CBH diagnosed in the 1990s and early 2000s were associated with mortality and severe neurodevelopmental impairment across multiple domains. In one stark example children with isolated CBH had a 66% rate of neurodevelopmental impairment relative to 5% in matched controls at mean age of 32 months.[8] The deficits spanned gross and fine motor, expressive and receptive language, cognition, and behavior. Behaviorally,

there was a higher frequency of internalizing behavior problems and abnormal autism spectrum disorder screening results. This cohort, however, included children born between 1998 and 2003 who had larger hemorrhages.

Previous reviews have described a wide range of outcomes in preterm newborns with CBH.[68] Two systematic reviews published recently concluded that CBH is associated with motor and cognitive outcomes.[16,17] One of the reviews included only 15 patients with punctate CBH and found that neonates with isolated punctate CBH had a frequency of neurodevelopmental impairment (13%–20%) that is similar to that of the general very preterm population[16,69] while the other review was unable to evaluate the effect of CBH size on outcome due to the small number of patients.[17] In addition most of the studies included in the systematic reviews began enrolling their cohorts in the 1990s and the mean age at follow-up in all the studies was less than 3 years of age.[16] Since the publication of these systematic reviews, Garfinkle et al. published a prospective cohort study evaluating the impact of CBH on 4.5-year neurodevelopmental outcomes.[13] It is also important to note that few reports of CBH and neurodevelopmental outcomes isolated the contribution of supratentorial injury to eventual outcomes.[68]

IMAGING CHARACTERISTICS AND THEIR RELATIONSHIP WITH OUTCOME

A distinction based on CBH size on MRI can be used to inform outcomes. In several studies punctate CBH detected on term-equivalent MRI were not associated with reduced neurodevelopmental scores at 2 years of age.[9,11,45] However a dichotomous distinction between punctate and larger CBH may not be sufficient to provide meaningful data to parents and clinicians. Another grading scheme classified CBH as punctate (≤4 mm), limited (>4 mm but <1/3 of the cerebellar hemisphere) or massive (≥1/3 of the cerebellar hemisphere).[15] Children with massive CBH had the highest rates of abnormal motor, cognitive, and behavioral outcomes at 2 years of age and had significantly reduced scores relative to children with limited CBH. However, massive CBH is rare in contemporary preterm survivors. In a recent prospective imaging cohort study enrolling newborns born between 2006 and 2012, only one of 36 newborns had a massive hemorrhage.[13] In this study, the precise 3- or 2-dimensional footprint of CBH was associated with motor, visuomotor, and behavioral outcomes.[13]

In addition to the size of CBH, the location of CBH may inform neurodevelopmental outcome. Most studies that have attempted to explore the complex relationship between CBH location and outcomes have categorized CBH according to the presence of injury to the cerebellar vermis. Indeed, the vast majority of preterm children with CBH involving the vermis have an adverse outcome.[16] In addition CBH that permeate more deeply within the cerebellar hemispheres were associated with motor, visuomotor, and behavioral dysfunction.[13] Embedded in the cerebellar hemispheric white matter are the dentate nuclei, which receive projections from the superficial cerebellar cortex and project to the contralateral cerebral cortex via the cerebello-thalamo-cortical tracts.[70] It is possible that injury to the deep cerebellar nuclei may have a more profound impact on neurodevelopment, but the current resolution of neonatal brain imaging makes it difficult to test this hypothesis.[71] It is important to note that the association between CBH location and outcomes may be confounded by size, as CBH involving the vermis and deeper aspects of the hemispheres are also typically large.

The age at which imaging is performed is another consideration relevant to the association between preterm CBH and outcome. A recent study reported that CBH was associated with outcome when evaluated on preterm MRI, but not on term-equivalent MRI, likely due to the involution of CBH over time. Indeed, the size of CBH decreased between early, preterm scans and scans repeated at term-equivalent age.[13]

MOTOR AND VISUOMOTOR OUTCOMES

Motor outcome in preterm children with large CBH is more likely to be impaired compared to preterm children without cerebellar injury.[8,50,72] CP has been described in preterm children with CBH.[50,73] However, the causal attribution of CBH to CP is ambiguous given the frequent co-occurrence of severe white matter injury. In one retrospective cohort study the frequency of CP was higher in those with CBH diagnosed by US compared to those without CBH. Of note, only cerebellar vermian hemorrhage, and not hemispheric hemorrhage, was associated with CP after adjustment for confounders.[50] Unfortunately, cohort studies of CBH have infrequently described the subtype of CP. Children with hypotonic or ataxic CP are often found to have injuries or malformations to the cerebellum, so it would be of interest to classify the type of CP identified in preterm children with CBH. A recent study found that four of 36 children with CBH had CP, two of whom had predominant hypotonia. Interestingly, all had Gross Motor Function Classification System Level I.

Contemporary cohort studies that have examined preterm children with only punctate CBH have not consistently identified an independent association with motor outcomes at 2 years.[9,45] Senden et al. examined 24 very preterm children with punctate CBH born between 2008 and 2013 at 2 years of age in a case-control study. They found no statistically significant differences on gross or fine motor assessment when comparing children with bilateral, unilateral, and no punctate CBH. Steggerda et al. evaluated a cohort of 108 very preterm children born between 2006 and 2007 at 2 years of age, of whom 16 had punctate CBH. There was no association between punctate CBH and abnormal fine or gross motor developmental outcome at 2 years of age. One cohort study with standardized neurologic examinations at 4 years found a higher rate of neurologic abnormalities, including tone, strength, and reflexes, on blinded neurologic exams.[11] Recently, a cohort study found an association between CBH size and both motor and visuomotor outcomes at 4.5 years of age, independent of supratentorial injury.[13]

The reduced motor function associated with CBH may be mediated by the interruption of interactions between the cerebellum and the cortex.[72] In the Limperopoulos cohort described above, preterm children were re-imaged at mean of 34 months of age and cortical volume was measured. They reported an association between the volume of the sensorimotor cortex contralateral to CBH and motor outcomes, thus linking secondary impairment in cerebral cortical growth and motor function in survivors of CBH.

COGNITIVE AND LANGUAGE OUTCOMES

Preterm children with large CBH have a higher frequency of cognitive and language impairment relative to those without.[8,50,72] Bilateral, large CBH may have the highest odds of cognitive dysfunction. In a retrospective cohort of extreme preterm neonates who underwent cranial US, CBH was associated with higher odds of mental impairment at 18 months.[50] In contrast, punctate CBH have not been associated with early cognition, even when there are multiple punctate bleeds.[9,13,45] Tam et al. evaluated cognition using the WPPSI-III at 4 years of age.[11] Mean Full Scale IQ (FSIQ) was not different between children with and without CBH after adjusting for supratentorial intraventricular hemorrhage and white matter injury (98 ± 6 and 99 ± 2, respectively). In addition Garfinkle et al. did not identify any association between the size of CBH and 4.5-year cognition after adjusting for confounders.[13]

BEHAVIORAL AND SOCIAL OUTCOMES

Few studies have examined childhood behavior in survivors of preterm CBH,[16] with varied associated findings reflecting the complex functions mediated by the cerebellum. The Limperopoulos cohort identified a high burden of internalizing but not externalizing problems in preterm children with CBH.[8] Neonates with CBH also scored significantly higher on the autism screening test (M-CHAT). Children with bilateral CBH and vermian involvement had the highest odds of an abnormal M-CHAT score. Decreased social-emotional capacities around 2 years of age have been reported in preterm children with large CBH detected on near-term MRI.[74] Another contemporary cohort study, on the other hand, did not find an association between CBH and behavioral outcomes on parental questionnaires at 2 years.[45] Recently, a cohort study demonstrated an association between CBH volume and externalizing but not internalizing behavior at 4.5 years after controlling for supratentorial injury.[74]

The association between preterm CBH and childhood behavioral and social outcomes is supported by the adult functional imaging data and lesion-symptom mapping reviewed above. Specifically, CBH primarily affects the posterior lobe, which is critical in nonmotor functions in adults.[75] In addition injury to the posterior lobe in adults results in CCAS, with dysregulated affect.[43]

Returning to the Case

Risk factors for AM to have CBH included low gestational age, low birth weight, intubation at birth, mechanical ventilation, early hypotension, and patent ductus arteriosus. His mother did not receive antenatal magnesium sulfate, which has been associated with reduced risk for CBH.

Imaging demonstrated large bilateral CBH resulting in severe cerebellar atrophy on follow-up. In addition to CBH, AM had severe IVH, posthemorrhagic ventricular dilatation, and periventricular leukomalacia (Fig. 5.2). CBH is expected to contribute to his increased risk for multiple neurodevelopmental impairments. Indeed, large CBH like those found in this child are associated with a high rate of severe neurodevelopmental impairment, especially due to the significant involvement of the cerebellar vermis. Due to the large, bilateral CBH, parents would be counseled to monitor for neurodevelopmental deficits, including motor, cognitive, and language impairments. From the CBH, neurological examination later in life could reveal hypotonic or ataxic CP. Childhood developmental follow-up should monitor for internalizing and externalizing behavioral problems, as well as screening for autism spectrum disorder.

Conclusions

CBH constitutes an increasingly recognized form of brain injury in preterm newborns. Diagnosis of CBH is important in informing the family about prognosis and large CBH is associated with problems in movement and behavior. Knowledge of cerebellar functional topography can inform our future understanding of the impact of CBH on outcome. Future research should better delineate the impact of smaller CBH on later neurodevelopment in regard to behavior and social cognition, especially in relation to how the location of hemorrhage relates to the functional topography of the cerebellum.

REFERENCES

1. Tam EWY. Cerebellar injury in preterm infants. *Handb Clin Neurol.* 2018;155:49-59.
2. Merrill JD, Piecuch RE, Fell SC, Barkovich AJ, Goldstein RB. A new pattern of cerebellar hemorrhages in preterm infants. *Pediatrics.* 1998;102:E62.
3. Volpe JJ. Cerebellum of the premature infant: rapidly developing, vulnerable, clinically important. *J Child Neurol.* 2009;24: 1085-1104.
4. Haldipur P, Dang D, Millen KJ. Embryology. *Handb Clin Neurol.* 2018;154:29-44.
5. Machold R, Fishell G. Math1 is expressed in temporally discrete pools of cerebellar rhombic-lip neural progenitors. *Neuron.* 2005;48:17-24.
6. Pape KE, Armstrong DL, Fitzhardinge PM. Central nervous system pathology associated with mask ventilation in the very low birthweight infant: a new etiology for intracerebellar hemorrhages. *Pediatrics.* 1976;58:473-483.
7. Perlman JM, Nelson JS, McAlister WH, Volpe JJ. Intracerebellar hemorrhage in a premature newborn: diagnosis by real-time ultrasound and correlation with autopsy findings. *Pediatrics.* 1983;71:159-162.
8. Limperopoulos C, Bassan H, Gauvreau K, et al. Does cerebellar injury in premature infants contribute to the high prevalence of long-term cognitive, learning, and behavioral disability in survivors? *Pediatrics.* 2007;120:584-593.
9. Senden REM, Keunen K, van der Aa NE, et al. Mild cerebellar injury does not significantly affect cerebral white matter microstructural organization and neurodevelopmental outcome in a contemporary cohort of preterm infants. *Pediatr Res.* 2018;83: 1004-1010.
10. Gano D, Ho ML, Partridge JC, et al. Antenatal exposure to magnesium sulfate is associated with reduced cerebellar hemorrhage in preterm newborns. *J Pediatr.* 2016;178:68-74.
11. Tam EW, Rosenbluth G, Rogers EE, et al. Cerebellar hemorrhage on magnetic resonance imaging in preterm newborns associated with abnormal neurologic outcome. *J Pediatr.* 2011; 158:245-250.
12. Steggerda SJ, Leijser LM, Wiggers-de Bruïne FT, van der Grond J, Walther FJ, van Wezel-Meijler G. Cerebellar injury in preterm infants: incidence and findings on US and MR Images. *Radiology.* 2009;252:190-199.
13. Garfinkle J, Guo T, Synnes A, et al. Location and size of preterm cerebellar hemorrhage and childhood development. *Ann Neurol.* 2020;88:1095-1108.
14. Kidokoro H, Anderson PJ, Doyle LW, Woodward LJ, Neil JJ, Inder TE. Brain injury and altered brain growth in preterm infants: predictors and prognosis. *Pediatrics.* 2014;134:e444-e453.
15. Boswinkel V, Steggerda SJ, Fumagalli M, et al. The CHOPIn Study: a multicenter study on cerebellar hemorrhage and outcome in preterm infants. *Cerebellum.* 2019;18:989-998.
16. Hortensius LM, Dijkshoorn ABC, Ecury-Goossen GM, et al. Neurodevelopmental consequences of preterm isolated cerebellar hemorrhage: a systematic review. *Pediatrics.* 2018;142:e20180609.
17. Villamor-Martinez E, Fumagalli M, Alomar YI, et al. Cerebellar hemorrhage in preterm infants: a meta-analysis on risk factors and neurodevelopmental outcome. *Front Physiol.* 2019;10:800.
18. Chang CH, Chang FM, Yu CH, Ko HC, Chen HY. Assessment of fetal cerebellar volume using three-dimensional ultrasound. *Ultrasound Med Biol.* 2000;26:981-988.

19. Azevedo FAC, Carvalho LRB, Grinberg LT, et al. Equal numbers of neuronal and nonneuronal cells make the human brain an isometrically scaled-up primate brain. *J Comp Neurol.* 2009; 513:532-541.
20. ten Donkelaar HJ, Lammens M, Wesseling P, Thijssen HO, Renier WO. Development and developmental disorders of the human cerebellum. *J Neurol.* 2003;250:1025-1036.
21. Haldipur P, Aldinger KA, Bernardo S, et al. Spatiotemporal expansion of primary progenitor zones in the developing human cerebellum. *Science.* 2019;366:454-460.
22. Martinez S, Andreu A, Mecklenburg N, Echevarria D. Cellular and molecular basis of cerebellar development. *Front Neuroanat.* 2013;7:18.
23. Carletti B, Rossi F. Neurogenesis in the cerebellum. *Neuroscientist.* 2007;14:91-100.
24. De Luca A, Parmigiani E, Tosatto G, et al. Exogenous sonic hedgehog modulates the pool of GABAergic interneurons during cerebellar development. *Cerebellum.* 2015;14:72-85.
25. Padget D. The development of the cranial arteries in the human embryo. Contributions to embryology. *Carnegie Inst.* 1948;32: 205-262.
26. Macchi V, Porzionato A, Guidolin D, Parenti A, De Caro R. Morphogenesis of the posterior inferior cerebellar artery with three-dimensional reconstruction of the late embryonic vertebrobasilar system. *Surg Radiol Anat.* 2005;27:56-60.
27. Amarenco P. The spectrum of cerebellar infarctions. *Neurology.* 1991;41:973-979.
28. Haines KM, Wang W, Pierson CR. Cerebellar hemorrhagic injury in premature infants occurs during a vulnerable developmental period and is associated with wider neuropathology. *Acta Neuropathol Commun.* 2013;1:69.
29. Delion M, Dinomais M, Mercier P. Arteries and veins of the cerebellum. *Cerebellum.* 2017;16:880-912.
30. Rhoton AL Jr. The posterior fossa veins. *Neurosurgery.* 2000; 47:S69-S92.
31. Strick PL, Dum RP, Fiez JA. Cerebellum and nonmotor function. *Ann Rev Neurosci.* 2009;32:413-434.
32. Ashida R, Cerminara NL, Brooks J, Apps R. Principles of organization of the human cerebellum: macro- and microanatomy. *Handb Clin Neurol.* 2018;154:45-58.
33. Stoodley CJ, Schmahmann JD. Evidence for topographic organization in the cerebellum of motor control versus cognitive and affective processing. *Cortex.* 2010;46:831-844.
34. Diedrichsen J, Balsters JH, Flavell J, Cussans E, Ramnani N. A probabilistic MR atlas of the human cerebellum. *NeuroImage.* 2009;46:39-46.
35. Park MT, Pipitone J, Baer LH, et al. Derivation of high-resolution MRI atlases of the human cerebellum at 3T and segmentation using multiple automatically generated templates. *NeuroImage.* 2014;95:217-231.
36. Schmahmann JD. The cerebellum and cognition. *Neurosci Lett.* 2019;688:62-75.
37. Stoodley CJ, Schmahmann JD. Functional topography in the human cerebellum: a meta-analysis of neuroimaging studies. *NeuroImage.* 2009;44:489-501.
38. Argyropoulos GPD, van Dun K, Adamaszek M, et al. The cerebellar cognitive affective/Schmahmann syndrome: a task force paper. *Cerebellum.* 2020;19:102-125.
39. Buckner RL, Krienen FM, Castellanos A, Diaz JC, Yeo BT. The organization of the human cerebellum estimated by intrinsic functional connectivity. *J Neurophysiol.* 2011;106:2322-2345.

40. Herzmann CS, Snyder AZ, Kenley JK, Rogers CE, Shimony JS, Smyser CD. Cerebellar functional connectivity in term- and very preterm-born infants. *Cereb Cortex.* 2019;29:1174-1184.

41. Tedesco AM, Chiricozzi FR, Clausi S, Lupo M, Molinari M, Leggio MG. The cerebellar cognitive profile. *Brain.* 2011;134: 3672-3686.

42. De Cocker LJ, Geerlings MI, Hartkamp NS, et al. Cerebellar infarct patterns: The SMART-Medea Study. *Neuroimage Clin.* 2015;8:314-321.

43. Stoodley CJ, MacMore JP, Makris N, Sherman JC, Schmahmann JD. Location of lesion determines motor vs. cognitive consequences in patients with cerebellar stroke. *Neuroimage Clin.* 2016;12:765-775.

44. Parodi A, Rossi A, Severino M, et al. Accuracy of ultrasound in assessing cerebellar haemorrhages in very low birthweight babies. *Arch Dis Child Fetal Neonatal Ed.* 2015;100:F289-F292.

45. Steggerda SJ, De Bruine FT, van den Berg-Huysmans AA, et al. Small cerebellar hemorrhage in preterm infants: perinatal and postnatal factors and outcome. *Cerebellum.* 2013;12:794-801.

46. Fumagalli M, Parodi A, Ramenghi L, et al. Ultrasound of acquired posterior fossa abnormalities in the newborn. *Pediatr Res.* 2020;87:25-36.

47. Kim H, Gano D, Ho ML, et al. Hindbrain regional growth in preterm newborns and its impairment in relation to brain injury. *Hum Brain Mapp.* 2016;37:678-688.

48. Rakic P, Sidman RL. Histogenesis of cortical layers in human cerebellum, particularly the lamina dissecans. *J Comp Neurol.* 1970;139:473-500.

49. Limperopoulos C, Benson CB, Bassan H, et al. Cerebellar hemorrhage in the preterm infant: ultrasonographic findings and risk factors. *Pediatrics.* 2005;116:717-724.

50. Zayek MM, Benjamin JT, Maertens P, Trimm RF, Lal CV, Eyal FG. Cerebellar hemorrhage: a major morbidity in extremely preterm infants. *J Perinatol.* 2012;32:699-704.

51. Vesoulis ZA, Herco M, El Ters NM, Whitehead HV, Mathur A. Cerebellar hemorrhage: a 10-year evaluation of risk factors. *J Matern Fetal Neonatal Med.* 2020;33:3680–3688.

52. Schendel DE, Berg CJ, Yeargin-Allsopp M, Boyle CA, Decoufle P. Prenatal magnesium sulfate exposure and the risk for cerebral palsy or mental retardation among very-low-birth-weight children aged 3 to 5 years. *JAMA.* 1996;276:1805-1810.

53. Wolf HT, Huusom LD, Henriksen TB, Hegaard HK, Brok J, Pinborg A. Magnesium sulphate for fetal neuroprotection at imminent risk for preterm delivery: a systematic review with meta-analysis and trial sequential analysis. *BJOG.* 2020;127: 1180-1188.

54. Magee L, Sawchuck D, Synnes A, von Dadelszen P. SOGC clinical practice guideline. Magnesium sulphate for fetal neuroprotection. *J Obstet Gynaecol Can.* 2011;33:516-529.

55. Marret S, Marpeau L, Zupan-Simunek V, et al. Magnesium sulphate given before very-preterm birth to protect infant brain: the randomised controlled PREMAG trial. *BJOG.* 2007;114:310-318.

56. Rouse DJ, Hirtz DG, Thom E, et al. A randomized, controlled trial of magnesium sulfate for the prevention of cerebral palsy. *N Engl J Med.* 2008;359:895-905.

57. Crowther CA, Hiller JE, Doyle LW, Haslam RR. Effect of magnesium sulfate given for neuroprotection before preterm birth: a randomized controlled trial. *JAMA.* 2003;290:2669-2676.

58. Murata T, Dietrich HH, Horiuchi T, Hongo K, Dacey RG Jr. Mechanisms of magnesium-induced vasodilation in cerebral penetrating arterioles. *Neurosci Res.* 2016;107:57-62.

59. Galinsky R, Davidson JO, Drury PP, et al. Magnesium sulphate and cardiovascular and cerebrovascular adaptations to asphyxia in preterm fetal sheep. *J Physiol.* 2016;594:1281-1293.

60. Pierson CR, Al Sufiani F. Preterm birth and cerebellar neuropathology. *Sem Fetal Neonatal Med.* 2016;21:305-311.

61. Yoo JY, Mak GK, Goldowitz D. The effect of hemorrhage on the development of the postnatal mouse cerebellum. *Exp Neurol.* 2014;252:85-94.

62. Tremblay S, Pai A, Richter L, et al. Systemic inflammation combined with neonatal cerebellar haemorrhage aggravates long-term structural and functional outcomes in a mouse model. *Brain Behav Immun.* 2017;66:257-276.

63. Limperopoulos C, Soul JS, Haidar H, et al. Impaired trophic interactions between the cerebellum and the cerebrum among preterm infants. *Pediatrics.* 2005;116:844-850.

64. Zwicker JG, Miller SP, Grunau RE, et al. Smaller cerebellar growth and poorer neurodevelopmental outcomes in very preterm infants exposed to neonatal morphine. *J Pediatr.* 2016;172: 81-87.e82.

65. Ranger M, Zwicker JG, Chau CM, et al. Neonatal pain and infection relate to smaller cerebellum in very preterm children at school age. *J Pediatr.* 2015;167:292-298.e291.

66. Bouyssi-Kobar M, du Plessis AJ, McCarter R, et al. Third trimester brain growth in preterm infants compared with in utero healthy fetuses. *Pediatrics.* 2016;138:e20161640.

67. Andescavage NN, du Plessis A, McCarter R, et al. Complex trajectories of brain development in the healthy human fetus. *Cereb Cortex.* 2017;27:5274-5283.

68. Brossard-Racine M, Limperopoulos C. Cerebellar injury in premature neonates: imaging findings and relationship with outcome. *Semin Perinatol.* 2021;45:151470.

69. Pascal A, Govaert P, Oostra A, Naulaers G, Ortibus E, Van den Broeck C. Neurodevelopmental outcome in very preterm and very-low-birthweight infants born over the past decade: a meta-analytic review. *Dev Med Child Neurol.* 2018;60:342–355.

70. Bernard JA, Peltier SJ, Benson BL, et al. Dissociable functional networks of the human dentate nucleus. *Cereb Cortex.* 2014; 24:2151-2159.

71. Hernandez-Castillo CR, Limperopoulos C, Diedrichsen J. A representative template of the neonatal cerebellum. *Neuroimage.* 2019;184:450-454.

72. Limperopoulos C, Chilingaryan G, Sullivan N, Guizard N, Robertson RL, du Plessis AJ. Injury to the premature cerebellum: outcome is related to remote cortical development. *Cereb Cortex.* 2014;24:728-736.

73. Johnsen SD, Bodensteiner JB, Lotze TE. Frequency and nature of cerebellar injury in the extremely premature survivor with cerebral palsy. *J Child Neurol.* 2005;20:60-64.

74. Duncan AF, Bann CM, Dempsey A, Peralta-Carcelen M, Hintz S. Behavioral deficits at 18–22 months of age are associated with early cerebellar injury and cognitive and language performance in children born extremely preterm. *J Pediatr.* 2019; 204:148-156.e144.

75. Schmahmann JD, Guell X, Stoodley CJ, Halko MA. The theory and neuroscience of cerebellar cognition. *Ann Rev Neurosci.* 2019;42:337-364.

Chapter 6

Posthemorrhagic Hydrocephalus Management Strategies

Andrew Whitelaw and Linda S. de Vries

Chapter Outline

Hemorrhage into the ventricles of the brain is one of the most serious complications of premature birth despite improvements in the survival of premature infants. Severe intraventricular hemorrhage (IVH) has a high risk of neurologic disability, and approximately 50% of children with a severe IVH go on to have progressive ventricular dilation.[1,2] Severe IVH is classified as grade III, a hemorrhage filling more than 50% of the ventricle and causing acute ventricular dilatation, or periventricular hemorrhagic infarction (PVHI),

previously referred to as grade IV. Increasing survival of extremely premature infants is associated with an increased number of infants with posthemorrhagic ventricular dilation (PHVD), with associated high morbidity and considerable mortality.[2] In the 1980s and 1990s, approximately two-thirds of these children had cerebral palsy (CP) and about one-third had multiple impairments.[3,4] Recent data show that around 40% to 60% of those with PVHI and 10% to 20% of those with a grade III without associated white matter injury (WMI) develop CP,

101

mostly unilateral spastic CP.[5-7] The term posthemorrhagic hydrocephalus (PHH) is generally reserved for cases in which PHVD is persistent, progressive, and associated with excessive head enlargement. Adams-Chapman[8] reported that CP, cognitive impairment, and visual impairment were considerably more frequent in infants who required surgery for PHH than infants without hydrocephalus, with the same grade of IVH and in the same weight range. Advances in our understanding of the pathophysiology and evidence from clinical trials in PHVD allow us to propose guidelines on its assessment and management, in addition, to identifying gaps in knowledge where further advances are needed.

Case History: Infant A

A mother in her first pregnancy had an uncomplicated pregnancy and received the first dose of corticosteroids 4 hours prior to an emergency Caesarean section at a gestation of 30 weeks and 5 days, because of suspected intra-uterine infection with fetal tachycardia and decelerations on the CTG. A female infant was born weighing 1400 g at delivery. Her Apgar scores were 3, 6, and 8 at 1, 5, and 10 minutes, respectively. Her respiration was supported with nasal continuous positive airway pressure and she received surfactant using the minimally invasive surfactant therapy (MIST) procedure. Her CRP was 118 mg/L on the second day after birth. Listeria monocytogenes was cultured from her blood culture. There was no pleocytosis (<7 10⁶/L white cells) in the CSF. Amoxicillin was given intravenously for 3 weeks. Her initial cranial ultrasound scan was unremarkable (Fig. 6.1A) but a repeat scan on day 4 showed bilateral IVH grade II–III (Fig. 6.1B). She was then scanned twice a week. Ventricular dimensions progressively enlarged and LPs were performed from day 10 onward (see Fig. 6.1C). These were successful and 10 mL/kg of port wine–colored cerebrospinal fluid (CSF) could be obtained each time.

As there was a need for repeated tapping of CSF and repeated LPs were becoming impractical, an Ommaya reservoir (ventricular access device) was inserted frontally in the right ventricle with the patient under general anesthesia. The reservoir was tapped daily, at 10 mL/kg/day for 4 days. Thereafter, the reservoir was tapped 7.5 mL/kg twice a day as the

ventricular dimensions did not decrease sufficiently. Tapping was increased to 15 mL/kg twice a day for 3 days and finally to 20 mL/kg twice a day. This increase in CSF removal was based on ventricular measurements on daily cranial ultrasound scans.

CSF protein was initially 1.7 g/L. Tapping the reservoir continued to be necessary for 7 weeks, and it was then decided to insert a ventriculoperitoneal low-pressure shunt when Infant A reached full-term equivalent age. Postoperatively, there was no pulmonary problem, CSF leak, or infection. Magnetic resonance imaging (MRI) at term showed very mild ventricular dilation.

Question 1: What Measurements of Ventricular Size Are Used in Diagnosis of PHVD?

The likelihood of progressive ventricular dilation increases with the amount of blood visible in the ventricles. With a small grade II intraventricular hemorrhage,[6] measurement of ventricular size once a week for 4 weeks and then at discharge is appropriate; with a large grade III or IV IVH,[9] twice-weekly ultrasonography is needed as a minimum because dilatation is likely and may be rapid. Although large, balloon-shaped ventricles are obvious without formal measurements, quantitative documentation is essential for decision making. Reference ranges for measurement of the width (midline to lateral border) of the lateral ventricles at the midcoronal level were first published in 1981.[10] Since 1984, an "action line," defined as width 4 mm higher than the 97th centile width for age, has been used as a definition of serious PHVD in therapeutic trials[3,4] and as a secondary outcome in randomized trials of neonatal intensive care interventions (Fig. 6.2). This measurement has the advantage that it is highly reproducible among observers because it is relatively unaffected by anterior or posterior angulation of the scan head as the lateral wall of the ventricle in this orientation runs fairly parallel to the midline. However, ventricular enlargement is not always sideways, and sometimes the most marked change is posterior enlargement or a change from thin slit to round balloon. With this in mind, Davies and colleagues[11] published reference ranges for anterior horn width (to capture the change in shape to balloon)

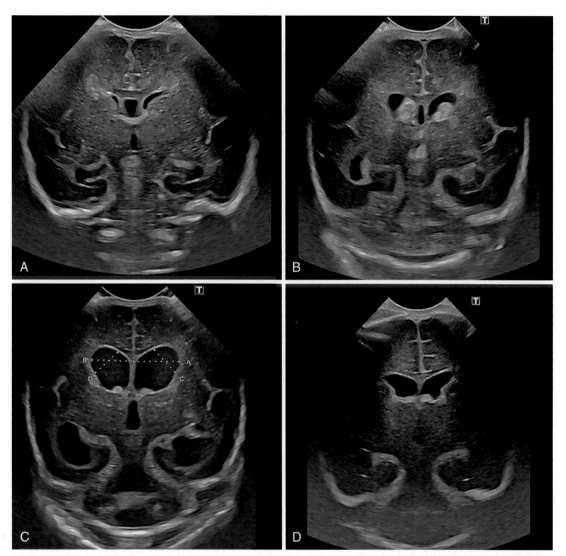

Fig. 6.1 Cranial ultrasound scans, coronal views from Infant A (Case History). A, Day 2, no IVH, mild periventricular echogenicity (PVE); B, day 4, bilateral IVH and PVE, left > right; C, day 10, day first LP, PHVD with balloon shape of the ventricles and enlarged temporal horns; D, 2 days post VP shunt placement.

(95th centile approximately 3 mm), thalamo-occipital width (to capture posterior enlargement) (95th centile approximately 25 mm), and third ventricle width (95th centile approximately 2 mm). New graphs have become available including infants below 26 weeks' gestation. An electronic spreadsheet is available to be downloaded, stored in secure servers, and used for individual patients in two formats: one is for postmenstrual age 24–42 weeks (https://tinyurl.com/PHVD-Measures-1)

and another for postmenstrual age 24–29 weeks (https://tinyurl.com/PHVD-Measures-2).[12] The fronto-temporal or fronto-occipital horn ratio (FTHR or FOHR; widest distance of the frontal horns plus temporal or occipital horns, respectively, divided by twice the largest bi-parietal distance) are also used.[13,14] A recent study showed that the intra-observer and inter-observer reliability are best for the VI and AHW and that the AHW best predicted subsequent development of PHVD

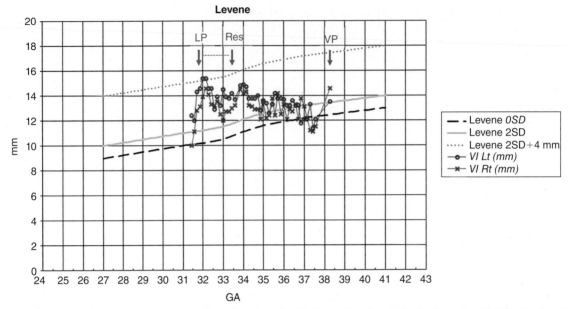

Fig. 6.2 97th centile for ventricular width with the 97th centile + 4-mm line ("action line") as the criterion for diagnosis of PHVD. Ventricular width plotted in the graph of Levene; daily LPs were performed between annotation LP and Res. VP shunt inserted as taps were still needed at 38 weeks. (Modified from Levene M. Measurement of the growth of the lateral ventricles in preterm infants with real-time ultrasound. *Arch Dis Child.* 1981;56:900–904.)

requiring neurosurgical intervention.[14] A combination of ventricular width over 97th centile and anterior horn width over 6 mm was used as eligibility for the ELVIS trial.[15]

Question 2: How Can Ventricular Dilation Driven by Cerebrospinal Fluid Under Pressure Be Distinguished From Ventricular Dilation Due to Loss of Periventricular White Matter?

To distinguish between CSF under pressure and loss of periventricular white matter as the cause of ventricular dilation is important because removing fluid that has accumulated as a replacement for dead brain (ex vacuo dilatation) is unlikely to improve outcome.

CSF-driven ventricular enlargement can be slow or rapid, it is characterized by balloon-shaped lateral ventricles, and if CSF pressure is measured, it is found to be raised or near the upper limit of normal, mean 3 mm Hg, upper limit 6 mm Hg.[16] Furthermore, head circumference growth over time is accelerated, although it may

lag behind ventricular enlargement by 1 to 2 weeks. In contrast, ventricular enlargement from atrophy is always slow, it is more irregular in outline rather than balloon shaped, and if CSF pressure is measured, it is found not to be raised. Head circumference velocity is either normal or slow but is not accelerated. There may also be notable accumulation of extra-axial fluid such as fluid between the hemispheres and between the cortical surface and the skull. Nonprogressive mild ventricular dilation at term is common and a marker of white matter injury.

Question 3: How Is Excessive Head Enlargement Defined?

Head circumference normally enlarges by approximately 1 mm per day between 26 weeks of gestation and 32 weeks, and about 0.7 mm per day between 32 and 40 weeks.[11] We regard a persistent increase of 2 mm per day as excessive. Measuring head circumference accurately, although "low-tech," is not as easy as it sounds. The relevant measurement is the maximum fronto-occipital circumference. Detecting a difference of 1 mm from day to day is difficult, and we do not react to a difference of 2 mm from one day to the next unless there is other evidence of raised intracranial pressure. However, an increase of 4 mm over 2 days is more likely to be real, and an increase of 14 mm over 7 days or less is definitely excessive. This is, however, a late sign of PHVD and poor correlation between head circumference and cranial ultrasound findings in premature infants with intraventricular hemorrhage has been reported.[17] It is therefore not recommended to wait for rapid increase in head-circumference for a decision to start with intervention.

Question 4: How Is Raised Intracranial Pressure Recognized?

It is possible to detect a change in palpation of the fontanelle from concave to bulging and to document excessive head enlargement. The preterm skull is very compliant and can easily accommodate an increase in CSF by expanding with separation of the sutures. When CSF pressure was measured with an electronic transducer in infants in whom ventricles were expanding after IVH, the mean CSF pressure was approximately 9 mm Hg, three times the mean in normal infants.[16] There was a considerable range, with ventricle and head expansion in some infants at a pressure of 5 to 6 mm Hg, and in a small number with CSF pressure around 15 mm Hg. A CSF pressure of 9 mm Hg does not necessarily produce clinical signs but may be associated with an increase in apnea or vomiting, hypotonia, hypertonia, or decreased alertness. A structured neurological examination such as that published by Dubowitz is recommended.[18]

Obtaining serial calculations of the Doppler flow-velocity resistance index (RI) on the anterior cerebral artery is a useful and practical way of detecting impairment of cerebral perfusion by raised intracranial pressure and can easily be done during ultrasound imaging. The resistance index is calculated as follows: (systolic velocity − diastolic velocity)/systolic velocity. This measurement is independent of the angle of insonation. If intracranial pressure rises to a level exceeding the infant's compensation, end-diastolic velocity tends to decrease, eventually becoming zero (RI is then 1.0) (Fig. 6.3). Serial increases in RI above 0.85 while the ventricles are rapidly expanding would be evidence that pressure is rising.[19] This statement assumes that the infant does not have a significant left-to-right shunt at the ductal level and that Pco_2 has not

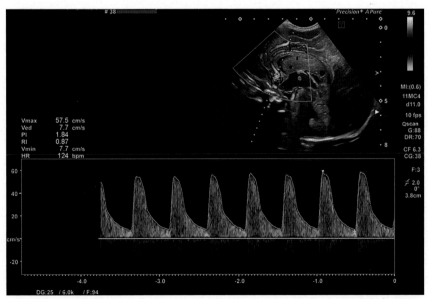

Fig. 6.3 Cerebral blood flow velocity spectra performed on the day after reservoir insertion. The RI (0.9) is slightly increased with increased systolic velocity.

decreased recently, because both of these physiologic changes could increase RI. Severe intracranial hypertension may cause reversed end-diastolic velocities. The sensitivity of resistance index can be increased by applying pressure to the fontanelle during the examination. An infant who is close to the limit of cranial compliance responds with a large decrease in end-diastolic velocities—that is, an increase in RI.[20] Somatosensory evoked potentials[21] and amplitude-integrated electroencephalography (EEG) may show a deterioration, with electroencephalographic activity becoming less frequent as dilation increases and improving with effective CSF drainage.[22] Several groups have shown that repeated near-infrared spectroscopy (NIRS) demonstrated deteriorating cerebral oxygen saturation with increasing ventricular size and improvement after decompression.[23-25] We regard all these signs of pressure as late in the development of PHVD and do recommend to start intervention before these signs have occurred.

Question 5: What Is Infant A's Prognosis?

The prognosis at diagnosis of PHVD using the preceding criteria is influenced by the presence of identifiable parenchymal lesions. The Ventriculomegaly and PHVD Drug Trials used the 4 mm + 97th centile definition of PHVD and had standardized follow-up. Of children in whom ultrasonographic examination shows no persistent periventricular echodensities or echolucencies (cysts), approximately 40% had cerebral palsy.[3,4] In the DRIFT trial, using the same treatment criteria, follow-up at 10 years of age in infants having similar management to A showed mean developmental quotient without hemorrhagic infarction to be 71 (+/–36) with 37% having cerebral palsy, 46% having extra educational resources and 23% at special schools.[26] In the more recent ELVIS trial where intervention started before or just after crossing the 4 mm + 97th centile, less than 10% of the infants with a grade III hemorrhage developed CP.[6] In the infants enrolled in the Preterm Erythropoietin Neuroprotection Trial, who were less mature, 19% of those with grade III developed CP.[7] Magnetic resonance imaging (MRI) at term can reveal parenchymal injury which cannot be easily detected with ultrasound, such as noncystic white matter injury, grey matter abnormality, and cerebellar hemorrhage and/or atrophy.[27]

Question 6: What Is the Mechanism of PHVD?

Following a large IVH, multiple blood clots can obstruct the ventricular system or channels of reabsorption, initially leading to a phase of CSF accumulation.[28] Although tissue plasminogen activator can be demonstrated in posthemorrhagic CSF, fibrinolysis is very inefficient in the CSF, which has low levels of plasminogen and high levels of plasminogen activator inhibitor.[29,30] This potentially reversible obstruction by thrombi may lead to a chronic obliterative, fibrosing arachnoiditis, and subependymal gliosis[31] involving deposition of extracellular matrix proteins such as laminin in the foramina of the fourth ventricle and the subarachnoid space (Fig. 6.4A and B).

Transforming growth factor-β (TGF-β) is involved in the initiation of wound healing and fibrosis and is likely to be one mediator of this process.[32] TGF-β elevates the expression of genes encoding fibronectin, various types of collagen,[33,34] and other extracellular matrix components,[35] and is involved in a number of serious diseases in which there is excessive deposition of collagen, including diabetic nephropathy and cirrhosis.[36] TGF-β1 is stored in platelets and thus provides a store of TGF-β1 for many weeks in the CSF after IVH. TGF-β is elevated in the CSF of adults with hydrocephalus after subarachnoid hemorrhage, and intrathecal administration of TGF-β to mice resulted in hydrocephalus.[37,38] TGF-β1 and TGF-β2 concentrations in CSF from infants with posthemorrhagic ventricular dilation are 10 to 20 times those in nonhemorrhagic CSF and the concentration of TGF-β in CSF is higher in those shunted later.[39] A product of TGF-β, aminoterminal propeptide of type 1 collagen is elevated in CSF from PHVD.[40] Chow and associates have demonstrated elevation of TGF-β2 and nitrated chondroitin sulfate proteoglycans (an extracellular matrix protein) in CSF from preterm infants with posthemorrhagic hydrocephalus.[41]

A rat pup model of PHVD has also provided evidence of the involvement of TGF-β and its downstream products, fibronectin, laminin, and vitronectin.[42,43] Transgenic mice that overexpress TGF-β1 in the central nervous system are born with hydrocephalus.[44] Thus there is a strong possibility of a role for the

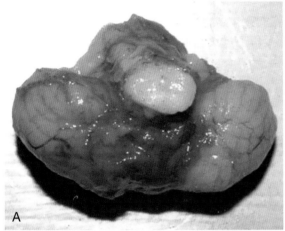

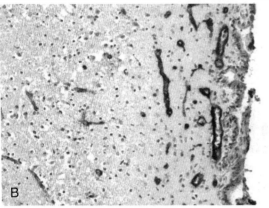

Fig. 6.4 A, Brainstem and cerebellum of an infant with posthemorrhagic ventricular dilation (PHVD) who died at age 2 months. In addition, to the staining from old blood, there are gray strands of connective tissue wrapped around the brainstem. B, Histologic section from the subependymal region of the brain of another infant with PHVD who also died at age 2 months. Immunostaining shows increased perivascular deposition of the extracellular matrix protein laminin.

TGF-βs in the development and/or maintenance of hydrocephalus after ventricular hemorrhage. However, two drugs that inhibit production of TGF-β, pirfenidone and losartan, did not reduce ventricular size or improve neuromotor performance in a rat pup model of PHVD.[45]

Amyloid precursor protein (APP) and L1 cell adhesion molecule (L1CAM) were also noted to be increased in infants with PHVD and were significantly related to fractional anisotropy in the corpus callosum.[46]

Question 7: How Can PHVD Injure White Matter?

Damage to periventricular white matter is probably exacerbated by ischemia due to raised intracranial pressure and parenchymal compression, by oxidative stress due to the generation of free radicals, and by the actions of inflammatory cytokines.

RAISED INTRACRANIAL PRESSURE, PARENCHYMAL COMPRESSION, AND ISCHEMIA

PHVD raises CSF pressure to, on average, three times normal.[16] Fig. 6.3 shows that in an infant with severe PVHD, a decrease can be seen in cerebral blood flow during diastole; when the ICP is increased further there may be absent flow during diastole with impaired cerebral perfusion. A reduction of perfusion of this magnitude raises the risk of ischemic injury.

Maximal ventricular size correlates inversely with cognitive, language, and motor Bayley scores at 2 years of age.[47-49] As some very immature infants can dilate with very modest pressure, these findings may indicate that physical distortion affects periventricular myelination independent of ischemia. Recent diffusion tensor imaging (DTI) studies do support this,[50] especially a recent study using diffusion basis spectrum imaging (DBSI).[51] They were able to show that PHH was associated with diffuse white matter injury, including tract-specific patterns of axonal and myelin injury.

FREE RADICAL–MEDIATED INJURY

Non–protein-bound iron is readily detectable in the CSF of neonates with PHVD.[52] Hemoglobin that enters the CSF releases large amounts of iron, which is likely to exceed the protein-binding capacity of the CSF and lead to the generation of hydroxyl free radicals from hydrogen peroxide via the Fenton reaction. Inder and coworkers[53] demonstrated products of lipid peroxidation in the CSF of infants with periventricular leukomalacia. Further evidence of potential oxidative stress comes from the finding of raised concentrations of hypoxanthine in the CSF of infants with PHVD.[54] Under conditions of ischemia, xanthine dehydrogenase is modified to form xanthine oxidase, which uses oxygen as the electron acceptor.[55] On restoration of cerebral perfusion, xanthine oxidase–mediated oxidation of xanthine and hypoxanthine generates superoxide and hydrogen peroxide, which cause oxidative damage. Oligodendrocyte progenitors, abundant in the periventricular white matter of premature infants, are highly susceptible to oxidative damage.[56] A recent study reported that higher CSF ferritin was significantly associated with larger ventricle size at permanent CSF diversion.[57]

INFLAMMATION

Clinical evidence suggests that inflammation causes damage to immature white matter.[58] The concentration of tumor necrosis factor α, interleukin-1β, interleukin-6, interleukin-8, and interferon-γ are significantly elevated in the CSF of infants with PHVD.[59] Tumor necrosis factor α and interleukin-1β have both been implicated in the development of periventricular leukomalacia,[60] and it seems likely that these proinflammatory cytokines also contribute to white matter damage in PHVD.

LOSS OF WHITE MATTER AND GRAY MATTER

In the rat model of PHVD, there is a significant negative correlation between the extent of ventricular dilatation and the thickness of both the corpus callosum and the frontal cortex.[61] The development of hydrocephalus is associated with a mean reduction in the thickness of the corpus callosum of 48%, and of the frontal cortex of 31%. Loss of white matter is also marked in the lateral periventricular region; loss of myelin and axons is associated with a reduced density of oligodendrocytes.[61] In a small observational study, PHVD was noted to be negatively related to deep gray matter and cerebellar volumes, while white matter ADC values were significantly higher on TEA-MRI, despite early intervention for PHVD in the majority of these infants.[62]

Question 8: What Interventions Have Been Used in PHVD? When Should Intervention Be Started and Is There Evidence of Improved Outcome?

Box 6.1 lists therapeutic interventions that have been used in infants with PHVD.

VENTRICULOPERITONEAL SHUNT SURGERY

Ventriculoperitoneal (VP) shunt surgery is the conventional approach to other types of established

BOX 6.1 THERAPEUTIC INTERVENTIONS THAT HAVE BEEN USED IN INFANTS WITH POSTHEMORRHAGIC HYDROCEPHALUS

- Repeated early lumbar punctures/ventricular taps
- Diuretic drugs to reduce cerebrospinal fluid (CSF) production
- Intraventricular fibrinolytic therapy
- External ventricular drain
- Ventricular reservoir and repeated taps
- Ventriculo-subgaleal shunt
- Third ventriculostomy
- Choroid plexus coagulation
- Ventricular lavage/neuroendoscopic lavage (NEL)
- Ventriculoperitoneal shunt after CSF clears and CSF protein level <1.5 g/L

hydrocephalus. Treatment of PHVD is more difficult than other types of hydrocephalus because the large amount of blood in the ventricles combined with the small size and instability of the patient make an early VP shunt operation impossible. In an early series of 19 infants with PHVD requiring shunt surgery, there were 29 shunt blockages and 12 infections.[63] The risk of shunt blockage was increased if the CSF protein concentration was more than 1.5 g/L at the time of shunt insertion. In a series of 36 infants who underwent shunt placement for PHVD, shunt blockage and infection occurred only in those operated before 35 days of age.[64] There is a considerable complication rate throughout a child's life from VP shunt surgery, and the child might be permanently dependent on the shunt system. A VP shunt is a treatment but not a cure, and the child is vulnerable to shunt dysfunction. Shunt blockage after the cranial sutures have fused can rapidly raise intracranial pressure, resulting in permanent cerebral damage. Sudden blindness and death have been recorded in such circumstances. Repeated shunt revisions are associated with a worsening of neurologic outcome.[65] Shunt infection is another complication that can further injure the developing brain.

OBJECTIVES IN TREATING PHVD

The objectives of treatment for PHVD are as follows:
1. To reduce secondary injury to the brain from pressure, distortion, free radicals, and inflammation.

2. To minimize iatrogenic injury from interventions, especially in those infants in whom PHVD resolves after a period of weeks.
3. To minimize the need for a VP shunt.

When Should Intervention Be Started?

There has been an ongoing debate whether intervention should be initiated based on clinical symptoms (bulging fontanel, splaying sutures, rapid increase in head circumference, sunsetting, apneas, and bradycardia) or based on increasing ventricular width and anterior horn width measured with serial cranial ultrasound. As clinical symptoms occur rather late, due to the presence of a large extracerebral space in the preterm infant, the ventricles are often quite large when symptoms develop. In an observational study, data from three centers were compared.[66] Two Dutch centers started early, based on ultrasound measures and the third center first started intervention following the onset of clinical symptoms. Two-year outcome was significantly better in infants treated before clinical symptoms occurred and more complications due to neurosurgical intervention were noted among the infants treated following development of clinical symptoms. A recent small single-center observational study in 25 infants with PHH showed that a smaller cumulative ventricle size from birth to permanent CSF diversion was associated with larger right hippocampal volumes and improved cognitive, motor, and language outcomes.[67]

A meta-analysis by Lai and colleagues supported these findings and on meta-regression, older age at temporary neurosurgical procedure (TNP) was a significant predictor of conversion to VP shunt and neurodevelopmental impairment.[48]

REPEATED LUMBAR PUNCTURES OR VENTRICULAR TAPS

Repeated lumbar punctures (LPs) were suggested as a way of controlling pressure, preventing progressive ventricular enlargement, and removing some of the red cells and protein from the CSF. Kreusser and associates[68] showed that a minimum of 10 mL/kg needed to be removed for the removal to have a significant effect on ventricular size. In our experience, only a minority of infants with PHVD have consistently communicating PHVD with a sufficient yield of CSF. A policy of repeated early tapping of lumbar or ventricular CSF for PHVD has been tested in four controlled clinical trials.[69] Overall, there was no evidence that this approach reduced the rate of VP shunt surgery or disability, and there was a 7% infection rate among the infants who underwent repeated tapping in the Ventriculomegaly Trial.[3] Performing a few LPs is, however, worth trying as some infants will improve and not need further neurosurgical intervention and in others the LPs will give time to consult the neurosurgeon and plan neurosurgical intervention. However, when the ventricles are very dilated or if there is a discrepancy between the third and fourth ventricles, suggesting blockade of the aqueduct, it is best to proceed directly to a ventricular access device. Ventricular taps are not recommended as they will result in needle tracks.

DRUG TREATMENT TO REDUCE CSF PRODUCTION

Acetazolamide had been in clinical use for benign intracranial hypertension and appeared to have acceptable adverse effects as long as electrolyte and acid-base balances were monitored. Uncontrolled reports were positive about the effect of acetazolamide in PHVD. Experimentally, acetazolamide produced an initial increase in cerebral blood flow mediated by an increase in tissue CO_2 and inhibition of respiratory elimination of CO_2.[70] Clinical investigation of infants with chronic lung disease of prematurity showed that acetazolamide produced an increase in Pco_2.[71] Eventually a large multicenter randomized trial of acetazolamide combined with furosemide (which also reduces CSF production) was carried out. Not only was there no clinical benefit, but the group receiving the combined drug treatment had significantly worse outcome in terms of shunt surgery and death or disability.[72]

INTRAVENTRICULAR FIBRINOLYTIC THERAPY

The idea of injecting a fibrinolytic agent intraventricularly grew out of Pang's experimental PHVD model, in which blood was injected intraventricularly into dogs. In this model, hydrocephalus developed in 80% of subjects, but if urokinase was injected intraventricularly, only 10% demonstrated hydrocephalus.[73] The idea was supported by laboratory work showing that there was weak endogenous fibrinolytic activity in posthemorrhagic CSF and by the relative safety of low-dose fibrinolytic therapy administered locally. A number of small nonrandomized trials of intraventricular streptokinase, urokinase, and tissue plasminogen activator, as well as two small randomized trials, have collectively shown that there is no reduction in VP shunt surgery and there is a risk of secondary intraventricular bleeding in infants receiving these agents.[74]

EXTERNAL VENTRICULAR DRAIN

The insertion of an external ventricular drain is a logical way of providing continuous relief from raised pressure, preventing distortion from ventricular enlargement, and removing protein and red blood cells. This approach has certainly been used in a small number of centers, but to our knowledge it has not been tested in a randomized trial.[75] The concern among neurosurgeons has been the risk of infection from prolonged presence of a ventricular drain. One recent study combined early external ventricular drainage with intermittent intraventricular injections of urokinase (every 3–6 hours) for a period of 14 days.[76] All but three of the 21 infants who were treated like this, did not need a VP shunt and outcome at 36 months was significantly better in the early intervention group. No rebleeds or infections occurred.

TAPPING VIA A VENTRICULAR RESERVOIR (ACCESS DEVICE)

The most widely used approach we have encountered in neonatal units that treat a considerable number of infants with PHVD is the insertion of ventricular access device, for example, an Ommaya reservoir, in those cases in which repeated tapping is necessary to control excessive head enlargement and suspected raised pressure (Fig. 6.5). This approach approximates that used in the standard "arm" of the DRIFT trial and is now, regarded as standard treatment. It is to be recommended to consult the neurosurgeon before infants with PHVD demonstrate excessive head enlargement or signs of raised pressure. Once it becomes obvious that repeated CSF tapping is necessary, the surgically inserted reservoir enables it to be done whenever the need arises but preferably in a tertiary care neonatal unit with pediatric neurosurgeons on site. Complications are not common and the infection rate is between 4% and 8% when the procedure is

performed under hygienic conditions, using gloves, mask, and gown. Wound dehiscence or catheter blockage are rarely seen. Care should be taken to perform the tap slowly at around 1 mL/min or over a 15-minute period. When the ventricular width is reduced too fast, periventricular or subcortical hemorrhages can occur.[77]

The Early v Late Ventricular Intervention Study (ELVIS) trial[78] compared low-threshold intervention (ventricular width over the 97th centile and frontal horn over 6 mm) with high-threshold intervention (ventricular width 4 mm over the 97th centile and frontal horn over 10 mm). One hundred twenty-six infants were randomized. The low threshold group had mean maximum ventricular width 2.8 mm over 97th centile and anterior horn 3 mm over 6 mm, versus ventricular width 4.2 mm over 97th centile and anterior horn 5 mm over 6 mm in the high threshold group. First intervention was, on average, 5 days later in the high threshold group.[78] It is important to point out that both interventions in ELVIS were early, relative to previous trials in which there was no upper limit to ventricular size for eligibility and many of the infants had huge ventricles at entry.

MR imaging at term equivalent age showed lower brain injury scores and smaller ventricles in the low threshold group.[79] At 2 years, the low threshold group had significantly better composite outcome of cerebral palsy, low cognitive score, or death after adjusting for GA and hemorrhage severity.[80] Infants in the low threshold group with a ventriculoperitoneal shunt, had cognitive and motor scores similar to those without a shunt, whereas, in the high threshold group, those with a ventriculoperitoneal shunt had significantly lower scores than those without a ventriculoperitoneal shunt. This is consistent with the hypothesis that late shunting allows more time for pressure and distortion to injure the brain.

Ventriculo-subgaleal Shunt

This procedure involves insertion of a ventricular catheter with a subcutaneous reservoir connected to a distal catheter ending in the subgaleal space. There is usually no valve in a subgaleal shunt. Ventricular fluid can then accumulate outside the skull but under the skin. Absorption of CSF is slow from this site and a

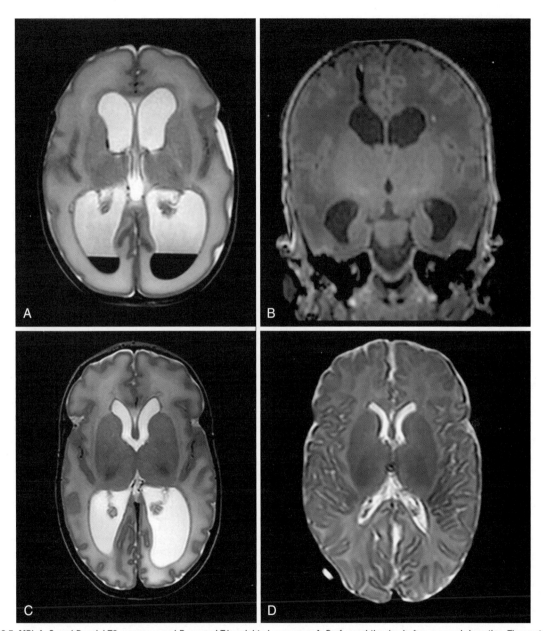

Fig. 6.5 MRI, A, C, and D: axial T2 sequence and B coronal T1 weighted sequence. A, Performed the day before reservoir insertion. The ventricles are enlarged with blood seen in the occipital horns. The signal intensity is increased especially in the occipital lobes. Note the reduced cortical folding and reduced extracerebral space. B, Needle track of the reservoir inserted in the right ventricle. Note a punctate white matter lesion in the left periventricular white matter. C, Performed the day before VP shunt insertion. The occipital horns are still dilated and the signal intensity is still increased especially in the left occipital lobe. D, Fast sequence performed at 4 months of age. The ventricles are no longer dilated and myelination is seen in the posterior limb bilaterally.

marked swelling becomes obvious on one side of the skull. This procedure is seen as an alternative to an Ommaya ventricular reservoir. The advantage is that ventricular drainage and control of intracranial pressure can occur continuously whereas drainage and control of pressure are intermittent with tapping a ventricular reservoir. One advantage of using a reservoir is that the frequency and volume of taps can be increased or decreased according to need. This cannot be done with a subgaleal shunt. The subcutaneous swelling can sometimes interfere with measuring changes in head circumference so interpretation has to allow for this and frequent scans are needed.

Limbrick et al.[81] reviewed 95 infants with PHVD treated either with a ventricular reservoir or a subgaleal shunt. One of 30 subgaleal shunts became infected against 4 of 65 ventricular reservoirs. There was no difference in the proportion requiring a permanent VP shunt. Similar observations were made in a more recent study, with conversion to VP shunt required in 63.5% for subgaleal shunt and 74.0% for ventricular reservoir.[82]

THIRD VENTRICULOSTOMY

Third ventriculostomy is carried out endoscopically and can be a good treatment for other types of hydrocephalus, especially aqueduct stenosis. The endoscope is inserted into the ventricular system and then into the third ventricle. A hole is made in the midline of the floor of the third ventricle, with care to avoid the arteries on either side. This communication between the third ventricle and the subarachnoid space allows CSF to bypass obstruction in the aqueduct and foramina of the fourth ventricle. However, in PHVD, the problem is mainly reabsorption of CSF and is not usually restricted to the aqueduct and fourth ventricle. Experience with third ventriculostomy in PHVD has been limited, and the results disappointing, especially in those who were less than 6 months of age when intervention took place.[83]

CHOROID PLEXUS COAGULATION

Choroid plexus coagulation is carried out endoscopically and is based on most CSF production coming from the choroid plexus within the lateral ventricles and third ventricle. Because the problem with PHVD is primarily failed reabsorption and not overproduction of

CSF, it would seem unlikely that this approach would be successful in PHVD. Choroid plexus coagulation has never been subjected to a controlled trial in PHVD.[84]

Ventricular Lavage

Drainage, irrigation, and fibrinolytic therapy (DRIFT), a form of ventricular lavage, is an approach that grew out of the unsatisfactory results of the preceding treatments and the emerging evidence that free radical injury and inflammation result from intraventricular blood and injure the brain over many weeks. The objectives were to remove as much as possible of the intraventricular blood and to gently decompress the ventricles earlier.

The procedure involves insertion of right frontal and left occipital ventricular catheters. Tissue plasminogen activator (TPA) was injected intraventricularly at a dose 0.5 mg/kg that is insufficient to produce a systemic effect, and it was left for approximately 8 hours. The occipital ventricular catheter was connected to a sterile close ventricular drainage system, and the height of the drainage reservoir was adjusted to keep intracranial pressure below 7 mm Hg. Artificial Cerebrospinal Fluid (Torbay Pharmaceutical Manufacturing Unit) was then pumped into the frontal ventricular catheter at 20 mL/hr with continuous intracranial pressure monitoring. The drainage fluid initially looked like cola but gradually cleared to look like white wine, at which point irrigation was stopped and the catheters were removed. This process commonly took 72 hours but could require up to 7 days.

DRIFT has been tested in a randomized trial that recruited 77 preterm infants with PHVD; 39 received DRIFT and 38 received standard treatment (LP followed by ventricular reservoir to be tapped to control expansion and pressure). There was no reduction in the proportion of either group who underwent surgical shunt placement or died.[85] All survivors were followed up at 2 years corrected age. Of the 39 patients in the DRIFT group, 21 (54%) were severely disabled or dead, compared with 27 of the 38 (71%) in the standard treatment group. Eleven of 35 survivors assessed with the Bayley scale (31%) in the DRIFT group had severe cognitive disability, compared with 19 of 32 (59%) in the standard group.[86] There was significantly more secondary intraventricular bleeding in the DRIFT group, but the bleeding was not associated with increased disability.

At 10 years of age, mean cognitive quotient was 69 in the DRIFT group compared to 54 in the standard group. 21 of 32 (66%) who received DRIFT were alive with no severe cognitive disability compared to only 11 of 30 (37%) in the standard group.[87] This difference in cognitive development (69 vs. 54) corresponds to well over a year, educationally important. This can be seen as proof of principle that ventricular lavage can reduce brain injury. DRIFT is a demanding and invasive procedure requiring close collaboration between neonatologist, intensive care nursing, and neurosurgeon for several days and is probably not suitable for general dissemination.

A simpler method of ventricular lavage, using a neuroendoscope in the operating room has been described in 50 neonates in Berlin with PHVD by Schulz et al.[88] and 46 infants in Seville.[89,90] They lavaged both lateral and the third ventricles with 2 to 3 liters of Ringer's solution in a single session. This technique is being disseminated, as the TROPHY survey in June 2021 reported an average of 3 procedures annually in 22 pediatric neurosurgical centers in 15 different countries.[91] Ventricular lavage can be combined with insertion of a subgaleal shunt or ventricular reservoir in a single session. In most infants, lavage was performed once, but in about 20% a repeat lavage was performed. When a third lavage was needed, septostomy was performed to also clean the contralateral ventricle.[89] This technique was, however, used when the VI was far above the p97 + 4 mm line.[88]

Although there are good grounds for wanting to remove harmful substances in CSF by ventricular lavage, the possibility of also removing necessary substances such as growth factors exists. Injection of stem cells at the end of ventricular lavage offers a possible solution.

Stem Cell Therapy

Using a rat model of IVH, Ahn et al. have shown that intraventricular injection of umbilical cord-derived mesenchymal stem cells reduces PHVD and inflammatory markers while improving myelination and neuromotor function when administered 2 days, but not 7 days, after IVH.[92,93] This impressive effect may be due to upregulation of brain-derived neurotrophic factor (BDNF). This group is now conducting a trial of intraventricular human umbilical cord-derived mesenchymal stem cells in infants within 7 days of diagnosis of grade IV IVH and has found the technique to be safe and well tolerated.[94,95]

Conclusions on Clinical Management

1. Posthemorrhagic hydrocephalus is characterized by inflammation and deposition of extracellular matrix proteins weeks after intraventricular hemorrhage.
2. Frequent cranial ultrasound scanning with measurement of ventricular width, anterior horn, and thalamo-occipital dimensions is necessary for decision making. Fronto-temporal horn ratio can also be used.
3. Raised intracranial pressure, distortion, inflammation, and free radical injury from iron are mechanisms by which periventricular white matter can be progressively injured.
4. Reducing pressure and distortion via lumbar puncture and ventricular reservoir earlier than was previously thought necessary has been shown to improve outcome developmentally and on MR brain imaging. Treatment thresholds of ventricular width over 97th centile, anterior horn over 6 mm, and thalamo-occipital over 25 mm with repeated tapping of 10 mL/kg to bring ventricular measurements back to the 97th centiles are evidence based as in the low threshold group in the ELVIS Trial.
5. Ventricular lavage, in the DRIFT trial, reduced cognitive disability, but is too complicated and lengthy for general practical use. Neuroendoscopic ventricular lavage can be combined with reservoir or subgaleal shunt placement in the operating room, is simpler and can be disseminated.

Areas Where Further Research Is Needed

1. Does combining ventricular lavage with placement of a reservoir or subgaleal shunt improve developmental outcome?
2. Can neuroprotective medication or stem cell therapy early after IVH reduce PHVD and its consequences?

REFERENCES

1. Inder T, Perlman JM, Volpe JJ. Preterm intraventricular hemorrhage/posthemorrhagic hydrocephalus. In: *Neurology of the Newborn*. 6th ed. Philadelphia: WB Saunders; 2018:607-698.
2. Murphy BP, Inder TE, Rooks V, et al. Posthemorrhagic ventricular dilatation in the premature infant: natural history and predictors of outcome. *Arch Dis Child*. 2002;87:F37-F41.
3. Ventriculomegaly Trial Group. Randomised trial of early tapping in neonatal posthaemorrhagic ventricular dilatation. *Arch Dis Child*. 1990;65:3-10.
4. International PHVD Drug Trial Group. International randomised trial of acetazolamide and furosemide in posthaemorrhagic ventricular dilatation. *Lancet*. 1998;352:433-440.
5. Cizmeci MN, de Vries LS, Ly LG, et al. Periventricular hemorrhagic infarction in very preterm infants: characteristic sonographic findings and association with neurodevelopmental outcome at age 2 years. *J Pediatr*. 2020;217:79-85.e1. doi:10.1016/j.jpeds.2019.09.081.
6. Cizmeci MN, Groenendaal F, Liem KD, et al. Randomized Controlled Early versus Late Ventricular Intervention Study in posthemorrhagic ventricular dilatation: outcome at 2 years. *J Pediatr*. 2020;226:28-35.e3. doi:10.1016/j.jpeds.2020.08.014.
7. Law JB, Wood TR, Gogcu S, et al. Intracranial hemorrhage and 2-year neurodevelopmental outcomes in infants born extremely preterm. *J Pediatr*. 2021;238:124-134.e10. doi:10.1016/j.jpeds.2021.06.071.
8. Adams-Chapman I, Hansen NI, Stoll BJ, et al. Neurodevelopmental outcome of extremely low birth weight infants with posthemorrhagic hydrocephalus requiring shunt insertion. *Pediatrics*. 2008;121(5):e1167-e1177.
9. Papile LA, Burstein J, Burstein R, Koffler H. Incidence and evolution of subependymal and intraventricular hemorrhage: a study of infants with birth weights less than 1,500 gm. *J Pediatr*. 1978;92:529-534.
10. Levene M. Measurement of the growth of the lateral ventricle in preterm infants with real-time ultrasound. *Arch Dis Child*. 1981;56:900-904.
11. Davies MW, Swaminathan M, Chuang SL, et al. Reference ranges for linear dimensions of intracranial ventricles in preterm neonates. *Arch Dis Child*. 2000;82:F218-F223.
12. El-Dib M, Limbrick DD Jr, Inder T, et al. Management of posthemorrhagic ventricular dilatation in the infant born preterm. *J Pediatr*. 2020;226:16-27.e3. doi:10.1016/j.jpeds.2020.07.079.
13. Radhakrishnan R, Brown BP, Kralik SF, et al. Frontal occipital and frontal temporal horn ratios: comparison and validation of head ultrasound-derived indexes with MRI and ventricular volumes in infantile ventriculomegaly. *AJR Am J Roentgenol*. 2019;213(4):925-931. doi:10.2214/AJR.19.21261.
14. Leijser LM, Scott JN, Roychoudhury S, et al. Post-hemorrhagic ventricular dilatation: inter-observer reliability of ventricular size measurements in extremely preterm infants. *Pediatr Res*. 2021;90(2):403-410. doi:10.1038/s41390-020-01245-0.
15. de Vries LS, Groenendaal F, Liem KD, et al. Treatment thresholds for intervention in posthaemorrhagic ventricular dilation: a randomised controlled trial. *Arch Dis Child Fetal Neonatal Ed*. 2019;104(1):F70-F75.
16. Kaiser A, Whitelaw A. Cerebrospinal fluid pressure during posthemorrhagic ventricular dilatation in newborn infants. *Arch Dis Child*. 1985;60:920-923.
17. Ingram MC, Huguenard AL, Miller BA, Chern JJ. Poor correlation between head circumference and cranial ultrasound findings in premature infants with intraventricular hemorrhage.

J Neurosurg Pediatr. 2014;14(2):184-189. doi:10.3171/2014.5.PEDS13602.
18. Dubowitz L, Dubowitz V, Mercuri E. *The Neurological Assessment of the Preterm and Full-Term Newborn Infant*. 2nd ed. London: MacKeith Press; 1999.
19. Quinn MW, Ando Y, Levene MI. Cerebral arterial and venous flow-velocity measurements in post-haemorrhagic ventricular dilatation. *Dev Med Child Neurol*. 1992;34:863-869.
20. Taylor GA, Madsen JR. Neonatal hydrocephalus: hemodynamic response to fontanelle compression: correlation with intracranial pressure and need for shunt placement. *Radiology*. 1996;201:685-689.
21. De Vries LS, Pierrat V, Minami T, Smet M, Casaer P. The role of short latency somatosensory evoked responses in infants with rapidly progressive ventricular dilatation. *Neuropediatrics*. 1990;21(3):136-139.
22. Olischar M, Klebermass K, Hengl B, et al. Cerebrospinal fluid drainage in posthaemorrhagic ventricular dilatation leads to improvement in amplitude-integrated electroencephalographic activity. *Acta Paediatr*. 2009;98:1002-1009.
23. Norooz F, Urlesberger B, Giordano V, et al. Decompressing posthaemorrhagic ventricular dilatation significantly improves regional cerebral oxygen saturation in preterm infants. *Acta Paediatr*. 2015;104(7):663-669.
24. Kochan, M, McPadden J, Bass WT, et al. Changes in cerebral oxygenation in preterm infants with progressive posthemorrhagic ventricular dilatation. *Pediatr Neurol*. 2017;73:57-63.
25. June A, Heck T, Shah TA, Vazifedan T, Bass WT. Decreased cerebral oxygenation in premature infants with progressive posthemorrhagic ventricular dilatation may help with timing of intervention. *Am J Perinatol*. October 21, 2021. doi:10.1055/s-0041-1736533.
26. Luyt K, Jary SL, Lea CL, et al. Drainage, irrigation and fibrinolytic therapy (DRIFT) for posthaemorrhagic ventricular dilatation: 10-year follow-up of a randomized controlled trial. *Arch Dis Child Fetal Neonatal Ed*. 2020;105(5):466-473.
27. Inder TE, de Vries LS, Ferriero DM, et al. Neuroimaging of the preterm brain: review and recommendations. *J Pediatr*. 2021;237:276-287.e4. doi:10.1016/j.jpeds.2021.06.014.
28. Hill A, Shackelford GD, Volpe JJ. A potential mechanism of pathogenesis for early post-hemorrhagic hydrocephalus in the premature newborn. *Pediatrics*. 1984;73:19-21.
29. Whitelaw A, Mowinckel MC, Abildgaard U. Low levels of plasminogen in cerebrospinal fluid after intraventricular haemorrhage: a limiting factor for clot lysis? *Acta Paediatr*. 1995;84:933-936.
30. Hansen A, Whitelaw A, Lapp C, Brugnara C. Cerebrospinal fluid plasminogen activator inhibitor-1: a prognostic factor in posthaemorrhagic hydrocephalus. *Acta Paediatr*. 1997;86:995-998.
31. Larroche JC. Posthemorrhagic hydrocephalus in infancy. *Biol Neonate*. 1972;20:287-299.
32. Beck LS, Chen TL, Amman AJ, et al. Accelerated healing of ulcer wounds in the rabbit ear by recombinant human transforming growth factor beta-1. *Growth Factors*. 1990;2:273-282.
33. Ignotz RA, Massague J. Transforming growth factor beta stimulates the expression of fibronectin and collagen and their incorporation into the extracellular matrix. *J Biol Chem*. 1986;261:4337-4345.
34. Roberts AB, Sporn MB, Assoian RK, et al. Transforming growth factor type β: rapid induction of fibrosis and angiogenesis in vivo and stimulation of collagen formation in vitro. *Proc Natl Acad Sci U S A*. 1986;83:4167-4171.

35. Border WA, Ruoslahti E. Transforming growth factor-beta 1 induces extracellular matrix formation in glomerulonephritis. *Cell Differ Dev.* 1990;32:425-431.

36. Castilla A, Prieto J, Fausto N. Transforming growth factors beta 1 and alpha in chronic liver disease. Effects of interferon alfa therapy. *N Engl J Med.* 1991;324:933-940.

37. Kitazawa K, Tada T. Elevation of transforming growth factor beta-1 level in cerebrospinal fluid of patients with communicating hydrocephalus after subarachnoid hemorrhage. *Stroke.* 1994;25:1400-1404.

38. Tada T, Kanaji M, Kobayashi S. Induction of communicating hydrocephalus in mice by intrathecal injection of human recombinant transforming growth factor beta-1. *J Neuroimmunol.* 1994;50:153-158.

39. Whitelaw A, Christie S, Pople I. Transforming growth factor β-1: a possible signal molecule for post-hemorrhagic hydrocephalus? *Pediatr Res.* 1999;46:576-580.

40. Heep A, Bartmann P, Stoffel-Wagner B, et al. Cerebrospinal fluid obstruction and malabsorption in human neonatal hydrocephaly. *Childs Nerv Syst.* 2006;22:1249-1255.

41. Chow LC, Soliman A, Zandian M, et al. Accumulation of transforming growth factor-beta2 and nitrated chondroitin sulfate proteoglycans in cerebrospinal fluid correlates with poor neurologic outcome in preterm hydrocephalus. *Biol Neonate.* 2005;88:1-11.

42. Cherian SS, Love S, Silver IA, et al. Posthemorrhagic ventricular dilation in the neonate: development and characterization of a rat model. *J Neuropathol Exp Neurol.* 2003;62:292-303.

43. Cherian S, Thoresen M, Silver IA, et al. Transforming growth factor-betas in a rat model of neonatal posthaemorrhagic hydrocephalus. *Neuropathol Appl Neurobiol.* 2004;30:585-600.

44. Wyss-Coray T, Feng L, Masliah E, et al. Increased central nervous system production of extracellular matrix components and development of hydrocephalus in transgenic mice overexpressing transforming growth factor-beta 1. *Am J Pathol.* 1995; 147:53-67.

45. Aquilina K, Hobbs C, Tucker A, et al. Do drugs that block transforming growth factor beta reduce posthaemorrhagic ventricular dilatation in a neonatal rat model? *Acta Paediatr.* 2008; 97:1181-1186.

46. Morales DM, Smyser CD, Han RH, et al. Tract-specific relationships between cerebrospinal fluid biomarkers and periventricular white matter in posthemorrhagic hydrocephalus of prematurity. *Neurosurgery.* 2021;88(3):698-706. doi:10.1093/neuros/nyaa466.

47. Srinivasakumar P, Limbrick D, Munro R, et al. Posthemorrhagic ventricular dilatation-impact on early neurodevelopmental outcome. *Am J Perinatol.* 2013;30:207-214.

48. Lai GY, Chu-Kwan W, Westcott AB, Kulkarni AV, Drake JM, Lam SK. Timing of temporizing neurosurgical treatment in relation to shunting and neurodevelopmental outcomes in posthemorrhagic ventricular dilatation of prematurity: a meta-analysis. *J Pediatr.* 2021;234:54-64.e20. doi:10.1016/j.jpeds.2021.01.030.

49. El-Dib M, Limbrick DD Jr, Inder T, et al. Management of posthemorrhagic ventricular dilatation in the infant born preterm. *J Pediatr.* 2020;226:16-27.e3. doi:10.1016/j.jpeds.2020.07.079.

50. Nieuwets A, Cizmeci MN, Groenendaal F, et al. Post-hemorrhagic ventricular dilatation affects white matter maturation in extremely preterm infants. *Pediatr Res.* August 26, 2021. doi:10.1038/s41390-021-01704-2.

51. Isaacs AM, Neil JJ, McAllister JP, et al. Microstructural periventricular white matter injury in post-hemorrhagic ventricular dilatation. *Neurology.* 2021;98(4):e364-e375. doi:10.1212/WNL.0000000000013080.

52. Savman K, Nilsson UA, Blennow M, et al. Non-protein-bound iron is elevated in cerebrospinal fluid from preterm infants with posthemorrhagic ventricular dilatation. *Pediatr Res.* 2001;49:208-212.

53. Inder T, Mocatta T, Darlow B, et al. Elevated free radical products in the cerebrospinal fluid of VLBW infants with cerebral white matter injury. *Pediatr Res.* 2002;52:213-218.

54. Bejar R, Saugstad OD, James H, Gluck L. Increased hypoxanthine concentrations in cerebrospinal fluid of infants with hydrocephalus. *J Pediatr.* 1983;103:44-48.

55. Nishino T, Tamura I. The mechanism of conversion of xanthine dehydrogenase to oxidase and the role of the enzyme in reperfusion injury. *Adv Exp Med Biol.* 1991;309A:327-333.

56. Back SA, Luo NL, Borenstein NS, et al. Late oligodendrocyte progenitors coincide with the developmental window of vulnerability for human perinatal white matter injury. *J Neurosci.* 2001;21:1302-1312.

57. Strahle JM, Mahaney KB, Morales DM, et al. Longitudinal CSF iron pathway proteins in posthemorrhagic hydrocephalus: associations with ventricle size and neurodevelopmental outcomes. *Ann Neurol.* 2021;90(2):217-226. doi:10.1002/ana.26133.

58. Leviton A, Paneth N, Reuss ML, et al. Maternal infection, fetal inflammatory response, and brain damage in very low birth weight infants. *Pediatr Res.* 1999;46:566-575.

59. Savman K, Blennow M, Hagberg H, et al. Cytokine responses in cerebrospinal fluid from preterm infants with posthaemorrhagic ventricular dilatation. *Acta Paediatr.* 2002;91:1357-1363.

60. Kadhim H, Tabarki B, Verellen G, et al. Inflammatory cytokines in the pathogenesis of periventricular leukomalacia. *Neurology.* 2001;56:1278-1284.

61. Cherian S, Whitelaw A, Thoresen M, Love S. The pathogenesis of neonatal post-hemorrhagic hydrocephalus. *Brain Pathol.* 2004;14:305-311.

62. Brouwer MJ, de Vries LS, Kersbergen KJ, et al. Effects of posthemorrhagic ventricular dilatation in the preterm infant on brain volumes and white matter diffusion variables at term-equivalent age. *J Pediatr.* 2016;168:41-49.e1.

63. Hislop JE, Dubowitz LM, Kaiser AM, et al. Outcome of infants shunted for post-haemorrhagic ventricular dilatation. *Dev Med Child Neurol.* 1988;30:451-456.

64. Taylor AG, Peter JC. Advantages of delayed VP shunting in post-haemorrhagic hydrocephalus seen in low-birth-weight infants. *Childs Nerv Syst.* 2001;17:328-333.

65. Tuli S. Risk factors for repeated cerebrospinal shunt failures in pediatric patients with hydrocephalus. *J Neurosurg.* 2000;92:31-38.

66. Leijser LM, Miller SP, van Wezel-Meijler G, et al. Posthemorrhagic ventricular dilatation in preterm infants: when best to intervene? *Neurology.* 2018;90(8):e698-e706. doi:10.1212/WNL.0000000000004984.

67. Paturu M, Triplett RL, Thukral S, et al. Does ventricle size contribute to cognitive outcomes in posthemorrhagic hydrocephalus? Role of early definitive intervention. *J Neurosurg Pediatr.* October 15, 2021. doi:10.3171/2021.4.PEDS212.

68. Kreusser KL, Tarby TJ, Kovnar E, et al. Serial lumbar punctures for at least temporary amelioration of neonatal posthemorrhagic hydrocephalus. *Pediatrics.* 1985;75:719-724.

69. Whitelaw A. Repeated lumbar or ventricular punctures in newborns with intraventricular hemorrhage. *Cochrane Database Syst Rev.* 2001;1:CD000216.

70. Thoresen M, Whitelaw A. Effect of acetazolamide on cerebral blood flow velocity and CO2 elimination in normotensive and hypotensive newborn piglets. *Biol Neonate*. 1990;58:200-207.

71. Cowan F, Whitelaw A. Acute effects of acetazolamide on cerebral blood flow velocity and pCO2 in the newborn infant. *Acta Paediatr Scand*. 1991;80:22-27.

72. Whitelaw A, Kennedy CR, Brion LP. Diuretic therapy for newborn infants with posthemorrhagic ventricular dilatation. *Cochrane Database Syst Rev*. 2001;2:CD002270.

73. Pang D, Sclabassi RJ, Horton JA. Lysis of intraventricular blood clot with urokinase in a canine model: part 3. Effects of intraventricular urokinase on clot lysis and posthemorrhagic hydrocephalus. *Neurosurgery*. 1986;19:553-572.

74. Whitelaw A, Odd DE. Intraventricular streptokinase after intraventricular hemorrhage in newborn infants. *Cochrane Database Syst Rev*. 2007;4:CD000498.

75. Berger A, Weninger M, Reinprecht A, et al. Long-term experience with subcutaneously tunneled external ventricular drainage in preterm infants. *Childs Nerv Syst*. 2000;16:103-109.

76. Park YS, Kotani Y, Kim TK, et al. Efficacy and safety of intraventricular fibrinolytic therapy for post-intraventricular hemorrhagic hydrocephalus in extreme low birth weight infants: a preliminary clinical study. *Childs Nerv Syst*. 2021;37(1):69-79. doi:10.1007/s00381-020-04766-5.

77. Cizmeci MN, de Vries LS, Tataranno ML, et al. Intraparenchymal hemorrhage after serial ventricular reservoir taps in neonates with hydrocephalus and association with neurodevelopmental outcome at 2 years of age. *J Neurosurg Pediatr*. 2021:1-8. doi:10.3171/2021.6.PEDS21120.

78. de Vries LS, Groenendaal F, Liem KD, et al. Treatment thresholds for intervention in posthaemorrhagic ventricular dilation: a randomised controlled trial. *Arch Dis Child Fetal Neonatal Ed*. 2019;104(1):F70-F75. doi:10.1136/archdischild-2017-31420659.

79. Cizmeci MN, Khalili N, Claessens NHP, et al. Assessment of brain injury and brain volumes after posthemorrhagic ventricular dilatation: a nested substudy of the randomized controlled ELVIS Trial. *J Pediatr*. 2019;208:191-197.

80. Cizmeci MN, Groenendaal F, Liem KD, et al. Randomized controlled early versus late ventricular intervention study in posthemorrhagic ventricular dilatation: outcome at 2 years. *J Pediatr*. 2020;226:28-35.e3.

81. Limbrick DD Jr, Mathur A, Johnston JM, et al. Neurosurgical treatment of progressive posthemorrhagic ventricular dilation in preterm infants: a 10-year single-institution study. *J Neurosurg Pediatr*. 2010;6(3):224-230.

82. Wellons JC, Shannon CN, Holubkov R, et al. Shunting outcomes in posthemorrhagic hydrocephalus: results of a Hydrocephalus Clinical Research Network prospective cohort study. *J Neurosurg Pediatr*. 2017;20(1):19-29. doi:10.3171/2017.1.PEDS16496.

83. Zaben M, Manivannan S, Sharouf F, et al. The efficacy of endoscopic third ventriculostomy in children 1 year of age or younger: a systematic review and meta-analysis. *Eur J Paediatr Neurol*. 2020;26:7-14.

84. Pople IK, Edwards RJ, Aquilina K. Endoscopic methods of hydrocephalus treatment. *Neurosurg Clin N Am*. 2001;12:719-735.

85. Whitelaw A, Evans D, Carter M, et al. Randomized clinical trial of prevention of hydrocephalus after intraventricular hemorrhage in preterm infants: brain-washing versus tapping fluid. *Pediatrics*. 2007;119:e1071-e1078.

86. Whitelaw A, Jary S, Kmita G, et al. Randomized trial of drainage, irrigation and fibrinolytic therapy for premature infants with posthemorrhagic ventricular dilatation: developmental outcome at 2 years. *Pediatrics*. 2010;125:e852-e858.

87. Luyt K, Jary SL, Lea CL, et al. Drainage, irrigation and fibrinolytic therapy (DRIFT) for posthaemorrhagic ventricular dilatation: 10-year follow-up of a randomized controlled trial. *Arch Dis Child Fetal Neonatal Ed*. 2020;105(5):466-473.

88. Schulz M, Bührer C, Pohl-Schickinger A, et al. Neuroendoscopic lavage for the treatment of intraventricular hemorrhage and hydrocephalus in neonates. *J Neurosurg Pediatr*. 2014;13(6):626-635.

89. Tirado-Caballero J, Rivero-Garvia M, Arteaga-Romero F, et al. Neuroendoscopic lavage for the management of posthemorrhagic hydrocephalus in preterm infants: safety, effectivity, and lessons learned. *J Neurosurg Pediatr*. 2020;15:1-10.

90. Tirado-Caballero J, Herreria-Franco J, Rivero-Garvía M, et al. Technical nuances in neuroendoscopic lavage for germinal matrix hemorrhage in preterm infants: twenty tips and pearls after more than one hundred procedures. *Pediatr Neurosurg*. 2021;56(4):392-400. doi:10.1159/000516183.

91. Thomale UW, Auer C, Spennato P, et al. TROPHY registry-status report. *Childs Nerv Syst*. June 29, 2021. doi:10.1007/s00381-021-05258-w. Epub ahead of print.

92. Park WS, Sung SI, Ahn SY, et al. Optimal timing of mesenchymal stem cell therapy for neonatal intraventricular hemorrhage. *Cell Transplant*. 2016;25(6):1131-1144.

93. Ahn SY, Chang YS, Sung DK, et al. Pivotal role of brain derived neurotrophic factor secreted by mesenchymal stem cells in severe intraventricular hemorrhage in the newborn rats. *Cell Transplant*. 2017;26(1):145-150.

94. Ahn SY, Chang YS, Park WS. Stem cells for neonatal brain disorders. *Neonatology*. 2016;109(4):377-383.

95. Ahn SY, Chang YS, Sung SI, Park WS. Mesenchymal stem cells for severe intraventricular hemorrhage in preterm infants: Phase I Dose-Escalation Clinical Trial. *Stem Cells Transl Med*. 2018;7(12):847-856.

Recent Trials for Hypoxic-Ischemic Encephalopathy: Extending Hypothermia to Infants Not Previously Studied

Lina Chalak and Abbot R. Laptook

Chapter Outline

Key Points

- Hypothermia remains the sole therapy for evolving HIE that is associated with a significant reduction in death or disability.
- A longer duration of cooling or a lower temperature for cooling when treating hypoxic-ischemic encephalopathy is not recommended as it can be associated with harm.
- Rewarming is associated with an increase in electrographic seizures that is associated with worse neurodevelopmental outcomes.
- Cooling on transport is effective when performed with a device that can control core temperature.
- There is little data to indicate benefit from hypothermia for hypoxic-ischemic encephalopathy among infants with a mild encephalopathy, preterm infants, or infants in low or middle-income countries.

Introduction

Therapeutic hypothermia (TH) is an effective therapy for neonatal encephalopathy when the likelihood of a hypoxic-ischemic origin is high. Multiple randomized trials have demonstrated that relatively small reductions in core temperature either alone, or in combination with reduced head temperature, reduced death or disability at 18 months.[1-6] The Cochrane metaanalysis indicates that TH reduced death or major neurodevelopmental disability in survivors from 61% in non-cooled infants compared with 46% in infants treated with hypothermia, yielding a risk ratio of 0.75 (95% confidence interval [CI] 0.68–0.83), along with decreased death from 34% to 25% (risk ratio 0.75, 95% CI 0.64–0.88), and decreased long term disability from 24.9% to 19.2% (risk ratio 0.77, 95% CI 0.63–0.94).[7] Neuroprotective effects of TH persisted even at 6 to 7 years.[8,9] Given the beneficial effects of hypothermia, the Committee on the Fetus and Newborn of the

American Academy of Pediatrics has provided an overview of the available data and expectations for centers that provide this therapy.[11] The importance of this therapy extends beyond the benefits provided to infants and their families; it signifies that hypoxic-ischemic brain injury is modifiable (Fig. 7.1) and has accelerated testing other potential neuroprotective interventions either with or without TH.[10]

It has been almost two decades since TH has become the standard treatment to treat moderate to severe neonatal encephalopathy of hypoxic-ischemic origin, a masterpiece of translational research which remains the single effective therapy. However, questions remain regarding whether hypothermia treatment can be improved and whether it can be extended to other patient cohorts, such as preterm infants, infants with mild encephalopathy, and infants born in low- and middle-income countries. This updated review addresses the preclinical and clinical evidence behind these questions.

Hypothermia regimens have multiple components: induction, maintenance, and rewarming. Induction represents the time from initiation of cooling to reaching target temperature; maintenance represents the duration of keeping the infant at the target temperature; and rewarming represents the reestablishment of a normothermic temperature. The initial trials of hypothermia[1-6] used remarkably similar cooling regimens. Specifically, the age of initiation was always less than 6 hours after birth, the extent of temperature reduction was 33.5°C for whole-body cooling and 34.5°C for head combined with body cooling, the duration of cooling was 72 hours, and the rate of rewarming was 0.5°C/hr. The similarity in hypothermia regimens facilitated metaanalyses of multiple trials to provide more accurate estimates of patient outcomes.[7] The only major component of cooling regimens that differed among the initial trials was the mode of cooling: whole-body versus head with body cooling. Metaanalysis indicated that outcomes are similar irrespective of the mode of cooling.[7]

Rationale for Further Investigations of Therapeutic Hypothermia

There are several justifications to perform further studies of hypothermia.[1-6] First, the Cochrane metaanalysis indicated that 46% of infants treated with hypothermia continue to either die or are diagnosed with moderate or severe disability.[7] Data from the National Institute of Child Health and Human Development (NICHD) Neonatal Research Network (NRN), Optimizing Cooling Trial enrolled a more recent cohort of infants with moderate to severe hypoxic-ischemic encephalopathy (HIE)

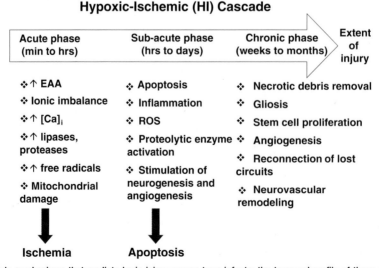

Fig. 7.1 There are multiple mechanisms that mediate brain injury among term infants; the temporal profile of these mechanisms overlaps but extends for periods from the initial hours to weeks following a hypoxic-ischemic event.

and reported that death or disability occurred in 29%.[1] Even though clinicians and NICUs have more experience caring for infants with HIE, care practices continue to evolve and outcomes have improved over the last decade, there is still much room for improvement in outcomes.[2] Clearly, further investigations of hypothermia are needed in that it was studied in a specific group of newborns—that is, those with a diagnosis of presumed hypoxia-ischemia presenting at less than 6 hours of age and with a gestational age of at least 36 weeks in high-income countries. These trials did not address other cohorts of newborns (preterm, mild encephalopathy, or cooling in low-resource countries).[3,54-56]

This chapter addresses important gaps concerning the use of TH for HIE. Some of the gaps have been addressed, some are currently under study, and some remain to be investigated.

What Is the Optimal Temperature and Duration for Therapeutic Hypothermia?

The depth of temperature reduction used in the first series of hypothermia trials[1-6] was extrapolated from preclinical investigation and pilot studies in newborns. Recognition that small changes in brain temperature modified the extent of hypoxic-ischemic brain injury in adult animals[13] prompted perinatal animal investigations to examine the effects of depth and duration of "modest hypothermia" at varying times after brain hypoxia-ischemia. Modest hypothermia encompassed a range of temperature reductions from as little as 2°C to as much as 5°C using newborn swine, rat pups, and fetal sheep.[14-18] This range reflected concerns regarding a possible trade-off between the potential benefit of lower temperature and adverse effects of hypothermia, which increase with greater reductions in core temperature.[19] The optimal temperature to use for hypothermic intervention in clinical trials was not known but was guided by existing animal data and the assessment of incremental reductions in core temperature in pilot human studies of head cooling combined with body cooling[20,21] and whole-body cooling.[22] Based on this body of work, clinical trials of head cooling combined with body cooling and whole-body cooling alone were conducted at a rectal temperature of 34.5°C and an esophageal temperature of 33.5°C, respectively.[1,2]

The optimal duration of hypothermia was also uncertain when the first series of clinical trials of hypothermia were undertaken in newborn infants.[1-6] Available data were derived primarily from adult animals and indicated that increasing the duration of hypothermia reduced brain injury compared with shorter cooling intervals.[23-25] Although not studied as extensively in newborn animals, 21-day-old rat pups subjected to hypoxia-ischemia had reduced brain injury when cooling was extended to 72 hours compared with 6 hours.[26] In preparation for clinical trials, pilot studies of hypothermia after brain ischemia in fetal sheep by Gunn et al. indicated rebound epileptiform activity when cooling was stopped after 48 hours but not if cooling was continued for 72 hours.[17] Based on these studies, clinical trials of head cooling with mild body cooling and whole-body cooling used a 72-hour cooling intervention.[27,28]

In response to these knowledge gaps, the NICHD NRN conducted a randomized clinical trial of cooling to a lower temperature and for a longer duration (Optimizing Cooling Trial, NCT 01192776).[29] The Optimizing Cooling Trial was a randomized 2 × 2 factorial design performed at 18 centers to determine if longer cooling (120 hours), deeper cooling (32.0°C), or both initiated before 6 hours of age are superior to cooling at 33.5°C for 72 hours among infants of at least 36 weeks' gestation with moderate or severe HIE. The esophageal profiles of each group are plotted in Fig. 7.2 demonstrating the different interventions. The primary outcome was death or disability at 18 to 22 months adjusted for center and level of encephalopathy. The trial was closed to patient enrollment after 364 of a planned 726 infants were enrolled based on recommendations of an independent Data Safety Monitoring Committee due to a trend of higher deaths with longer and deeper cooling and futility. In-hospital mortality rates for cooling of 72 compared with 120 hours' duration were 11% and 16%, respectively (adjusted risk ratio [aRR] 1.37, 95% CI 0.92–2.04). In-hospital mortality rates for cooling at 33.5°C compared with 32.0°C were 12% and 16%, respectively (aRR 1.24, 95% CI 0.69–2.25). Although not statistically different, the risk ratio and boundary of the 95% CI suggest that longer cooling maybe associated with an increase in mortality. Cooling for 120 hours was associated with more arrhythmias, anuria, and a

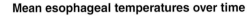

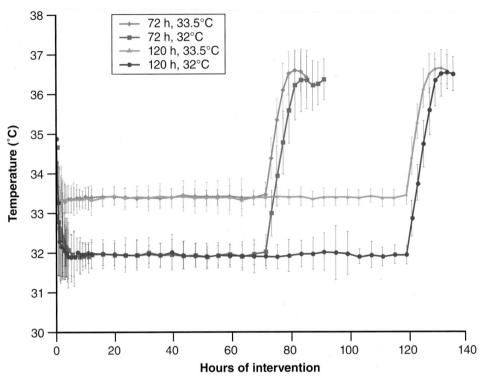

Fig. 7.2 Infants who met criteria for therapeutic hypothermia (biochemical and/or clinical criteria followed by moderate or severe encephalopathy on neurologic examination) were randomly assigned to one of four groups in a factorial design to study lower or longer durations of hypothermia. The temporal profile of esophageal temperature is plotted for infants assigned to cooling of 33.5°C for 72 hours, 33.5°C for 120 hours, 32.0°C for 72 hours, and 32.0°C for 120 hours.

longer length of hospital stay compared with 72 hours of cooling, whereas cooling to 32.0°C was associated with a higher use of inhaled nitric oxide, extracorporeal membrane oxygenation, longer use of supplemental oxygen, and a higher incidence of bradycardia compared with cooling to 33.5°C. The results at 18-month follow-up confirmed the concern for futility; specifically, death or disability occurred in 32% of infants cooled for 72 hours and 32% for infants cooled for 120 hours (aRR 0.92, 95% CI 0.68–1.25), and 32% of infants cooled to 33.5°C and 31% for infants cooled to 32.0°C (aRR 0.92, 95% CI 0.68–1.26).[30]

The results of this trial indicate that among infants of at least 36 weeks' gestation with HIE, longer cooling was not superior to 72 hours of cooling, and deeper cooling was not superior to cooling to 33.5°C. The Optimizing Cooling Trial supports the continued

practice of whole-body hypothermia at 33.5°C for 72 hours and drifts from this practice could be associated with increased mortality and morbidity.

Does Rewarming Affect Neuroprotection?[12]

The clinical guidelines and all trials to date recommend that infants be rewarmed at a rate of 0.5°C per hour, but this is not based on strong evidence.[4] The effect of rewarming on seizures and neurodevelopmental outcome has not been well studied. There are no randomized controlled trials investigating the optimal rate of rewarming after TH for infants with HIE. The rewarming regimen was uniformly set in all neonatal hypothermia trials to increase the core body temperature by 0.5°C per hour until normothermia is achieved despite the absence of data to support such a regimen.[5,6] The importance of monitoring for seizures during rewarming is underscored by studies demonstrating that even brief increases in brain temperature following ischemia increase neuronal injury.[7,8] Rebound electrical seizures during rewarming after 72 hours of hypothermia have been reported in clinical practice.[9-11]

The Systematic Monitoring of EEG in Asphyxiated Newborns during Rewarming after Hypothermia Therapy (SMaRT) study is a nested cohort of the Optimizing Cooling trial. SMaRT used continuous recordings of amplitude-integrated electroencephalogram (aEEG) with a validated raw EEG method of visual confirmation to assess the frequency of electrographic seizures before and during rewarming initiated at 72 hours versus 120 hours.[12] Key study findings were twice higher odds of electrographic seizures during rewarming after 72 hours of TH which was associated with a significantly higher risk of the composite outcome of death or moderate to severe disability at 18 to 22 months of age.[12]

The study showed that 23% of infants had seizures during rewarming and that a longer duration of cooling to 120 hours did not reduce the incidence of seizures. Most concerning was the increased relative risk of abnormal 18 to 22 months outcomes in infants who had seizures during rewarming even after adjusting for baseline severity of encephalopathy, as well as for center. These observations along with other studies[13,14] point to the need to monitor and treat seizures that occur during rewarming.

Potentially, rewarming could reactivate inflammatory responses that have been suppressed during hypothermia. Alternatively, rewarming could also lead to reversal of hypothermic suppression of oxidative stress and excitotoxin release.[15,16] There is no data, however, to demonstrate that rewarming at a slower rate may modify the increase in seizures noted with rewarming at 0.5°C/hr. Furthermore, there is no consensus among studies on what constitutes a "rapid" or "slow" rate of rewarming in preclinical models which largely depends on the species, their baseline temperature and cooling.[4] Future clinical translational studies following the recent SMaRT publication[12] should evaluate the effects of different rates of rewarming.

How Late Can Hypothermia Be Initiated?

The time of initiation of hypothermia represents the component of a hypothermia regimen studied in the most systematic fashion in preclinical investigations. Gunn et al. performed a series of fetal sheep studies where 30 minutes of brain ischemia was followed by 72 hours of hypothermia (cooling cap positioned on the fetal head in utero) initiated at 1.5, 5.5, and 8.5 hours following ischemia.[17,31,32] A neuronal loss score in different brain regions was assessed at 48 hours after completion of hypothermia and demonstrated that the extent of neuroprotection was time sensitive. Earlier cooling was neuroprotective (initiation at 1.5 more so than 5.5 hours) but later cooling (initiation at 8.5 hours) was not. These experiments provided the rationale for initiation of cooling within 6 hours of birth in the first series of human cooling trials.[1-6] These trials, however, could not determine if initiation of cooling earlier in the 6-hour window is more effective since the vast majority of enrolled infants had hypothermia initiated between 4 and 5 hours. In the TOBY trial, there was a trend for a reduction in the primary outcome (survival with neurodevelopmental disability) among infants randomized prior to 4 hours (relative risk 0.77, 95% CI 0.44–1.04) in contrast to infants randomized between 4 and 6 hours after birth (relative risk 0.95, 95% CI 0.72–1.25).[17] A more recent single-center retrospective cohort analysis of hypothermia reported that initiation of cooling at 3 hours or earlier is associated with higher psychomotor developmental scores using the Bayley II Scales of Infant Development compared with cooling initiated after 3 hours.[33] Despite the lack of direct evidence from clinical trials, many embrace the goal of initiating TH as early as possible after birth for optimal effectiveness.[18]

Although these data suggest that studying initiation of hypothermia after 6 hours of age would be of lesser benefit, there is strong biologic and clinical rationale for further investigation. Even when cooling was initiated at 8.5 hours after ischemia in fetal sheep, a time when seizures occur in this model, there are areas of the brain that have reduced neuronal loss with hypothermia.[19] Furthermore, data from animal models may not be readily extrapolated to newborns. Specifically, a well-defined hypoxic-ischemia event in terms of severity, duration, and timing relative to an intervention in a laboratory setting, may be considerably different from scenarios encountered in neonatal intensive care units. A therapeutic window of 6 hours in fetal sheep is established, but there is no information of the duration of the therapeutic window in newborns with HIE because all cooling trials initiated hypothermia by 6 hours.[7] Whether in utero preconditioning events prolong the therapeutic window is unknown.[34,35] Enrollment in clinical trials of hypothermia at less than 6 hours of age assumes that hypoxic-ischemic events occur proximate to delivery. However, precise timing of hypoxic-ischemia in utero among newborns with HIE may be inaccurate in the absence of a sentinel event, and prior trials likely enrolled infants beyond 6 hours from hypoxia-ischemia. Other important considerations are births in rural communities remote from centers that provide hypothermia, evolution of encephalopathy after 6 hours of age, and late recognition of encephalopathy. All these variables may limit application of hypothermia within a putative narrow therapeutic window of 6 hours following birth.

Given the knowledge gap concerning initiation of hypothermia beyond 6 hours, the NRN has conducted a randomized trial to obtain an unbiased estimate of the probability of benefit or harm from "late" initiation of hypothermia. https://clinicaltrials.gov/ct2/show/NCT00614744 (Fig. 7.3).[67]

Infants at least 36 weeks of gestational age with moderate or severe HIE assessed at or after 6 hours up to 24 hours of age were randomly assigned to an esophageal temperature of 33.5°C maintained for 96 hours, compared with an esophageal temperature maintained at 37.0°C to determine the risk of death or disability at 18 months. A major challenge for this trial was determination of the sample size given the anticipated limited number of infants who may qualify for study. In most clinical trials, a frequentist analytic approach is used to determine the probability of the observed data or more extreme data if the null hypothesis is true. An alternative approach is to use a Bayesian analysis, which provides different information for hypothesis testing and was prespecified in this trial. A Bayesian analysis provides the probability that the hypothesis is true based on the observed data. It is a

formal statistical method to assess the range of treatment effects compatible with the best available evidence and is recommended for trials with limited sample size.[37] In contrast to a traditional frequentist analysis, a Bayesian analysis uses preexisting data (pilot studies, clinical trials, observational reports, and animal work) to establish a prior distribution representing the probability of a hypothesized treatment effect. To be conservative, a neutral prior distribution was used to indicate an equal probability of benefit or harm of late initiation of hypothermia and reflects the absence of data on this issue. The prior distribution is then combined with the observed data from the trial to yield a posterior probability of treatment effect. The latter can be characterized by the area under the curve less than aRR of 1.0 and represents the posterior probability of a treatment benefit (e.g., reduction in death or disability).

Eighty-three hypothermic infants were maintained at 33.5°C for 96 hours and then rewarmed while eighty-five noncooled infants were maintained at 37.0°C. The primary outcome of death and disability occurred in 24.4% of hypothermic and 27.9% of the noncooled group (unadjusted absolute risk difference, 3.5%). Bayesian analysis indicated a 76% posterior probability of reduced death or disability with hypothermia relative to the noncooled group (adjusted posterior risk ratio of 0.86, 95% credible interval 0.58–1.29) (Fig. 7.2). The probability that death or disability in cooled infants was at least 1%, 2%, or 3% less than noncooled infants was 71%, 64%, and 56%, respectively. The results of this trial indicate less neuroprotection by hypothermia compared to starting hypothermia at <6 hours of age and suggest the importance of early identification of at-risk infants and implementation of cooling. This trial provides the most rigorous assessment of cooling beyond 6 hours of age given the random allocation of infants, similar baseline characteristics, and follow-up assessments at 18 to 22 months by certified examiners masked to treatment with minimal loss to follow-up. Given the uncertainty of the results, some may choose not to use hypothermia beyond 6 hours of age. Others may view the results as the best available evidence to provide cooling beyond 6 hours given the probability of some reduction in death or disability,

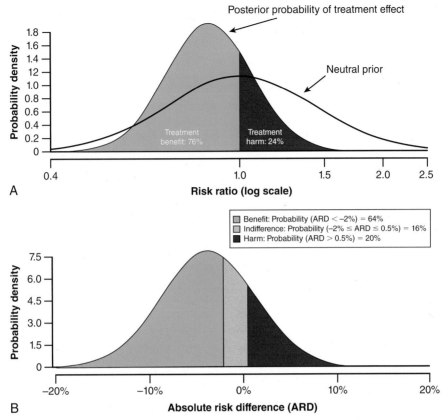

Fig. 7.3 Posterior probability results for late hypothermia initiated between 6 and 24 hours of age. Prior distribution representing the probability of a hypothesized treatment effect. A neutral prior distribution centered at a risk ratio of 1.0 was used to reflect the absence of data and indicates an equal number of infants would be expected to be benefited or harmed by the treatment. The posterior probability of the treatment effect was derived by combining the prior distribution with the trial results and demonstrates a shift to the left of a risk ratio of 1.0 and is characterized by an adjusted point estimate of 0.86. The area under the curve that is less than a risk ratio on 1.0 represents the posterior probability of the reduction in death or disability; for late initiation of hypothermia, it was 76%.

the absence of harm, and the seriousness of the potential outcome.

Should Infants With Mild HIE Receive Hypothermia Therapy?

Neonatal HIE affects 4 million infants worldwide annually, with more than half of these infants presenting within the mild range of the HIE spectrum.[1] These neonates were excluded from prior randomized controlled trials of TH which focused on moderate and severe HIE.[1-6] Early data of 226 infants ≥37 weeks'

gestation with evidence of HIE born between 1974 and 1979 from western Canada[38] demonstrated the relationship between stage of encephalopathy (mild n = 79, moderate n = 119, severe n = 28) and neurodevelopmental and school-age follow-up based on the most *severe stage* during the first week of life. Among infants with mild HIE, there were no deaths or handicap (cerebral palsy, sensory impairment, cognitive delay, or severe seizures) at 3.5 years. However, a delay of more than 6 months in gross motor skills occurred in 5% of mild HIE survivors, indicating the potential for subtle injury. At 8 years, assessments were compared among 56 of the 79 children who had mild HIE and a peer group of 155 children and there were no differences for intelligence quotients (IQs), visual motor integration, receptive vocabulary, and delays in reading, spelling, and math.[39] Subsequent reports indicate that children with mild encephalopathy may have subtle differences from infants who did not experience mild HIE; infants with mild HIE had lower mean IQ scores (Wechsler Intelligence Scale) than controls (99 ± 17 vs. 109 ± 12, respectively).[40] Children with mild encephalopathy assessed at 9 to 10 years were reported to have more problematic behavior compared with controls, including social problems, anxiety and depression, attention regulation, and thought problems.[41]

Following completion of the initial hypothermia trials,[1-6] retrospective studies reported that some infants not provided hypothermia had adverse short-term outcomes, including seizures, feeding difficulties, and abnormal magnetic resonance imaging (MRI) scans.[42-44] These observations prompted some centers to provide TH for infants with mild HIE despite the absence of clinical trials to justify treatment.[43,45] Furthermore, none of these publications provided early childhood neurodevelopmental assessments. Although not intended, two of the first series of hypothermia trials enrolled a limited number of infants with mild HIE.[54,56] Death or disability occurred in one trial[5] but not the other[6] among infants with mild HIE, making it difficult to reconcile these observations. The recognition of morbidities associated with mild HIE in the era of hypothermia compared to prehypothermia may reflect designation of the level of encephalopathy at less than 6 hours following birth compared with the worst stage of encephalopathy in the first week (prehypothermia) since progression of encephalopathy is known to occur. Alternatively, the limitations of retrospective reports, lack of definitions for mild HIE, and variability in the assessment of encephalopathy may also contribute to reports of morbidities associated with mild HIE.

Prospective data regarding mild HIE determined at less than 6 hours of age is limited but provocative. A multicenter international research initiative (Prospective Research of Infants with Mild Encephalopathy [PRIME]) described the short-term outcomes of infants with mild HIE following perinatal acidosis and/or resuscitation at birth without hypothermia treatment.[20,46] This investigation used a standardized definition of mild HIE and used trained examiners to promote consistency among centers. Fifty-four infants had complete data and twenty-eight infants (52%) had abnormalities of any of the following predefined short-term outcomes: an aEEG before 9 hours of age, an MRI scan, and a discharge neurologic examination. Brain MRI abnormalities (17%) were mostly limited to focal changes in the cerebral cortex, except in two infants who showed abnormalities in the basal ganglia/thalamus. The majority of the discharge examination abnormalities represented persistent features of encephalopathy (22 of 54, 41%). The PRIME cohort has been followed to 18 to 22 months of age and a Bayley III score of <85 was observed in 16%, 14%, and 32% in the cognitive, motor, and language domains, respectively.[20] The median and interquartile range for the composite cognitive score in mild HIE was 95 (90–106).[20] A prospective observational cohort from Ireland evaluated cognitive function at 5 years among infants of at least 37 weeks' gestation with a history of mild neonatal HIE (n = 22) and showed lower cognitive outcome than control infants (n = 30) for full-scale IQ (median, interquartile range, 99 [94–112] vs. 117 [110–124], p = .001), verbal IQ (105 [99–111] vs. 116 [112–125], p = .001), and performance IQ (103 [98–112] vs. 115 [107–124], p = .004).[47,48]

There has been recent therapeutic creep with many centers using hypothermia for mild HIE and resulting in *variable practice and the absence of a standard of care for mild HIE*.[21-25] The assumption of therapeutic benefit of TH has reduced equipoise to conduct a randomized trial. Not only is it unknown if hypothermia provides benefit for mild HIE, but treatment with TH includes risk of bradycardia, thrombocytopenia, coagulopathy, disrupted maternal-infant bonding, decreased breastfeeding, prolonged length of stay, and increased stress potentially offsetting positive treatment effects in this unstudied population. The fundamental question of optimal management of mild HIE remains unanswered. This has been a topic of yearly commentaries[7-10] and loss of equipoise for conducting a clinical trial grows each year.[26]

There are ongoing planned trials based on the PRIME definition of mild HIE in the first 6 hours.

Thayill et al. published on a subset of neonates with mild HIE who were enrolled in an MRI biomarkers study (Marble Study NCT01309711).[27] There were 32 babies with mild HIE who were cooled, and 15 who were either not cooled (n = 10) or cooled for <12 hours (n = 5). White matter injury was seen in 29 of 47 infants: 16 of 32 (50%) who were cooled and 13 of 15 (87%) who were not cooled or cooled for <12 hours.[27] The COMET Study (NCT03409770) (n = 140) is now randomizing infants with mild HIE to normothermia or hypothermia for either 48 hours or 72 hours. The TIME Study (NCT04176471) (n = 68), a feasibility pilot RCT for mild HIE in California, aims to determine feasibility of randomization and short-term neurodevelopmental outcomes at 1 year of age of hypothermia versus normothermia. The COOL PRIME (NCT04621279) is a planned prospective registry that aims to follow the trajectory of follow-up outcomes in infants recruited at multiple centers that is expected to start recruitment in 2023. The COOL PRIME design is a comparative effectiveness trial of cooling versus normothermia for mild HIE as allocated per standard of care at each center.

Should Hypothermia Be Used in Preterm Infants With HIE?

Extending the use of TH to preterm infants has many questions reflecting a greater susceptibility of preterm infants to the adverse effects of hypothermia and ongoing maturational changes in the neurological assessment. Data about diagnosis, frequency, severity, and outcome of HIE in infants 33 to 35 weeks GA are sparse. These gaps need further study as these infants were not included in prior hypothermia trials.[28]

Currently, there is no validated neurological examination to identify and classify encephalopathy among preterm infants. While the modified Sarnat exam has been used extensively in the evaluation of term newborns at risk for encephalopathy, its interrater reliability in preterm infants needs testing. Pavageau et al. conducted a recent prospective evaluation of 86 late preterm newborns, to determine the reliability of the neurologic exam between study investigators and other neonatologists. The interrater kappa score was good to excellent (k > 0.72) in most categories except for Moro and tone which had fair agreement.[28] These

findings are encouraging for the conduct of neuroprotective trials among preterm infants since the neurological examination is typically an inclusion criterion.

The importance of temperature for low birth weight infants was demonstrated by Silverman et al.[29] who demonstrated a survival advantage for infants nursed in incubators over 5 days with an air temperature of 31.1°C to 32.1°C compared to 28.3°C to 29.4°C. In spite of this, multiple reports indicate therapeutic creep with TH provided to infants <36 weeks gestation in clinical practice; among registry data up to 2.4% of infants receiving TH were late preterm infants at 33 to 35 weeks, although these infants were not well represented in randomized trials.[17] Rao et al. reported a small retrospective cohort study of 31 preterm infants, 34 to 35 weeks gestational age, and reported increased mortality compared to term infants.[30] In another retrospective report, 31 infants born between 33^0 and 35^6 weeks with HIE underwent cooling; 17% had an IVH and 65% had death or disability at follow-up but there was no comparison group.[31] Without a comparison group, it will not be possible to ascertain the safety profile of TH applied to moderate and late preterm infants. The propensity for brain hemorrhagic complications remains a concern when caring for sick preterm infants (Fig. 7.4).[49]

A major knowledge gap that may impact the efficacy of TH in a clinical trial among moderate and late preterm infants is the absence of definitive data on the neuropathology of hypoxic-ischemic brain injury in this gestational age group. Is the pathology similar to that of a term infant, dominated by selective neuronal necrosis and parasagittal cerebral injury?[49] Alternatively, is it mainly white matter injury and arrest of the oligodendrocyte lineage?[50,51,52] Despite this knowledge gap, there is biologic rationale for considering TH as a treatment option for preterm infants. Brain ischemia followed by hypothermia in fetal sheep at preterm gestations indicated that cooling protects oligodendrocytes, the critical target for brain injury in preterm infants.

Based on these considerations, the NICHD NRN has undertaken and completed enrollment in a trial of TH among infants 33^0 to 35^6 weeks in which infants with moderate or severe HIE were randomly allocated to an esophageal temperature of 33.5°C or 36.5°C to 37.3°C. https://clinicaltrials.gov/ct2/show/NCT01793129.

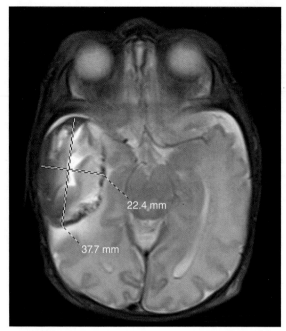

Fig. 7.4 Example of brain MRI large intraparenchymal hemorrhage in a preterm 34-week preterm with HIE who had received hypothermia.[49]

The primary outcome is death or moderate to severe disability at 18 to 22 months corrected age. The trial has completed enrollment of 168 infants who are now undergoing follow-up with the hope it will provide evidence to support use of cooling among preterm infants born at 33 to 35 weeks gestation.

How Should Cooling on Transport Be Conducted?

HIE affects births in Level I facilities owing to obstetric events that cannot be anticipated (e.g., placental abruption, ruptured uterus, maternal trauma). TH should not be performed in every hospital because HIE is characterized by multisystem organ dysfunction and requires neonatal intensive care units with the necessary expertise, consultants, and diagnostic services to manage the full spectrum of morbidities associated with encephalopathy. The therapeutic window during which hypothermia is most effective is time sensitive and necessitates close working relationships between tertiary centers and referral institutions for proper stabilization and recognition of encephalopathy.

Geographic constraints and postnatal age of recognition may limit application of hypothermia and have led to initiation of hypothermia during transport.

Initial attempts at cooling on transport involved either passive cooling (removal of exogenous heat sources) or active cooling (application of gel packs or ice to the body). Although this approach allows a higher percentage of infants to have therapy initiated before 6 hours of age, only 44% of infants had core temperatures within the targeted range for TH on admission to tertiary centers using a statewide database.[57] Some admission temperatures were exceedingly low and risk hazard while other temperatures were negligibly reduced with presumably little neuroprotective benefit. Other methods of cooling have been used (mattresses with phase-changing material, cooling fans) with unsatisfactory results.[58] In contrast, investigators in the United Kingdom developed consensus guidelines for passive cooling at referring hospitals and on transport that were prospectively evaluated.[59] They demonstrated that 67% of infants were in the target range of 33°C to 34°C on arrival at the tertiary center. Although guidelines for passive cooling represent a step forward to initiate hypothermia earlier and more effectively, they will still be challenging for many referral hospitals and transport teams. This reflects that moderate or severe HIE is an uncommon event in community hospitals given an occurrence of 1.5 per 1000 live births in population-based studies.[60]

Continuous monitoring and the ability to regulate core temperature are critical to initiating effective and safe hypothermia on transport. A clinical trial of cooling on transport for infants with HIE has been performed among nine neonatal intensive care units in California (NCT 01683383).[61] Infants were randomly assigned to receive cooling according to usual center practices compared with servo control of temperature using the Tecotherm Neo (Inspiration Healthcare, Leicester, United Kingdom, FDA approved). Usual center practices included passive cooling (removing exogenous heat sources) and/or active cooling (ice or gel packs), and rectal or esophageal temperatures were recorded at 15-minute intervals using indwelling temperature probes. The Tecotherm device was used to continuously adjust either rectal or esophageal temperature via indwelling probes. The percent of all core temperatures recorded within the target range of 33°C to 34°C indicated large group differences: the median and interquartile range for the device arm was 73% (17%–88%) compared with 0% (0%–52%) for the usual center practices (Fig. 7.5). Servo control of temperature is markedly more effective than nondevice methods of initiating hypothermia on transport.

Another important aspect of transport is whether infants are appropriate candidates for the treatment and manifest moderate or severe encephalopathy.[1-6] Training transport teams to recognize HIE is critical, but geographic constraints may limit the opportunity of transport teams to assess infants before 6 hours. Outreach education for referring providers is used by many centers. However, distinguishing subtle aspects of encephalopathy may be challenging for examiners who encounter such infants every 1 to 3 years even with intermittent education refreshers. Harnessing technology by the use of video conferencing and smartphones can enable real-time communication between referring providers and personnel at tertiary centers to improve decisions regarding initiation of cooling on transport.[32]

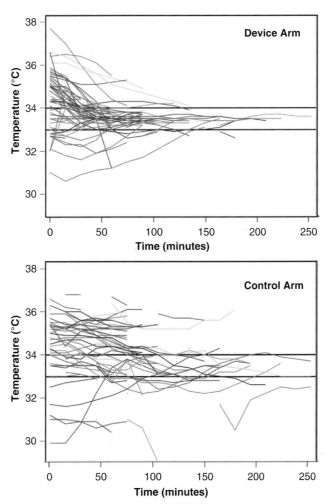

Fig. 7.5 Core temperature (rectal or esophageal) patterns during transport of infants whose temperature was adjusted with a servo-controlled device (device arm, *upper panel*) or via usual care practices using either passive or active cooling without a device (control arm, *lower panel*). The target temperature range was 33.0°C to 34.0°C; each infant is represented by an individual line. (Reprinted with permission from Akula VP, Joe P, Thusu K, et al. A randomized clinical trial of therapeutic hypothermia mode during transport for neonatal encephalopathy. *J Pediatr.* 2015;166(4):856-861.)

Is Therapeutic Hypothermia Neuroprotective When Used in Low- and Middle-Income Countries?

The primary causes of neonatal mortality worldwide are prematurity (28%), infections (26%), and hypoxia-ischemia (23%, commonly termed asphyxia). It is estimated that approximately one million newborns die each year from neonatal encephalopathy in low- and middle-income countries.[62,63] Unfortunately, there may be limitations to direct extrapolation from clinical trials of TH performed in high-income countries[1-6] to low- and middle-income countries. This reflects differences in prenatal care, obstetric monitoring and interventions during labor, and the infrastructure to care for the multiorgan system dysfunction characteristic of HIE available in high-income countries compared to low- to middle-income countries.

Seven small RCTs of TH performed in low- and middle-income countries and have been pooled for metaanalysis (n = 567 infants).[64] Most infants did not receive any mechanical ventilation and cooling devices (cooling caps, gel packs, ice water bottles, and mattresses with phase-changing material). Cooling therapy was not associated with a reduction in neonatal mortality. Only three trials reported neurodevelopmental outcome; follow-up rates were poor and the confidence intervals of reported outcomes were wide such that important clinical differences could not be excluded. Although hypothermia treatment achieved group differences in temperature among these trials, the benefit of cooling remains unclear.

A larger, rigorous randomized trial has been completed using centers in India, Sri Lanka, and Bangladesh (Hypothermia for Encephalopathy in Low- and Middle-Income Countries trial [HELIX trial], NCT 02387385[33]). From 2015 to 2019, 408 infants with moderate or severe HIE were enrolled and 202 were assigned to hypothermia (target rectal temperature 33.5°C for 72 hours) and 206 to the control group. Follow-up at 18 to 22 months for the primary outcome (death or moderate to severe disability) was achieved in 97% of each study arm. Death or disability occurred in 50% of the hypothermia group and 94 47% in the control group (risk ratio 1.06, 95% CI 0.87–1.30, $p = 0.55$). Death occurred in 84 infants (42%) in the hypothermia group and 63 infants in the control group (31%, $p = 0.02$). This was a well-planned

trial including randomization, an appropriate sample size for the postulated effect size, baseline characteristics that largely did not differ between groups, compliance with the intervention, and minimal loss to follow-up.[34] The results do not support the use of TH among infants with HIE in low- and middle-income countries, although this was a single study heavily weighted for India representation and not representative of global low and middle countries overall.

Use of Adjunct Erythropoietin Therapy: High Dose Erythropoietin for Asphyxia and Encephalopathy (HEAL) Updates

Recombinant human erythropoietin is a cytokine with possible neuroregenerative effects in neonatal hypoxia-ischemia (Fig. 7.1).[35-40] Erythropoietin 1000 U/kg given intravenously has emerged as a promising adjuvant neuroprotection agent based on animal data.[41] In a phase II trial of 50 infants undergoing TH randomized to 5 doses of erythropoietin 1000 U/kg or placebo, the treated group had better neonatal brain MRI and improved motor function at 1 year of age.[42] The High Dose Erythropoietin for Asphyxia and Encephalopathy (HEAL), a phase III randomized, double-blind, placebo-controlled trial, was completed in 2022 to determine the safety and efficacy of high doses of erythropoietin in conjunction with TH for neuroprotection in term and near-term infants with HIE and did not find any significant differences in MRI,[43] death and or neurodevelopmental impairment at age 22 to 36 months occurred (Accepted PAS Virtual Platform 2022).[66]

Conclusions

It is tempting to extrapolate from clinical trials that established efficacy and safety of hypothermia for HIE[1-6] to other clinical scenarios related to HIE. There have been multiple editorials[44,53,65] suggesting the extension of the use of TH for indications outside clinical trials. This is understandable given the associated mortality and lifelong, serious morbidity associated with HIE. However, well-designed, carefully performed clinical trials of hypothermia to determine if (1) there are better hypothermia regimens or (2) cooling works in other groups of infants with similar efficacy and safety profiles are needed to prevent drifts in practice without evidence and unintended adverse effects. The lessons learned from the NRN Optimizing Cooling Trial are a strong reminder that extrapolation to conditions thought to provide greater neuroprotection, lower temperature, and/or longer cooling had unexpectedly worse outcomes. As demonstrated by the HELIX trial, extrapolation of TH among infants with HIE in low- to middle-income countries maybe without benefit and possibly with harm. The message is very clear: until new information is available and critically reviewed, the use of TH should follow published, evidence-based protocols.

REFERENCES

1. Gluckman PD, Wyatt JS, Azzopardi D, et al. Selective head cooling with mild systemic hypothermia after neonatal encephalopathy: multicentre randomised trial. *Lancet*. 2005;365(9460):663-670.
2. Shankaran S, Laptook AR, Ehrenkranz RA, et al. Whole-body hypothermia for neonates with hypoxic-ischemic encephalopathy. *N Engl J Med*. 2005;353(15):1574-1584.
3. Azzopardi DV, Strohm B, Edwards AD, et al. Moderate hypothermia to treat perinatal asphyxial encephalopathy. *N Engl J Med*. 2009;361(14):1349-1358.
4. Simbruner G, Mittal RA, Rohlmann F, Muche R. Systemic hypothermia after neonatal encephalopathy: outcomes of neo. nEURO.network RCT. *Pediatrics*. 2010;126(4):e771-e778.
5. Jacobs SE, Morley CJ, Inder TE, et al. Whole-body hypothermia for term and near-term newborns with hypoxic-ischemic encephalopathy: a randomized controlled trial. *Arch Pediatr Adolesc Med*. 2011;165(8):692-700.
6. Zhou WH, Cheng GQ, Shao XM, et al. Selective head cooling with mild systemic hypothermia after neonatal hypoxic-ischemic encephalopathy: a multicenter randomized controlled trial in China. *J Pediatr*. 2010;157(3):367-372, 372.e361-e363.
7. Jacobs SE, Berg M, Hunt R, Tarnow-Mordi WO, Inder TE, Davis PG. Cooling for newborns with hypoxic ischaemic encephalopathy. *Cochrane Database Syst Rev*. 2013;1:CD003311.
8. Shankaran S, Pappas A, McDonald SA, et al. Childhood outcomes after hypothermia for neonatal encephalopathy. *N Engl J Med*. 2012;366(22):2085-2092.
9. Azzopardi D, Strohm B, Marlow N, et al. Effects of hypothermia for perinatal asphyxia on childhood outcomes. *N Engl J Med*. 2014;371(2):140-149.
10. Robertson NJ, Tan S, Groenendaal F, et al. Which neuroprotective agents are ready for bench to bedside translation in the newborn infant? *J Pediatr*. 2012;160(4):544-552.e4.
11. Committee on Fetus and Newborn. Hypothermia and neonatal encephalopathy. *Pediatrics*. 2014;133(6):1146-1150.
12. Chalak LF, Pappas A, Tan S, et al. Association between increased seizures during rewarming after hypothermia for neonatal hypoxic ischemic encephalopathy and abnormal neurodevelopmental outcomes at 2-year follow-up: A Nested Multisite Cohort Study. *JAMA Neurol*. 2021;78(12):1484-1493.
13. Busto R, Dietrich WD, Globus MY, Valdes I, Scheinberg P, Ginsberg MD. Small differences in intraischemic brain temperature critically determine the extent of ischemic neuronal injury. *J Cereb Blood Flow Metab*. 1987;7(6):729-738.
14. Laptook AR, Corbett RJ, Sterett R, Burns DK, Garcia D, Tollefsbol G. Modest hypothermia provides partial neuroprotection when used for immediate resuscitation after brain ischemia. *Pediatr Res*. 1997;42(1):17-23.
15. Thoresen M, Bagenholm R, Loberg EM, Apricena F, Kjellmer I. Posthypoxic cooling of neonatal rats provides protection against brain injury. *Arch Dis Child Fetal Neonatal Ed*. 1996;74(1):F3-F9.
16. Trescher WH, Ishiwa S, Johnston MV. Brief post-hypoxic-ischemic hypothermia markedly delays neonatal brain injury. *Brain Dev*. 1997;19(5):326-338.
17. Gunn AJ, Gunn TR, de Haan HH, Williams CE, Gluckman PD. Dramatic neuronal rescue with prolonged selective head cooling after ischemia in fetal lambs. *J Clin Invest*. 1997;99(2):248-256.
18. Bona E, Hagberg H, Loberg EM, Bagenholm R, Thoresen M. Protective effects of moderate hypothermia after neonatal hypoxia-ischemia: short- and long-term outcome. *Pediatr Res*. 1998;43(6):738-745.
19. Schubert A. Side effects of mild hypothermia. *J Neurosurg Anesthesiol*. 1995;7(2):139-147.
20. Gunn AJ, Gluckman PD, Gunn TR. Selective head cooling in newborn infants after perinatal asphyxia: a safety study. *Pediatrics*. 1998;102(4 Pt 1):885-892.
21. Battin MR, Penrice J, Gunn TR, Gunn AJ. Treatment of term infants with head cooling and mild systemic hypothermia (35.0 degrees C and 34.5 degrees C) after perinatal asphyxia. *Pediatrics*. 2003;111(2):244-251.
22. Shankaran S, Laptook A, Wright LL, et al. Whole-body hypothermia for neonatal encephalopathy: animal observations as a basis for a randomized, controlled pilot study in term infants. *Pediatrics*. 2002;110(2 Pt 1):377-385.
23. Carroll M, Beek O. Protection against hippocampal CA1 cell loss by post-ischemic hypothermia is dependent on delay of initiation and duration. *Metab Brain Dis*. 1992;7(1):45-50.
24. Colbourne F, Corbett D. Delayed and prolonged post-ischemic hypothermia is neuroprotective in the gerbil. *Brain Res*. 1994;654(2):265-272.
25. Coimbra C, Wieloch T. Moderate hypothermia mitigates neuronal damage in the rat brain when initiated several hours following transient cerebral ischemia. *Acta Neuropathol*. 1994;87(4):325-331.
26. Sirimanne ES, Blumberg RM, Bossano D, et al. The effect of prolonged modification of cerebral temperature on outcome after hypoxic-ischemic brain injury in the infant rat. *Pediatr Res*. 1996;39(4 Pt 1):591-597.
27. Ferriero DM. Neonatal brain injury. *N Engl J Med*. 2004;351(19):1985-1995.
28. Yenari MA, Han HS. Neuroprotective mechanisms of hypothermia in brain ischaemia. *Nat Rev Neurosci*. 2012;13(4):267-278.
29. Shankaran S, Laptook AR, Pappas A, et al. Effect of depth and duration of cooling on deaths in the NICU among neonates with hypoxic ischemic encephalopathy: a randomized clinical trial. *JAMA*. 2014;312(24):2629-2639.
30. Shankaran S, Laptook AR, Pappas A, McDonald SA, Das A, Tyson JE, et al. Effect of Depth and Duration of Cooling on Death or Disability at Age 18 Months Among Neonates With Hypoxic-Ischemic Encephalopathy: A Randomized Clinical Trial. *JAMA*. 2017;318(1):57-67.
31. Gunn AJ, Gunn TR, Gunning MI, Williams CE, Gluckman PD. Neuroprotection with prolonged head cooling started before postischemic seizures in fetal sheep. *Pediatrics*. 1998;102(5):1098-1106.
32. Gunn AJ, Bennet L, Gunning MI, Gluckman PD, Gunn TR. Cerebral hypothermia is not neuroprotective when started after

postischemic seizures in fetal sheep. *Pediatr Res.* 1999;46(3): 274-280.

33. Thoresen M, Tooley J, Liu X, et al. Time is brain: starting therapeutic hypothermia within three hours after birth improves motor outcome in asphyxiated newborns. *Neonatology.* 2013; 104(3):228-233.

34. Galle AA, Jones NM. The neuroprotective actions of hypoxic preconditioning and postconditioning in a neonatal rat model of hypoxic-ischemic brain injury. *Brain Res.* 2013;1498:1-8.

35. Hassell KJ, Ezzati M, Alonso-Alconada D, Hausenloy DJ, Robertson NJ. New horizons for newborn brain protection: enhancing endogenous neuroprotection. *Arch Dis Child Fetal Neonatal Ed.* 2015;100(6):F541-F552.

36. Azzopardi D, Strohm B, Linsell L, et al. Implementation and conduct of therapeutic hypothermia for perinatal asphyxial encephalopathy in the UK—analysis of national data. *PLoS One.* 2012;7(6):e38504.

37. Lilford RJ, Thornton JG, Braunholtz D. Clinical trials and rare diseases: a way out of a conundrum. *BMJ.* 1995;311(7020): 1621-1625.

38. Robertson C, Finer N. Term infants with hypoxic-ischemic encephalopathy: outcome at 3.5 years. *Dev Med Child Neurol.* 1985;27(4):473-484.

39. Robertson CM, Finer NN, Grace MG. School performance of survivors of neonatal encephalopathy associated with birth asphyxia at term. *J Pediatr.* 1989;114(5):753-760.

40. van Kooij BJ, van Handel M, Nievelstein RA, Groenendaal F, Jongmans MJ, de Vries LS. Serial MRI and neurodevelopmental outcome in 9- to 10-year-old children with neonatal encephalopathy. *J Pediatr.* 2010;157(2):221-227.e2.

41. van Handel M, Swaab H, de Vries LS, Jongmans MJ. Behavioral outcome in children with a history of neonatal encephalopathy following perinatal asphyxia. *J Pediatr Psychol.* 2010;35(3):286-295.

42. DuPont TL, Chalak LF, Morriss MC, Burchfield PJ, Christie L, Sanchez PJ. Short-term outcomes of newborns with perinatal acidemia who are not eligible for systemic hypothermia therapy. *J Pediatr.* 2013;162(1):35-41.

43. Massaro AN, Murthy K, Zaniletti I, et al. Short-term outcomes after perinatal hypoxic ischemic encephalopathy: a report from the Children's Hospitals Neonatal Consortium HIE focus group. *J Perinatol.* 2015;35(4):290-296.

44. Gagne-Loranger M, Sheppard M, Ali N, Saint-Martin C, Wintermark P. Newborns referred for therapeutic hypothermia: association between initial degree of encephalopathy and severity of brain injury (what about the newborns with mild encephalopathy on admission?). *Am J Perinatol.* 2016;33(2):195-202.

45. Kracer B, Hintz SR, Van Meurs KP, Lee HC. Hypothermia therapy for neonatal hypoxic ischemic encephalopathy in the state of California. *J Pediatr.* 2014;165(2):267-273.

46. Garfinkle J, Chalak LF, Prempunpong C, et al. Prospective research in infants with mild encephalopathy—the PRIME study. *Pediatric.* 2016;153. Academic Societies' meeting abstracts, Abstract#4116.

47. Murray DM, O'Connor CM, Ryan CA, Korotchikova I, Boylan GB. Early EEG grade and outcome at 5 years after mild neonatal hypoxic ischemic encephalopathy. *Pediatrics.* 2016;138(4):e20160659.

48. Eicher DJ, Wagner CL, Katikaneni LP, et al. Moderate hypothermia in neonatal encephalopathy: efficacy outcomes. *Pediatr Neurol.* 2005;32(1):11-17.

49. Volpe JJ. *Neurology of the Newborn.* 5th ed. Philadelphia, PA: Saunders Elsevier; 2008.

50. Back SA, Riddle A, McClure MM. Maturation-dependent vulnerability of perinatal white matter in premature birth. *Stroke.* 2007;38(suppl 2):724-730.

51. Volpe JJ, Kinney HC, Jensen FE, Rosenberg PA. The developing oligodendrocyte: key cellular target in brain injury in the premature infant. *Int J Dev Neurosci.* 2011;29(4):423-440.

52. Bennet L, Roelfsema V, George S, Dean JM, Emerald BS, Gunn AJ. The effect of cerebral hypothermia on white and grey matter injury induced by severe hypoxia in preterm fetal sheep. *J Physiol.* 2007;578(Pt 2):491-506.

53. Austin T, Shanmugalingam S, Clarke P. To cool or not to cool? Hypothermia treatment outside trial criteria. *Arch Dis Child Fetal Neonatal Ed.* 2013;98(5):F451-F453.

54. Smit E, Liu X, Jary S, Cowan F, Thoresen M. Cooling neonates who do not fulfil the standard cooling criteria—short- and long-term outcomes. *Acta Paediatr.* 2015;104(2):138-145.

55. Walsh WF, Butler D, Schmidt JW. Report of a pilot study of cooling four preterm infants 32–35 weeks gestation with HIE. *J Neonatal Perinatal Med.* 2015;8:47-51.

56. Rao R, Trivedi S, Vesoulis Z, Liao SM, Smyser CD, Mathur AM. Safety and short-term outcomes of therapeutic hypothermia in preterm neonates 34–35 weeks gestational age with hypoxic-ischemic encephalopathy. *J Pediatr.* 2017;183: 37-42.

57. Akula VP, Gould JB, Davis AS, Hackel A, Oehlert J, Van Meurs KP. Therapeutic hypothermia during neonatal transport: data from the California Perinatal Quality Care Collaborative (CPQCC) and California Perinatal Transport System (CPeTS) for 2010. *J Perinatol.* 2013;33(3):194-197.

58. Robertson NJ, Kendall GS, Thayyil S. Techniques for therapeutic hypothermia during transport and in hospital for perinatal asphyxial encephalopathy. *Semin Fetal Neonatal Med.* 2010; 15(5):276-286.

59. Kendall GS, Kapetanakis A, Ratnavel N, Azzopardi D, Robertson NJ. Passive cooling for initiation of therapeutic hypothermia in neonatal encephalopathy. *Arch Dis Child Fetal Neonatal Ed.* 2010;95(6):F408-F412.

60. Kurinczuk JJ, White-Koning M, Badawi N. Epidemiology of neonatal encephalopathy and hypoxic-ischaemic encephalopathy. *Early Hum Dev.* 2010;86(6):329-338.

61. Akula VP, Joe P, Thusu K, et al. A randomized clinical trial of therapeutic hypothermia mode during transport for neonatal encephalopathy. *J Pediatr.* 2015;166(4):856-861.e612.

62. Lawn JE, Cousens S, Zupan J. Lancet Neonatal Survival Steering Team. 4 million neonatal deaths: When? Where? Why? *Lancet.* 2005;365(9462):891-900.

63. Liu L, Oza S, Hogan D, et al. Global, regional, and national causes of child mortality in 2000–13, with projections to inform post-2015 priorities: an updated systematic analysis. *Lancet.* 2015;385(9966):430-440.

64. Pauliah SS, Shankaran S, Wade A, Cady EB, Thayyil S. Therapeutic hypothermia for neonatal encephalopathy in low- and middle-income countries: a systematic review and meta-analysis. *PLoS One.* 2013;8(3):e58834.

65. Saliba E. Should we extend the indications for therapeutic hypothermia? *Acta Paediatr.* 2015;104(2):114-115.

66. Wu YW, Comstock BA, Gonzalez FF, Mayock DE, Goodman AM, Maitre NL, et al. Trial of erythropoietin for hypoxic-ischemic encephalopathy in newborns. *N Engl J Med.* 2022;387(2):148-159.

67. Laptook AR, Shankaran S, Tyson JE, Munoz B, Bell EF, Goldberg RN, et al. Effect of therapeutic hypothermia initiated after 6 hours of age on death or disability among newborns with hypoxic-ischemic encephalopathy: A randomized clinical trial. *JAMA.* 2017;318(16):1550-1560.

Chapter 8

General Supportive Management of the Term Infant With Neonatal Encephalopathy Following Intrapartum Hypoxia-Ischemia

Ericalyn Kasdorf and Jeffrey M. Perlman

Chapter Outline

Key Points

- Early identification of the infant at risk for evolving hypoxic-ischemic brain injury and initiation of therapeutic hypothermia is critical in overall management.
- Glucose should be checked shortly after birth and corrected promptly as needed.
- Carbon dioxide should be maintained within a normal range to avoid exacerbation of brain injury.
- Judicious fluid management is necessary in this population at risk for acute kidney injury and oliguria.
- Hyperthermia should be avoided, and passive or active cooling may be considered for infants traveling long distances to a cooling center.
- Adjunctive therapies for therapeutic hypothermia are needed.

Case History

Infant was a 3200 g, 38-week gestation male infant born to a 28-year-old G2P1 (gravida 2, para 1) mother following an uncomplicated pregnancy. Labor was complicated by a maternal temperature of 38.5°C and fetal tachycardia for which the mother received antibiotics, a prolonged second stage of labor associated with variable decelerations, and a bradycardic episode that resulted in an emergency cesarean section. Meconium staining of the amniotic fluid was noted. The infant was hypotonic at delivery and without respiratory effort. Resuscitation included intubation and positive-pressure ventilation (PPV). The initial heart rate was 50 beats/min but increased rapidly to >100 beats/min within 30 seconds of the start of PPV. The infant's color improved, and he took a first gasp at 4 minutes and made a first respiratory effort at 8 minutes. Rectal temperature in the delivery room was 38.2°C. The Apgar scores were 1, 4, and 7 at 1, 5, and 10 minutes, respectively. The infant was transferred to the neonatal intensive care unit (NICU) for further management. The cord arterial blood gas analysis revealed a partial pressure of carbon dioxide (Pco_2) of 101 mm Hg, pH of 6.78, and base deficit of −23 mEq/L. The initial arterial blood gas analysis at 30 minutes revealed a Pao_2 of 146 mm Hg (on 50% oxygen), Pco_2 of 30 mm Hg, and pH of 7.12. The initial blood glucose level was 32 mg/dL. The hypoglycemia was treated with a 2 mL/kg bolus of dextrose 10% in water ($D_{10}W$), and subsequent glucose concentration was 84 mg/dL. The initial clinical assessment revealed a lethargic infant with a low-level sensory response. The anterior fontanel was soft. The capillary refill time was approximately 2 seconds. Pertinent cardiovascular findings were a heart rate of 134 beats/min and blood pressure of 44/24 mm Hg with a mean of 34 mm Hg. The infant was intubated and placed on modest ventilator support with equal but coarse breath sounds. The central nervous examination revealed pupils that were 3 mm and reactive. There were weak gag and suck reflexes, along with central hypotonia with proximal weakness. The reflexes were present and symmetric. The encephalopathy at this stage was categorized as Sarnat Stage 2. Because of the history and clinical findings, the infant underwent an amplitude-integrated electroencephalography (aEEG) examination that revealed a moderately suppressed pattern without seizure activity. The infant met criteria for therapeutic hypothermia, which was initiated at approximately 4 hours of age. At 12 hours of age the infant began to exhibit subtle seizure activity with blinking of the eyes, mouth smacking, and horizontal eye deviation associated with desaturation episodes. A clinical diagnosis of seizures was

made, and the infant was treated with a total of 40 mg/kg phenobarbital. The seizures persisted over the next 12 hours and the infant was started on a midazolam infusion and treated with one additional dose of phenobarbital before control of the clinical as well as the electrographic seizures was achieved. The encephalopathy peaked on day of life (DOL) 2, and the infant remained in Sarnat Stage 2 encephalopathy. The initial urine output was less than 1 mL/kg/hour for the first 24 hours but increased thereafter, and by DOL 3 the infant was in a diuretic phase. Sodium was initially 136 mEq/L, reached a nadir of 128 mEq/L on DOL 3, but corrected over the next 36 hours. The initial serum bicarbonate level was 18 mEq/L with an anion gap of 16. Both resolved spontaneously by DOL 3. The infant received assisted ventilation until DOL 3, and the Pco_2 values ranged between 40 and 50 mm Hg. Additional abnormalities included low calcium and magnesium levels (DOL 2) and mildly elevated liver enzymes. Low-dose dopamine treatment was started for approximately 24 hours for a low mean blood pressure. The infant was treated with antibiotics for 48 hours, with subsequent negative blood cultures. Parenteral nutrition was initiated on DOL 3, and the infant was able to achieve full oral feedings by DOL 14. The neurologic findings improved, although they were still abnormal with central hypotonia and increased deep tendon reflexes at the time of discharge. Magnetic resonance imaging (MRI) on DOL 7 revealed marked hyperintensity on the diffusion-weighted images within the putamen and thalamus bilaterally. Findings of repeat electroencephalography (EEG) were pertinent for mild background slowing. Finally, the placental pathology was consistent with acute chorioamnionitis. The infant was discharged to home on DOL 16.

This case illustrates typical evolving encephalopathy following intrapartum hypoxia-ischemia against the background of placental inflammation. The brain injury that develops is an evolving process that is initiated during the insult and extends into a recovery period, the latter being referred to as the "reperfusion phase" of injury.[1-3] Management of such an infant should be initiated in the delivery room with effective resuscitation and continued throughout their entire stay including planning of discharge services, such as therapy services. Management consists of the early identification of the infant being at high risk for brain injury, supportive therapy to facilitate adequate perfusion and nutrients to the brain, and neuroprotective strategies, including therapeutic hypothermia as well as therapy targeted at the cellular level to ameliorate the processes that may exacerbate ongoing brain injury (see Chapter 4). These management components are briefly discussed in this chapter.

Introduction

Hypoxic-ischemic encephalopathy (HIE) is an infrequent event with a range of reported incidences, with a rate of 1.5 per 1000 live births in one report.[4] HIE secondary to intrapartum asphyxia is a widely recognized cause of long-term neurologic sequelae, including cerebral palsy.[5] Severe and prolonged interruption of placental blood flow will ultimately lead to asphyxia, the biochemical process characterized by worsening hypoxia, hypercarbia, and acidosis (in the more severe cases defined as an umbilical arterial cord pH ≤ 7.00).[6] During the acute phase of asphyxia, the ability to autoregulate cerebral blood flow (CBF) to maintain cerebral perfusion is lost. When this state occurs, CBF becomes entirely dependent on blood pressure to maintain perfusion pressure, a term known as a *pressure-passive cerebral circulation*.[3] With interruption of placental blood flow the fetus will attempt to maintain CBF by redistributing cardiac output not only to the brain but also to the adrenal glands and myocardium. This redistribution occurs at the expense of blood flow to kidneys, intestine, and skin.[6] Despite such redistribution efforts, even a moderate decrease in blood pressure at this stage could lead to severely compromised CBF. With ongoing hypoxia-ischemia, CBF declines, leading to deleterious cellular effects. With oxygen depletion, a number of cellular alterations occur including replacement of oxidative phosphorylation with anaerobic metabolism, diminution of adenosine triphosphate (ATP), intracellular acidosis, and accumulation particularly of calcium. The ultimate deleterious effects include the release of excitatory neurotransmitters, such as glutamate, free radical production from fatty acid peroxidation, and nitric oxide (NO)–mediated neurotoxicity, all resulting in cell death.[5,6] Following resuscitation and the reestablishment of CBF and oxygenation, a phase of secondary energy failure occurs. In the experimental paradigm this phase transpires from

6 to 48 hours after the initial insult and is thought to be related to extension of the preceding mechanisms, leading to mitochondrial dysfunction.[1] It is clear that during asphyxia, not only the brain but also many other vital organs are at risk for injury. For this reason, postresuscitation management of the infant who has suffered intrapartum hypoxia-ischemia must also focus on supporting those systemic organs that may have been injured. Future therapies must also target the cellular injury that occurs following asphyxia.

Delivery Room Management

The use of room air or supplemental oxygen in the delivery room has been previously identified as a gap in knowledge that is crucial to resolve. Resuscitation of the depressed newborn infant is aimed at restoring blood flow and oxygen delivery to the tissues. The most current international guidelines continue to recommend initiation of resuscitation with room air for term and late preterm infants ≥ 35 weeks' gestation and to avoid use of 100% oxygen in this population as it has been associated with excess mortality.[7,8] The exception to this, is the recommendation to increase to 100% oxygen if the infant's heart rate remains less than 60 beats/min after at least 30 seconds of PPV that moves the chest, and as chest compressions are initiated.[9] Monitoring should take place via pulse oximeter, with the goal of achieving oxygen saturations in the interquartile range of preductal saturations measured in healthy term babies born vaginally at sea level (Table 8.1).[10,11] Notably, a 2019 meta-analysis of five randomized controlled trials (RCTs) and five quasi-RCTs showed a decrease in short-term mortality when using room air versus 100% oxygen for resuscitation of infants ≥ 35 weeks' gestation (risk ratio [RR] = 0.73, 95% confidence interval [CI] 0.57–0.94).[12] Two of these aforementioned RCTs showed no difference in neurodevelopmental impairment in survivors at 1 to 3 years of age, and five RCTs showed no significant difference in rates of Sarnat Stage 2–3 HIE.[12] The mechanisms contributing to mortality in the oxygen group are unclear and important to determine. Interestingly, use of 100% oxygen has been associated with increased biochemical markers of oxidative stress in asphyxiated term neonates, as well as delay to first cry and sustained respiration.[13]

TABLE 8.1   Targeted Pre-ductal SpO$_2$ After Birth

Time After Birth (min)	SpO$_2$ Level (%)
1	60–65
2	65–70
3	70–75
4	75–80
5	80–85
10	85–95

Adapted from Wyckoff MH, Aziz K, Escobedo MB, et al. Part 13: neonatal resuscitation: 2015 American Heart Association guidelines update for cardiopulmonary resuscitation and emergency cardiovascular care. Reprinted with permission. *Circulation.* 2015;132:S543-S560. ©2015 American Heart Association, Inc.

There have been few studies comparing room air with 100% oxygen, specifically during resuscitation of infants with HIE. One study performed in the era before cooling demonstrated increased risk of adverse outcome, defined as death or severe neurodevelopmental disability, by 24 months of age in infants diagnosed with asphyxia and exposed to severe hyperoxemia in the first 2 hours of life (defined as arterial partial pressure of oxygen [Pao$_2$] >200 mm Hg).[14] Another study of infants with perinatal acidemia or an acute perinatal event, in addition to a 10-minute Apgar score of five or less or ongoing need for assisted ventilation at 10 minutes and hyperoxemia on admission (defined as a Pao$_2$ >100 mm Hg), demonstrated an association with moderate-severe HIE and abnormal brain MRI. This population included both infants treated with whole-body hypothermia as well as controls, and importantly more infants in the hyperoxemia group developed signs of moderate-severe encephalopathy, qualifying them for whole-body hypothermia.[15] These data support ongoing judicious use of oxygen during resuscitation.

Early Identification of Infants at Highest Risk for Development of Hypoxic-Ischemic Brain Injury

The initial step in management is early identification of those infants at greatest risk for progression to HIE. This is a highly relevant issue because the therapeutic window, the interval following hypoxia-ischemia during which interventions might be efficacious in reducing the severity of ultimate brain injury, is likely to be short. It is estimated on the basis of experimental studies to vary from soon after the insult to approximately 6 hours.[16–18] Given this presumed short window of opportunity, infants must be identified as soon as possible after delivery to facilitate the implementation of early interventions as described in the case history. Studies exploring initiation of treatment between 6 and 24 hours following birth suggest there may be some benefit to this strategy; however, uncertainty remains regarding its effectiveness and more research is needed in this area.[19] What put the infant presented in this case at high risk for neurologic injury? There was clinical evidence of chorioamnionitis, fetal bradycardia, and perinatal depression with need for resuscitation in the delivery room, including intubation and PPV, and there was evidence of severe fetal acidemia, followed by evidence of early abnormal neurologic findings and abnormal cerebral function as demonstrated by amplitude-integrated EEG.[20–22] Indeed, the infant progressed to stage 2 encephalopathy with seizures.

Supportive Care

A summary of supportive management is given in Fig. 8.1.

VENTILATION

Assessment of adequate respiratory function is critical in the infant with HIE. Inadequate ventilation and frequent apneic episodes are not uncommon in severely affected infants, necessitating assisted ventilation. Changes in carbon dioxide (CO$_2$) are important to monitor carefully as hypercarbia increases and hypocarbia decreases CBF.[23] Some experimental animal studies had previously suggested that a modest elevation in Paco$_2$ (50–55 mm Hg) at the time of hypoxia-ischemia was associated with better outcome than when the Paco$_2$ is within the normal (mid-30s) range.[24] However, this is a complex issue as it has been shown that progressive hypercarbia in ventilated premature infants, for example, is associated with loss of autoregulation.[25] Moreover, in the management of preterm infants with respiratory distress

---

Delivery Room

- Resuscitation beginning with room air or 100% oxygen if initiating CPR

Temperature

- Avoid hyperthermia

Ventilation

- Maintain Pco_2 in normal range

Perfusion

- Promptly treat hypotension
- Avoid hypertension

Fluid and Metabolic Status

- Adjust fluid and electrolytes to individual needs
- Follow serum sodium concentration and fluid balance
- Follow serial glucoses and correct promptly when abnormal

Fig. 8.1 Summary of supportive management for neonatal encephalopathy after hypoxia-ischemia.

---

syndrome (RDS), the presence of hypocarbia, particularly when prolonged, has been associated with periventricular leukomalacia (PVL) (see Chapter 2). In term infants, there is also evidence that hypocarbia is associated with adverse outcome, especially in the setting of HIE. In a study of term infants diagnosed with intrapartum asphyxia, severe hypocapnia (defined as $Paco_2$ <20 mm Hg) increased risk of adverse outcome defined as death or severe neurodevelopmental disability at 12 months of age.[14] A secondary study of the National Institute of Child Health and Human Development (NICHD) whole-body hypothermia trial demonstrated an association of minimum $Paco_2$ and cumulative exposure to $Paco_2$ less than 35 mm Hg with adverse neurodevelopmental outcome at 18 to 22 months of age.[26] A post hoc analysis of the Cool Cap Study showed similar results, with hypocapnia in the first 72 hours after randomization (defined as $Paco_2$ <30 mm Hg) associated with an increased risk of death or severe neurodevelopmental disability at 18 months of age.[27] The authors of this study speculated that the etiology for frequent hypocapnia is unclear; it may be related to less CO_2 production in the setting of severe brain injury versus excessive support with mechanical

ventilation and/or resuscitation. Additionally, a retrospective cohort study of 198 term infants with moderate to severe HIE treated with therapeutic hypothermia showed an association of lowest Pco_2 averaged over days 1 to 4 of life with identification of brain injury on MRI (odds ratio [95% CI] 1.07 [1.00–1.14]; $P = 0.04$).[28] With these data in mind, it is recommended that CO_2 be maintained in the normal range in mechanically ventilated infants at risk for HIE. This goal may be difficult to achieve in clinical practice as infants with HIE often demonstrate hypocapnia. In a study of 52 term infants with HIE, only 11.5% of infants were normocapnic through the first 3 days of life; 29% were moderately hypocapnic and 5.8% were severely hypocapnic.[29]

MAINTENANCE OF ADEQUATE PERFUSION

Given the presence of a pressure-passive cerebral circulation, as discussed earlier, management strategy should aim to maintain the arterial blood pressure within a normal range for age and gestation. It is not uncommon for infants with hypoxia-ischemia to exhibit hypotension which may be related to myocardial dysfunction, endothelial cell damage, or rarely to volume loss. The treatment should be directed toward the cause—that is, inotropic support should be given for myocardial dysfunction, and volume replacement for intravascular depletion.[30] Hemodynamics may also be affected by treatment with therapeutic hypothermia and subsequent rewarming. One small observational study of infants with HIE treated with hypothermia demonstrated an increase in mean arterial blood pressure by median of 8 mm Hg and a decline in heart rate by 32 beats/min during the cooling process.[31] Another observational study of 20 infants with HIE treated with therapeutic hypothermia demonstrated that both heart rate and cardiac output increased during the rewarming process following hypothermia.[32] Interestingly, in this study while mean arterial blood pressure was noted to decline with rewarming, middle cerebral artery systolic flow velocity increased during this time. Additionally, a recent systematic review and meta-analysis of the effect of hypothermia on renal and myocardial function suggests possible short-term myocardial benefits of cooling as measured by level of brain natriuretic peptide, cardiac troponin, and creatine kinase MB as well as less frequent evidence of myocardial dysfunction on EKG, echocardiogram, and tissue doppler measurements.[33] It is unclear whether these short-term cardioprotective effects will confer long-term benefit.

FLUID STATUS

Hypoxic-ischemic infants often progress to a fluid overload state. The fluid overload seen after delivery may be related to renal failure secondary to acute tubular necrosis or to the syndrome of inappropriate antidiuretic hormone release (SIADH). Clinically such infants present with an increase in weight, low urine output, and hyponatremia. Indeed, in our case example, all these findings were present until diuresis was achieved. While fluid restriction is common practice for treatment of infants with HIE, the most recent Cochrane review of this subject highlights the need for further studies to assess whether this practice impacts morbidity and mortality in infants with HIE.[34] A 2018 randomized controlled trial of 80 neonates with HIE treated with whole-body cooling showed no difference in death or neurodevelopmental disability at 6 months of life between infants randomized to normal fluid intake and those to restricted fluid intake (defined as 2/3 of normal intake) in the first 4 days of life.[35] Fluid and electrolyte administration should be individualized to the need of each patient.

RENAL FUNCTION

A 2021 meta-analysis assessing renal function in term and near-term infants with asphyxia showed a significant difference between the incidence of acute kidney injury in infants treated with therapeutic hypothermia compared to controls (RR = 0.81; 95% CI 0.67–0.98, $P = 0.03$).[33] In one randomized controlled trial included in this meta-analysis, the incidence of acute kidney injury was 32% in the group of term infants with encephalopathy treated with therapeutic hypothermia, compared to 60% of those infants randomized to standard treatment and not treated with therapeutic hypothermia ($P < 0.05$).[36] The mechanism of this potential protective effect is not entirely understood and warrants further investigation. Renal perfusion does appear to be dynamic during the cooling and rewarming process, with renal saturation (Rsat) increasing and renal oxygen

extraction levels decreasing in one study, as measured by near-infrared spectroscopy, after rewarming in infants with HIE treated with hypothermia.[37] The authors noted that Rsat started to increase even before the rewarming process, which they hypothesize may be in part due to the natural evolution of renal reperfusion following asphyxia, followed by an increase in cardiac output and vasodilation, which occurs after rewarming.

Past studies have assessed the treatment of oliguria, which often occurs in encephalopathic infants with theophylline, on the theory that adenosine acts as a vasoconstrictive metabolite following hypoxia-ischemia, which contributes to a decreased glomerular filtration rate. In two randomized controlled studies, asphyxiated infants received a single 8 mg/kg dose of theophylline within the first hour of life in an attempt to block this vasoconstriction. Theophylline was associated with a decrease in serum creatinine and urinary β_2-microglobulin concentrations as well as enhancement of creatinine clearance.[38,39] A meta-analysis of four studies, including these two, assessing the use of prophylactic theophylline for the prevention of renal dysfunction in term infants with asphyxia showed a reduced incidence of severe renal dysfunction.[40] These studies, however, were conducted before the era of therapeutic hypothermia and theophylline levels were not measured in two of the four studies. One recent pharmacokinetic study in term infants with HIE treated with therapeutic hypothermia demonstrated low clearance of theophylline, with a 50% longer half-life compared to full-term infants without HIE and normothermia.[41] A 2018 systematic review and meta-analysis including six trials with a total of 436 term infants with birth asphyxia showed a 60% reduction in the risk of acute kidney injury treated with a single dose of aminophylline, albeit with only moderate quality of evidence.[42] Cleary more data are needed to better assess pharmacokinetics and potential side effects, as well as to understand the drugs' effects in conjunction with therapeutic hypothermia.

CONTROL OF BLOOD GLUCOSE CONCENTRATION

In the context of cerebral hypoxia-ischemia, experimental studies suggest that both hyperglycemia and hypoglycemia may exacerbate brain damage. In adult experimental models as well as in humans, hyperglycemia accentuates brain damage, whereas in immature animals subjected to cerebral hypoxia-ischemia, significant hyperglycemia to a blood glucose concentration of 600 mg/dL entirely prevented brain damage.[43] Conversely, the effects of hypoglycemia in experimental neonatal models vary, as do the mechanisms of the hypoglycemia. Thus insulin-induced hypoglycemia is detrimental to immature rat brain subjected to hypoxia-ischemia. However, if fasting induces hypoglycemia, a high degree of protection is noted.[44] This protective effect is thought to be secondary to the increased concentrations of ketone bodies, which presumably serve as alternative substrates to the immature brain.

In the clinical setting, hypoglycemia when associated with hypoxia-ischemia is detrimental to the brain. Thus term infants delivered in the presence of severe fetal acidemia (umbilical arterial pH <7.0) who presented with an initial blood glucose concentration lower than 40 mg/dL were 18 times more likely to progress to moderate or severe encephalopathy compared with infants with a glucose greater than 40 mg/dL.[45] In another post hoc analysis of the Cool Cap Study, unfavorable outcome at 18 months was seen more commonly in infants with hypoglycemia (≤40 mg/dL) and hyperglycemia (≥150 mg/dL) within the first 12 hours following randomization.[46] Interestingly, multiorgan dysfunction, as measured by liver and renal function and hematologic studies, was more severely abnormal in the hypoglycemic population.[46] Additionally, after adjusting for Sarnat stage and 5-minute Apgar score, only hyperglycemic infants randomized to hypothermia had a reduced risk of death and/or severe disability at 18 months of age (adjusted RR = 0.8, 95% CI: 0.66–0.99), infants with hypoglycemia or normoglycemia did not benefit significantly from treatment.[47] Derangements in glucose levels have also been associated with varying patterns of brain injury on MRI. Thus a prospective study of 179 infants with moderate-to-severe HIE treated with therapeutic hypothermia showed that infants with hypoglycemia and labile glucoses had higher adjusted odds of watershed or focal-multifocal strokes, as well as basal ganglia or watershed injury on MRI obtained at a median of 9 days of life, compared with infants with normal glucose values.[48] Hypoglycemia was another risk factor for adverse outcome in our case as the infant presented with an initial blood glucose

concentration of 32 mg/dL. In the ongoing management of hypoxia-ischemia, a glucose level should be screened shortly after birth, corrected promptly as needed, and monitored closely.

TEMPERATURE

In both animal and human studies, ischemic brain injury has been shown to be influenced by temperature; elevation either during or following the insult exacerbates brain injury, whereas a modest reduction in temperature reduces the extent of injury (see Chapter 4).[49] The potential risks associated with an elevated temperature were highlighted in an observational secondary study of the NICHD whole-body cooling trial.[50] This study found that an increased temperature in the control group following hypoxia-ischemia was associated with a higher risk of adverse outcome. The odds ratio of death or disability at 18 to 22 months of age was increased 3.6- to 4-fold for each 1°C increase in the highest quartile of skin or esophageal temperatures (see also Chapter 4).[50] In this same cohort, this effect persisted into childhood, with an increased odds of death or IQ less than 70 at age 6 to 7 years for infants with an average esophageal or skin temperature in the upper quartile in the first 3 days of life.[51] Therefore it is important to pay close attention to temperature in the infant with a hypoxic-ischemic event. At the time of delivery, the infant's temperature may be in the normal range or may be elevated in the context of clinical chorioamnionitis with maternal fever, making temperature a highly relevant issue. This raises the important question of how to manage temperature immediately following resuscitation of a near-term or term infant. Should the goal be to maintain the temperature in a normal range until it is evident that the neonate is a potential candidate for therapeutic hypothermia? On the other hand, the clinician could consider initiating passive cooling even at the time of delivery, with discontinuation of use of the radiant warmer in the delivery room. In a study of passive cooling initiated before and during transport to a referral center for evaluation for therapeutic hypothermia, passive cooling resulted in initiation of therapy 4.6 hours earlier than if therapy had been started at the cooling center.[52] This concept is especially relevant because many infants who may be treated with therapeutic hypothermia are born at referring centers.

Thus in a study of 45 term infants with moderate or severe HIE treated at a single center with selective head cooling, 96% were outborn, and the time to initiate cooling was 4.69 ± 0.79 hours.[53] Another study comparing active cooling with a servo-controlled mattress to passive cooling during transport demonstrated a later age at cooling and greater temperature instability in the passively cooled group; 27% of infants in the passive group did not achieve the target temperature and 34% of infants were overcooled.[54] An additional study comparing passive cooling to active cooling with a servo-controlled device showed a significantly lower heart rate in the actively cooled group (140 vs. 124 beats/min on admission), without any significant differences in coagulation profiles, rate of pulmonary artery hypertension, or other vital sign changes.[55] Given these results, transport teams traveling long distances with infants to a cooling center may consider development of protocols for the transfer of such infants, so as to avoid a delay in cooling and to improve temperature stability.[54]

SEIZURES

Hypoxic-ischemic cerebral injury is one of the most common causes of early-onset neonatal seizures. Although seizures are a consequence of the underlying brain injury, seizure activity in itself may also contribute to ongoing injury. Experimental evidence strongly suggests that repetitive seizures disturb brain growth and development as well as increase the risk for subsequent epilepsy.[56,57] Human studies, however, show conflicting evidence. Glass et al. demonstrated that clinical seizures in the setting of HIE in the era before therapeutic hypothermia were associated with worse cognitive and motor outcome at age 4 years.[58] The Cool Cap Study also demonstrated that the presence of aEEG seizures at time of enrollment was independently associated with an unfavorable outcome, defined as death or severe disability at 18 months.[59] It remains unclear if seizures may be truly damaging to the newborn brain or if they are simply reflective of the degree of brain injury. In contrast, a secondary analysis of the NICHD whole-body cooling trial demonstrated that the presence of clinical seizures at any time during the hospitalization was not associated with death or moderate or severe disability at 18 months of life.[60] This conflicting evidence may be

secondary to the fact that electrographic seizures frequently do not have a clinical correlate, and some clinical events suspected to be related to seizures may be nonepileptic in origin.[61] It is recommended that all infants at risk for seizures, such as the infant in our case or infants undergoing therapeutic hypothermia, undergo continuous EEG to accurately characterize seizures, although this remains challenging in many NICU settings.[62]

The optimal therapeutic approach for seizures in the neonatal period in the setting of HIE remains unclear (see also Chapter 7).[63–65] In many centers clinical and/or electrographic seizures are treated with an anticonvulsant, commonly phenobarbital as a first-line agent, and treatment is continued if seizures persist until the anticonvulsant therapy (e.g., phenobarbital, fosphenytoin, midazolam, or levetiracetam) has been optimized. Wide variation in antiepileptic drug use has been reported between centers treating infants with HIE with therapeutic hypothermia. A review of the Children's Hospital Neonatal Database and Pediatric Health Information Systems data for 1658 neonates treated with therapeutic hypothermia from 20 NICUs showed that 95% of patients with electrographic seizures received antiepileptic treatment, most commonly phenobarbital (97.6%), followed by levetiracetam (16.9%), and phenytoin/fosphenytoin (15.6%).[66] A recent small randomized controlled trial demonstrated phenobarbital to be more effective in neonatal seizure cessation compared to levetiracetam (80% vs. 28%, $P < 0.001$) due to any cause.[67] Large RCTs are still warranted to guide evidence-based management for monitoring and management of seizures associated with HIE.

Prophylactic Barbiturates

The prophylactic administration of high-dose barbiturates to infants at highest risk for developing HIE was evaluated in small studies before the era of therapeutic hypothermia and the results were conflicting. In one randomized study, the administration of thiopental initiated within 2 hours of birth and infused for 24 hours did not alter the frequency of seizures, intracranial pressure, or short-term neurodevelopmental outcome at 12 months.[68] Of importance was the observation that systemic hypotension occurred significantly more often in the treated group. In another randomized study, 40 mg/kg body weight of phenobarbital administered intravenously to asphyxiated infants between 1 and 6 hours of life was associated with subsequent neuroprotection. In this study there was no difference in the frequency of seizures between the two groups in the neonatal period; however, 73% of the pretreated infants compared with 18% of the control group ($P < 0.05$) demonstrated normal neurodevelopmental outcome at 3-year follow-up. No adverse effect of phenobarbital administration was observed.[69] There have been additional studies demonstrating a decrease in the incidence of seizures in infants treated with prophylactic phenobarbital. In one small study of term and near-term asphyxiated infants, phenobarbital administered within 6 hours of life resulted in a seizure frequency of 8% in the treatment group versus 40% in the control group ($P = 0.01$). Mortality and neurologic outcome at discharge were not different between the two groups.[70] Similarly, in another study, infants who were given 40 mg/kg of prophylactic phenobarbital during whole-body cooling had fewer clinical seizures than a control group of infants (15% vs. 82%, $P < 0.0001$). There was, however, no reduction in neurodevelopmental impairment at follow-up (range 18–49 months).[71] The most recent Cochrane review of prophylactic barbiturate administration following perinatal asphyxia demonstrated an overall reduction in seizures with treatment, but with no significant change in mortality.[72] This review also highlighted the paucity of data regarding long-term outcome and concluded that prophylactic phenobarbital administration could not be recommended but is a promising area of research.

Coagulopathy

Known adverse effects of therapeutic hypothermia in newborns include a significant increase in thrombocytopenia.[73] Infants with prolonged hypoxia often demonstrate a trend toward moderate thrombocytopenia, which may be compounded by alterations in platelet activation and aggregation seen with hypothermia.[74] One meta-analysis of a wide spectrum of patients treated with therapeutic hypothermia demonstrated an increased risk of thrombocytopenia and transfusion requirements, without a resultant increased risk of hemorrhage.[75] Hematologic parameters should be monitored closely and appropriate blood products administered as needed.

Potential Neuroprotective Strategies Aimed at Ameliorating Secondary Brain Injury

In addition to hypothermia (see Chapter 4), the following potential neuroprotective strategies have been considered.

ERYTHROPOIETIN

Erythropoietin (Epo) is a glycoprotein hormone most recognized for its role in erythropoiesis. However, it has also been shown to naturally increase during hypoxia-ischemia, along with an increase in Epo receptors. Epo is thought to provide a neuroprotective adaptive response during hypoxia-ischemia because of this effect.[3] Suggested protective mechanisms of action include antioxidant and antiinflammatory responses, induction of antiapoptotic factors, and decreased nitric oxide–mediated injury and susceptibility to glutamate toxicity.[76] Both stroke and hypoxic-ischemic animal models have demonstrated histologic protection with recombinant human Epo treatment.[77–80] In the neonatal rat stroke model, treated animals also performed better in most components of spatial learning and memory performance.[77]

Epo has also shown a beneficial effect in a study of term infants with moderate-severe HIE who were not treated with therapeutic hypothermia. In this study, infants were randomly assigned to receive recombinant Epo (rEpo) at either 300 U/kg or 500 U/kg every other day for 2 weeks beginning at less than 48 hours after birth. The rate of death or moderate-severe disability at 18 months was significantly reduced, occurring in 43.8% in the control group versus 24.6% in the rEpo group (RR 0.62, 95% CI 0.41–0.94). Benefit was seen in infants with moderate ($P = 0.001$) but not severe HIE ($P = 0.227$). There was no difference in primary outcome between doses used in this study and Epo was well tolerated.[81] In a multicenter phase 1 study of infants of at least 36 weeks' gestation with HIE, Epo (1000 U/kg) administered in conjunction with therapeutic hypothermia was safe and resulted in plasma concentrations that were neuroprotective in animal studies.[82] Follow-up of infants enrolled in this pharmacokinetics study between 8 and 34 months of age (mean 22 months) reported no deaths and moderate-severe developmental disability in only 1 of 22 patients available for follow-up, though this study was not designed to determine efficacy.[83] A larger phase II double-blinded trial of 50 infants treated with hypothermia and randomly assigned to either placebo or five total doses of Epo at 1000 U/kg per dose showed fewer infants treated with Epo with brain injury on MRI performed at 4 to 7 days of age and improved motor outcome at 1 year of life.[84] The High-Dose Erythropoietin for Asphyxia and Encephalopathy (HEAL) trial, a phase III randomized, placebo-controlled trial of Epo in infants with moderate to severe HIE treated with therapeutic hypothermia and multiple doses of Epo (1000 U/kg/dose) compared to placebo enrolled 500 infants $\geq$36 weeks' gestation, with primary composite outcome of death or mild, moderate or severe neurodevelopmental impairment at 2 years of life.[85] There was no significant difference in mortality or two year neurodevelopmental outcomes recently reported, and additionally Epo was associated with a higher number of serious adverse events.[86]

OXYGEN FREE RADICAL INHIBITORS AND SCAVENGERS

Another proposed therapeutic approach for the elimination of oxygen free radicals generated during and after hypoxia-ischemia is to administer specific enzymes, such as allopurinol, known to degrade highly reactive radicals to a nonreactive component.[3] In a clinical study, asphyxiated infants who received allopurinol demonstrated lower blood concentrations of oxygen free radicals than control infants.[87] However, a 2012 Cochrane review of three trials, involving 114 infants with encephalopathy treated with allopurinol, concluded there was no significant difference between treated and control groups in the risk of death during infancy or of neonatal seizures.[88] With such a small number of patients included, larger studies may be needed to determine whether there is truly lack of benefit. Follow-up from two of these randomized studies showed no difference in long-term outcomes at 4 to 8 years of age between treated infants and controls.[89] Melatonin has also been suggested as a potential adjunctive therapy because of its antioxidant properties. Aly et al. described a small study of 30 term infants with HIE and 15 controls. Half of the infants with HIE were randomly assigned to the 10 mg/kg enteral melatonin plus hypothermia group and the other half to hypothermia alone. The melatonin/hypothermia group had

fewer seizures on follow-up EEG at 2 weeks and fewer white matter abnormalities on MRI obtained after 2 weeks of life compared with the hypothermia group alone.[90] A more recent small randomized-controlled trial of 25 infants with hypoxia-ischemia randomized 12 infants to hypothermia plus a daily 5 mg/kg IV dose of melatonin and 13 to hypothermia plus placebo. Infants in the hypothermia plus melatonin group were found to score significantly higher on the Bayley III cognitive testing at 18 months of life (101 vs. 85, $P = 0.05$).[91] A 2021 systematic review and meta-analysis of melatonin for neuroprotection in neonatal encephalopathy confirms there is a paucity of data with these small studies, with a total of only 215 infants from five randomized-controlled trials, including the trial just described.[92] This meta-analysis highlights the need for larger clinical trials studying melatonin in this population.

EXCITATORY AMINO ACID ANTAGONISTS

Given the important role of excessive stimulation of neuronal surface receptors by glutamate in promoting a cascade of events leading to cellular death, it has been logical to identify pharmacologic agents that would either inhibit glutamate release or block its postsynaptic action.[3] Glutamate receptor antagonists (i.e., N-methyl-D-aspartate [NMDA] subtypes) have been extensively investigated in experimental animals. Noncompetitive antagonists provided a reduction in brain damage in adult animals even when administered up to 24 hours after the insult. The available NMDA antagonists include dizocilpine (MK-801), magnesium, xenon, phencyclidine (PCP), dextromethorphan, and ketamine.[3] Most of the previously mentioned NMDA antagonists are not widely used, however, magnesium and xenon will be discussed further in the following sections.

Magnesium

Magnesium is an NMDA antagonist, blocking neuronal influx of Ca^{2+} within the ion channel, and is also thought to potentially have antioxidant, anticytokine, and antiplatelet effects in the setting of perinatal asphyxia.[3] One large multicenter trial of infants born to women treated with magnesium sulfate who were at imminent risk for delivery between 24 and 31 weeks' gestation demonstrated that moderate or severe cerebral palsy occurred significantly less frequently in the magnesium-treated group (1.9% vs. 3.5%; RR 0.55, 95% CI 0.32–0.95).[93]

With this promise of neuroprotection with magnesium in preterm infants, there has been additional investigation in term asphyxiated infants. In a study performed by Bhat et al., term infants with severe perinatal asphyxia received three doses of magnesium (250 mg/kg per dose) within 6 hours of birth and at 24-hour intervals. An abnormal neurologic examination at discharge, performed by a clinician blinded to group assignment, was found in 22% of the treatment group compared with 56% of the placebo group ($P = 0.04$).[94] This is an interesting finding and is supported by a clinical study in which low plasma magnesium (<0.76 mmol/L) in the first 3 days of life was associated with impaired brain metabolism as measured by magnetic resonance spectroscopy in 65 term infants with HIE.[95] Despite these observations, there is a paucity of data with long-term outcome of magnesium administration to term infants with HIE. A meta-analysis of five clinical studies, including the study by Bhat et al., demonstrated a reduction in adverse short-term outcome with no difference in mortality or seizures.[96] There have been several studies assessing feasibility of therapeutic hypothermia administration in addition to magnesium sulfate. One small study of nine neonatal patients with HIE treated infants with therapeutic hypothermia, as well as combination therapy of Epo with magnesium, without any adverse events.[97] Clearly larger clinical studies are needed with long-term follow-up assessing the combined effect of magnesium with hypothermia.

Xenon

Xenon, an inhaled anesthetic, has been investigated as another adjunctive therapy with hypothermia, as it acts as a noncompetitive antagonist of the NMDA subtype of the glutamate receptor in the brain and rapidly crosses the blood-brain barrier.[3,76] While some preclinical studies of xenon showed great potential, results of the first randomized clinical study in term newborns with HIE have not been as promising. The Total Body hypothermia plus Xenon (TOBY-Xe) trial assessed a total of 92 infants, 46 treated with cooling alone and 46 with cooling plus 30% inhaled xenon administered within 12 hours of life for a duration of 24 hours.

There were no differences in biomarkers of cerebral damage, including a lactate-to-N-acetyl aspartate ratio in the thalamus and fractional anisotropy in the posterior limb of the internal capsule. This finding was thought to potentially be related to the late administration of xenon (median 10 hours), the lack of power to detect a difference in the N-acetyl aspartate ratio, or the possibility that infants in this cohort were too severely affected at enrollment.[98] Larger clinical studies are still needed to determine the time window in which xenon could be administered with hypothermia, the dose and duration of treatment needed, and xenon's effect on long-term neurodevelopmental outcomes.

Conclusions

The discovery of the benefits of therapeutic hypothermia has been one of the greatest advancements in newborn neuroprotection over the past 2 decades. There are many aspects of care the clinician can tailor to their individualized patient to optimize outcome, including judicious oxygen and fluid administration. There are many adjunctive therapies on the horizon that may also provide benefit and continue to be investigated on an ongoing basis (Fig. 8.2).

Gaps in Knowledge

1. Will the infant with HIE displaying milder forms of neonatal encephalopathy benefit from therapeutic hypothermia? If so, should duration or depth of hypothermia differ?
2. Will the short-term renal and cardioprotective effects seen with therapeutic hypothermia translate

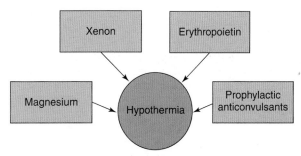

Fig. 8.2 Potential strategies to evaluate in high-risk infants treated with therapeutic hypothermia.

to long-term benefit? What is optimal anticonvulsant management in infants with seizures in the setting of HIE? Can larger high-quality studies assessing the use of prophylactic anticonvulsants be performed given that up to 50% of infants exhibit early seizures, with reports of decreased frequency of approximately 25% for those infants with moderate encephalopathy treated with therapeutic hypothermia?[59,99–101]

3. Are there benefits to the addition of melatonin as an adjunct to therapeutic hypothermia?

4. Are there other adjunctive agents that could improve outcomes in infants with HIE, such as modulators of neuroinflammation and repair/regeneration? If so, how can they be investigated in an animal model or early-phase trial for efficacy?

REFERENCES

1. Perlman JM. Intervention strategies for neonatal hypoxic-ischemic cerebral injury. *Clin Ther.* 2006;28(9):1353-1365.
2. Shalak L, Perlman JM. Hypoxic-ischemic brain injury in the term infant-current concepts. *Early Hum Dev.* 2004;80(2):125-141.
3. Volpe JJ, ed. *Volpe's Neurology of the Newborn.* 6th ed. Philadelphia: Elsevier; 2018.
4. Kurinczuk JJ, White-Koning M, Badawi N. Epidemiology of neonatal encephalopathy and hypoxic-ischaemic encephalopathy. *Early Hum Dev.* 2010;86(6):329-338.
5. Perlman JM. Summary proceedings from the neurology group on hypoxic-ischemic encephalopathy. *Pediatrics.* 2006;117 (3 Pt 2):S28-S33.
6. Stola A, Perlman J. Post-resuscitation strategies to avoid ongoing injury following intrapartum hypoxia-ischemia. *Semin Fetal Neonatal Med.* 2008;13(6):424-431.
7. Wyckoff MH, Wyllie J, Aziz K, et al. Neonatal life support 2020 International Consensus on Cardiopulmonary Resuscitation and Emergency Cardiovascular Care Science with treatment recommendations. *Resuscitation.* 2020;156:A156-A187.
8. Escobedo MB, Aziz K, Kapadia VS, et al. 2019 American Heart Association focused update on neonatal resuscitation: an update to the American Heart Association guidelines for cardiopulmonary resuscitation and emergency cardiovascular care. *Pediatrics.* 2020;145(1).
9. Weiner GM, Zaichkin J, eds. *Textbook of Neonatal Resuscitation.* 8th ed. American Academy of Pediatrics: 2021.
10. Aziz K, Lee HC, Escobedo MB, et al. Part 5: Neonatal resuscitation: 2020 American Heart Association guidelines for cardiopulmonary resuscitation and emergency cardiovascular care. *Circulation.* 2020;142(16 suppl 2):S524-S550.
11. Wyckoff MH, Aziz K, Escobedo MB, et al. Part 13: Neonatal resuscitation: 2015 American Heart Association guidelines update for cardiopulmonary resuscitation and emergency cardiovascular care. *Circulation.* 2015;132(18 suppl 2):S543-S560.
12. Welsford M, Nishiyama C, Shortt C, et al. Room air for initiating term newborn resuscitation: a systematic review with meta-analysis. *Pediatrics.* 2019;143(1):e20181825. doi:10.1542/peds.2018-1825.
13. Vento M, Asensi M, Sastre J, Garcia-Sala F, Pallardo FV, Vina J. Resuscitation with room air instead of 100% oxygen prevents oxidative stress in moderately asphyxiated term neonates. *Pediatrics.* 2001;107(4):642-647.
14. Klinger G, Beyene J, Shah P, Perlman M. Do hyperoxaemia and hypocapnia add to the risk of brain injury after intrapartum asphyxia? *Arch Dis Child Fetal Neonatal Ed.* 2005;90(1):F49-F52.
15. Kapadia VS, Chalak LF, DuPont TL, Rollins NK, Brion LP, Wyckoff MH. Perinatal asphyxia with hyperoxemia within the first hour of life is associated with moderate to severe hypoxic-ischemic encephalopathy. *J Pediatr.* 2013;163(4):949-954.
16. Gunn AJ, Bennet L, Gunning MI, Gluckman PD, Gunn TR. Cerebral hypothermia is not neuroprotective when started after postischemic seizures in fetal sheep. *Pediatr Res.* 1999;46(3):274-280.
17. Gunn AJ, Gunn TR, Gunning MI, Williams CE, Gluckman PD. Neuroprotection with prolonged head cooling started before postischemic seizures in fetal sheep. *Pediatrics.* 1998;102(5):1098-1106.
18. Gunn AJ. Cerebral hypothermia for prevention of brain injury following perinatal asphyxia. *Curr Opin Pediatr.* 2000;12(2):111-115.
19. Laptook AR, Shankaran S, Tyson JE, et al. Effect of therapeutic hypothermia initiated after 6 hours of age on death or disability among newborns with hypoxic-ischemic encephalopathy: a randomized clinical trial. *JAMA.* 2017;318(16):1550-1560.
20. Hellstrom-Westas L, Rosen I, Svenningsen NW. Predictive value of early continuous amplitude integrated EEG recordings on outcome after severe birth asphyxia in full term infants. *Arch Dis Child Fetal Neonatal Ed.* 1995;72(1):F34-F38.
21. al Naqeeb N, Edwards AD, Cowan FM, Azzopardi D. Assessment of neonatal encephalopathy by amplitude-integrated electroencephalography. *Pediatrics.* 1999;103(6 Pt 1):1263-1271.
22. Shalak LF, Laptook AR, Velaphi SC, Perlman JM. Amplitude-integrated electroencephalography coupled with an early neurologic examination enhances prediction of term infants at risk for persistent encephalopathy. *Pediatrics.* 2003;111(2):351-357.
23. Rosenberg AA, Jones MD Jr, Traystman RJ, Simmons MA, Molteni RA. Response of cerebral blood flow to changes in PCO2 in fetal, newborn, and adult sheep. *Am J Physiol.* 1982;242(5):H862-H866.
24. Vannucci RC, Brucklacher RM, Vannucci SJ. Effect of carbon dioxide on cerebral metabolism during hypoxia-ischemia in the immature rat. *Pediatr Res.* 1997;42(1):24-29.
25. Kaiser JR, Gauss CH, Williams DK. The effects of hypercapnia on cerebral autoregulation in ventilated very low birth weight infants. *Pediatr Res.* 2005;58(5):931-935.
26. Pappas A, Shankaran S, Laptook AR, et al. Hypocarbia and adverse outcome in neonatal hypoxic-ischemic encephalopathy. *J Pediatr.* 2011;158(5):752-758.e1.
27. Lingappan K, Kaiser JR, Srinivasan C, Gunn AJ. Relationship between PCO2 and unfavorable outcome in infants with moderate-to-severe hypoxic ischemic encephalopathy. *Pediatr Res.* 2016;80(2):204-208.
28. Lopez Laporte MA, Wang H, Sanon PN, et al. Association between hypocapnia and ventilation during the first days of life and brain injury in asphyxiated newborns treated with hypothermia. *J Matern Fetal Neonatal Med.* 2019;32(8):1312-1320.
29. Nadeem M, Murray D, Boylan G, Dempsey EM, Ryan CA. Blood carbon dioxide levels and adverse outcome in neonatal

hypoxic-ischemic encephalopathy. *Am J Perinatol.* 2010;27(5): 361-365.

30. Wyckoff MH, Perlman JM, Laptook AR. Use of volume expansion during delivery room resuscitation in near-term and term infants. *Pediatrics.* 2005;115(4):950-955.

31. Thoresen M, Whitelaw A. Cardiovascular changes during mild therapeutic hypothermia and rewarming in infants with hypoxic-ischemic encephalopathy. *Pediatrics.* 2000;106(1 Pt 1):92-99.

32. Wu TW, Tamrazi B, Soleymani S, Seri I, Noori S. Hemodynamic changes during rewarming phase of whole-body hypothermia therapy in neonates with hypoxic-ischemic encephalopathy. *J Pediatr.* 2018;197:68-74.e2.

33. van Wincoop M, de Bijl-Marcus K, Lilien M, van den Hoogen A, Groenendaal F. Effect of therapeutic hypothermia on renal and myocardial function in asphyxiated (near) term neonates: a systematic review and meta-analysis. *PLoS One.* 2021;16(2):e0247403.

34. Kecskes Z, Healy G, Jensen A. Fluid restriction for term infants with hypoxic-ischaemic encephalopathy following perinatal asphyxia. *Cochrane Database Syst Rev.* 2005;(3):CD004337.

35. Tanigasalam V, Plakkal N, Vishnu Bhat B, Chinnakali P. Does fluid restriction improve outcomes in infants with hypoxic ischemic encephalopathy? A pilot randomized controlled trial. *J Perinatol.* 2018;38(11):1512-1517.

36. Tanigasalam V, Bhat V, Adhisivam B, Sridhar MG. Does therapeutic hypothermia reduce acute kidney injury among term neonates with perinatal asphyxia?—a randomized controlled trial. *J Matern Fetal Neonatal Med.* 2016;29(15):2545-2548.

37. Chock VY, Frymoyer A, Yeh CG, Van Meurs KP. Renal saturation and acute kidney injury in neonates with hypoxic ischemic encephalopathy undergoing therapeutic hypothermia. *J Pediatr.* 2018;200:232-239.e1.

38. Jenik AG, Ceriani Cernadas JM, Gorenstein A, et al. A randomized, double-blind, placebo-controlled trial of the effects of prophylactic theophylline on renal function in term neonates with perinatal asphyxia. *Pediatrics.* 2000;105(4):E45.

39. Bhat MA, Shah ZA, Makhdoomi MS, Mufti MH. Theophylline for renal function in term neonates with perinatal asphyxia: a randomized, placebo-controlled trial. *J Pediatr.* 2006;149(2): 180-184.

40. Al-Wassia H, Alshaikh B, Sauve R. Prophylactic theophylline for the prevention of severe renal dysfunction in term and post-term neonates with perinatal asphyxia: a systematic review and meta-analysis of randomized controlled trials. *J Perinatol.* 2013;33(4):271-277.

41. Frymoyer A, Van Meurs KP, Drover DR, Klawitter J, Christians U, Chock VY. Theophylline dosing and pharmacokinetics for renal protection in neonates with hypoxic-ischemic encephalopathy undergoing therapeutic hypothermia. *Pediatr Res.* 2020;88(6):871-877.

42. Bhatt GC, Gogia P, Bitzan M, Das RR. Theophylline and aminophylline for prevention of acute kidney injury in neonates and children: a systematic review. *Arch Dis Child.* 2019;104(7):670-679.

43. Vannucci RC, Mujsce DJ. Effect of glucose on perinatal hypoxic-ischemic brain damage. *Biol Neonate.* 1992;62(4):215-224.

44. Yager JY. Hypoglycemic injury to the immature brain. *Clin Perinatol.* 2002;29(4):651-674, vi.

45. Salhab WA, Wyckoff MH, Laptook AR, Perlman JM. Initial hypoglycemia and neonatal brain injury in term infants with severe fetal acidemia. *Pediatrics.* 2004;114(2):361-366.

46. Basu SK, Kaiser JR, Guffey D, et al. Hypoglycaemia and hyperglycaemia are associated with unfavourable outcome in infants with hypoxic ischaemic encephalopathy: a post hoc analysis of the CoolCap Study. *Arch Dis Child Fetal Neonatal Ed.* 2016; 101(2):F149-F155.

47. Basu SK, Salemi JL, Gunn AJ, Kaiser JR, CoolCap Study Group. Hyperglycaemia in infants with hypoxic-ischaemic encephalopathy is associated with improved outcomes after therapeutic hypothermia: a post hoc analysis of the CoolCap Study. *Arch Dis Child Fetal Neonatal Ed.* 2017;102(4):F299-F306.

48. Basu SK, Ottolini K, Govindan V, et al. Early glycemic profile is associated with brain injury patterns on magnetic resonance imaging in hypoxic ischemic encephalopathy. *J Pediatr.* 2018; 203:137-143.

49. Laptook AR, Corbett RJ. The effects of temperature on hypoxic-ischemic brain injury. *Clin Perinatol.* 2002;29(4):623-649, vi.

50. Laptook A, Tyson J, Shankaran S, et al. Elevated temperature after hypoxic-ischemic encephalopathy: risk factor for adverse outcomes. *Pediatrics.* 2008;122(3):491-499.

51. Laptook AR, McDonald SA, Shankaran S, et al. Elevated temperature and 6- to 7-year outcome of neonatal encephalopathy. *Ann Neurol.* 2013;73(4):520-528.

52. Kendall GS, Kapetanakis A, Ratnavel N, Azzopardi D, Robertson NJ, Cooling on Retrieval Study Group. Passive cooling for initiation of therapeutic hypothermia in neonatal encephalopathy. *Arch Dis Child Fetal Neonatal Ed.* 2010;95(6):F408-F412.

53. Takenouchi T, Cuaycong M, Ross G, Engel M, Perlman JM. Chain of brain preservation—a concept to facilitate early identification and initiation of hypothermia to infants at high risk for brain injury. *Resuscitation.* 2010;81(12):1637-1641.

54. Chaudhary R, Farrer K, Broster S, McRitchie L, Austin T. Active versus passive cooling during neonatal transport. *Pediatrics.* 2013;132(5):841-846.

55. Lumba R, Mally P, Espiritu M, Wachtel EV. Therapeutic hypothermia during neonatal transport at Regional Perinatal Centers: active vs. passive cooling. *J Perinat Med.* 2019;47(3):365-369.

56. Dzhala V, Ben-Ari Y, Khazipov R. Seizures accelerate anoxia-induced neuronal death in the neonatal rat hippocampus. *Ann Neurol.* 2000;48(4):632-640.

57. Holmes GL, Gairsa JL, Chevassus-Au-Louis N, Ben-Ari Y. Consequences of neonatal seizures in the rat: morphological and behavioral effects. *Ann Neurol.* 1998;44(6):845-857.

58. Glass HC, Glidden D, Jeremy RJ, Barkovich AJ, Ferriero DM, Miller SP. Clinical neonatal seizures are independently associated with outcome in infants at risk for hypoxic-ischemic brain injury. *J Pediatr.* 2009;155(3):318-323.

59. Gluckman PD, Wyatt JS, Azzopardi D, et al. Selective head cooling with mild systemic hypothermia after neonatal encephalopathy: multicentre randomised trial. *Lancet.* 2005;365 (9460):663-670.

60. Kwon JM, Guillet R, Shankaran S, et al. Clinical seizures in neonatal hypoxic-ischemic encephalopathy have no independent impact on neurodevelopmental outcome: secondary analyses of data from the neonatal research network hypothermia trial. *J Child Neurol.* 2011;26(3):322-328.

61. Pressler RM, Cilio MR, Mizrahi EM, et al. The ILAE classification of seizures and the epilepsies: modification for seizures in the neonate. Position paper by the ILAE Task Force on Neonatal Seizures. *Epilepsia.* 2021;62(3):615-628.

62. Shellhaas RA, Chang T, Tsuchida T, et al. The American clinical neurophysiology society's guideline on continuous electroencephalography monitoring in neonates. *J Clin Neurophysiol.* 2011;28(6):611-617.

63. Scher MS, Aso K, Beggarly ME, Hamid MY, Steppe DA, Painter MJ. Electrographic seizures in preterm and full-term neonates:

clinical correlates, associated brain lesions, and risk for neurologic sequelae. *Pediatrics.* 1993;91(1):128-134.
64. Mizrahi EM. Consensus and controversy in the clinical management of neonatal seizures. *Clin Perinatol.* 1989;16(2):485-500.
65. van Rooij LG, Hellstrom-Westas L, de Vries LS. Treatment of neonatal seizures. *Semin Fetal Neonatal Med.* 2013;18(4):209-215.
66. Dizon MLV, Rao R, Hamrick SE, et al. Practice variation in antiepileptic drug use for neonatal hypoxic-ischemic encephalopathy among regional NICUs. *BMC Pediatr.* 2019;19(1):67.
67. Sharpe C, Reiner GE, Davis SL, et al. Levetiracetam versus phenobarbital for neonatal seizures: a randomized controlled trial. *Pediatrics.* 2020;145(6):e20193182. doi:10.1542/peds.2019-3182. Erratum in: Pediatrics. 2021;147(1).
68. Goldberg RN, Moscoso P, Bauer CR, et al. Use of barbiturate therapy in severe perinatal asphyxia: a randomized controlled trial. *J Pediatr.* 1986;109(5):851-856.
69. Hall RT, Hall FK, Daily DK. High-dose phenobarbital therapy in term newborn infants with severe perinatal asphyxia: a randomized, prospective study with three-year follow-up. *J Pediatr.* 1998;132(2):345-348.
70. Singh D, Kumar P, Narang A. A randomized controlled trial of phenobarbital in neonates with hypoxic ischemic encephalopathy. *J Matern Fetal Neonatal Med.* 2005;18(6):391-395.
71. Meyn DF Jr, Ness J, Ambalavanan N, Carlo WA. Prophylactic phenobarbital and whole-body cooling for neonatal hypoxic-ischemic encephalopathy. *J Pediatr.* 2010;157(2):334-336.
72. Young L, Berg M, Soll R. Prophylactic barbiturate use for the prevention of morbidity and mortality following perinatal asphyxia. *Cochrane Database Syst Rev.* 2016;5:CD001240.
73. Jacobs SE, Berg M, Hunt R, Tarnow-Mordi WO, Inder TE, Davis PG. Cooling for newborns with hypoxic ischaemic encephalopathy. *Cochrane Database Syst Rev.* 2013;(1):CD003311.
74. Wood T, Thoresen M. Physiological responses to hypothermia. *Semin Fetal Neonatal Med.* 2015;20(2):87-96.
75. Wang CH, Chen NC, Tsai MS, et al. Therapeutic hypothermia and the risk of hemorrhage: a systematic review and meta-analysis of randomized controlled trials. *Medicine (Baltimore).* 2015;94(47):e2152.
76. Kelen D, Robertson NJ. Experimental treatments for hypoxic ischaemic encephalopathy. *Early Hum Dev.* 2010;86(6):369-377.
77. Gonzalez FF, Abel R, Almli CR, Mu D, Wendland M, Ferriero DM. Erythropoietin sustains cognitive function and brain volume after neonatal stroke. *Dev Neurosci.* 2009;31(5):403-411.
78. Aydin A, Genc K, Akhisaroglu M, Yorukoglu K, Gokmen N, Gonullu E. Erythropoietin exerts neuroprotective effect in neonatal rat model of hypoxic-ischemic brain injury. *Brain Dev.* 2003;25(7):494-498.
79. Kellert BA, McPherson RJ, Juul SE. A comparison of high-dose recombinant erythropoietin treatment regimens in brain-injured neonatal rats. *Pediatr Res.* 2007;61(4):451-455.
80. Fan X, Heijnen CJ, van der KM, Groenendaal F, van Bel F. Beneficial effect of erythropoietin on sensorimotor function and white matter after hypoxia-ischemia in neonatal mice. *Pediatr Res.* 2011;69(1):56-61.
81. Zhu C, Kang W, Xu F, et al. Erythropoietin improved neurologic outcomes in newborns with hypoxic-ischemic encephalopathy. *Pediatrics.* 2009;124(2):e218-e226.
82. Wu YW, Bauer LA, Ballard RA, et al. Erythropoietin for neuroprotection in neonatal encephalopathy: safety and pharmacokinetics. *Pediatrics.* 2012;130(4):683-691.
83. Rogers EE, Bonifacio SL, Glass HC, et al. Erythropoietin and hypothermia for hypoxic-ischemic encephalopathy. *Pediatr Neurol.* 2014;51(5):657-662.
84. Wu YW, Mathur AM, Chang T, et al. High-dose erythropoietin and hypothermia for hypoxic-ischemic encephalopathy: a phase II trial. *Pediatrics.* 2016;137(6):e20160191. doi:10.1542/peds.2016-0191.
85. Juul SE, Comstock BA, Heagerty PJ, et al. High-dose erythropoietin for asphyxia and encephalopathy (HEAL): a randomized controlled trial—background, aims, and study protocol. *Neonatology.* 2018;113(4):331-338.
86. Wu YW, Mathur AM, Chang T, et al., eds. *Randomized Controlled Trial of Erythropoietin for Neonatal Hypoxic-Ischemic Encephalopathy.* Denver, CO: Pediatric Academic Societies; 2022.
87. Van Bel F, Shadid M, Moison RM, et al. Effect of allopurinol on postasphyxial free radical formation, cerebral hemodynamics, and electrical brain activity. *Pediatrics.* 1998;101(2):185-193.
88. Chaudhari T, McGuire W. Allopurinol for preventing mortality and morbidity in newborn infants with hypoxic-ischaemic encephalopathy. *Cochrane Database Syst Rev.* 2012;(7):CD006817.
89. Kaandorp JJ, van Bel F, Veen S, et al. Long-term neuroprotective effects of allopurinol after moderate perinatal asphyxia: follow-up of two randomised controlled trials. *Arch Dis Child Fetal Neonatal Ed.* 2012;97(3):F162-F166.
90. Aly H, Elmahdy H, El-Dib M, et al. Melatonin use for neuroprotection in perinatal asphyxia: a randomized controlled pilot study. *J Perinatol.* 2015;35(3):186-191.
91. Jerez-Calero A, Salvatierra-Cuenca MT, Benitez-Feliponi A, et al. Hypothermia plus melatonin in asphyctic newborns: a randomized-controlled pilot study. *Pediatr Crit Care Med.* 2020;21(7):647-655.
92. Ahmed J, Pullattayil SA, Robertson NJ, More K. Melatonin for neuroprotection in neonatal encephalopathy: a systematic review & meta-analysis of clinical trials. *Eur J Paediatr Neurol.* 2021;31:38-45.
93. Rouse DJ, Hirtz DG, Thom E, et al. A randomized, controlled trial of magnesium sulfate for the prevention of cerebral palsy. *N Engl J Med.* 2008;359(9):895-905.
94. Bhat MA, Charoo BA, Bhat JI, Ahmad SM, Ali SW, Mufti MU. Magnesium sulfate in severe perinatal asphyxia: a randomized, placebo-controlled trial. *Pediatrics.* 2009;123(5):e764-e769.
95. Chakkarapani E, Chau V, Poskitt KJ, et al. Low plasma magnesium is associated with impaired brain metabolism in neonates with hypoxic-ischaemic encephalopathy. *Acta Paediatr.* 2016;105(9):1067-1073.
96. Tagin M, Shah PS, Lee KS. Magnesium for newborns with hypoxic-ischemic encephalopathy: a systematic review and meta-analysis. *J Perinatol.* 2013;33(9):663-669.
97. Nonomura M, Harada S, Asada Y, et al. Combination therapy with erythropoietin, magnesium sulfate and hypothermia for hypoxic-ischemic encephalopathy: an open-label pilot study to assess the safety and feasibility. *BMC Pediatr.* 2019;19(1):13.
98. Azzopardi D, Robertson NJ, Bainbridge A, et al. Moderate hypothermia within 6 h of birth plus inhaled xenon versus moderate hypothermia alone after birth asphyxia (TOBY-Xe): a proof-of-concept, open-label, randomised controlled trial. *Lancet Neurol.* 2016;15(2):145-153.
99. Shankaran S, Laptook AR, Ehrenkranz RA, et al. Whole-body hypothermia for neonates with hypoxic-ischemic encephalopathy. *N Engl J Med.* 2005;353(15):1574-1584.
100. Azzopardi DV, Strohm B, Edwards AD, et al. Moderate hypothermia to treat perinatal asphyxial encephalopathy. *N Engl J Med.* 2009;361(14):1349-1358.
101. Gano D, Orbach SA, Bonifacio SL, Glass HC. Neonatal seizures and therapeutic hypothermia for hypoxic-ischemic encephalopathy. *Mol Cell Epilepsy.* 2014;1(3):e88. doi:10.14800/mce.88.

Chapter 9

Diagnosis and Management of Acute Symptomatic Seizures in Neonates

Jennifer C. Keene and Hannah C. Glass

Chapter Outline

Neonatal Seizures—Introduction

Seizures occur during the neonatal period in approximately 2 to 4 per 1000 live births.[1–4] Seizures are a neurologic emergency: they are often caused by acute brain injury or treatable underlying conditions and rapid, appropriate treatment can improve treatment success.[5,6] Seizure management includes rapid and thorough diagnostic evaluation, as seizures are frequently the presenting symptom for electrolyte abnormalities, infection, hypoxic-ischemic injury, and intracranial hemorrhage. Seizures in this age group have unique features requiring an age-appropriate approach to classification and diagnosis using an electroencephalogram (EEG). An appreciation for the multifactorial effects of antiseizure medications (ASMs) and seizure burden on the rapidly developing brain is essential.

This chapter will focus on seizure diagnosis and classification in the neonatal population, diagnostic, treatment, and prognostic considerations in confirmed neonatal seizures, and the ongoing controversies associated with each of these topics.

Diagnosis

ELECTROENCEPHALOGRAM

EEG is an essential tool for seizure diagnosis in neonates. Neonates often exhibit paroxysmal movements, which can be difficult for even skilled providers to distinguish from seizures clinically. When experienced neonatal healthcare providers evaluated standardized videos of seizures and seizure mimics, they identified seizures correctly only 50% of the time.[7] Furthermore, prospective cohort studies have demonstrated that up to 80% of neonatal seizure burden may be electrographic only.[8,9] Significant underdiagnosis occurs if seizures are diagnosed using only clinical observation. Electrographic seizures can persist when clinical manifestations resolve, even when clinical neonatal seizures are appropriately identified and treated. This phenomenon has been termed *electroclinical uncoupling* and is estimated to occur in up to 25% of neonates.[10] Recent evidence suggests that early identification and treatment of electrographic seizures may increase the odds of successful seizure treatment.[5,6]

In 2011, the American Clinical Neurophysiology Society developed guidelines for monitoring and diagnosing neonates at risk for seizures. These guidelines recommend long-term conventional video EEG monitoring for multiple neonatal populations, including neonates with unexplained paroxysmal events, encephalopathy, central nervous system infection or trauma, suspected perinatal stroke or hemorrhage, suspected inborn errors of metabolism or genetic epilepsies, and children who require cardiopulmonary bypass.[11]

Historically, a seizure in neonates has been defined as sudden, repetitive, rhythmic, evolving EEG activity with a minimum of 2 μV peak-to-peak voltage that lasts a minimum of 10 seconds.[12] More recently, the International League Against Epilepsy (ILAE) expanded the definition to include shorter events if the duration is sufficient to demonstrate clear onset, evolution of the frequency and morphology, and resolution of the abnormal discharge.[13] Discharges without clear evolution of the rhythmic activity are considered to be brief rhythmic discharges (BRDs). BRDs are thought to confer an increased seizure risk. The traditional definition of status epilepticus in older children and adults, which includes a failure to return to baseline cognitive function, is difficult to apply to neonates. Neonatal status epilepticus has instead been operationally defined as seizures lasting greater than 50% of any 1-hour epoch of EEG recording.[11]

Conventional Versus Amplitude-Integrated EEG

The American Clinical Neurophysiology Society guidelines recommend conventional video EEG (cEEG) as the gold standard for seizure diagnosis in neonates. Amplitude-integrated EEG (aEEG) is a simplified brain-monitoring tool that has been widely adopted in many units for ease of bedside monitoring.

In neonates, the International 10–20 system for EEG is simplified to approximately 20 scalp electrodes accompanied by an electrocardiogram lead and respiratory belt.[12] Interpretation requires specialized education to learn preterm and term neonates' normal patterns in wakefulness and sleep and the appearance of important pathologies, including seizures. EEG technologists and bedside nursing staff are essential to help identify the plethora of potential artifacts commonly observed on cEEG recordings.

aEEG is a widely available bedside tool that is easy to apply and interpret at the bedside.[14] It uses a limited montage (usually 1–3 channels to cover the frontal and central or parietal regions). The maximum and minimum amplitude recorded during a specified time epoch are plotted on a compressed time scale and semilogarithmic y-axis for amplitude to display a trend tracing for each electrode pair.[15] A seizure is suspected when a sudden and sustained increase in amplitude is noted on both upper and lower margins of the aEEG tracing. A concurrent review of the raw EEG signal is helpful to confirm an evolving, monomorphic waveform consistent with seizure.[16] Limitations of aEEG include low sensitivity to detect low amplitude, brief, or very focal seizures occurring in an area not directly adjacent to the electrodes. In 125 neonates greater than 34 weeks postmenstrual age who were evaluated with concurrent cEEG and aEEG, neonatologists were able to use aEEG to identify between 12% and 38% of the individual seizures seen on cEEG, and overall aEEG use identified between 22% and 57% of neonates with seizures.[17]

Common EEG and aEEG artifacts include patting, sucking, intravascular line drips, ventilation artifact, and extracorporeal membrane oxygenation artifact.[15,18] Artifacts may be more difficult to distinguish from seizures on aEEG due to limited channels, lack of video, and absent technologist input to resolve electrical artifacts. Prospective cohort studies have found dramatically differing rates of events concerning for seizures depending on the type of neurophysiology monitoring used, particularly in the preterm neonatal population. In two similar prospective cohorts of preterm neonates, 48% of children had seizures when aEEG was used for diagnosis[19] compared with 5% of children when gold standard cEEG was used for diagnosis.[20] Such divergent results suggest that, while aEEG may serve as an excellent screening tool (especially in resource-limited settings), gold-standard cEEG is necessary for optimal seizure management.[21,22]

For most monitoring systems, aEEG can be displayed at the bedside (using the leads placed for the full montage recording) while the cEEG is recorded and made available for remote access by the neurophysiologist.[21] This approach has the advantage of providing both a bedside tool for immediate use by the neonatology team and the gold-standard recording for definitive seizure identification. Furthermore, using the same machine and recording for both the aEEG and traditional EEG display can facilitate communication between teams as annotations regarding clinical condition or medication administration by the bedside team can be communicated easily with the neurophysiologist and vice versa.

Automated Seizure Detection

Quantitative EEG (qEEG) has been increasingly used to predict and aid in identifying neonatal seizures. qEEG analysis, including relative and absolute spectral analysis, has been used to evaluate neonatal EEG seizure risk in neonates with encephalopathy.[23] Ongoing work is focused on translating qualitative use of EEG background to predict seizure risk[24,25] into quantified and more easily applied metrics.

Seizure detection algorithms developed in adults have low accuracy for detecting seizures in neonates.[26] Recent efforts to develop neonatal-specific seizure detection algorithms have demonstrated decreased time to treatment and seizure burden when partnered with physician review.[27] Initial neonatal qEEG development has focused on term and near-term neonates, but efforts are underway to develop qEEG techniques specific for preterm neonates.[18]

CLASSIFICATION OF SEIZURES

There have been multiple historical classification systems for neonatal seizures, which typically do not fit neatly into the seizure classifications used for older children or adults. In 2021, the ILAE published an updated framework to classify neonatal seizures[13] (Fig. 9.1). The updated classification system emphasizes the need to incorporate EEG evaluation and explicitly recognizes electrographic-only seizures due to their high frequency and importance in neonates.[10,28,29] Generalized seizures are not included in the classification as seizure onset is always focal in neonates.[30] Electroclinical seizures are categorized as motor seizures, nonmotor seizures (autonomic changes or behavioral arrest), sequential seizures, or unclassified (Table 9.1).

Motor Seizure

Automatisms

Neonatal seizures with automatisms usually consist of oral-lingual-buccal movements and are frequently accompanied by alternations of consciousness.[13] They may be associated with fluctuations in blood pressure, heart rate, and oxygen saturation but are often clinically subtle unless accompanied by other seizure types.

Clonic Seizures

Clonic seizures consist of rhythmic movements, which are nonsuppressible and unaltered by repositioning. Focal clonic seizures are the most consistently correctly

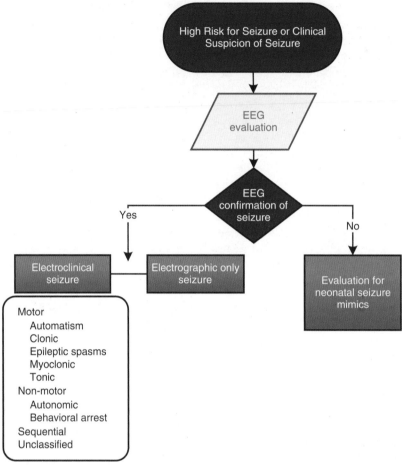

Fig. 9.1 **Diagnostic framework for neonatal seizure diagnosis and classification as outlined in the 2021 ILAE guideline.** (Adapted from Pressler RM, Cilio MR, Mizrahi EM, et al. The ILAE classification of seizures and the epilepsies: modification for seizures in the neonate. Position paper by the ILAE task force on neonatal seizures. *Epilepsia* 2021;62(3):615–628.)

identified type of neonatal seizure[7] and are often associated with injury localized to a specific site, such as a perinatal stroke or other cerebrovascular event.[31–34] Multifocal clonic seizures are more common in neonates with multifocal or generalized brain injury such as hypoxic-ischemic encephalopathy. Clonic seizures in a neonate may be mistaken for nonepileptic tremor, jitteriness, or clonus.

Myoclonic Seizures
Myoclonic movements are extremely rapid (<100 msec) jerks of one or multiple limbs. Myoclonus can represent seizure or originate at more distal regions of the central nervous system, including the brainstem and spinal cord. Myoclonic seizures are most commonly seen in neonatal-onset genetic epilepsies and inborn errors of metabolism.[31,35–38]

Epileptic Spasms
Epileptic spasms in neonates are rare. Their clinical presentation is similar to older-onset infantile spasms (which typically present around 6 months of age), with sudden flexion or extension of the proximal and truncal muscles. Spasms are longer than myoclonic movements but briefer than tonic seizures and usually occur in clusters. Subtle forms can consist of clusters of abnormal eye movements or head nodding.[13] This rare seizure type is classically associated with inborn errors of metabolism.[35–44]

TABLE 9.1 ILAE Seizure Classification for Neonates and Common Nonepileptic Mimics		
Seizure Type	Characteristics	Nonepileptic Mimics
Electrographic only	• No clinical manifestations • Requires EEG diagnosis	• None
Motor: automatisms	• Uninterruptible rhythmic orofacial, movements, which may be associated with impaired consciousness	• Nonepileptic sucking and oromotor movements
Motor: clonic	• Focal, nonsuppressible rhythmic movements, which may involve one or more body areas	• Clonus • Tremor/jitter • Sleep myoclonus
Motor: epileptic spasms	• Rapid extension or flexion of the extremities and trunk, typically occurring in clusters lasting seconds to minutes	• Nonepileptic myoclonus • Head bobbing • Gastroesophageal reflux
Motor: myoclonic	• Nonsuppressible, extremely rapid jerk of one or multiple extremities, may or may not occur in clusters	• Nonepileptic myoclonus • Sleep myoclonus
Motor: tonic	• Stiffening of one or more extremities with associated EEG decrement or another ictal pattern	• Dystonia • Gastroesophageal reflux
Nonmotor: autonomic	• Paroxysmal alteration of respiratory, cardiovascular, pupillary function, or flushing with ictal EEG correlate	• Nonepileptic apnea, tachycardia, or autonomic fluctuation
Nonmotor: behavioral arrest	• Arrest in normal neonatal movements with ictal EEG correlate	• Typical behavioral fluctuation in movement
Sequential	• Variable progression of multiple motor and nonmotor ictal features with an EEG correlate	• Normal neonatal movement

Tonic Seizures

Tonic seizures are marked by sustained flexion or extension lasting seconds to minutes. Tonic seizures can include neck or head version, forced eye deviation, or trunk and limb involvement.[13] Neonatal tonic seizures are highly variable, including focal, unilateral, or bilateral asymmetric, and are typically associated with early infantile-onset epileptic encephalopathies.[31,37,44,45]

Nonmotor Seizure

Autonomic Seizure

Autonomic seizures are paroxysmal alterations in cardiovascular, respiratory, vasomotor, or pupillary function with EEG epileptic correlate. Isolated autonomic abnormalities are rarely caused by seizure; less than 5% of studies obtained for isolated apnea have an ictal correlate.[46] Autonomic seizures are usually associated with intraventricular hemorrhage, temporal lobe or occipital lesions, and occasionally with early-onset epileptic encephalopathies.[29,39,47,48]

Behavioral Arrest

Ictal behavioral arrest is rare in isolation. More commonly, a behavioral arrest is part of a sequential seizure.[31,39]

Sequential Seizure

Neonatal seizures are sequential when the ictal pattern progresses through a series of phases associated with EEG changes.[13] Within the individual ictal event, the lateralization and composition of ictal features may vary. This type of seizure is associated with genetic epilepsies, particularly KCNQ2 encephalopathy.[45,49–52]

NONEPILEPTIC MIMICS OF SEIZURES IN NEONATES

Neonates have a wide array of paroxysmal movements, which can be easily mistaken for seizures.[7] The most common mimics include tremulousness, nonepileptic myoclonus, dystonic movements, and more rarely hyperekplexia.

Tremor or Jitteriness

Tremor and jitteriness can occur in both ill and healthy neonates. The movements are characterized by rhythmic oscillation of varying amplitudes and stereotypy. Tremor may be asymmetric and either spontaneous or induced by stimulation or movement.[53] Tremor and jitteriness may be differentiated from seizure by suppression with flexion, restraint, or repositioning. Tremor and jitteriness can occur in neonates with hypothermia, or secondary to metabolic derangements, particularly hypoglycemia and hypocalcemia. Tremor and jitteriness are also seen in neonates exposed to some maternal medications classes, including selective serotonin reuptake inhibitors (SSRI), cocaine, and marijuana.[54–56]

Myoclonus Without Electrographic Correlate

Nonepileptic myoclonus, like myoclonic seizures, is characterized by rapid ($<$100 msec) jerks of one or more areas of the body.[57] In the preterm neonate, benzodiazepines may cause medication-induced myoclonus thought to be due to developmental differences in the γ-aminobutyric acid (GABA) receptors, which abate as neonates mature.[58,59] Nonepileptic myoclonus has been described in the setting of intracranial infection, intracranial hemorrhage, periventricular leukomalacia, and genetic and metabolic disorders.[41,42,60,61]

In an otherwise healthy neonate with a normal neurologic exam and jerking movements occurring only during sleep, benign neonatal sleep myoclonus should be considered. Benign neonatal sleep myoclonus is arrhythmic, may increase with attempts to physically suppress the movements, occurs at all sleep stages, and stops when the child is wakened.[62] Benign neonatal sleep myoclonus will typically resolve by 3 months of age, although a few infants may have movements up to a year of age.[62]

Dystonia

Dystonia is a sustained involuntary contraction of opposing muscle groups, often resulting in a twisted or abnormal posture.[57] In neonates, dystonia or opisthotonic posturing is most commonly seen in encephalopathic neonates who have sustained an injury to the basal ganglia.[63] Less common causes include inborn error of metabolism (e.g., monoamine neurotransmitter disorders, maple syrup urine disease[64,65]). Nonepileptic bilateral tonic extension not having a correlate on EEG may represent "brainstem release" in the setting of extensive cortical dysfunction or posterior fossa pathology.[29]

Hyperekplexia

Hyperekplexia is a rare but important cause of hyperkinetic paroxysmal events in neonates that is characterized by nonextinguishable exaggerated startle reflex accompanied by hyperreflexia and hypertonia. Hyperekplexia is most commonly associated with mutations of the glycine receptor, but can also be seen in molybdenum cofactor deficiency.[66,67]

Untreated hyperekplexia is associated with death secondary to apneic spells, which can be mitigated using scheduled benzodiazepines.[68,69]

CONTROVERSIES IN DIAGNOSIS

Clinical versus EEG Diagnosis of Seizures

- Based on the high rate of misdiagnosis using clinical features alone,[7] frequency of electrographic-only seizures and emerging evidence regarding the importance of early seizure treatment,[5] the American Clinical Neurophysiology Society recommends cEEG for definitive seizure diagnosis and monitoring of high-risk neonates. cEEG should also be used to manage ASMs and to determine resolution of acute provoked seizures (operationally defined as at least 24 hours without EEG seizures). There is ongoing controversy regarding safe seizure management in lower resource settings without access to cEEG.

aEEG versus cEEG

- aEEG is easy to apply and interpret at the bedside, but lacks the sensitivity and specificity of cEEG, particularly in the hands of inexperienced users.[17,70] A safe and efficient balance between utilizing these tools is a topic of ongoing discussion.

EEG Seizure Duration Definition

- The duration of both an individual seizure and neonatal status epilepticus have historically been arbitrarily defined. Recent ILAE guidelines[13] suggest duration should not be included in neonatal seizure definitions, particularly as several uncommon seizure types have a duration substantially shorter than the historical seizure definition of 10 seconds. However, defining seizures shorter than 10 seconds based on feature evolution alone is challenging and may decrease interrater reliability. Future work may focus on determining which definition(s) of seizure best correlate with clinical outcomes.

Frequency of Seizures in Preterm Infants

- Depending on the type of monitoring (cEEG vs. aEEG vs. clinical) and individual cohort composition, a widely divergent frequency of preterm seizures has been reported. The optimal indications, duration, and type of EEG monitoring for preterm infants remain an area of active research.

Seizure Causes in Neonates

DIAGNOSTIC EVALUATION OF ETIOLOGY IN NEONATES WITH SEIZURES

The underlying cause for seizures in neonates should be rapidly and systematically evaluated with an early focus on identifying reversible and treatable causes. A thorough history and exam will often reveal important seizure risk factors. Essential information includes birth history suggesting a risk of hypoxic-ischemic injury, infectious risk factors, drug exposure, known congenital malformations, or a family history of seizures in infancy. All neonates should be screened for electrolyte derangements, including hypoglycemia, hypocalcemia, and hyponatremia.[71] History of fetal distress or advanced resuscitation, laboratory evaluation suggesting global hypoxia-ischemia (i.e., acidotic cord or blood gas, elevation in liver enzymes), and encephalopathic exam can be used to identify neonates with risk of a hypoxic injury. A thorough infectious workup, including lumbar puncture, should be considered in the correct clinical context to evaluate for treatable infectious causes of seizure. A viral cause of seizure may be identified through standard testing; metagenomic sequencing can be used to augment the diagnostic yield.[72] Urine toxicologic evaluation may be indicated based on history. Urgent neuroimaging with head ultrasound scans (HUS) may identify hemorrhagic, and in some cases ischemic, stroke. Neuroimaging with brain magnetic resonance imaging (MRI) can accurately identify the seizure etiology in most cases. All neonates with seizures should receive MRI, even if a reversible cause is suspected. MRI timing should be tailored to the presumed cause (e.g., 4–7 days for suspected ischemic injury or as soon as medically safe for other causes).

Genetic and metabolic evaluation should be pursued when no clear etiology has been identified after evaluating for acute provoked and transient causes, or if seizures remain refractory to ASM longer than 3 days. An infantile epilepsy panel or whole exome sequencing is recommended as the first-line evaluation for suspected genetic epilepsy. If screening labs suggest inborn error of metabolism (e.g., high ammonia, high lactate in the absence of a hypoxic-ischemic insult), genetic-metabolic screening (including ammonia, lactate, pyruvate, serum amino acids, urine organic acids, carnitine, and acylcarnitine profiles) and consultation with a genetic-metabolic specialist is indicated.

ACUTE PROVOKED SEIZURES

The majority of seizures in neonates are due to an acute provoked (also called "acute symptomatic") cause, such as hypoxic-ischemic encephalopathy, ischemic stroke, or intracranial hemorrhage (Fig. 9.2; Box 9.1). Once a diagnosis of seizure has been established, care is focused on rapidly treating ongoing seizures and, just as importantly, identifying the underlying cause.

Hypoxic-ischemic Encephalopathy (HIE)

HIE is the most common cause of seizures in neonates, accounting for 38% in a recent prospective cohort.[28] The frequency of seizure in neonates with moderate HIE has decreased by approximately half since therapeutic hypothermia was established as the standard of care by multiple randomized controlled trials.[73–75] The onset of seizures in HIE varies but is typically within the first 24 hours[74] after birth, with recent data suggesting it is rare to have seizure onset after 24 hours in the setting of a normal or mildly abnormal EEG background.[24] The majority of seizures in neonates due to HIE will abate within 72 hours.[76]

Ischemic and Hemorrhagic Stroke

Ischemic stroke of either venous or arterial origin and intracranial hemorrhage are common and important causes of seizures in neonates. Up to 90% of neonates with perinatal arterial ischemic infarct present with seizures,[77] most often focal clonic seizures.[31] Neonates with perinatal arterial ischemic infarcts may be otherwise well appearing. Bland and hemorrhagic infarcts associated with neonatal cerebral venous sinus thrombosis are more commonly seen after complicated pregnancy or delivery, sepsis, or dehydration and frequently have seizures as a presenting symptom.[78] Intraventricular hemorrhage is the most common cause of seizures in the very preterm neonate (<32 weeks).[79] Term neonates with intraventricular hemorrhage should be evaluated for cerebral venous sinus thrombosis.

Neonates requiring early repair of congenital heart defects or extracorporeal membrane oxygenation have unique risk factors for cerebrovascular injury leading to seizures.[80] Approximately 10% of neonates monitored with cEEG after repair of the congenital heart defect have clinical or subclinical seizures.[81–83] Up to 30% of children undergoing extracorporeal membrane oxygenation have seizures.[84,85] Imaging suggests that seizures are secondary to a mix of injuries, including hypotensive hypoxic injuries, embolic infarction, and

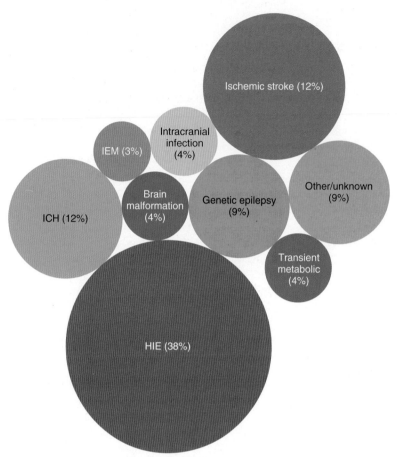

Seizure Etiology and % of Total Percent. Color shows details about Seizure Etiology. Size shows sum of Percent. The marks are labeled by Seizure Etiology and % of Total Percent.

Fig. 9.2 Relative frequencies of seizure cause in neonates. *HIE,* Hypoxic ischemic encephalopathy; *ICH,* intracranial hemorrhage; *IEM,* inborn error of metabolism. (Based on Glass HC, Shellhaas RA, Wusthoff CJ, et al. Contemporary profile of seizures in neonates: a prospective cohort study. *J Pediatr* 2016;174:98–103.e1.)

BOX 9.1   DIFFERENTIAL DIAGNOSIS FOR ACUTE PROVOKED SEIZURES AND NEONATAL-ONSET EPILEPSY

ACUTE PROVOKED/TRANSIENT SEIZURES
- Hypoxic-ischemic encephalopathy
- Ischemic stroke
- Intracranial infection
- Intracranial hemorrhage
- Transient metabolic (e.g., hypoglycemia, hypocalcemia)

NEONATAL-ONSET EPILEPSIES
- Genetic epilepsy (e.g., KCNQ2)
- Inborn error of metabolism
- Brain malformation

an increased risk of intracranial hemorrhage in the setting of anticoagulation.[82–84]

Infection

Viral and bacterial meningitis are important causes of neonatal encephalopathy and seizures. Neonatal herpes encephalitis[86,87] and enteroviruses (and particularly parechovirus)[88,89] are the most common causes of seizures due to viral infection. Bacterial meningitis is also directly implicated in seizures and is frequently complicated by arterial stroke, cerebral venous sinus thrombosis, and cerebral abscess, which may further contribute to seizure burden and injury.[90]

Metabolic Derangements

Metabolic derangements that cause seizures include hypoglycemia, hypocalcemia, hyponatremia, and hypernatremia. Hypoglycemia is associated with seizures, jitteriness, and abnormal tone. Profound hypoglycemia can result in parieto-occipital predominant injury, particularly if prolonged.[91] Parenchymal injury may lead to seizures even after reversing the initial hypoglycemia.[92] Symptomatic hypocalcemia can occur at an ionized calcium level of less than 4.8 mg/dL (1.2 mmol/L) in term infants and less than 4.0 mg/dL (1 mmol/L) in premature infants.[93] Symptomatic neonates may experience myoclonic jerks, exaggerated startle, and seizures until calcium is appropriately repleted.[94,95] Both hypo and hypernatremic seizures are rare in the neonate and are typically seen in the setting of excess maternal water intake during labor, endocrine abnormalities, infection, dehydration, or iatrogenic causes and are treated with judicious correction of the electrolyte abnormality and the underlying cause.[96]

Drug Withdrawal and Intoxication

Prenatal exposure to a variety of substances can put neonates at risk for seizures and common seizure mimics. Maternal opiate and alcohol ingestion can both result in seizures due to substance withdrawal.[54,97] Maternal cocaine use can cause seizures through several mechanisms, including acute intoxication, withdrawal, and increased risk of neonatal stroke.[55,98]

Maternal SSRI use has been associated with neonatal withdrawal syndrome, that includes neonatal convulsions, tremor, jitteriness, and disturbed state regulation, which can also mimic seizures.[99] Most children with convulsions due to maternal SSRI use do not have EEG seizures and do not require treatment with ASM therapy. A common clue that the etiology is SSRI withdrawal is the presence of very early convulsions, within the first hours after birth. Similarly, withdrawal from prenatal exposure to methamphetamines is associated with tremor, jitteriness, and exaggerated startle, which may be easily mistaken for seizures.[56]

NEONATAL-ONSET EPILEPSY

Epilepsy is defined as a tendency to have recurrent, unprovoked seizures. Although the vast majority of seizures in neonates are due to an acute provoked cause, approximately 15% of cases are due to neonatal-onset epilepsy (Fig. 9.2; Box 9.1).[28] Early identification of seizures that are not due to acute illness is important as their management differs significantly from that of acute provoked seizures. In contrast to acute provoked seizures, neonates with epilepsy typically require ongoing ASM therapy,[100] sometimes tailored to the underlying etiology. The most common causes of neonatal-onset epilepsy are genetic epilepsies, brain malformations, and inborn errors of metabolism.

Genetic Epilepsies

Neonatal-onset familial genetic epilepsies and epileptic encephalopathies are individually rare, but collectively account for more than half of neonatal-onset epilepsy.[100] They are clinically heterogeneous, and can be associated with myoclonic seizures, tonic seizures, epileptic spasms, or sequential seizures,[13,31,35–37,101] with at least one study citing tonic seizures as a key seizure semiology.[101]

Benign neonatal familial seizures are associated with a normal interictal EEG and neurological examination, and seizures that respond readily to ASM. Neonatal-onset epileptic encephalopathies present with a severely abnormal EEG background, neurological examination,[51] and limited response to phenobarbital (PB). Mutations in potassium and sodium channels can cause both benign familial and epileptic encephalopathy phenotypes. *KCNQ2*, *KCNQ3*, and *SCN2A* are among the most common channelopathies presenting in the neonatal period.[102–104] Neonates with early-onset genetic epilepsies often respond favorably to sodium channel blockers such as oxcarbazepine.[105]

For neonates without an acute provoked etiology for seizures, genetic testing is increasingly considered standard of care.[106,107] Although specific EEG patterns and physical findings may suggest a particular genetic etiology, neonatal-onset genetic epilepsies as a whole have a high degree of phenotypic overlap. Therefore, broad genetic testing with an infantile epilepsy panel, or whole exome/genome testing is warranted.[108–110]

Brain Malformation

Between 4% and 9% of neonates diagnosed with seizures have an underlying brain malformation.[28,111] Of these, a subset may be identified on prenatal ultrasound and referred for advanced prenatal imaging and neurological counseling. Malformations that are readily identified on prenatal imaging include holoprosencephaly,

Dandy Walker-associated malformations, and some disorders of neuronal migration and organization.[100,112] Many malformations associated with seizures go undetected prenatally and are diagnosed after birth. Cerebral malformations that are associated with epilepsy include polymicrogyria, focal cortical dysplasias, schizencephalies, and grey matter heterotopias.[100] Brain malformations may accompany additional physical findings, including congenital heart disease and ophthalmologic findings[100] but are more commonly isolated alterations in neuronal proliferation and migration unique to the brain. Neonatal encephalopathy secondary to diffuse malformations may be mistaken for or accompanied by hypoxic-ischemic injury, but magnetic resonance neuroimaging is well suited for differentiating between these etiologies.

Inborn Errors of Metabolism

Inborn errors of metabolism are identified in only 1% to 4% of neonates with seizures[28,113] but are crucial to identify promptly due to the availability of specific treatments for some disorders.[114] An inborn error of metabolism may initially be diagnosed as (or coexist with) HIE.[115] Clinicians should maintain a high level of suspicion, particularly in the setting of consanguinity or family history of neonatal-onset seizures, prenatal onset of seizures, or progressive worsening of seizures and EEG background without explanation.[116] Examples of inborn errors of metabolism that present with seizures in the neonatal period include glycine encephalopathy,[41,42] pyridoxine-dependent epilepsy,[115] glucose transporter type 1 deficiency,[117] and molybdenum cofactor deficiency.[118]

CONTROVERSIES IN DETERMINING ETIOLOGY

Timing and Choice of Genetic Testing for Suspected Epilepsy

An acute provoked or transient metabolic cause is identified in more than 70% of neonates with seizures. Genetic epilepsy should be suspected in the setting of: a family history of epilepsy or early life seizures, when no acute cause of seizures is identified (and particularly when the MRI is normal), uncommon seizure types are present (i.e., myoclonic, tonic, or epileptic spasms), seizures continue beyond 72 hours, or the EEG background is severely disorganized without a clear

etiology. Advances in genetic testing have led to the widespread availability and rapid turnaround for infantile-onset epilepsy panels[119] (available through commercial vendors) and whole exome sequencing. Recent studies support early use of whole exome[108,109] or whole genome sequencing[110,120] as a first-line study for acutely ill infants, including children with suspected epileptic encephalopathy.

Timing of Screening for Inborn Error of Metabolism

Even when limited to screening for treatable inborn errors of metabolism, testing is complex, costly, and can take days to weeks to result. Indications for early testing and trial of therapeutic intervention (including pyridoxine trial,[115] dietary restriction,[114] and consideration for recently approved molybdenum cofactor biosynthetic precursor[118]) are similar to those listed above for genetic epilepsies (myoclonic seizures or spasms, refractory seizures, or severely disorganized EEG background without a clear etiology). Additional red flags include abnormal screening lab results (persistent lactate/acidosis, high ammonia) and clinical deterioration (the clinical course is typically one of improvement in the setting of acute injuries such as HIE or stroke). Even when an acute provoked etiology is suspected, genetic and metabolic testing and therapeutic interventions may be warranted for refractory seizures.[115]

Seizure Treatment

Rapid initiation of seizure treatment should begin concurrently with the evaluation for underlying etiology. Treatment with ASM may result in electroclinical dissociation with suppression of clinical seizure manifestations. As such, neonates should be monitored using cEEG during seizure treatment until at least 24 hours after the last seizure.[11] When an easily correctable metabolic or toxic etiology is identified, treatment should focus on correcting the underlying cause.

Although more than 20 years have elapsed since the first high-quality randomized controlled trial,[121] there is no consensus on the treatment of neonates with seizures.[71] The development of evidence-based guidelines has been stymied by the inherent difficulty of rigorous trials in neonates with seizures,[122] resulting in a paucity of randomized controlled trials.[123,124] The 2011 ILAE seizure management guideline in neonates offered limited guidance on specific medications or dosing,[71] with current practice primarily driven by physician preference.[125] Despite these challenges, a study comparing the treatment pathways for seizures in neonates at level IV neonatal intensive care units (NICUs) with expertise in neonatal neurocritical care across the US demonstrated many similarities in approach.[126] There was a clear consensus around the need for continuous EEG monitoring, use of PB as a first-line agent, treatment escalation for ongoing electrographic seizures, use of midazolam infusion for refractory seizures, and discontinuation of ASMs prior to discharge for neonates with acute provoked seizures. There is also widespread support for rapid initiation of ASM, as seizures are easier to treat early in the clinical course,[121,127] and adverse outcomes are associated with higher burden of seizures.[128] Novel approaches to expedite medication administration include automated seizure detection with bedside alerts,[27] and implementation of a seizure rescue process that includes bedside pharmacy support.[129] However, there remains a clear need for improved therapeutic options, clarity around the relative efficacy of currently available second-line medications, and neonate-specific dosing optimization.

ASM OPTIONS AND EFFICACY

First-Line ASM Treatment

PB is the most commonly used first-line ASM in neonates.[125,130,131] PB is a barbiturate that enhances GABA action at the GABA receptor. PB has a long duration of action, between 45 and 200 hours,[132] and is typically dosed as a 20 mg/kg loading bolus with repeated dosing for ongoing seizures. In vitro studies have suggested that PB may be neuroapoptotic[133] and has several clinical side effects, including hypotension[134] and hemodynamic lability, and PB may contribute to deleterious developmental effects when used long term.[135]

In most studies, PB leads to seizure resolution in approximately 50% of neonates,[121,127,136] although a recent prospective randomized trial demonstrated a 70% success rate[124] after a first PB loading dose. The recent trial's higher rate of seizure cessation may be due to prospective

seizure monitoring and rapid treatment initiation, which is associated with overall treatment efficacy.[5] Concern regarding side effects and incomplete efficacy of PB has led to the off-label use of multiple other ASMs. The only two randomized controlled trials for first-line ASM compared PB with fosphenytoin (FOS, Painter trial)[121] and PB with levetiracetam (LEV, NEOLEV2).[124] These trials demonstrated that PB has similar efficacy to FOS[121] with superior neonatal pharmacokinetic properties[137] and that PB was more effective than LEV[124] at trialed doses. Interest remains in developing alternative first-line neonatal ASMs, but PB is likely to remain the treatment of choice for the near future.

Second-Line ASM Treatment

Second-line treatment choices are guided primarily by physician preference, with FOS and LEV being the most common choices.[28,125,126,130,138] There have been no randomized controlled trials directly comparing the efficacy of these agents to treat seizures in neonates. Based on extrapolated data from the Painter[121] and NEOLEV2 trials,[124] many clinicians have suggested that FOS is more likely than LEV to lead to seizure resolution when used second line. A randomized controlled trial comparing FOS and LEV for second-line treatment of convulsive status epilepticus in older children demonstrated no significant difference in efficacy.[139]

FOS is a prodrug of phenytoin with fewer infusion side effects than phenytoin that is typically loaded at 20 mg phenytoin equivalents/kg.[140] It can be used as a bolus infusion and as a maintenance medication, although phenytoin levels are often difficult to maintain in neonates, which makes it most appropriate for short-term use.[137] Similar to PB, in vitro studies have suggested that phenytoin may be neuroapoptotic,[133] although little is known about the long-term neurodevelopmental effects. We favor short-term use (24–72 hours after resolution of seizures) of FOS when used as a second-line agent for acute provoked cause of seizures in a neonate.

LEV has been increasingly used in the neonatal population since receiving Food and Drug Administration (FDA) orphan drug status for neonatal use in 2010.[141–143] LEV is an attractive option due to few adverse side effects in neonates,[144–146] animal models suggesting it may have a neuroprotective effect,[147,148] and retrospective studies suggesting noninferiority of seizure cessation relative to PB.[144] However, LEV's significantly worse efficacy compared to PB in the NEOLEV2 trial[124] has led many clinicians to limit its use. LEV is still often favored in clinical situations where the hemodynamic side effects of PB and FOS may not be well tolerated.[126]

Infusion ASM Treatment

Infusion medications are typically used for refractory seizures and status epilepticus in neonates. Most centers use midazolam infusion as the third- or fourth-line agent of choice after PB and FOS or LEV.[126] Midazolam is the most commonly used infusion medication in the United States[28] and has been studied for safety and efficacy in small cohorts of neonates.[149,150] Lidocaine infusion is more commonly utilized for refractory seizures in Europe.[151-153] A large, retrospective European-based cohort of neonates found that lidocaine was significantly more effective than midazolam as a second-line agent.[153] However, concerns remain regarding cardiac adverse effects, particularly arrhythmias, and lidocaine should not be combined with FOS.[154]

Less Common ASM Options

Multiple other ASMs have been used in the neonatal population, either for targeted treatment of genetic epilepsy or to treat refractory seizures. Carbamazepine and oxcarbazepine have good efficacy for genetic neonatal-onset epilepsies (particularly KCNQ2 benign familial neonatal epilepsy and epileptic encephalopathy).[155] Topiramate use has been described, but there is no currently available intravenous formulation.[156] There is an ongoing trial for intravenous lacosamide use.[157] A European randomized controlled trial of bumetanide versus PB was halted early due to poor efficacy and concern for hearing loss.[158] However, a US randomized, double-blind phase 1/2 trial comparing bumetanide add-on therapy to standard PB monotherapy therapy found no increased burden of side effects and a significant benefit of bumetanide therapy. Results of this trial were limited by small size and a chance imbalance of seizure severity among groups. Further investigation of bumetanide as an adjunctive treatment may be warranted.[159]

Pyridoxine

Although pyridoxine-dependent seizures are a very rare cause of neonatal-onset epilepsy,[160] it is important to consider a treatment trial in neonates with refractory seizures. A recent international consensus recommends a trial of 100 mg intravenous pyridoxine over 5 minutes with close evaluation of EEG response and consideration for additional 100 mg doses up to a total of 500 mg in nonresponders.[115]

DISCONTINUATION OF ASM

Timing of ASM discontinuation after resolution of acute provoked seizures has historically been variable, with ASM prescribed for days to months or even years.[161] Accumulating evidence now strongly supports discontinuation of ASMs before hospital discharge in most cases.[162-166] Acute provoked seizures are typically transient, and ongoing ASM therapy, particularly with PB, may impair neonatal feeding and state regulation secondary to sedative properties. Long-term PB use has also been associated with neurodevelopmental delay in early childhood.[135,167] Both retrospective and large prospective cohorts have demonstrated a low risk of early seizure recurrence and that a long duration of therapy does not lower the risk of epilepsy or provide neurodevelopmental benefit.[162,163,165] For the bedside clinician who is uncertain about the safety of discontinuing ASMs for a particular child, careful consideration is warranted. First, is the seizure cause confirmed to be acute provoked (i.e., HIE, ischemic stroke, hemorrhage, or other brain injury)? Second, have the seizures resolved on EEG for at least 24 hours? Third, have the parents been taught what to do in case of suspected seizures? If the answer to all three questions is "yes," ASM can be safely discontinued.

CONTROVERSIES IN SEIZURE TREATMENT

Threshold for Seizure Treatment and Escalation in Neonates

While the medical community has reached a consensus that seizures require treatment, the threshold for treatment initiation and escalation remains inconsistent across sites. A recent international working group set a minimum threshold of 30 sec/hr for inclusion in future ASM trials for seizures in neonates.[122] In pediatric patients, a seizure burden of greater than

12 min/hr is associated with worse developmental outcomes,[168] and in the neonatal population, a maximum hourly seizure burden of greater than 13 min/hr is similarly associated with an eightfold-increased odds of an adverse neurodevelopmental outcome.[128] In current clinical practice, most centers escalate treatment to second-line therapy for all electrographic seizures if a neonate has failed to respond to first-line treatment.[126] The threshold for further escalation to third-line and infusion treatments may be based upon an individualized clinical evaluation of risks and benefits; we favor escalating treatment for acute provoked seizures until they have been abolished.[126]

Second-Line ASM Choice

Although 20% to 50% of seizures are refractory to first-line ASM treatment, second- and third-line treatment choices remain dictated primarily by individual physician preference rather than strong evidence. FOS and LEV are both frequently used[126] but have not been directly compared for second-line treatment. Indirect evidence from the crossover phase of randomized controlled trials comparing each to PB demonstrated that neonates who failed PB therapy achieved seizure cessation 27% of the time with FOS[121] and 17% of the time with LEV.[124] Altogether, the evidence points to higher likelihood of treatment response to FOS; however, this comparison is limited by very small numbers, different methodologies of seizure diagnosis, and over 20 years between studies.

Timing of ASM Discontinuation

Recommendations to continue ASM for at least 3 months after resolution of seizures in the setting of abnormal neurological examination and EEG were developed before the advent of MRI and genetic testing to determine the cause of seizures and routine continuous video EEG monitoring to accurately determine seizure resolution. Newer data strongly support discontinuation of ASMs before discharge for neonates with acute provoked seizures; however, this approach represents a practice change for many providers.[162] The optimal duration of ASM therapy after resolution of seizures is not known. The median duration of PB treatment was 4 days in a study where children were safely discontinued prior to discharge home.[162] Continued work will be needed to implement this practice change and to understand whether specific subpopulations would benefit from shorter or more prolonged ASM therapy.

Preterm versus Term Treatment Strategies

It is widely recognized that pharmacokinetics, hepatic and renal function, and CNS development rapidly change as neonates grow from preterm to term, suggesting that the ASM approach should ideally be tailored to developmental age. However, ASMs have not been well studied in the preterm population, and there are no evidence-based approaches currently available to optimize preterm seizure treatment. Most clinical providers use similar seizure treatment guidelines for preterm and term neonates.[79,169]

Therapeutic Trial Design for Seizures in Neonates

While there is consensus that there is a need for effective ASMs with low side-effect profiles to treat seizures in neonates, developing rigorous yet practical trials remains a challenge. Challenges include the variable timing of onset of acute provoked seizures, need for timely EEG diagnosis, diverse opinions regarding the best way to define efficacy (e.g., complete seizure cessation vs. alteration in seizure burden), and limited willingness of parents and clinicians to enroll newborns in randomized trials.[122] Work is underway to develop an international consensus on the approach to clinical trial design.

Prognosis

DEVELOPMENTAL OUTCOMES

The prognosis of neonates diagnosed with seizures varies widely depending on the underlying etiology. For neonates with acute provoked seizures, the severity of the ischemic, hemorrhagic, or infectious insult resulting in seizures plays a key role in determining outcome,[164] as does the location of injury for focal insults.

There is no direct, high-quality evidence to determine the extent to which seizures in neonates alter neurodevelopmental outcomes. However, multiple lines of preclinical and clinical studies support evidence of harm secondary to seizures strongly enough that it would be ethically unacceptable to withhold treatment of seizures, for example, in the setting of a placebo-controlled trial. Multiple preclinical studies inform our understanding of the mechanism by which seizures are detrimental to the injured developing brain.[170,171] Neonatal clinical studies have shown that a higher seizure burden is independently associated with imaging markers of neuronal injury[172] and with increased neurodevelopmental disability.[28,128,173] Given this evidence, there is clinical consensus that treatment of seizures in the setting of underlying brain injury may be an important neuroprotective strategy.

Multiple studies have examined risk factors for poor neurodevelopmental outcome after seizures and encephalopathy in neonates. Serial EEG evaluation has demonstrated that rapid evolution to normal or nearly normal background within 24 to 36 hours after the injury portends a reassuring developmental outcome.[174,175] Other studied prognostic factors include method of delivery, birth weight, Apgar score at 1 minute, neurologic examination at seizure onset, neuroimaging findings, time of seizure onset, presence of status epilepticus, interictal EEG background, and seizure etiology.[128,176–178] Combinations of these risk factors have been analyzed by regression analysis and machine learning to predict outcome with sensitivity and specificity of >80%.[177] In clinical practice, discussion of prognosis is typically based on an individualized evaluation of global history, EEG data, imaging, and serial clinical exam. Prognostic information is complex and challenging to communicate.[179] Recent research has focused on partnering with families to build tools and enhance best communication practices (Box 9.2).[180–182]

POSTNEONATAL EPILEPSY

Neonates who experience acute provoked seizures are at an increased risk of developing recurrent unprovoked seizures (epilepsy) months to years later. Approximately 15% to 25% of neonates will develop postneonatal epilepsy.[183–187] In a recent cohort, approximately one-third of neonates who developed

BOX 9.2 KEY STRATEGIES TO ENHANCE COMMUNICATION WITH PARENTS OF NEONATES WITH SEIZURE[a]

EFFECTIVE FAMILY COMMUNICATION
- Communicate consistently across teams
- Provide comprehensive, balanced prognostic information
- Be prepared to repeat information as needed
- Acknowledge uncertainty

VALIDATE AND EMPOWER PARENTS
- Elicit and provide information that matches parental needs
- Validate parent concerns
- Engage parents in both decision making and daily clinical care

PROVIDE FAMILY RESOURCES
- Acknowledge and support the need for parental care
- Connect parents with peer support
- Empower parents to seek education
- Provide concrete support for navigating complex care

---

[a]Adapted from Lemmon ME, Glass HC, Shellhaas RA, et al. Family-centered care for children and families impacted by neonatal seizures: advice from parents. *Pediatr Neurol* 2021;124:26–32. Based on interviews with parents of neonates with seizures.

epilepsy after acute provoked neonatal seizures presented with infantile spasms, and one-third were diagnosed with medically intractable epilepsy by 24 months of age.[187] Factors predicting later development of epilepsy include severely abnormal background EEG pattern in the NICU and >3 days of EEG confirmed seizures, while normal versus abnormal EEG at 3 months did not help predict epilepsy development.[187,188] More than 50% of children with three key risk factors developed infantile spasms: (1) severely abnormal EEG background or 3 or more days of EEG seizures, (2) MRI injury in the deep grey nuclei or brainstem, and (3) abnormal tone at discharge.[188]

CONTROVERSIES IN PROGNOSIS
Optimizing Prognostic Communication

Prognostic outcomes for neonates with seizures are nearly always uncertain, making clear communication with families challenging for even the best communicators. Parents and clinicians appreciate the opportunity to enhance communication with customized tools, including a neonatal question prompt list.[180]

Parents appreciate accurate and compassionately communicated information that is consistent between team members. Parents also value when providers validate the parent experience and actively provide parents with support and resources.[181] Enhancing communication and support for families grappling with seizures in their neonates will remain an ongoing opportunity for improvement.

Conclusions

Rapidly diagnosing and treating seizures in neonates are fundamental skills needed to optimize brain care for the ill neonate. Controversies in diagnosis include constant need to improve seizure diagnosis in the preterm neonate and optimal utilization of aEEG versus cEEG. The initial evaluation of underlying etiology is focused on determining whether the seizures are due to a transient metabolic derangement, acute provoked cause, or neonatal-onset epilepsy. Advanced genetic testing has revolutionized rapid diagnosis of genetic epilepsies and enhanced the ability to rapidly identify treatable metabolic conditions. There is consensus that rapid and appropriate treatment of electrographic and electroclinical seizures is essential. However, the choice of ASMs for neonates with refractory seizures remains controversial. The developmental implications of seizures in neonates are multifactorial and remain an essential facet of neonatal care and parental communication. Overall, the care of neonates with seizures continues to evolve and improve. Three of the key recent advances in the care of neonates with seizures include:

- Increasing availability and use of cEEG for more rapid, accurate evaluation of seizures in neonates.
- Increased availability of diagnostic tools including MRI, genetic testing, and enhanced evaluation for infectious diseases.
- Recognition that ASM therapy can be safely discontinued during acute hospitalization for neonates with acute provoked seizures.

REFERENCES

1. Lanska MJ, Lanska DJ, Baumann RJ, Kryscio RJ. A population-based study of neonatal seizures in Fayette County, Kentucky. *Neurology.* 1995;45(4):724-732. doi:10.1212/WNL.45.4.724.

2. Ronen GM, Penney S, Andrews W. The epidemiology of clinical neonatal seizures in Newfoundland: a population-based study. *J Pediatr.* 1999;134(1):71-75. doi:10.1016/S0022-3476(99)70374-4.

3. Saliba RM, Annegers JF, Waller DK, Tyson JE, Mizrahi EM. Incidence of neonatal seizures in Harris County, Texas, 1992–1994. *Am J Epidemiol.* 1999;150(7):763-769. doi:10.1093/oxfordjournals.aje.a010079.

4. Glass HC, Pham TN, Danielsen B, Towner D, Glidden D, Wu YW. Antenatal and intrapartum risk factors for seizures in term newborns: a population-based study, California 1998–2002. *J Pediatr.* 2009;154(1):24-28.e1. doi:10.1016/j.jpeds.2008.07.008.

5. Wusthoff CJ, Sundaram V, Abend NS, et al. Seizure control in neonates undergoing screening vs confirmatory EEG monitoring. *Neurology.* 2021;97(6):e587-e596. doi:10.1212/WNL.0000000000012293.

6. Pavel AM, Rennie JM, de Vries LS, et al. Neonatal seizure management—is the timing of treatment critical? *J Pediatr.* 2022;243:61-68.e2. doi:10.1016/J.JPEDS.2021.09.058.

7. Malone A, Anthony Ryan C, Fitzgerald A, Burgoyne L, Connolly S, Boylan GB. Interobserver agreement in neonatal seizure identification. *Epilepsia.* 2009;50(9):2097-2101. doi:10.1111/j.1528-1167.2009.02132.x.

8. Murray DM, Boylan GB, Ali I, Ryan CA, Murphy BP, Connolly S. Defining the gap between electrographic seizure burden, clinical expression and staff recognition of neonatal seizures. *Arch Dis Child Fetal Neonatal Ed.* 2008;93(3):F187-F191. doi:10.1136/adc.2005.086314.

9. Clancy RR, Legido A, Lewis D. Occult neonatal seizures. *Epilepsia.* 1988;29(3):256-261. doi:10.1111/j.1528-1157.1988.tb03715.x.

10. Scher MS, Alvin J, Gaus L, Minnigh B, Painter MJ. Uncoupling of EEG-clinical neonatal seizures after antiepileptic drug use. *Pediatr Neurol.* 2003;28(4):277-280. doi:10.1016/S0887-8994(02)00621-5.

11. Shellhaas RA, Chang T, Tsuchida T, et al. The American Clinical Neurophysiology Society's guideline on continuous electroencephalography monitoring in neonates. *J Clin Neurophysiol.* 2011;28(6):611-617. doi:10.1097/WNP.0b013e31823e96d7.

12. Tsuchida TN, Wusthoff CJ, Shellhaas RA, et al. American Clinical Neurophysiology Society standardized EEG terminology and categorization for the description of continuous EEG monitoring in neonates: report of the American Clinical Neurophysiology Society critical care monitoring committee. *J Clin Neurophysiol.* 2013;30(2):161-173. doi:10.1097/WNP.0b013e3182872b24.

13. Pressler RM, Cilio MR, Mizrahi EM, et al. The ILAE classification of seizures and the epilepsies: modification for seizures in the neonate. Position paper by the ILAE task force on neonatal seizures. *Epilepsia.* 2021;62(3):615-628. doi:10.1111/epi.16815.

14. Shah D, Mathur A. Amplitude-integrated EEG and the newborn infant. *Curr Pediatr Rev.* 2014;10(1):11-15. doi:10.2174/1573396310011140408115859.

15. El-Dib M, Chang T, Tsuchida TN, Clancy RR. Amplitude-integrated electroencephalography in neonates. *Pediatr Neurol.* 2009;41(5):315-326. doi:10.1016/j.pediatrneurol.2009.05.002.

16. Shah DK, Mackay MT, Lavery S, et al. Accuracy of bedside electroencephalographic monitoring in comparison with simultaneous continuous conventional electroencephalography for seizure detection in term infants. *Pediatrics.* 2008;121(6):1146-1154. doi:10.1542/PEDS.2007-1839.

17. Shellhaas RA, Soaita AI, Clancy RR. Sensitivity of amplitude-integrated electroencephalography for neonatal seizure detection. *Pediatrics.* 2007;120(4):770-777. doi:10.1542/peds.2007-0514.

18. O'Toole JM, Boylan GB. Quantitative preterm EEG analysis: the need for caution in using modern data science techniques. *Front Pediatr.* 2019;7:174. doi:10.3389/fped.2019.00174.

19. Vesoulis ZA, Inder TE, Woodward LJ, Buse B, Vavasseur C, Mathur AM. Early electrographic seizures, brain injury, and neurodevelopmental risk in the very preterm infant. *Pediatr Res.* 2014;75(4):564-569. doi:10.1038/pr.2013.245.

20. Lloyd RO, O'Toole JM, Pavlidis E, Filan PM, Boylan GB. Electrographic seizures during the early postnatal period in preterm infants. *J Pediatr.* 2017;187:18-25.e2. doi:10.1016/j.jpeds.2017.03.004.

21. Glass HC, Wusthoff CJ, Shellhaas RA. Amplitude-integrated electro-encephalography: the child neurologist's perspective. *J Child Neurol.* 2013;28(10):1342-1350. doi:10.1177/0883073813488663.

22. Fernández IS, Loddenkemper T. aEEG and cEEG: two complementary techniques to assess seizures and encephalopathy in neonates: Editorial on "Amplitude-integrated EEG for detection of neonatal seizures: a systematic review" by Rakshasbhuvankar et al. *Seizure.* 2015;33:88-89. doi:10.1016/j.seizure.2015.10.010.

23. Jain SV, Mathur A, Srinivasakumar P, et al. Prediction of neonatal seizures in hypoxic-ischemic encephalopathy using electroencephalograph power analyses. *Pediatr Neurol.* 2017;67:64-70.e2. doi:10.1016/j.pediatrneurol.2016.10.019.

24. Benedetti GM, Vartanian RJ, McCaffery H, Shellhaas RA. Early electroencephalogram background could guide tailored duration of monitoring for neonatal encephalopathy treated with therapeutic hypothermia. *J Pediatr.* 2020;221:81-87.e1. doi:10.1016/j.jpeds.2020.01.066.

25. Glass HC, Wusthoff CJ, Shellhaas RA, et al. Risk factors for EEG seizures in neonates treated with hypothermia. *Neurology.* 2014;82(14):1239-1244. doi:10.1212/WNL.0000000000000282.

26. Sharpe C, Davis SL, Reiner GE, et al. Assessing the feasibility of providing a real-time response to seizures detected with continuous long-term neonatal electroencephalography monitoring. *J Clin Neurophysiol.* 2019;36(1):9-13. doi:10.1097/WNP.0000000000000525.

27. Pavel AM, Rennie JM, de Vries LS, et al. A machine-learning algorithm for neonatal seizure recognition: a multicentre, randomised, controlled trial. *Lancet Child Adolesc Heal.* 2020;4(10):740-749. doi:10.1016/S2352-4642(20)30239-X.

28. Glass HC, Shellhaas RA, Wusthoff CJ, et al. Contemporary profile of seizures in neonates: a prospective cohort study. *J Pediatr.* 2016;174:98-103.e1. doi:10.1016/j.jpeds.2016.03.035.

29. Mizrahi EM, Kellaway P. Characterization and classification of neonatal seizures. *Neurology.* 1987;37(12):1837-1844. doi:10.1212/wnl.37.12.1837.

30. Nagarajan L, Ghosh S, Palumbo L. Ictal electroencephalograms in neonatal seizures: characteristics and associations. *Pediatr Neurol.* 2011;45(1):11-16. doi:10.1016/J.PEDIATRNEUROL.2011.01.009.

31. Nunes ML, Yozawitz EG, Zuberi S, et al. Neonatal seizures: is there a relationship between ictal electroclinical features and etiology? A critical appraisal based on a systematic literature review. *Epilepsia Open.* 2019;4(1):10-29. doi:10.1002/epi4.12298.

32. Low E, Mathieson SR, Stevenson NJ, et al. Early postnatal EEG features of perinatal arterial ischaemic stroke with seizures. *PLoS One.* 2014;9(7):e100973. doi:10.1371/journal.pone.0100973.

33. Nunes ML, Martins MP, Barea BM, Wainberg RC, Da Costa JC. Neurological outcome of newborns with neonatal seizures: a cohort study in a tertiary university hospital. *Arq Neuropsiquiatr.* 2008;66(2A):168-174. doi:10.1590/S0004-282X2008000200005.

34. Schulzke S, Weber P, Luetschg J, Fahnenstich H. Incidence and diagnosis of unilateral arterial cerebral infarction in newborn infants. *J Perinat Med.* 2005;33(2):170-175. doi:10.1515/JPM.2005.032.

35. Ohtahara S, Yamatogi Y. Ohtahara syndrome: with special reference to its developmental aspects for differentiating from early myoclonic encephalopathy. *Epilepsy Res.* 2006;70(suppl 1):58-67. doi:10.1016/j.eplepsyres.2005.11.021.

36. Kobayashi K, Inoue T, Kikumoto K, et al. Relation of spasms and myoclonus to suppression-burst on EEG in epileptic encephalopathy in early infancy. *Neuropediatrics.* 2007;38(5):244-250. doi:10.1055/s-2008-1062716.

37. Watanabe K, Miura K, Natsume J, Hayakawa F, Furune S, Okumura A. Epilepsies of neonatal onset: seizure type and evolution. *Dev Med Child Neurol.* 2007;41(5):318-322. doi:10.1111/j.1469-8749.1999.tb00609.x.

38. Djukic Aleksandra A, Ladoa FA, Shinnar S, Moshé SL. Are early myoclonic encephalopathy (EME) and the Ohtahara syndrome (EIEE) independent of each other? *Epilepsy Res.* 2006;70(suppl 1):68-76. doi:10.1016/j.eplepsyres.2005.11.022.

39. Nagarajan L, Palumbo L, Ghosh S. Classification of clinical semiology in epileptic seizures in neonates. *Eur J Paediatr Neurol.* 2012;16(2):118-125. doi:10.1016/j.ejpn.2011.11.005.

40. Beniczky S, Conradsen I, Pressler R, Wolf P. Quantitative analysis of surface electromyography: biomarkers for convulsive seizures. *Clin Neurophysiol.* 2016;127(8):2900-2907. doi:10.1016/j.clinph.2016.04.017.

41. Cusmai R, Martinelli D, Moavero R, et al. Ketogenic diet in early myoclonic encephalopathy due to non ketotic hyperglycinemia. *Eur J Paediatr Neurol.* 2012;16(5):509-513. doi:10.1016/j.ejpn.2011.12.015.

42. Dalla Bernardina B, Aicardi J, Goutieres F, Plouin P. Glycine encephalopathy. *Neuropadiatrie.* 1979;10(3):209-225. doi:10.1055/s-0028-1085326.

43. Porri S, Fluss J, Plecko B, Paschke E, Korff CM, Kern I. Positive outcome following early diagnosis and treatment of pyridoxal-5′-phosphate oxidase deficiency: a case report. *Neuropediatrics.* 2014;45(1):64-68. doi:10.1055/s-0033-1353489.

44. Milh M, Villeneuve N, Chouchane M, et al. Epileptic and nonepileptic features in patients with early onset epileptic encephalopathy and STXBP1 mutations. *Epilepsia.* 2011;52(10):1828-1834. doi:10.1111/j.1528-1167.2011.03181.x.

45. Olson HE, Kelly M, LaCoursiere CM, et al. Genetics and genotype-phenotype correlations in early onset epileptic encephalopathy with burst suppression. *Ann Neurol.* 2017;81(3):419-429. doi:10.1002/ana.24883.

46. Dang LT, Shellhaas RA. Diagnostic yield of continuous video electroencephalography for paroxysmal vital sign changes in pediatric patients. *Epilepsia.* 2016;57(2):272-278. doi:10.1111/epi.13276.

47. Castro Conde JR, González-Hernández T, González Barrios D, González Campo C. Neonatal apneic seizure of occipital lobe origin: continuous video-EEG recording. *Pediatrics.* 2012;129(6):1616-1620. doi:10.1542/peds.2011-2447.

48. Sirsi D, Nadiminti L, Packard MA, Engel M, Solomon GE. Apneic seizures: a sign of temporal lobe hemorrhage in full-term neonates. *Pediatr Neurol.* 2007;37(5):366-370. doi:10.1016/j.pediatrneurol.2007.06.004.

49. Hirsch E, Velez A, Sellal F, et al. Electroclinical signs of benign neonatal familial convulsions. *Ann Neurol.* 1993;34(6):835-841. doi:10.1002/ana.410340613.

50. Ronen GM, Rosales TO, Connolly M, Anderson VE, Leppert M. Seizure characteristics in chromosome 20 benign familial

neonatal convulsions. *Neurology.* 1993;43(7):1355-1360. doi:10.1212/wnl.43.7.1355.

51. Weckhuysen S, Mandelstam S, Suls A, et al. KCNQ2 encephalopathy: emerging phenotype of a neonatal epileptic encephalopathy. *Ann Neurol.* 2012;71(1):15-25. doi:10.1002/ana.22644.

52. Wolff M, Brunklaus A, Zuberi SM. Phenotypic spectrum and genetics of SCN 2A related disorders, treatment options, and outcomes in epilepsy and beyond. *Epilepsia.* 2019;60(S3):S59-S67. doi:10.1111/epi.14935.

53. Collins M, Young M. Benign neonatal shudders, shivers, jitteriness, or tremors: early signs of vitamin D deficiency. *Pediatrics.* 2017;140(2):e20160719. doi:10.1542/PEDS.2016-0719.

54. Pierog S, Chandavasu O, Wexler I. Withdrawal symptoms in infants with the fetal alcohol syndrome. *J Pediatr.* 1977; 90(4):630-633. doi:10.1016/S0022-3476(77)80387-9.

55. Chiriboga CA, Bateman DA, Brust JCM, Allen Hauser W. Neurologic findings in neonates with intrauterine cocaine exposure. *Pediatr Neurol.* 1993;9(2):115-119. doi:10.1016/0887-8994(93)90045-E.

56. Hudak ML, Tan RC, Frattarelli DAC, et al. Neonatal drug withdrawal. *Pediatrics.* 2012;129(2):e540-e560. doi:10.1542/peds.2011-3212.

57. Sanger TD, Chen D, Fehlings DL, et al. Definition and classification of hyperkinetic movements in childhood. *Mov Disord.* 2010;25(11):1538-1549. doi:10.1002/mds.23088.

58. Magny JF, D'Allest AM, Nedelcoux H, Zupan V, Dehan M. Midazolam and myoclonus in neonate. *Eur J Pediatr.* 1994;153(5): 389-390. doi:10.1007/BF01956430.

59. Ozcan B, Kavurt S, Yucel H, Bas AY, Demirel N. Rhythmic myoclonic jerking induced by midazolam in a preterm infant. *Pediatr Neurol.* 2015;52(6):e9. doi:10.1016/J.PEDIATRNEUROL.2015.02.019.

60. Scher MS. Pathologic myoclonus of the newborn: electrographic and clinical correlations. *Pediatr Neurol.* 1985;1(6):342-348. doi:10.1016/0887-8994(85)90068-2.

61. Mulkey SB, Ben-Zeev B, Nicolai J, et al. Neonatal nonepileptic myoclonus is a prominent clinical feature of KCNQ2 gain-of-function variants R201C and R201H. *Epilepsia.* 2017;58(3): 436-445. doi:10.1111/epi.13676.

62. Maurer VO, Rizzi M, Bianchetti MG, Ramelli GP. Benign neonatal sleep myoclonus: a review of the literature. *Pediatrics.* 2010;125(4):919-924. doi:10.1542/peds.2009-1839.

63. Scher MS. Neonatal hypertonia: differential diagnosis and proposed neuroprotection. *Pediatr Neurol.* 2008;39(6):373-380. doi:10.1016/j.pediatrneurol.2008.09.009.

64. Hyland K. Presentation, diagnosis, and treatment of the disorders of monoamine neurotransmitter metabolism. *Semin Perinatol.* 1999;23(2):194-203. doi:10.1016/S0146-0005(99)80051-2.

65. Stauss K, Puffenberger E, Morton D. Maple syrup urine disease. 2006 Jan 20 [Updated 2013 May 9]. In: Pagon R, Adam M, Ardinger H, eds. *Gene Reviews.* University of Washington, Seattle; 2020. Availablea t: http://www.ncbi.nlm.nih.gov/books/NBK1319/. Accessed February 26, 2021.

66. Zhou L, Chillag KL, Nigro MA. Hyperekplexia: a treatable neurogenetic disease. *Brain Dev.* 2002;24(7):669-674. doi:10.1016/S0387-7604(02)00095-5.

67. Macaya A, Brunso L, Fernández-Castillo N, et al. Molybdenum cofactor deficiency presenting as neonatal hyperekplexia: a clinical, biochemical and genetic study. *Neuropediatrics.* 2005;36(6):389-394. doi:10.1055/S-2005-872877/ID/33.

68. Nigro MA, Lim HCN. Hyperekplexia and sudden neonatal death. *Pediatr Neurol.* 1992;8(3):221-225. doi:10.1016/0887-8994(92)90073-8.

69. Balint B, Thomas R. Hereditary hyperekplexia overview. 2007 July 7 [Updated 2019 Dec 19]. In: *Gene Reviews.* University of Washington, Seattle; 2019. Available at: https://www.ncbi.nlm.nih.gov/books/NBK1260/. Accessed March 23, 2021.

70. Karamian AGS, Wusthoff CJ. How helpful is aEEG? Context and user experience matter. *Am J Perinatol.* 2022;39(10):1132-1137. doi:10.1055/S-0040-1721711.

71. World Health Organization. *Guidelines on Neonatal Seizures.* 2011. Available at: https://apps.who.int/iris/handle/10665/77756. Accessed May 8, 2021.

72. Ge M, Gan M, Yan K, et al. Combining metagenomic sequencing with whole exome sequencing to optimize clinical strategies in neonates with a suspected central nervous system infection. *Front Cell Infect Microbiol.* 2021;11:671109. doi:10.3389/FCIMB.2021.671109/FULL.

73. Orbach SA, Bonifacio SL, Kuzniewicz MW, Glass HC. Lower incidence of seizure among neonates treated with therapeutic hypothermia. *J Child Neurol.* 2014;29(11):1502-1507. doi:10.1177/0883073813507978.

74. Low E, Boylan GB, Mathieson SR, et al. Cooling and seizure burden in term neonates: an observational study. *Arch Dis Child Fetal Neonatal Ed.* 2012;97(4):F267-F272. doi:10.1136/archdischild-2011-300716.

75. Jacobs SE, Berg M, Hunt R, Tarnow-Mordi WO, Inder TE, Davis PG. Cooling for newborns with hypoxic ischaemic encephalopathy. *Cochrane Database Syst Rev.* 2013;2013(1):CD003311. doi:10.1002/14651858.CD003311.pub3.

76. Lynch NE, Stevenson NJ, Livingstone V, et al. The temporal characteristics of seizures in neonatal hypoxic ischemic encephalopathy treated with hypothermia. *Seizure.* 2015;33:60-65. doi:10.1016/J.SEIZURE.2015.10.007.

77. Grunt S, Mazenauer L, Buerki SE, et al. Incidence and outcomes of symptomatic neonatal arterial ischemic stroke. *Pediatrics.* 2015;135(5):e1220-e1228. doi:10.1542/peds.2014-1520.

78. Moharir MD, Shroff M, Pontigon AM, et al. A Prospective outcome study of neonatal cerebral sinovenous thrombosis. *J Child Neurol.* 2011;26(9):1137-1144. doi:10.1177/0883073811408094.

79. Glass HC, Shellhaas RA, Tsuchida TN, et al. Seizures in preterm neonates: a multicenter observational cohort study. *Pediatr Neurol.* 2017;72:19-24. doi:10.1016/j.pediatrneurol.2017.04.016.

80. Massey SL, Glass HC, Shellhaas RA, et al. Characteristics of neonates with cardiopulmonary disease who experience seizures: a multicenter study. *J Pediatr.* 2022;242:63-73. doi:10.1016/J.JPEDS.2021.10.058.

81. Gaynor JW, Nicolson SC, Jarvik GP, et al. Increasing duration of deep hypothermic circulatory arrest is associated with an increased incidence of postoperative electroencephalographic seizures. *J Thorac Cardiovasc Surg.* 2005;130(5):1278-1286. doi:10.1016/J.JTCVS.2005.02.065.

82. Naim MY, Gaynor JW, Chen J, et al. Subclinical seizures identified by postoperative electroencephalographic monitoring are common after neonatal cardiac surgery. *J Thorac Cardiovasc Surg.* 2015;150(1):169-180. doi:10.1016/J.JTCVS.2015.03.045.

83. Clancy RR, Sharif U, Ichord R, et al. Electrographic neonatal seizures after infant heart surgery. *Epilepsia.* 2005;46(1):84-90. doi:10.1111/j.0013-9580.2005.22504.x.

84. Cook RJ, Rau SM, Lester-Pelham SG, et al. Electrographic seizures and brain injury in children requiring extracorporeal membrane oxygenation. *Pediatr Neurol.* 2020;108:77-85. doi:10.1016/j.pediatrneurol.2020.03.001.

85. Piantino JA, Wainwright MS, Grimason M, et al. Nonconvulsive seizures are common in children treated with extracorporeal cardiac life support. *Pediatr Crit Care Med*. 2013;14(6):601-609. doi:10.1097/PCC.0b013e318291755a.

86. Mizrahi EM, Tharp BR. A characteristic EEG pattern in neonatal herpes simplex encephalitis. *Neurology*. 1982;32(11):1215-1220. doi:10.1212/wnl.32.11.1215.

87. Mikati MA, Feraru E, Krishnamoorthy K, Lombroso CT. Neonatal herpes simplex meningoencephalitis: EEG investigations and clinical correlates. *Neurology*. 1990;40(9):1433-1437. doi:10.1212/wnl.40.9.1433.

88. Verboon-Maciolek MA, Krediet TG, Gerards LJ, Fleer A, van Loon TM. Clinical and epidemiologic characteristics of viral infections in a neonatal intensive care unit during a 12-year period. *Pediatr Infect Dis J*. 2005;24(10):901-904. doi:10.1097/01.inf.0000180471.03702.7f.

89. Britton PN, Dale RC, Nissen MD, et al. Parechovirus encephalitis and neurodevelopmental outcomes. *Pediatrics*. 2016;137(2):e20152848. https://doi.10.1542/peds.2015-2848.

90. Fitzgerald KC, Golomb MR. Neonatal arterial ischemic stroke and sinovenous thrombosis associated with meningitis. *J Child Neurol*. 2007;22(7):818-822. doi:10.1177/0883073807304200.

91. Montassir H, Maegaki Y, Ogura K, et al. Associated factors in neonatal hypoglycemic brain injury. *Brain Dev*. 2009;31(9):649-656. doi:10.1016/J.BRAINDEV.2008.10.012.

92. Tam EWY, Widjaja E, Blaser SI, MacGregor DL, Satodia P, Moore AM. Occipital lobe injury and cortical visual outcomes after neonatal hypoglycemia. *Pediatrics*. 2008;122(3):507-512. doi:10.1542/peds.2007-2002.

93. Levy-Shraga Y, Dallalzadeh K, Stern K, Paret G, Pinhas-Hamiel O. The many etiologies of neonatal hypocalcemic seizures. *Pediatr Emerg Care*. 2015;31(3):197-201. doi:10.1097/PEC.0000000000000380.

94. Keen JH. Significance of hypocalcaemia in neonatal convulsions. *Arch Dis Child*. 1969;44(235):356-361. doi:10.1136/adc.44.235.356.

95. Jain A, Agarwal R, Sankar MJ, Deorari A, Paul VK. Hypocalcemia in the newborn. *Indian J Pediatr*. 2010;77(10):1123-1128. doi:10.1007/s12098-010-0176-0.

96. Nardone R, Brigo F, Trinka E. Acute symptomatic seizures caused by electrolyte disturbances. *J Clin Neurol*. 2016;12(1):21-33. doi:10.3988/jcn.2016.12.1.21.

97. Herzlinger RA, Kandall SR, Vaughan HG. Neonatal seizures associated with narcotic withdrawal. *J Pediatr*. 1977;91(4):638-641. doi:10.1016/S0022-3476(77)80523-4.

98. Kramer LD, Locke GE, Ogunyemi A, Nelson L. Neonatal cocaine-related seizures. *J Child Neurol*. 1990;5(1):60-64. doi:10.1177/088307389000500115.

99. Sanz EJ, De-las-Cuevas C, Kiuru A, Bate A, Edwards R. Selective serotonin reuptake inhibitors in pregnant women and neonatal withdrawal syndrome: a database analysis. *Lancet*. 2005;365(9458):482-487. doi:10.1016/s0140-6736(05)17865-9.

100. Shellhaas RA, Wusthoff CJ, Tsuchida TN, et al. Profile of neonatal epilepsies. *Neurology*. 2017;89(9):893-899. doi:10.1212/WNL.0000000000004284.

101. Cornet MC, Morabito V, Lederer D, et al. Neonatal presentation of genetic epilepsies: early differentiation from acute provoked seizures. *Epilepsia*. 2021;62(8):1907-1920. doi:10.1111/epi.16957.

102. Berkovic SF, Heron SE, Giordano L, et al. Benign familial neonatal-infantile seizures: characterization of a new sodium channelopathy. *Ann Neurol*. 2004;55(4):550-557. doi:10.1002/ana.20029.

103. Heron SE, Cox K, Grinton BE, et al. Deletions or duplications in KCNQ2 can cause benign familial neonatal seizures. *J Med Genet*. 2007;44(12):791-796. doi:10.1136/jmg.2007.051938.

104. Grinton BE, Heron SE, Pelekanos JT, et al. Familial neonatal seizures in 36 families: clinical and genetic features correlate with outcome. *Epilepsia*. 2015;56(7):1071-1080. doi:10.1111/epi.13020.

105. Pisano T, Numis AL, Heavin SB, et al. Early and effective treatment of KCNQ2 encephalopathy. *Epilepsia*. 2015;56(5):685-691. doi:10.1111/epi.12984.

106. Novotny EJ. Early genetic testing for neonatal epilepsy. *Neurology*. 2017;89(9):880-881. doi:10.1212/WNL.0000000000004287.

107. Berg AT, Coryell J, Saneto RP, et al. Early-life epilepsies and the emerging role of genetic testing. *JAMA Pediatr*. 2017;171(9):863-871. doi:10.1001/jamapediatrics.2017.1743.

108. Stark Z, Tan TY, Chong B, et al. A prospective evaluation of whole-exome sequencing as a first-tier molecular test in infants with suspected monogenic disorders. *Genet Med*. 2016;18(11):1090-1096. doi:10.1038/gim.2016.1.

109. Stark Z, Schofield D, Alam K, et al. Prospective comparison of the cost-effectiveness of clinical whole-exome sequencing with that of usual care overwhelmingly supports early use and reimbursement. *Genet Med*. 2017;19(8):867-874. doi:10.1038/gim.2016.221.

110. Saunders CJ, Miller NA, Soden SE, et al. Rapid whole-genome sequencing for genetic disease diagnosis in neonatal intensive care units. *Sci Transl Med*. 2012;4(154):154ra135. doi:10.1126/scitranslmed.3004041.

111. Sheth RD, Hobbs GR, Mullett M. Neonatal seizures: incidence, onset, and etiology by gestational age. *J Perinatol*. 1999;19(1):40-43. doi:10.1038/sj.jp.7200107.

112. Edwards L, Hui L. First and second trimester screening for fetal structural anomalies. *Semin Fetal Neonatal Med*. 2018;23(2):102-111. doi:10.1016/J.SINY.2017.11.005.

113. Vasudevan C, Levene M. Epidemiology and aetiology of neonatal seizures. *Semin Fetal Neonatal Med*. 2013;18(4):185-191. doi:10.1016/j.siny.2013.05.008.

114. Pearl PL. Amenable treatable severe pediatric epilepsies. *Semin Pediatr Neurol*. 2016;23(2):158-166. doi:10.1016/j.spen.2016.06.004.

115. Coughlin CR, Tseng LA, Abdenur JE, et al. Consensus guidelines for the diagnosis and management of pyridoxine-dependent epilepsy due to α-aminoadipic semialdehyde dehydrogenase deficiency. *J Inherit Metab Dis*. 2021;44(1):178-192. doi:10.1002/jimd.12332.

116. Ficicioglu C, Bearden D. Isolated neonatal seizures: when to suspect inborn errors of metabolism. *Pediatr Neurol*. 2011;45(5):283-291. doi:10.1016/j.pediatrneurol.2011.07.006.

117. Leen WG, Klepper J, Verbeek MM, et al. Glucose transporter-1 deficiency syndrome: the expanding clinical and genetic spectrum of a treatable disorder. *Brain*. 2010;133(3):655-670. doi:10.1093/brain/awp336.

118. Schwahn BC, Van Spronsen FJ, Belaidi AA, et al. Efficacy and safety of cyclic pyranopterin monophosphate substitution in severe molybdenum cofactor deficiency type A: a prospective cohort study. *Lancet*. 2015;386(10007):1955-1963. doi:10.1016/S0140-6736(15)00124-5.

119. Dunn P, Albury CL, Maksemous N, et al. Next generation sequencing methods for diagnosis of epilepsy syndromes. *Front Genet*. 2018;9:20. doi:10.3389/fgene.2018.00020.

120. Dimmock D, Caylor S, Waldman B, et al. Project Baby Bear: rapid precision care incorporating rWGS in 5 California

children's hospitals demonstrates improved clinical outcomes and reduced costs of care. *Am J Hum Genet.* 2021;108(7):1231-1238. doi:10.1016/j.ajhg.2021.05.008.

121. Painter MJ, Scher MS, Stein AD, et al. Phenobarbital compared with phenytoin for the treatment of neonatal seizures. *N Engl J Med.* 1999;341(7):485-489. doi:10.1056/nejm199908123410704.

122. Soul JS, Pressler R, Allen M, et al. Recommendations for the design of therapeutic trials for neonatal seizures. *Pediatr Res.* 2019;85(7):943-954. doi:10.1038/s41390-018-0242-2.

123. Slaughter LA, Patel AD, Slaughter JL. Pharmacological treatment of neonatal seizures: a systematic review. *J Child Neurol.* 2013;28(3):351-364. doi:10.1177/0883073812470734.

124. Sharpe C, Reiner GE, Davis SL, et al. Levetiracetam versus phenobarbital for neonatal seizures: a randomized controlled trial. *Pediatrics.* 2020;145(6):e20193182. doi:10.1542/peds.2019-3182.

125. Bartha AI, Shen J, Katz KH, et al. Neonatal seizures: multicenter variability in current treatment practices. *Pediatr Neurol.* 2007;37(2):85-90. doi:10.1016/j.pediatrneurol.2007.04.003.

126. Keene JC, Morgan LA, Abend NS, et al. Treatment of neonatal seizures: comparison of treatment pathways from 11 neonatal intensive care units. *Pediatr Neurol.* 2022;128:67-74. doi:10.1016/J.PEDIATRNEUROL.2021.10.004.

127. Glass HC, Soul JS, Chu CJ, et al. Response to antiseizure medications in neonates with acute symptomatic seizures. *Epilepsia.* 2019;60(3):e20-e24. doi:10.1111/EPI.14671.

128. Kharoshankaya L, Stevenson NJ, Livingstone V, et al. Seizure burden and neurodevelopmental outcome in neonates with hypoxic–ischemic encephalopathy. *Dev Med Child Neurol.* 2016;58(12):1242-1248. doi:10.1111/dmcn.13215.

129. Kramer K, Bekmezian A, Nash K, Papp E, Glass HC. Expediting treatment of seizures in the intensive care nursery. *Pediatrics.* 2021;148(3):e2020013730. doi:10.1542/PEDS.2020-013730.

130. Blume HK, Garrison MM, Christakis DA. Neonatal seizures: treatment and treatment variability in 31 United States pediatric hospitals. *J Child Neurol.* 2009;24(2):148-154. doi:10.1177/0883073808321056.

131. Shellhaas RA, Chang T, Wusthoff CJ, et al. Treatment duration after acute symptomatic seizures in neonates: a multicenter cohort study. *J Pediatr.* 2017;181:298-301.e1. doi:10.1016/j.jpeds.2016.10.039.

132. Lockman LA, Kriel R, Zaske D, Thompson T, Virnig N. Phenobarbital dosage for control of neonatal seizures. *Neurology.* 1979;29(11):1445-1449. doi:10.1212/wnl.29.11.1445.

133. Bittigau P, Sifringer M, Ikonomidou C. Antiepileptic drugs and apoptosis in the developing brain. *Ann N Y Acad Sci.* 2003;993:103-114. doi:10.1111/j.1749-6632.2003.tb07517.x.

134. Filippi L, la Marca G, Cavallaro G, et al. Phenobarbital for neonatal seizures in hypoxic ischemic encephalopathy: a pharmacokinetic study during whole body hypothermia. *Epilepsia.* 2011;52(4):794-801. doi:10.1111/j.1528-1167.2011.02978.x.

135. Maitre NL, Smolinsky C, Slaughter JC, Stark AR. Adverse neurodevelopmental outcomes after exposure to phenobarbital and levetiracetam for the treatment of neonatal seizures. *J Perinatol.* 2013;33(11):841-846. doi:10.1038/jp.2013.116.

136. Booth D, Evans DJ. Anticonvulsants for neonates with seizures. *Cochrane Database Syst Rev.* 2004;3:CD004218. doi:10.1002/14651858.CD004218.pub2.

137. Painter MJ, Pippenger C, Wasterlain C, et al. Phenobarbital and phenytoin in neonatal seizures: metabolism and tissue distribution. *Neurology.* 1981;31(9):1107-1112. doi:10.1212/wnl.31.9.1107.

138. McNally MA, Hartman AL. Variability in preferred management of electrographic seizures in neonatal hypoxic ischemic encephalopathy. *Pediatr Neurol.* 2017;77:37-41. doi:10.1016/j.pediatrneurol.2017.06.006.

139. Dalziel SR, Borland ML, Furyk J, et al. Levetiracetam versus phenytoin for second-line treatment of convulsive status epilepticus in children (ConSEPT): an open-label, multicentre, randomised controlled trial. *Lancet.* 2019;393(10186):2135-2145. doi:10.1016/S0140-6736(19)30722-6.

140. Painter MJ, Pippenger C, MacDonald H, Pitlick W. Phenobarbital and diphenylhydantoin levels in neonates with seizures. *J Pediatr.* 1978;92(2):315-319. doi:10.1016/S0022-3476(78)80034-1.

141. Döring JH, Lampert A, Hoffmann GF, Ries M. Thirty years of orphan drug legislation and the development of drugs to treat rare seizure conditions: a cross sectional analysis. *PLoS One.* 2016;11(8):1-15. doi:10.1371/journal.pone.0161660.

142. Fürwentsches A, Bussmann C, Ramantani G, et al. Levetiracetam in the treatment of neonatal seizures: a pilot study. *Seizure.* 2010;19(3):185-189. doi:10.1016/j.seizure.2010.01.003.

143. Falsaperla R, Vitaliti G, Mauceri L, et al. Levetiracetam in neonatal seizures as first-line treatment: a prospective study. *J Pediatr Neurosci.* 2017;12(1):24-28. doi:10.4103/jpn.JPN_172_16.

144. Rao LM, Hussain SA, Zaki T, et al. A comparison of levetiracetam and phenobarbital for the treatment of neonatal seizures associated with hypoxic–ischemic encephalopathy. *Epilepsy Behav.* 2018;88:212-217. doi:10.1016/j.yebeh.2018.09.015.

145. Khan O, Cipriani C, Wright C, Crisp E, Kirmani B. Role of intravenous levetiracetam for acute seizure management in preterm neonates. *Pediatr Neurol.* 2013;49(5):340-343. doi:10.1016/j.pediatrneurol.2013.05.008.

146. Ramantani G, Ikonomidou C, Walter B, Rating D, Dinger J. Levetiracetam: safety and efficacy in neonatal seizures. *Eur J Paediatr Neurol.* 2011;15(1):1-7. doi:10.1016/j.ejpn.2010.10.003.

147. Kilicdag H, Daglioglu K, Erdogan S, et al. The effect of levetiracetam on neuronal apoptosis in neonatal rat model of hypoxic ischemic brain injury. *Early Hum Dev.* 2013;89(5):355-360. doi:10.1016/j.earlhumdev.2012.12.002.

148. Komur M, Okuyaz C, Celik Y, et al. Neuroprotective effect of levetiracetam on hypoxic ischemic brain injury in neonatal rats. *Childs Nerv Syst.* 2014;30(6):1001-1009. doi:10.1007/s00381-014-2375-x.

149. Sheth RD, Buckley DJ, Gutierrez AR, Gingold M, Bodensteiner JB, Penney S. Midazolam in the treatment of refractory neonatal seizures. *Clin Neuropharmacol.* 1996;19(2):165-170. doi:10.1097/00002826-199619020-00005.

150. Castro Conde JR, Hernández Borges AA, Doménech Martínez E, González Campo C, Perera Soler R. Midazolam in neonatal seizures with no response to phenobarbital. *Neurology.* 2005;64(5):876-879. doi:10.1212/01.WNL.0000152891.58694.71.

151. Shany E, Benzaqen O, Watemberg N. Comparison of continuous drip of midazolam or lidocaine in the treatment of intractable neonatal seizures. *J Child Neurol.* 2007;22(3):255-259. doi:10.1177/0883073807299858.

152. Lundqvist M, Ågren J, Hellström-Westas L, Flink R, Wickström R. Efficacy and safety of lidocaine for treatment of neonatal seizures. *Acta Paediatr.* 2013;102(9):863-867. doi:10.1111/apa.12311.

153. Weeke LC, Toet MC, van Rooij LGMM, et al. Lidocaine response rate in aEEG-confirmed neonatal seizures: retrospective study of 413 full-term and preterm infants. *Epilepsia.* 2016;57(2):233-242. doi:10.1111/epi.13286.

154. Malingré MM, Van Rooij LGM, Rademaker CMA, et al. Development of an optimal lidocaine infusion strategy for neonatal seizures. *Eur J Pediatr.* 2006;165(9):598-604. doi:10.1007/S00431-006-0136-X.

155. Sands TT, Balestri M, Bellini G, et al. Rapid and safe response to low-dose carbamazepine in neonatal epilepsy. *Epilepsia.* 2016;57(12):2019-2030. doi:10.1111/epi.13596.

156. Glass HC, Poulin C, Shevell MI. Topiramate for the treatment of neonatal seizures. *Pediatr Neurol.* 2011;44(6):439-442. doi:10.1016/j.pediatrneurol.2011.01.006.

157. *A Study to Evaluate the Efficacy, Safety, and Pharmacokinetics of Lacosamide in Neonates With Repeated Electroencephalographic Neonatal Seizures.* Full Text View. ClinicalTrials.gov. Available at: https://clinicaltrials.gov/ct2/show/NCT04519645. Accessed May 6, 2021.

158. Pressler RM, Boylan GB, Marlow N, et al. Bumetanide for the treatment of seizures in newborn babies with hypoxic ischaemic encephalopathy (NEMO): an open-label, dose finding, and feasibility phase 1/2 trial. *Lancet Neurol.* 2015;14(5):469-477. doi:10.1016/S1474-4422(14)70303-5.

159. Soul JS, Bergin AM, Stopp C, et al. A pilot randomized, controlled, double-blind trial of bumetanide to treat neonatal seizures. *Ann Neurol.* 2021;89(2):327-340. doi:10.1002/ana.25959.

160. Gospe Jr SM. Pyridoxine-dependent epilepsy. In: Adam MP, Ardinger HH, Pagon RA, et al., eds. *GeneReviews®* [Internet]. Seattle, WA: University of Washington; 1993-2021. Available at: https://www.ncbi.nlm.nih.gov/books/NBK1486/. Accessed April 29, 2021.

161. Guillet R, Kwon JM. Prophylactic phenobarbital administration after resolution of neonatal seizures: survey of current practice. *Pediatrics.* 2008;122(4):731-735. doi:10.1542/peds.2007-3278.

162. Glass HC, Soul JS, Chang T, et al. Safety of early discontinuation of antiseizure medication after acute symptomatic neonatal seizures. *JAMA Neurol.* 2021;78(7):817-825. doi:10.1001/jamaneurol.2021.1437.

163. Guillet R, Kwon J. Seizure recurrence and developmental disabilities after neonatal seizures: outcomes are unrelated to use of phenobarbital prophylaxis. *J Child Neurol.* 2007;22(4):389-395. doi:10.1177/0883073807301917.

164. Glass HC, Numis AL, Gano D, Bali V, Rogers EE. Outcomes after acute symptomatic seizures in children admitted to a neonatal neurocritical care service. *Pediatr Neurol.* 2018;84:39-45. doi:10.1016/j.pediatrneurol.2018.03.016.

165. Hellstrom-Westas L, Blennow G, Lindroth M, Rosen I, Svenningsen NW. Low risk of seizure recurrence after early withdrawal of antiepileptic treatment in the neonatal period. *Arch Dis Child.* 1995;72(suppl 2):97-98. doi:10.1136/fn.72.2.f97.

166. Fitzgerald MP, Kessler SK, Abend NS. Early discontinuation of antiseizure medications in neonates with hypoxic–ischemic encephalopathy. *Epilepsia.* 2017;58(6):1047-1053. doi:10.1111/EPI.13745.

167. Farwell JR, Lee YJ, Hirtz DG, Sulzbacher SI, Ellenberg JH, Nelson KB. Phenobarbital for febrile seizures—effects on intelligence and on seizure recurrence. *N Engl J Med.* 1990;322(6):364-369. doi:10.1056/nejm199002083220604.

168. Payne ET, Zhao XY, Frndova H, et al. Seizure burden is independently associated with short term outcome in critically ill children. *Brain.* 2014;137(5):1429-1438. doi:10.1093/brain/awu042.

169. Glass HC, Kan J, Bonifacio SL, Ferriero DM. Neonatal seizures: treatment practices among term and preterm infants. *Pediatr Neurol.* 2012;46(2):111-115. doi:10.1016/J.PEDIATRNEUROL.2011.11.006.

170. Dzhala V, Ben-Ari Y, Khazipov R. Seizures accelerate anoxia-induced neuronal death in the neonatal rat hippocampus. *Ann Neurol.* 2000;48(4):632-640.

171. Holmes GL. The long-term effects of neonatal seizures. *Clin Perinatol.* 2009;36(4):901-914. doi:10.1016/j.clp.2009.07.012.

172. Miller SP, Weiss J, Barnwell A, et al. Seizure-associated brain injury in term newborns with perinatal asphyxia. *Neurology.* 2002;58(4):542-548. doi:10.1212/WNL.58.4.542.

173. Srinivasakumar P, Zempel J, Trivedi S, et al. Treating EEG seizures in hypoxic ischemic encephalopathy: a randomized controlled trial. *Pediatrics.* 2015;136(5):e1302-e1309. doi:10.1542/peds.2014-3777.

174. Pressler RM, Boylan GB, Morton M, Binnie CD, Rennie JM. Early serial EEG in hypoxic ischaemic encephalopathy. *Clin Neurophysiol.* 2001;112(1):31-37. doi:10.1016/S1388-2457(00)00517-4.

175. Murray DM, Boylan GB, Ryan CA, Connolly S. Early EEG findings in hypoxic-ischemic encephalopathy predict outcomes at 2 years. *Pediatrics.* 2009;124(3):459-467. doi:10.1542/peds.2008-2190.

176. Pisani F, Sisti L, Seri S. A scoring system for early prognostic assessment after neonatal seizures. *Pediatrics.* 2009;124(4):e580-e587. doi:10.1542/PEDS.2008-2087.

177. Garfinkle J, Shevell MI. Prognostic factors and development of a scoring system for outcome of neonatal seizures in term infants. *Eur J Paediatr Neurol.* 2011;15(3):222-229. doi:10.1016/J.EJPN.2010.11.002.

178. Temko A, Doyle O, Murray D, Lightbody G, Boylan G, Marnane W. Multimodal predictor of neurodevelopmental outcome in newborns with hypoxic-ischaemic encephalopathy. *Comput Biol Med.* 2015;63:169-177. doi:10.1016/J.COMPBIOMED.2015.05.017.

179. Boss RD, Lemmon ME, Arnold RM, Donohue PK. Communicating prognosis with parents of critically ill infants: direct observation of clinician behaviors. *J Perinatol.* 2017;37(11):1224-1229. doi:10.1038/jp.2017.118.

180. Lemmon ME, Donohue PK, Williams EP, Brandon D, Ubel PA, Boss RD. No question too small: development of a question prompt list for parents of critically ill infants. *J Perinatol.* 2018;38(4):386-391. doi:10.1038/s41372-017-0029-z.

181. Lemmon ME, Glass HC, Shellhaas RA, et al. Family-centered care for children and families impacted by neonatal seizures: advice from parents. *Pediatr Neurol.* 2021;124:26-32. doi:10.1016/J.PEDIATRNEUROL.2021.07.013.

182. Barks MC, Schindler EA, Ubel PA, et al. Assessment of parent understanding in conferences for critically ill neonates. *Patient Educ Couns.* 2022;105(3):599-605. doi:10.1016/j.pec.2021.06.013.

183. Clancy RR, Legido A. Postnatal epilepsy after EEG-confirmed neonatal seizures. *Epilepsia.* 1991;32(1):69-76. doi:10.1111/j.1528-1157.1991.tb05614.x.

184. Pisani F, Piccolo B, Cantalupo G, et al. Neonatal seizures and postneonatal epilepsy: a 7-y follow-up study. *Pediatr Res.* 2012;72(2):186-193. doi:10.1038/pr.2012.66.

185. Pisani F, Leali L, Parmigiani S, et al. Neonatal seizures in preterm infants: clinical outcome and relationship with subsequent epilepsy. *J Matern Neonatal Med.* 2004;16(2):51-53. doi:10.1080/jmf.16.2.51.53.

186. Glass HC, Hong KJ, Rogers EE, et al. Risk factors for epilepsy in children with neonatal encephalopathy. *Pediatr Res.* 2011;70(5):535-540. doi:10.1203/PDR.0b013e31822f24c7.

187. Shellhaas RA, Wusthoff CJ, Numis AL, et al. Early-life epilepsy after acute symptomatic neonatal seizures: a prospective multicenter study. *Epilepsia.* 2021;62(8):1871-1882. doi:10.1111/EPI.16978.

188. Glass HC, Grinspan ZM, Li Y, et al. Risk for infantile spasms after acute symptomatic neonatal seizures. *Epilepsia.* 2020;61(12):2774-2784. doi:10.1111/EPI.16749.

Chapter 10

Glucose and Perinatal Brain Injury: Questions and Controversies

Sarbattama Sen and Jane E. Harding

Chapter Outline

Introduction

Neonatal hypoglycemia is the most common biochemical abnormality of the newborn, affecting 5%–15% of all infants and 50% of those with risk factors. Although severe hypoglycemia has been incontrovertibly linked with brain injury and impairment, the glucose thresholds below which injury occurs have not been clearly established, and in fact, may differ based on various host factors. In the absence of clear evidence of a causative link between mild or asymptomatic neonatal hypoglycemia and brain injury, committees have recommended that infants who are at high risk based on maternal or fetal physiology are screened and treated if their blood glucose drops below "operational thresholds," or concentration of blood glucose at which clinicians should consider intervention. These thresholds have been determined based on consensus opinion, incorporating a combination of norms in healthy infants, neuroglycopenic thresholds, and associations between early glycemia and later development from observational studies.

In this chapter, we will review key metabolic transitions that occur soon after birth that, when dysregulated, can result in neonatal hypoglycemia, summarize mechanisms that underlie the association between neonatal hypoglycemia and later outcomes, and review the animal and human studies that have investigated the link between hypoglycemia and neurodevelopment. We will also summarize current glycemic assessment modalities and prevention and treatment recommendations. Throughout, we will highlight unanswered questions and areas of controversy that urgently require further inquiry.

Perinatal Glucose Regulation

The primary source of energy for the fetus is glucose, which the fetus receives from its mother down a concentration gradient.[1–3] Insulin is secreted at lower glucose concentrations in utero compared to postnatally as its function during this time is primarily related to fetal growth rather than glucose regulation.[4] Just before delivery, maternal and fetal glucose concentrations increase[5] until clamping of the umbilical cord, when maternal glucose supply to the infant is interrupted and neonatal glucose concentrations decrease, reaching a nadir between 1 and 3 hours after birth. In response to falling glucose concentrations, the infant's insulin secretion should decrease while secretion of glucagon and catecholamines increase, stimulating glucose production through gluconeogenesis and glycogenolysis. Typically, these physiologic transitions, which involve "resetting" the threshold for glucose-stimulated insulin secretion by the pancreatic beta cell to the higher, adult glucose concentration range,[6] occur over the first 48 to 72 hours after birth, resulting in infants achieving normoglycemia by adult definitions by this time point.[7,8]

Established risk factors for neonatal hypoglycemia: Maternal, fetal, and neonatal conditions that predispose infants to a delayed or exaggerated glycemic transition fall into three broad categories: high in utero fetal insulin secretion, decreased insulin sensitivity, and decreased stores of glycogen. Current guidelines recommend screening infants for hypoglycemia based on the following risk factors that together result in approximately one-third of infants warranting screening for hypoglycemia, of whom approximately 50% experience hypoglycemia based on current definitions.[9] The risk factors that are identified include:

i. Prematurity: 10.1% of infants in the United States are born preterm (<37 weeks gestation).[10] Glycogen and adipose tissue accumulation accelerates in the third trimester, stimulated by relative maternal insulin resistance and hyperinsulinemia. Thus, in general, preterm infants have less glycogen and adipose tissue stores at birth than those born at term. In addition, the concentrations of the lynchpin enzyme for glycogenolysis, glucose-6-phosphatase, are lower in preterm infants than in term infants, rendering preterm infants less able to utilize available glycogen stores.[11] Lastly, preterm infants produce lower concentrations of ketones than term infants in the setting of hypoglycemia.[12,13]

ii. Growth restriction: 8% of infants are considered growth restricted.[14] Growth-restricted fetuses have increased production of catecholamines resulting in suppressed insulin secretion in utero, and postnatal compensations that result in inappropriately high insulin secretion.[15] In addition, growth-restricted fetuses have reduced glycogen stores related to limited nutrient supply across the placenta, and limited capacity for oxidation of free fatty acids.[16] Growth-restricted infants often have relative "head sparing," so that brain size is disproportionately large for their birthweight, further compounding the mismatch between glucose demand and supply.

iii. Infants born to women with diabetes: Diabetes affects approximately 10% of pregnancies in the United States and disproportionately impacts pregnant women with overweight or obesity.[17] Rates of diabetes in pregnancy have increased more than 50% in the past 10 years.[17] Throughout pregnancy, women experience a gradual decline in insulin sensitivity, influenced by factors including obesity, placental hormones, structural changes and dysfunction of the placenta, and changes in cytokine levels. This decreased insulin sensitivity is accompanied by an increase in insulin production by the pancreatic beta cells in pregnancies with typical glucose tolerance.[18] However, in pregnancies affected by diabetes, there is inadequate insulin production to accommodate the decreased insulin sensitivity, resulting in maternal and thus fetal hyperglycemia and leading to increased fetal insulin secretion.[19–21] Persistence of this increased insulin secretion after birth can lead to neonatal hypoglycemia, particularly in infants born to women with diabetes that is poorly controlled.

iv. Large-for-gestational-age infants: Infants who are large-for-gestational age but not born to women with diabetes are currently screened due to the theoretical concern that the large fetal size is a result of excess insulin production. In these infants, maternal hyperglycemia may not reach the threshold of clinical diabetes diagnosis, but the fetal exposure to excessive glucose supply and hence fetal insulin secretion predisposes them to impaired metabolic adaptation. It is reported that 16%–39% of large-for-gestational-age infants who were not born to women with diabetes developed hypoglycemia,[9] depending on the study population.[22]

v. Maternal β blocker exposure: Hypertensive disorders complicate 5%–10% of pregnancies and β blockers are commonly used in their treatment.[23] β Blockers cross the placenta and lead to fetal sympathetic blockade and increased insulin production. The risk of neonatal hypoglycemia in β blocker–exposed neonates was 4.3% versus 1.2% in unexposed infants.[24]

vi. Family history of hypoglycemic disorder, inborn error of metabolism, or genetic syndrome linked to hypoglycemia (Table 10.1): Infants who fall into these categories are at risk based on abnormalities of insulin secretion (hyperinsulinism), decreased production of cortisol and/or growth hormone, and inborn errors of metabolism that limit glucose production.

Mechanisms Underlying Hypoglycemia-induced Brain Injury

Brain energy metabolism (Fig. 10.1): Glucose is an essential metabolic fuel for the brain. In the newborn, the disproportionately large brain for body size requires approximately 2 to 3 times the rate of glucose consumption relative to body weight compared to an

TABLE 10.1   Genetic Disorders That Can Present as Neonatal Hypoglycemia and Examples or Candidate Genetic Defects

Congenital hyperinsulinism	ABCC8, KCNJ11, UCP2 mutation
Endocrinopathies	Panhypopituitarism
	Growth hormone deficiency
	Cortisol deficiency
	Hypothyroidism
Inborn errors of metabolism	Carbohydrate metabolism (e.g., galactosemia, glucose-6-phosphate deficiency)
	Glycogen storage disorders
	Organic acid metabolism (e.g., propionic acidemia, methylmalonic acidemia)
	Pyruvate carboxylase deficiency, Fatty acid oxidation disorders, mitochondrial disorders
Genetic syndrome	Beckwith-Wiedemann, Prader-Willi, Kabuki, Turner

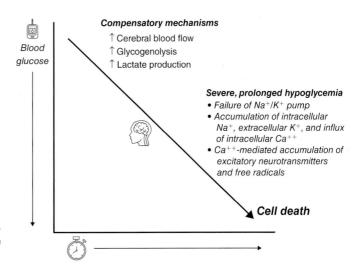

Fig. 10.1 Schematic of cerebral adaptations to hypoglycemia over time and postulated mechanisms that contribute to hypoglycemia-associated brain injury.

adult[25,26] and utilizes more than 30% of hepatic glucose output.[27] Glucose uptake from blood to the brain occurs via facilitated diffusion through energy-independent glucose transporters.[28–31] Twelve glucose transporters have been identified and labeled as GLUT 1 through 12.[32] Within the brain, GLUT 1 and 3 are predominant. All brain endothelial GLUT proteins are low during the first week of life and increase in the second and third postnatal weeks.[31] There is a regional developmental progression in cerebral glucose utilization. Animal and human studies have reported that in early development, the brain stem utilizes the highest proportion of glucose. Over the first year after birth, glucose utilization progressively increases and expands through the sensorimotor cortex, thalamus, parietal, temporal, and occipital cortices and lastly in the frontal cortex.[33] Unsurprisingly but of developmental importance, electroencephalographic studies have reported that the functional development of these regions coincides with increases in glucose utilization.[34]

In the brain, glucose is phosphorylated to glucose-6-phosphate by hexokinase. Glucose-6-phosphate can then be aerobically oxidized to generate adenosine triphosphate (ATP) through the citric acid cycle. Glucose-6-phosphate can also be stored as glycogen or shunted toward lipid production or nucleic acid synthesis. Low glucose concentrations are likely to result in inadequate brain energy delivery. Lactate provides a potential alternative fuel in the first 48 hours, as demonstrated by studies in the newborn dog reporting that 95% of the brain energy supply arises from glucose and 4% from lactate under normoglycemic conditions.[35] With hypoglycemia, the proportion of energy from lactate increases and there is evidence to suggest that the neonatal brain is better able to utilize lactate than an adult, although the energy produced is significantly lower than with glucose metabolism. Ketones can also provide an alternative to glucose for cerebral oxidative metabolism. However, ketone production remains low even under conditions of hypoglycemia, until 3 to 4 days after birth, likely related to persisting relatively hyperinsulinemic conditions.[36] With prolonged exposure to hypoglycemia, amino acid utilization also increases in the brain to preserve energy production.[47] A recent neonatal study reported that glucose contributed 72% to 84% of available potential ATP. Lactate contributed 25% of potential ATP

on the first day and remained the largest potential source of ATP other than glucose throughout the first 5 days. Ketones were most available on days 2 to 3 but still only contributed 7% of potential ATP. Total potential ATP available from these fuels was 17% lower on days 1 to 2 than on days 4 to 5.[37]

Cerebral adaptations and responses to hypoglycemia: Under conditions of hypoglycemia, brain energy delivery is partially preserved by recruitment of cerebral capillaries, resulting in increased cerebral blood flow. This adaptation was noted below a blood glucose threshold of 30 mg/dL in preterm infants[38] and was inversely correlated with cerebral regional oxygenation in term and preterm infants in another recent study.[39] Early data regarding the impact of hypoglycemia on cerebral blood flow was described from animal models and supported a compensatory increase in cerebral blood flow with low blood glucose concentrations.[40] Studies have since investigated the associations between glycemia and cerebral blood flow and oxygen saturations in infants. Recently, Matterberger et al. reported cross-sectional data in a cohort of 75 infants showing that one measured blood glucose concentration at 15 to 20 minutes after birth was negatively correlated with cerebral blood flow and oxygen saturations (r = −0.35 in term infants and −0.69 in preterm infants, both $p < 0.05$).[39] Similar findings have been reported in a cohort of 11 preterm infants, pairing continuous glucose monitoring with near-infrared spectroscopy (NIRS).[41] Data regarding the predictive value of high cerebral oxygen saturations has been limited to the population of infants with hypoxic-ischemic encephalopathy, where higher cerebral oxygen saturation is associated with brain injury on MRI in infants with hypoxic-ischemic encephalopathy.[42–44]

Other cerebral compensatory mechanisms during hypoglycemia include glycogenolysis to mobilize glucose from available stores and increased lactate utilization for energy production, as previously described. Although these mechanisms together may fully compensate for decreased glucose availability in many infants, the increased cerebral perfusion, and resultant hyperoxia and oxidative stress, particularly if experienced for longer periods, may contribute to brain injury.

With severe, prolonged hypoglycemia in adult animals, a failure of the neuronal energy-dependent Na$^+$/

K^+ pump results in accumulation of intracellular Na^+, extracellular K^+, and influx of intracellular Ca^{++}. Similar to neuronal injury induced by hypoxic conditions, Ca^{++}-mediated accumulation of excitatory neurotransmitters and free radicals contributes to the final pathway resulting in cell death.[28,34,45,46] In addition with prolonged exposure to hypoglycemia, ammonia levels increase markedly, likely related to use of amino acids as an energy source. A possible underlying cause of cellular injury in the newborn may, however, be related to the release of excitatory amino acids. In a preterm animal model of hyperinsulinemic hypoglycemia, decreasing blood glucose concentrations were strongly inversely correlated with concentrations of extracellular glutamate.[47] Similarly, in hypoglycemic newborns, lower blood glucose concentrations were associated with higher concentrations of glutamate and aspartate in cerebrospinal fluid.[48]

In vitro and animal models informing neuronal vulnerability to hypoglycemia: In vitro cell culture studies as well as animal models of pure hypoglycemia have been helpful in documenting the effects of significantly low blood glucose levels on brain pathology. In vitro nuclear magnetic resonance studies on energy metabolism of neurons and astroglia under various pathologic conditions have shown that hypoglycemia per se does not significantly alter the high-energy reserves of either neurons or glia.[49] Immature astrocytes exposed to a substrate-free medium (absence of glucose and amino acids) are able to survive for almost twice as long as the mature astrocytes, suggesting that immature neurons may have the ability to tolerate hypoglycemia better than adult neurons.[50] In adolescent primates with insulin-induced hypoglycemia, blood glucose concentrations <20 mg/dL for 2 hours or more led to neuronal necrosis throughout the cerebral cortices, with particular vulnerability in the parieto-occipital region, as well as the hippocampus, caudate, and putamen. Similar findings were present in primates exposed to prolonged (6 hours) hypoglycemia, with neuropathologic alterations occurring primarily in the basal ganglia, cerebral cortex, and hippocampus.[51] The adult rat has been used as a model for defining the neuropathologic consequences of severe hypoglycemia, although differences between the immature and mature brains must be considered in interpreting these studies. Several important features of hypoglycemic brain damage have

been described that distinguish it from typical patterns of ischemic injury, including a superficial to deep gradient of neuronal necrosis in the cerebral cortex, caudate putamen involvement near the white matter and near the angle of the lateral ventricle, and dense neuronal necrosis in the hippocampus at the crest of the dentate gyrus (which is always spared in ischemia).[52–54] Interestingly, white matter injury was not particularly addressed in these studies.

Taken together, the available data suggest that the newborn brain is capable of some compensatory mechanisms that help maintain brain fuel delivery under conditions of hypoglycemia. However, it is unclear which infants are or are not able to maintain adequate brain fuel delivery with these compensations, and how these compensations and their metabolic by-products, particularly if prolonged, can impact neural development during a time of extreme susceptibility.

Hypoglycemia and Neurologic Markers

A series of studies have identified a specific pattern of cerebral abnormality on neuroimaging after hypoglycemia involving the parieto-occipital cortex and underlying white matter. These imaging findings are consistent with the areas responsible for the observed neurodevelopmental associations (see below). Abnormal signal intensity with restricted diffusion is reported on MRI and is visualized better with diffusion-weighted imaging. Spectroscopy does not show significant elevations of lactate. About 10%–15% of these areas of restricted diffusion resolve, but some can result in volume loss of cortex and white matter. With severe hypoglycemia, a more diffuse pattern of cerebral cortical injury can occur.[55–60] A recent study highlighted the persistence of cerebral imaging differences in childhood. Nine-year-old children who experienced hypoglycemia as neonates had smaller deep grey matter brain regions and thinner occipital lobe cortices than children who did not experience neonatal hypoglycemia.[61]

One early study (n = 5 newborns; 17 infants total) reported that blood glucose <47 mg/dL was associated with a prolongation of latency and abnormal sensory evoked potentials.[62] However, a more recent study in neonates did not find that moderate hypoglycemia was associated with changes in amplitude-integrated EEG markers.[63] Severe and persistent hypoglycemia can also result in electroencephalographic and clinical seizures. A retrospective study of 36 children (age 6 months–15 years) with severe hypoglycemia and seizures in the neonatal period revealed posterior temporo-occipital (n = 23), multifocal or generalized spikes, polyspikes, and spike/wave discharges (n = 10) in the interictal period. Three patients had a normal initial EEG, and eight showed a hypsarrhythmic EEG associated with infantile spasms at seizure onset. Interictal EEG remained abnormal in 32 of 36 patients (88.8%). All of these infants had occipital brain injury on MRI in the neonatal period.[64]

Measurement of Blood Glucose in Neonates

There are three approaches to blood glucose measurement in the neonate: glucose oxidase-laboratory-based measurement, point-of-care whole blood glucose measurement, and enzymatic point-of-care analyzers. The gold standard for blood glucose measurement is the glucose oxidase method, typically performed in the laboratory. Due to red cell glycolysis, delays in processing blood samples and assaying glucose can reduce the glucose concentration by up to 6 mg/dL/h. Given the turn-around-time for these assays and the risk of delayed treatment, recommendations for the screening and treatment of neonatal hypoglycemia have commonly involved the use of point-of-care glucose meters for initial screening,[65] with a laboratory assay to confirm low point-of-care readings while treating the low glucose to prevent treatment delay.

Point-of-care devices were developed for adult diabetics and FDA guidance states that "95% of all values are within 12 mg/dL at glucose concentrations ≤75 mg/dL."[66] The accuracy of different devices used to measure glucose concentrations can vary substantially and overall, these devices tend to be somewhat inaccurate at the low glucose concentrations characteristic of newborns.[67] In addition, whole blood glucose values are approximately 15% lower than plasma glucose concentrations.

A third approach to blood glucose measurement is enzymatic point-of-care analyzers with specific glucose cartridges. The drawbacks of using these devices are that they are not universally available and they require more blood collected in a specific collection device, although they may be associated with overall cost savings related to decreasing the need for laboratory glucose measurement.[68]

A number of anticipated future advances in biochemical monitoring will likely improve care of the neonate at risk of neonatal hypoglycemia. These include the use of continuous interstitial glucose monitors, which have been shown to be safe and feasible in neonates[69,70] and provide information on direction and rate of change in glucose concentrations as well as duration of exposure to hypoglycemia. Despite their potential, these monitors are currently not approved for neonates, do not provide readings <40 mg/dL, and there are, as yet, few data on their clinical utility. Another much-needed advance is point-of-care devices that accurately measure glucose and alternative fuels, such as ketones and lactate, in very small samples, developed specifically for neonates. In the longer term, options for noninvasive glucose monitoring, including "pulse glucometers" analogous to pulse oximeters, are already in development.

Definitions of Hypoglycemia

Identifying an outcomes-derived definition of hypoglycemia is challenging given that glycemic regulation is dynamic and host factors undoubtedly contribute, so that adverse outcomes may result in one infant but not in another at the same blood glucose concentration. Given this uncertainty, two approaches have been proposed to define hypoglycemia: the statistical definition based on population norms and a neurophysiologic definition based on glycemic thresholds below which a neurophysiologic marker is affected.

The statistical approach defines hypoglycemia as a blood or plasma glucose concentration lower than two standard deviations below the mean (<5%). In term appropriate-for-gestational age healthy newborns, blood glucose concentrations can range between 25 and 110 mg/dL within the first few hours after birth; however, by about 72 hours of age, glucose concentrations typically reach at least 60 to 100 mg/dL.[4] In the GLOW study, the mean plasma glucose increased from a mean of 59 ± 11 mg/dL in the first 48 hours to 83 ± 14 mg/dL after 72 hours. The challenge with a statistical definition is that different populations of infants have different typical ranges that vary widely, making this difficult to translate to clinical practice.

The neurophysiologic definition has been used in informing current guidelines. Blood glucose concentrations <47 mg/dL have been associated with prolongation of neurosensory response latencies,[62] although only five of the 17 infants studied were newborns. Cerebral blood flow has been shown to increase with blood glucose <30 mg/dL and transport of cerebral glucose is limited at <54 mg/dL.

As a bridge between the statistical and the neurophysiologic thresholds, operational thresholds have been proposed as an approach to recommend clinician interventions at specific thresholds. Different operational thresholds have been adopted by national and international organizations (Fig. 10.2) based on interpretations of population-based norms and neurodevelopmental outcome studies. However, none of these approaches incorporate thresholds for neuronal injury that may be modulated based on host susceptibility.

A pragmatic trial (n = 278) of two thresholds (36 vs. 47 mg/dL) for treatment of mild-moderate hypoglycemia that was diagnosed within 24 hours after birth did not find that maintaining blood glucose at the higher threshold improved outcomes at 18 months. However, outcomes from this trial have not been reported to school age, when many of the developmental domains thought to be associated with hypoglycemia can be assessed.[71] Thus the controversy around definitions of hypoglycemia continues without data to support the impact of treatment at various thresholds on long-term outcomes.

Symptomatic hypoglycemia: Most (79%) hypoglycemic infants, by contemporary definitions, are asymptomatic.[9] If symptomatic, the most common features of hypoglycemic encephalopathy are an alteration in the level of consciousness, described as lethargy or somnolence. Irritability, jitteriness, high-pitched cry, or exaggerated primitive reflexes may also be present. If hypoglycemia is untreated, these symptoms can progress to seizures, apnea, hypotonia, and coma.[55] Hawdon suggested that symptomatic hypoglycemia suggests host susceptibility to lower brain glucose delivery and should be treated as pathologic, while asymptomatic hypoglycemia should be treated if prolonged.[72]

Hypoglycemia and Developmental Outcomes

SEVERITY OF HYPOGLYCEMIA

Given the complexities surrounding the definition and diagnosis of hypoglycemia in newborns and the challenges with follow-up until school age, when more subtle, but still functionally significant, neurodevelopmental sequelae are reliably recognized, it has been difficult to conclusively ascertain the neurodevelopmental sequelae of hypoglycemic exposures. We have summarized the populations, methods, and results of several key reports that have informed our understanding of this association in Table 10.2.

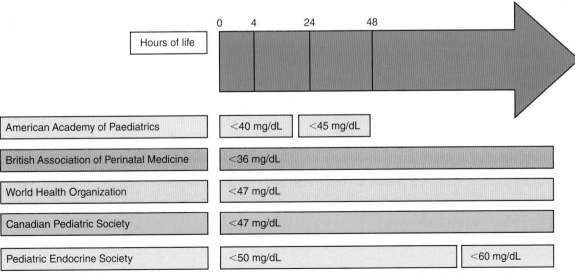

Fig. 10.2 Illustration of suggested glycemic operational thresholds by different organizations.

TABLE 10.2   Summary of Studies Examining Associations Between Neonatal Hypoglycemia and Neurodevelopmental Outcomes in Childhood

Author, Year	Design	n	Population	Exposure (NH definition)	Outcome	Age at Outcome	Key Findings of Infants with NH
McKinlay, 2017	Prospective cohort study	477 (280 with and 197 without NH)	Infants >32 weeks with 1 or more NH risk factor	BG <47 mg/dL	Neurosensory impairment (poor performance in one or more domains)	4.5 years	↑ Risk of low executive function; ↑ Risk of low visual motor function; No increased risk of neurosensory impairment
Goode, 2016	Secondary analysis of Randomized controlled trial	745 (461 with and 284 without NH)	Preterm, low birthweight infants (<37 weeks and <2500 g)	BG <45 mg/dL	Cognitive, academic, and behavioral measures	3, 8, 18 years	No significant difference in cognitive achievement; No significant difference in academic achievement; No significant difference in behavioral achievement
McKinlay, 2015	Prospective cohort study	404 (216 with and 188 without NH)	Infants >35 weeks with 1 or more NH risk factor	BG <47 mg/dL	Bayley, executive function, visual function	2 years	No increased risk of processing difficulty; No increased risk of neurosensory impairment
Kaiser, 2015	Retrospective cohort study	1395 (89 with and 1306 without NH)	All infants with at least 1 recorded glucose	BG <35 mg/dL	Academic performance	10 years	↓ Odds of proficiency on literacy and mathematics achievement tests
Kerstjens, 2012	Cohort study	832 (67 with and 765 without NH)	Moderately preterm infants (32-<36 weeks)	BG <30 mg/dL	Ages and Stages Questionnaire	43–49 months	↑ Risk of developmental delay (ASQ total-problems score)
Brand, 2005	Cohort study	75 (60 with and 15 without NH)	Term, LGA infants	BG <40 mg/dL	Development, intelligence, behavior	4 years	No significant difference in development; No significant difference in behavior; No significant difference in total IQ, but ↓ in reasoning IQ subscale
Duvanel, 1999	Cohort study	85 (62 with and 23 without NH)	Preterm, SGA infants	BG <47 mg/dL	Psychomotor development	6, 12, 18 months and 3.5, 5 years	↓ Scores in specific psychometric tests at 3.5 and 5 years

Study	Study type	Sample	Population	Glucose threshold	Outcomes measured	Age at follow-up	Results
Stenninger, 1998	Cohort study	28 (13 with and 15 without NH) IDM, 28 controls	Infants of diabetic mothers + infants of nondiabetic mothers (control infants)	BG <27 mg/dL	Minimal brain dysfunction, motor development, mental development	7–8 years	↑ Total scores in minimal brain dysfunction screening test compared to control infants; No significant differences in motor development compared to control infants; ↓ Total development quotient compared to normoglycemic IDM and control infants
Lucas, 1988	Cohort study	661 (433 with and 218 without NH)	Preterm infants	BG <46 mg/dL	Bayley motor and mental development scales	18 months	↓ Psychomotor development index in infants with 5 or more days of recorded NH; ↓ Mental development index in infants with 5 or more days of recorded NH
Pildes, 1974	Prospective cohort study	80 (39 with and 41 without NH)	All infants	BG <20 mg/dL	Physical growth, neurological, and EEG abnormalities	1–7 years	Significantly higher incidence of neurological abnormalities at 2, 3, and 6 years; No significant difference in EEG abnormalities; ↓ Mean IQ at 4 years
Koivisto, 1972	Retrospective cohort study	151 NH (77 symptomatic NH, 66 asymptomatic NH, 8 NH-related seizures) and 56 control (no NH)	All infants	BG <30 mg/dL	Motor functions, speech development, social behavior, sensory screening, and visual acuity	1–4 years	Symptomatic NH, particularly seizures, associated with increased risk of neurodevelopmental abnormalities
Griffiths, 1971	Cohort study	82 (41 with and 41 without NH)	Infants admitted to special care unit	BG <20 mg/dL	Cognitive, behavioral, and motor		No significant difference in IQ; No significant difference in locomotor scores; No significant difference in incidence of behavior disorders

Previous studies have reported that hypoglycemia in specific high-risk populations (preterm,[73] growth restricted,[74] infants of women with diabetes)[75,76] is associated with adverse neurodevelopmental outcomes. However, this association has not been detected in other studies, with particular controversy over large-for-gestational-age infants who are not born to women with diabetes.[77] A recent meta-analysis[78] of observational studies reported that exposure to neonatal hypoglycemia was not associated with neurodevelopmental impairment in early childhood (n = 1657 infants; OR = 1.16, 95% CI = 0.86–1.57) but was associated with visual-motor impairment (n = 508; OR = 3.46, 95% CI = 1.13–10.57) and executive dysfunction (n = 463; OR = 2.50, 95% CI = 1.20–5.22).[76,77,79–83] In the largest study to examine school-age outcomes (n = 473), children in the lowest quintile for interstitial glucose concentrations in the first 12 hours after birth had increased risk of neurosensory impairment at age 4.5 years.[80] The association of neonatal hypoglycemia with outcomes was dose-dependent, with the greatest risk of a low executive function score and a low visual motor integration score in children exposed to severe (<36 mg/dL) or recurrent (≥3 episodes) hypoglycemia. Clinically undetected hypoglycemia, determined to be present only by post-hoc blinded continuous glucose monitoring, was associated with higher risk of executive dysfunction. In this study, clinically detected hypoglycemia was treated to maintain blood glucose concentrations ≥47 mg/dL, whereas clinically undetected hypoglycemia was untreated.[80] Pooled results of small observational studies have not supported the association of neonatal hypoglycemia with epilepsy,[76,80,82] cognitive impairment,[80,82,84] emotional-behavioral difficulty,[76,80,84] or visual, hearing, or motor impairment.[79,80,82] Neonatal hypoglycemia was found to be associated with mid-childhood neurodevelopmental impairment in a small, pooled analysis (n = 54; OR = 3.62, 95% CI = 1.05–12.42),[75,81] and with low literacy (n = 1395; OR = 2.04, 95% CI = 1.20–3.47) and numeracy (n = 1395; OR = 2.04, 95% CI = 1.21–3.44) in a single study.[85] The extant literature is limited by the low number of quality studies (of the 1665 studies that were screened only 12 publications were included in the meta-analysis), small sample sizes, lack of follow-up beyond mid-childhood, and minimal information about maternal metabolic status, making it impossible to determine whether the outcomes were related to the in utero environment, neonatal hypoglycemia, or both. All of these studies were conducted in populations considered "at-risk" for hypoglycemia, so generalizability of these associations beyond these populations is also limited.

BLOOD GLUCOSE VARIABILITY

Data from a rat model of insulin-induced hypoglycemia show accentuation of neuronal injury after rapid overcorrection of hypoglycemia, likely through increased cerebral blood flow, glucose reperfusion, and formation of reactive oxygen species,[38,86] as discussed previously. In one study with continuous interstitial glucose monitoring (n = 404 at 2 years and 477 infants at 4.5 years), children who developed neurosensory impairment at 2 years were more likely to have a steeper rise in interstitial glucose concentrations after hypoglycemia, particularly among infants treated with dextrose. Similarly, children who developed neurosensory impairment between 2 and 4.5 years had a steeper rise in interstitial glucose concentration after hypoglycemia. Another study (n = 139) found that the risk of neurosensory impairment at 4.5 years increased with both shorter (<2.2 hours) and longer (>4.3 hours) time to reach maximum interstitial glucose concentrations.[87] A retrospective study comparing 13 neonates with and 45 without brain injury on MRI or EEG found that blood glucose variability, hypoglycemia severity, and duration of hypoglycemia were all related to the brain injury outcome.[88] It remains to be determined whether glucose instability is on the causal pathway of neuronal injury or is simply a marker of perinatal stress, but available data supports a judicious approach to correction of hypoglycemia.

Prevention and Treatment of Hypoglycemia

Current guidelines (Fig. 10.2) differ in the thresholds for recommended treatment and the definition of which infants are at risk for hypoglycemia. In general, guidelines support preventive measures such as skin-to-skin, early feeding, and temperature regulation to prevent hypoglycemia. Screening is recommended between 12 and 48 hours with intermittent blood glucose measurement for infants considered to be at risk, and longer screening for infants at risk for prolonged hypoglycemia. Most guidelines suggest feeding and buccal dextrose gel as the treatment for moderate or brief hypoglycemia and IV dextrose for severe or prolonged hypoglycemia.

Recent research has supported the use of dextrose gel for the treatment of hypoglycemia. The Sugar Babies trial randomized 242 infants to 200 mg/kg dextrose or placebo gel, followed by a feed. Infants who received dextrose gel were less likely to require IV dextrose and less likely to be admitted to the NICU for hypoglycemia.[89] The mean increase in blood glucose with gel was 11.7 (95% CI 10.4–12.8) mg/dL.[90] In addition, dextrose gel treatment decreased formula feeding[89] and decreased cost of care.[91,92] There was no impact of this intervention on neurodevelopment at 2 years of age.[93] Prevention of hypoglycemia in at-risk infants with dextrose gel is an area of ongoing investigation. At-risk infants randomized to prophylactic dextrose gel versus placebo given at 1 hour of age (n = 2149) were less likely to develop hypoglycemia,[94] did not experience more recurrent or severe episodes of hypoglycemia, and did not have higher maximum glucose concentrations.[95] Dextrose gel prophylaxis is also likely to be cost saving to the health care system.[96] The impact of prophylactic dextrose gel on neurodevelopmental outcome is currently being investigated.

Feeding is also recommended to prevent and treat hypoglycemia. Two retrospective, observational studies have found that formula feeding with or without dextrose gel was associated with a higher rise in blood glucose than breastfeeding, although breastfeeding was associated with a decreased need for repeat treatment with dextrose gel.[89,97] One of these studies reported that donor milk feeding with dextrose gel was associated with a similar rise in blood glucose to that after formula feeding, but only in preterm infants.[97]

Most current hypoglycemia guidelines recommend intravenous dextrose administration for infants whose blood glucose concentrations remain low after feeding and dextrose gel administration.[98–100] The recommended dose is an initial bolus of 200 mg/kg followed by intravenous dextrose infusion at 5–8 mg/kg/min.[98,99] However, given emerging data around the role of blood glucose variability in neurodevelopment,

a more judicious, graded approach to correcting hypoglycemia with intravenous dextrose after failure of enteral measures may also be considered. For example, a graded approach to intravenous dextrose has been reported to significantly decrease blood glucose variability, as well as decrease the need for intensive care admission and shorten the length and cost of hypoglycemia-related in-hospital care for neonates.[101]

The Pediatric Endocrine Society guideline recommends that infants who are at high risk for persistent hypoglycemia (those with associated genetic syndromes, family history of hypoglycemia, or infants who require prolonged intravenous dextrose) should maintain blood glucose >60 mg/dL through a feed/fast cycle (approximately 6 hours without feeding) before discharge home.[99]

Unanswered Questions and Key Controversies

Although the data clearly show that severe, recurrent, and prolonged hypoglycemia leads to adverse neurodevelopmental sequelae, significant knowledge gaps remain in our understanding of and approach to neonatal hypoglycemia that future studies should aim to address:

a. *Contribution of perinatal risk factors*: Few studies have addressed the role of maternal dysmetabolism during pregnancy on child outcomes. To disentangle the role of the maternal in utero environment and neonatal hypoglycemia on outcomes, studies must conduct thorough maternal metabolic assessments and rigorously account for these in analyzing the association with child developmental outcomes. In addition, as rates of obesity and diabetes have rapidly increased in reproductive-age women, groups such as infants born to women with obesity (when screened for another established indication) have been found in some studies to be at increased risk for hypoglycemia.[102–105] Studies are urgently needed to understand if silent, unrecognized hypoglycemia contributes to the adverse neurodevelopmental outcomes observed in this population.

b. *Integrating host factors into susceptibility*: The role of infant host factors, such as ability to produce alternate fuels, cerebral vasoreactivity, cellular antioxidant defense production, and genetics have been minimally investigated and are difficult to integrate into generalizable guidelines. However, development of proximal neurophysiologic markers that reflect the integration of glycemia and host factors is urgently needed to ascertain functional glycemic thresholds.

   c. *Outcome-based definitions of hypoglycemia*: Current definitions of hypoglycemia are operational thresholds, but treatment to maintain glucose above these thresholds has not been shown to necessarily improve outcomes. Future studies should randomize infants to treatment at different thresholds and examine school-age outcomes in domains thought to be affected by hypoglycemia, with sample sizes adequately powered for subgroup analyses within specific risk categories.

   d. *Optimizing glycemic measurement methodologies*: Current methods of glucose measurement are limited in their accuracy and do not provide information on length of exposure. Glycemic measurement technologies that are targeted to the unique physiology and anatomy of a neonate, provide continuous or frequent monitoring, and provide information on alternative fuels are urgently needed to improve care provision.

   e. *Role of blood glucose variability in outcome*: Convincing preclinical and clinical data suggest that rapid changes in glycemia can adversely impact outcome. Studies should address optimal rates for correction of hypoglycemia and clinical guidelines should seek to reflect this data.

   f. *Optimizing hypoglycemia prevention and treatment*: Prevention of hypoglycemia is most effective at limiting potential harm, so studies designed to evaluate the effectiveness of preventive strategies, such as pumping breastmilk before delivery to feed to the at-risk newborn and prophylactic dextrose gel, on school-age outcomes are needed to inform practice and policy.

Conclusions

Neonatal hypoglycemia is one of the most common diseases of the newborn and yet, one of the most controversial. Compelling extant data establish associations between hypoglycemia and adverse neurodevelopmental outcomes, but rigorous research is urgently needed to inform causal inference, advance our practice, and improve the health of future generations. Moving the field forward requires a multi-disciplinary and collaborative approach, keeping the long-term health of the child at the forefront.

REFERENCES

1. Schneider H, Reiber W, Sager R, Malek A. Asymmetrical transport of glucose across the in vitro perfused human placenta. *Placenta*. 2003;24(1):27-33.
2. Holme AM, Roland MCP, Lorentzen B, Michelsen TM, Henriksen T. Placental glucose transfer: a human in vivo study. *PLoS One*. 2015;10(2):e0117084.
3. Bozzetti P, Ferrari MM, Marconi AM, et al. The relationship of maternal and fetal glucose concentrations in the human from midgestation until term. *Metabolism*. 1988;37(4):358-363.
4. Güemes M, Rahman SA, Hussain K. What is a normal blood glucose? *Arch Dis Child*. 2016;101(6):569-574.
5. Hillman NH, Kallapur SG, Jobe AH. Physiology of transition from intrauterine to extrauterine life. *Clin Perinatol*. 2012;39(4):769-783.
6. Stanescu DL, Stanley CA. Advances in understanding the mechanism of transitional neonatal hypoglycemia and implications for management. *Clin Perinatol*. January 21, 2022. Available at: doi.org/10.1016/j.clp.2021.11.007.
7. Srinivasan G, Pildes RS, Cattamanchi G, Voora S, Lilien LD. Plasma glucose values in normal neonates: a new look. *J Pediatr*. 1986;109(1):114-117.
8. Harris DL, Weston PJ, Gamble GD, Harding JE. Glucose profiles in healthy term infants in the first 5 days: The Glucose in Well Babies (GLOW) Study. *J Pediatr*. 2020;223:34-41.e4.
9. Harris DL, Weston PJ, Harding JE. Incidence of neonatal hypoglycemia in babies identified as at risk. *J Pediatr*. 2012;161(5):787-791.
10. March-of-Dimes-2021-Full-Report-Card.pdf. https://www.marchofdimes.org/sites/default/files/2022-11/March-of-Dimes-2022-Full-Report-Card.pdf
11. Burchell A, Gibb L, Waddell ID, Giles M, Hume R. The ontogeny of human hepatic microsomal glucose-6-phosphatase proteins. *Clin Chem*. 1990;36(9):1633-1637.
12. Hawdon JM, Ward Platt MP, Aynsley-Green A. Patterns of metabolic adaptation for preterm and term infants in the first neonatal week. *Arch Dis Child*. 1992;67(4 Spec):357-365.
13. Jackson L, Burchell A, McGeechan A, Hume R. An inadequate glycaemic response to glucagon is linked to insulin resistance in preterm infants? *Arch Dis Child Fetal Neonatal Ed*. 2003;88(1):F62-F66.
14. McCowan LME, Roberts CT, Dekker GA, et al. Risk factors for small-for-gestational-age infants by customised birthweight centiles: data from an international prospective cohort study. *BJOG*. 2010;117(13):1599-1607.
15. Limesand SW, Rozance PJ. Fetal adaptations in insulin secretion result from high catecholamines during placental insufficiency. *J Physiol*. 2017;595(15):5103-5113.

16. Ward Platt M, Deshpande S. Metabolic adaptation at birth. *Semin Fetal Neonatal Med*. 2005;10(4):341-350.

17. Centers for Disease Control and Prevention. *Diabetes During Pregnancy*. January 16, 2019. Available at: https://www.cdc.gov/reproductivehealth/maternalinfanthealth/diabetes-during-pregnancy.htm. Accessed February 22, 2022.

18. Kampmann U, Knorr S, Fuglsang J, Ovesen P. Determinants of maternal insulin resistance during pregnancy: an updated overview. *J Diabetes Res*. 2019;2019:5320156.

19. Etomi O, Banerjee A. The management of pre-existing (type 1 and type 2) diabetes mellitus in pregnancy. *Medicine*. 2018; 46(12):731-737.

20. Farrar D. Hyperglycemia in pregnancy: prevalence, impact, and management challenges. *Int J Womens Health*. 2016;8:519-527.

21. Pedersen J. *The Pregnant Diabetic and Her Newborn*. Problems and Management. Philadelphia, PA: William & Wilkins; 1967.

22. Schaefer-Graf UM, Rossi R, Bührer C, et al. Rate and risk factors of hypoglycemia in large-for-gestational-age newborn infants of nondiabetic mothers. *Am J Obstet Gynecol*. 2002;187(4): 913-917.

23. Kuklina EV, Ayala C, Callaghan WM. Hypertensive disorders and severe obstetric morbidity in the United States. *Obstet Gynecol*. 2009;113(6):1299-1306.

24. Bateman BT, Patorno E, Desai RJ, et al. Late pregnancy β blocker exposure and risks of neonatal hypoglycemia and bradycardia. *Pediatrics*. 2016;138(3). Available at: /doi.org/10.1542/peds.2016-0731.

25. Sunehag AL, Haymond MW. Glucose extremes in newborn infants. *Clin Perinatol*. 2002;29(2):245-260.

26. Bier DM, Leake RD, Haymond MW, et al. Measurement of "true" glucose production rates in infancy and childhood with 6,6-dideuteroglucose. *Diabetes*. 1977;26(11):1016-1023.

27. Powers WJ, Rosenbaum JL, Dence CS, Markham J, Videen TO. Cerebral glucose transport and metabolism in preterm human infants. *J Cereb Blood Flow Metab*. 1998;18(6):632-638.

28. Yager JY. Hypoglycemic injury to the immature brain. *Clin Perinatol*. 2002;29(4):651-674, vi.

29. De Vivo DC, Trifiletti RR, Jacobson RI, Ronen GM, Behmand RA, Harik SI. Defective glucose transport across the blood-brain barrier as a cause of persistent hypoglycorrhachia, seizures, and developmental delay. *N Engl J Med*. 1991;325(10): 703-709.

30. Fishman RA. The glucose-transporter protein and glucopenic brain injury. *N Engl J Med*. 1991;325(10):731-732.

31. Vannucci SJ. Developmental expression of GLUT1 and GLUT3 glucose transporters in rat brain. *J Neurochem*. 1994;62(1): 240-246.

32. Simpson IA, Carruthers A, Vannucci SJ. Supply and demand in cerebral energy metabolism: the role of nutrient transporters. *J Cereb Blood Flow Metab*. 2007;27(11):1766-1791.

33. Chugani HT, Phelps ME. Maturational changes in cerebral function in infants determined by 18FDG positron emission tomography. *Science*. 1986;231(4740):840-843.

34. Nehlig A, Pereira de Vasconcelos A. Glucose and ketone body utilization by the brain of neonatal rats. *Prog Neurobiol*. 1993;40(2):163-221.

35. Hernández MJ, Vannucci RC, Salcedo A, Brennan RW. Cerebral blood flow and metabolism during hypoglycemia in newborn dogs. *J Neurochem*. 1980;35(3):622-628.

36. Harris DL, Weston PJ, Harding JE. Lactate, rather than ketones, may provide alternative cerebral fuel in hypoglycaemic newborns. *Arch Dis Child Fetal Neonatal Ed*. 2015;100(2):F161-F164.

37. Harris DL, Weston PJ, Harding JE. Alternative cerebral fuels in the first five days in healthy term infants: The Glucose in Well Babies (GLOW) Study. *J Pediatr*. 2021;231:81-86.e2.

38. Pryds O, Christensen NJ, Friis-Hansen B. Increased cerebral blood flow and plasma epinephrine in hypoglycemic, preterm neonates. *Pediatrics*. 1990;85(2):172-176.

39. Matterberger C, Baik-Schneditz N, Schwaberger B, et al. Blood glucose and cerebral tissue oxygenation immediately after birth—an observational study. *J Pediatr*. 2018;200:19-23.

40. Anwar M, Vannucci RC. Autoradiographic determination of regional cerebral blood flow during hypoglycemia in newborn dogs. *Pediatr Res*. 1988;24(1):41-45.

41. Vanderhaegen J, Vanhaesebrouck S, Vanhole C, Casaer P, Naulaers G. The effect of glycaemia on the cerebral oxygenation in very low birthweight infants as measured by near-infrared spectroscopy. *Adv Exp Med Biol*. 2010;662:461-466.

42. Szakmar E, Smith J, Yang E, Volpe JJ, Inder T, El-Dib M. Association between cerebral oxygen saturation and brain injury in neonates receiving therapeutic hypothermia for neonatal encephalopathy. *J Perinatol*. 2021;41(2):269-277.

43. Ancora G, Maranella E, Grandi S, et al. Early predictors of short term neurodevelopmental outcome in asphyxiated cooled infants. A combined brain amplitude integrated electroencephalography and near infrared spectroscopy study. *Brain Dev*. 2013; 35(1):26-31.

44. Lemmers PMA, Zwanenburg RJ, Benders MJNL, et al. Cerebral oxygenation and brain activity after perinatal asphyxia: does hypothermia change their prognostic value? *Pediatr Res*. 2013; 74(2):180-185.

45. Vannucci RC, Vannucci SJ. Cerebral carbohydrate metabolism during hypoglycemia and anoxia in newborn rats. *Ann Neurol*. 1978;4(1):73-79.

46. Wieloch T. Hypoglycemia-induced neuronal damage prevented by an N-methyl-D-aspartate antagonist. *Science*. 1985;230(4726): 681-683.

47. Silverstein FS, Simpson J, Gordon KE. Hypoglycemia alters striatal amino acid efflux in perinatal rats: an in vivo microdialysis study. *Ann Neurol*. 1990;28(4):516-521.

48. Aral YZ, Gücüyener K, Atalay Y, et al. Role of excitatory amino-acids in neonatal hypoglycemia. *Acta Paediatr Jpn*. 1998;40(4): 303-306.

49. Alves PM, Fonseca LL, Peixoto CC, Almeida AC, Carrondo MJ, Santos H. NMR studies on energy metabolism of immobilized primary neurons and astrocytes during hypoxia, ischemia and hypoglycemia. *NMR Biomed*. 2000;13(8):438-448.

50. Hertz L, Yager JY, Juurlink BH. Astrocyte survival in the absence of exogenous substrate: comparison of immature and mature cells. *Int J Dev Neurosci*. 1995;13(6):523-527.

51. Brierly JB, Brown AW, Meldrum BS. The neuropathology of insulin induced hypoglycemia in primate. In: Meldrum JB, Brierley BS, eds. *Brain Hypoxia*. Philadelphia, PA: JB Lippincott; 1971.

52. Auer RN, Kalimo H, Olsson Y, Siesjö BK. The temporal evolution of hypoglycemic brain damage. I. Light-and electron-microscopic findings in the rat cerebral cortex. *Acta Neuropathol*. 1985;67(1-2):13-24.

53. Auer RN, Kalimo H, Olsson Y, Siesjö BK. The temporal evolution of hypoglycemic brain damage. II. Light- and electron-microscopic findings in the hippocampal gyrus and subiculum of the rat. *Acta Neuropathol*. 1985;67(1-2):25-36.

54. Kalimo H, Auer RN, Siesjö BK. The temporal evolution of hypoglycemic brain damage. III. Light and electron microscopic findings in the rat caudoputamen. *Acta Neuropathol*. 1985;67(1-2):37-50.

55. Volpe JJ. *Neurology of the Newborn.* 4th ed. Philadelphia, PA: WB Saunders; 2001.

56. Montassir H, Maegaki Y, Ogura K, et al. Associated factors in neonatal hypoglycemic brain injury. *Brain Dev.* 2009;31(9): 649-656.

57. Montassir H, Maegaki Y, Ohno K, Ogura K. Long term prognosis of symptomatic occipital lobe epilepsy secondary to neonatal hypoglycemia. *Epilepsy Res.* 2010;88(2-3):93-99.

58. Tam EWY, Widjaja E, Blaser SI, Macgregor DL, Satodia P, Moore AM. Occipital lobe injury and cortical visual outcomes after neonatal hypoglycemia. *Pediatrics.* 2008;122(3):507-512.

59. Musson RE, Batty R, Mordekar SR, Wilkinson ID, Griffiths PD, Connolly DJA. Diffusion-weighted imaging and magnetic resonance spectroscopy findings in a case of neonatal hypoglycaemia. *Dev Med Child Neurol.* 2009;51(8):653-654.

60. Gataullina S, De Lonlay P, Dellatolas G, et al. Topography of brain damage in metabolic hypoglycaemia is determined by age at which hypoglycaemia occurred. *Dev Med Child Neurol.* 2013;55(2):162-166.

61. Nivins S, Kennedy E, Thompson B, et al. Associations between neonatal hypoglycaemia and brain volumes, cortical thickness and white matter microstructure in mid-childhood: an MRI study. *Neuroimage Clin.* 2022;33:102943.

62. Koh TH, Aynsley-Green A, Tarbit M, Eyre JA. Neural dysfunction during hypoglycaemia. *Arch Dis Child.* 1988;63(11): 1353-1358.

63. Harris DL, Weston PJ, Williams CE, et al. Cot-side electroencephalography monitoring is not clinically useful in the detection of mild neonatal hypoglycaemia. *J Pediatr.* 2011;159(5):755-760.e1.

64. Arhan E, Öztürk Z, Serdaroğlu A, Aydın K, Hirfanoğlu T, Akbaş Y. Neonatal hypoglycemia: a wide range of electroclinical manifestations and seizure outcomes. *Eur J Paediatr Neurol.* 2017;21(5):738-744.

65. Rozance PJ, Hay WW. Hypoglycemia in newborn infants: features associated with adverse outcomes. *Biol Neonate.* 2006; 90(2):74-86.

66. FDA Executive Summary: Measuring Blood Glucose Using Capillary Blood with Blood Glucose Meters in all Hospital Patients. Presented at: Clinical Chemistry and Clinical Toxicology Devices Panel; March 30, 2018. Available at: www.fda.gov/media/112158/download.

67. Beardsall K. Measurement of glucose levels in the newborn. *Early Hum Dev.* 2010;86(5):263-267.

68. Glasgow MJ, Harding JE, Edlin R, for the CHYLD Study Team. Cost analysis of cot-side screening methods for neonatal hypoglycaemia. *Neonatology.* 2018;114(2):155-162.

69. Galderisi A, Facchinetti A, Steil GM, et al. Continuous glucose monitoring in very preterm infants: a randomized controlled trial. *Pediatrics.* 2017;140(4). Available at: doi.org/10.1542/peds.2017-1162.

70. Harris DL, Battin MR, Weston PJ, Harding JE. Continuous glucose monitoring in newborn babies at risk of hypoglycemia. *J Pediatr.* 2010;157(2):198-202.e1. Available at: http://doi.org/10.1016/j.jpeds.2010.02.003.

71. van Kempen AAMW, Eskes PF, Nuytemans DHGM, et al. Lower versus traditional treatment threshold for neonatal hypoglycemia. *N Engl J Med.* 2020;382(6):534-544.

72. Hawdon JM. Definition of neonatal hypoglycaemia: time for a rethink? *Arch Dis Child Fetal Neonatal Ed.* 2013;98(5): F382-F383.

73. Lucas A, Morley R, Cole TJ. Adverse neurodevelopmental outcome of moderate neonatal hypoglycaemia. *BMJ.* 1988;297(6659): 1304-1308.

74. Duvanel CB, Fawer CL, Cotting J, Hohlfeld P, Matthieu JM. Long-term effects of neonatal hypoglycemia on brain growth and psychomotor development in small-for-gestational-age preterm infants. *J Pediatr.* 1999;134(4):492-498.

75. Stenninger E, Flink R, Eriksson B, Sahlèn C. Long-term neurological dysfunction and neonatal hypoglycaemia after diabetic pregnancy. *Arch Dis Child Fetal Neonatal Ed.* 1998;79(3): F174-F179.

76. Haworth JC, McRae KN, Dilling LA. Prognosis of infants of diabetic mothers in relation to neonatal hypoglycaemia. *Dev Med Child Neurol.* 1976;18(4):471-479.

77. Brand PLP, Molenaar NLD, Kaaijk C, Wierenga WS. Neurodevelopmental outcome of hypoglycaemia in healthy, large for gestational age, term newborns. *Arch Dis Child.* 2005;90(1):78-81.

78. Shah R, Harding J, Brown J, McKinlay C. Neonatal glycaemia and neurodevelopmental outcomes: a systematic review and meta-analysis. *Neonatology.* 2019;115(2):116-126.

79. McKinlay CJD, Alsweiler JM, Ansell JM, et al. Neonatal glycemia and neurodevelopmental outcomes at 2 years. *N Engl J Med.* 2015;373(16):1507-1518.

80. McKinlay CJD, Alsweiler JM, Anstice NS, et al. Association of neonatal glycemia with neurodevelopmental outcomes at 4.5 years. *JAMA Pediatr.* 2017;171(10):972-983.

81. Pildes RS, Cornblath M, Warren I, et al. A prospective controlled study of neonatal hypoglycemia. *Pediatrics.* 1974;54(1): 5-14.

82. Koivisto M, Blanco-Sequeiros M, Krause U. Neonatal symptomatic and asymptomatic hypoglycaemia: a follow-up study of 151 children. *Dev Med Child Neurol.* 1972;14(5):603-614.

83. Kerstjens JM, Bocca-Tjeertes IF, de Winter AF, Reijneveld SA, Bos AF. Neonatal morbidities and developmental delay in moderately preterm-born children. *Pediatrics.* 2012;130(2): e265-e272.

84. Griffiths AD, Bryant GM. Assessment of effects of neonatal hypoglycaemia. A study of 41 cases with matched controls. *Arch Dis Child.* 1971;46(250):819-827.

85. Kaiser JR, Bai S, Gibson N, et al. Association between transient newborn hypoglycemia and fourth-grade achievement test proficiency: a population-based study. *JAMA Pediatr.* 2015;169(10): 913-921.

86. Ennis K, Dotterman H, Stein A, Rao R. Hyperglycemia accentuates and ketonemia attenuates hypoglycemia-induced neuronal injury in the developing rat brain. *Pediatr Res.* 2015;77(1-1): 84-90.

87. Burakevych N, McKinlay CJD, Harris DL, Alsweiler JM, Harding JE. Factors influencing glycaemic stability after neonatal hypoglycaemia and relationship to neurodevelopmental outcome. *Sci Rep.* 2019;9(1):8132.

88. Lv Y, Zhu LL, Shu GH. Relationship between blood glucose fluctuation and brain damage in the hypoglycemia neonates. *Am J Perinatol.* 2018;35(10):946-950.

89. Harris DL, Weston PJ, Signal M, Chase JG, Harding JE. Dextrose gel for neonatal hypoglycaemia (the Sugar Babies Study): a randomised, double-blind, placebo-controlled trial. *Lancet.* 2013;382(9910):2077-2083.

90. Harris DL, Gamble GD, Weston PJ, Harding JE. What happens to blood glucose concentrations after oral treatment for neonatal hypoglycemia? *J Pediatr.* 2017;190:136-141.

91. Dextrose gel cost effective in neonates at risk of hypoglycaemia. *Pharmacoeconomics Outcomes News.* 2020;858(1):12. Available at: https://doi.org/10.1007/s40274-020-6985-0

92. Glasgow MJ, Harding JE, Edlin R, Children with Hypoglycemia and Their Later Development (CHYLD) Study Team. Cost

analysis of treating neonatal hypoglycemia with dextrose gel. *J Pediatr*. 2018;198:151-155.e1.

93. Harris DL, Alsweiler JM, Ansell JM, et al. Outcome at 2 years after dextrose gel treatment for neonatal hypoglycemia: follow-up of a randomized trial. *J Pediatr*. 2016;170:54-59.e1-e2.

94. Harding JE, Hegarty JE, Crowther CA, et al. Evaluation of oral dextrose gel for prevention of neonatal hypoglycemia (hPOD): a multicenter, double-blind randomized controlled trial. *PLoS Med*. 2021;18(1):e1003411.

95. Hegarty JE, Alsweiler JM, Gamble GG, Crowther CA, Harding JE. Effect of prophylactic dextrose gel on continuous measures of neonatal glycemia: secondary analysis of the pre-hPOD trial. *J Pediatr*. 2021;235:107-115.e4.

96. Glasgow MJ, Edlin R, Harding JE. Cost-utility analysis of prophylactic dextrose gel vs standard care for neonatal hypoglycemia in at-risk infants. *J Pediatr*. 2020;226:80-86.e1.

97. Sen S, Andrews C, Anderson E, Turner D, Monthé-Drèze C, Wachman EM. Type of feeding provided with dextrose gel impacts hypoglycemia outcomes: comparing donor milk, formula, and breastfeeding. *J Perinatol*. 2020;40(11):1705-1711.

98. Committee on Fetus and Newborn. postnatal glucose homeostasis in late-preterm and term infants. *Pediatrics*. 2011;127(3):575-579.

99. Thornton PS, Stanley CA, De Leon DD, et al. Recommendations from the pediatric endocrine society for evaluation and management of persistent hypoglycemia in neonates, infants, and children. *J Pediatr*. 2015;167(2):238-245.

100. *British Association of Perinatal Medicine. Identification and Management of Neonatal Hypoglycaemia in the Full Term Infant: Framework for Practice*. April 2017. Available at: https://hubble-live-assets.s3.amazonaws.com/bapm/file_asset/file/37/Identification_and_Management_of_Neonatal_Hypoglycaemia_in_the__full_term_infant_-_A_Framework_for_Practice_revised_Oct_2017.pdf.

101. Sen S, Cherkerzian S, Turner D, Monthé-Drèze C, Abdulhayoglu E, Zupancic JAF. A graded approach to intravenous dextrose for neonatal hypoglycemia decreases blood glucose variability, time in the neonatal intensive care unit, and cost of stay. *J Pediatr*. 2021;231:74-80. doi:10.1016/j.jpeds.2020.12.025. Available at: https://pubmed.ncbi.nlm.nih.gov/33338495/.

102. Turner D, Monthé-Drèze C, Cherkerzian S, Gregory K, Sen S. Maternal obesity and cesarean section delivery: additional risk factors for neonatal hypoglycemia? *J Perinatol*. 2019;39(8):1057-1064.

103. Blomberg M. Maternal obesity, mode of delivery, and neonatal outcome. *Obstet Gynecol*. 2013;122(1):50-55. Available at: doi.org/10.1097/aog.0b013e318295657f.

104. Neumann K, Indorf I, Härtel C, Cirkel C, Rody A, Beyer D. C-section prevalence among obese mothers and neonatal hypoglycemia: a cohort analysis of the Department of Gynecology and Obstetrics of the University of Lübeck. *Geburtshilfe Frauenheilkd*. 2017;77(5):487-494.

105. Suk D, Kwak T, Khawar N, et al. Increasing maternal body mass index during pregnancy increases neonatal intensive care unit admission in near and full-term infants. *J Matern Fetal Neonatal Med*. 2016;29(20):3249-3253.

Chapter 11

Neonatal Meningitis: Current Treatment Options—An Update

David A. Kaufman, Santina A. Zanelli and Pablo J. Sánchez

Chapter Outline

Summary

- As many as 40% of infants with meningitis do not have a positive blood culture at the time of their diagnosis.
- Infants with uncomplicated meningitis due to group B streptococcus should receive a 14-day course of antimicrobial therapy. A minimum of a 4-week treatment course is recommended for infants with complicated courses (e.g., abscess).
- The treatment of gram-negative meningitis initially includes the addition of a third- or fourth-generation cephalosporin such as cefotaxime or cefepime for early-onset meningitis and cefepime for late-onset meningitis. Depending on

susceptibilities, a carbapenem antibiotic such as meropenem can be used if resistance to third- and fourth-generation cephalosporins is present.

- For meningitis due to gram-negative bacilli, the duration of antimicrobial therapy is a minimum of 21 days.
- Among infants with meningitis, approximately 10% of affected infants die, and neurologic sequelae are found in up to 50% of survivors.
- Polymerase chain reaction for the detection of bacterial, viral and fungal DNA/RNA ultimately may improve detection of CSF pathogens.

BOX 11.1 CAUSATIVE AGENTS OF NEONATAL MENINGITIS

1. **Bacteria:**
   Aerobic:
   Gram-positive: group B streptococcus, group A strepto-coccus, *Enterococcus* sp., *Streptococcus bovis,* viridans streptococci, *Staphylococcus aureus,* coagu-lase-negative staphylococci, *Listeria monocytogenes, Streptococcus pneumoniae*
   Gram-negative: *Escherichia coli, Klebsiella* spp., *Entero-bacter* spp., *Serratia* spp., *Proteus* spp., *Citrobacter* spp., *Salmonella* spp., *Pseudomonas aeruginosa, Haemophilus influenzae, Neisseria gonorrhoeae, Neisseria meningitidis*
   Anaerobic:
   Gram-positive: *Clostridium* spp., *Peptostreptococcus* spp.

   Gram-negative: *Bacteroides fragilis*
   Genital mycoplasmas: *Ureaplasma* spp., *Mycoplasma hominis*
   Spirochetes: *Treponema pallidum, Borrelia burgdorferi*
   Mycobacteria: *Mycobacteria tuberculosis*
2. **Viruses:** Herpes simplex virus, cytomegalovirus, enteroviruses, human immunodeficiency virus, varicella-zoster virus, rubella virus, human parvovirus B19, lymphocytic choriomeningitis virus, Zika virus
3. **Fungi:** *Candida* spp., *Malassezia* spp., *Aspergillus* spp., *Trichosporon beigelis, Cryptococcus, Coccidiodes immitis*
4. **Protozoa:** *Toxoplasma gondii*

Bacterial meningitis occurs in approximately 0.4 neonates per 1000 live births. It is defined as inflammation of the meninges that is manifested by an elevated number of white blood cells in the cerebrospinal fluid (CSF). It often is associated with elevated protein content and a low glucose concentration in CSF. Meningitis generally results as a consequence of hematogenous dissemination of bacteria via the choroid plexus and into the central nervous system (CNS) during a sepsis episode. Invasion of the meninges occurs in about 1% to 2% of infants evaluated for sepsis and is increased to about 10% with bacteremia. Rarely, meningitis develops secondary to extension from infected skin through the soft tissues and skull as may occur with an infected cephalohematoma or direct spread from skin surfaces, as in infants with myelomeningoceles or other congenital malformations of the neural tube. In addition, ventriculoperitoneal shunts or ventricular reservoirs may be the primary site of infection. A potential but infrequent complication of meningitis is brain abscess that results from hematogenous spread of bacteria into tissue that has incurred anoxic injury or severe vasculitis with hemorrhage or infarction.

Virtually all organisms that cause neonatal infection or sepsis can result in CNS disease with severe consequences for the developing brain.[1-3] A list of the more commonly reported pathogens is provided in Box 11.1. It is imperative that a correct and timely diagnosis with a specific organism be made because treatment decisions vary by causative agent.

The case of a preterm infant is presented and discussed to highlight the multifaceted nature of this disease. The objective of this chapter is to review the current management of neonatal bacterial meningitis, in the hope of ameliorating the destructive nature of many of these organisms and ultimately improving the outcome of these high-risk infants.

Case History

A preterm infant weighing 1004 g was born at 28 weeks' gestation to a 24-year-old mother by cesarean section. The pregnancy was complicated by premature rupture of membranes 2 weeks before delivery, and the mother developed intrapartum fever and was diagnosed with an intraamniotic infection. She received antenatal steroids and antimicrobial therapy consisting of ampicillin and gentamicin. At delivery, the infant was floppy with poor respiratory effort, and he required intubation and admission to the neonatal intensive care unit (NICU). Apgar scores were 3 at 1 minute and 7 at 5 minutes. The infant's vital signs were normal, and antimicrobial therapy with ampicillin and gentamicin was initiated after a blood culture was obtained. Respiratory distress syndrome was diagnosed and the infant received exogenous surfactant therapy.

Question 1: What Risk Factors Predispose This Infant to Have Early-Onset Bacterial Meningitis?

Because meningitis is a complication of bacteremia, the risk factors are similar to those that contribute to neonatal sepsis—namely prematurity, prolonged rupture of fetal membranes ($\geq$18 hours), preterm premature rupture of membranes, maternal urinary tract infection, and maternal intrapartum fever or intraamniotic infection (chorioamnionitis).[4–6] Immune dysfunction as well as lack of transplacentally acquired maternal immunoglobulin G (IgG) antibodies in premature infants also may increase risk of sepsis and CNS infection. Recently, lower neonatal 25-hydroxyvitamin D levels have been associated with early-onset sepsis in term infants.[7]

Likewise, clinical signs suggestive of bacterial meningitis are similar to those of neonatal sepsis. In the full-term infant, fever, lethargy, hypotonia, irritability, apnea, poor feeding, high-pitched cry, emesis, seizures, and bulging fontanelle are prominent clinical signs, whereas in preterm infants, respiratory decompensation consisting of an increased number of apneic episodes predominates. Neonates with meningitis are never "asymptomatic."

The widespread and routine use of intrapartum antibiotic prophylaxis (IAP) since 1996 has significantly reduced the rate of early-onset group B streptococcal (GBS) infection by more than 70%.[8] While there has not been a reciprocal increase in early-onset bacterial infections among full-term infants caused by gram-negative organisms in the United States, there has been a shift toward more gram-negative infections in preterm infants. Several studies over the past decades from the NICUs comprising the National Institute of Child Health and Human Development (NICHD) Neonatal Research Network centers have helped inform our clinical practice by examining rates, pathogens and resistance patterns. IAP resulted in a significant decrease in early-onset GBS infection. The rate of infections caused by Escherichia coli (E. coli) initially increased significantly in infants <1500 g from 3 (1991–1993) to 7 (1998–2000) cases per 1000 live birth, then stabilized at 5.07 per 1000 live births (2006–2009) and most recently (2015–2017) increased again to 8.68 per 1000 live births.[9–11] The overall rate of early-onset sepsis in the most recent time period (2015–2017), defined as a positive blood or CSF bacterial culture at less than 72 hours of age, was 1.16 infections per 1000 live births with rates inversely related to birth weight (BW; 401–1500 g BW, 15.05/1000; 1501–2500 g BW, 1.78/1000; >2500 g BW, 0.63/1000).[11] Among cases of

early-onset meningitis, around 50% are due to E. coli and 50% are due to GBS. In a study of 721 infants from 69 centers with early-onset or late-onset E. coli blood, urine or CSF infection, 66.7% of infections had resistant or intermediate susceptibility to ampicillin, 16.6% to aminoglycosides, and 4.9% to extended-spectrum β-lactamase phenotype antibiotics.[12] All were susceptible to carbapenems. Nonsusceptibility to both ampicillin and gentamicin was present in 10.1% (22 of 218) early-onset infections.

Question 2: Do Infants With Meningitis Have Positive Blood Cultures?

As many as 40% of infants with meningitis who have a gestational age of 34 weeks or more do not have a positive blood culture at the time of their diagnosis. Similarly, among VLBW infants, almost one-half of cases of meningitis occur with sterile blood cultures. Therefore it is imperative that a lumbar puncture be performed if sepsis or meningitis are highly suspected. Evaluation of CSF indices and Gram stain not only will establish a diagnosis but also will help guide initial therapy. Normal CSF indices are provided in Table 11.1.[13,14]

Meningitis with early-onset sepsis evaluations in preterm infants admitted to the NICU with respiratory distress syndrome is very uncommon.[11] Therefore, performance of a lumbar puncture in these infants in whom sepsis is not suspected is not mandatory. Similar data are available for full-term infants. However, if the blood culture yields a pathogenic organism with either early or late-onset sepsis, then evaluation of CSF should be done. There is variation in this practice when bacteremia is due to coagulase-negative staphylococcus (CoNS).[15] A lumbar puncture is contraindicated when there is cardiorespiratory instability. Delay in performing a lumbar puncture only delays a potential diagnosis of meningitis and can lead to prolonged and possibly inappropriate antibiotic use.[15,16] If there is delay in performing a lumbar puncture, meningitis/encephalitis multiplex panel polymerase chain reaction (PCR) assays may help to identify CSF pathogens after antimicrobial initiation.[17]

While awaiting culture results, unless there are CSF abnormalities suggestive of meningitis, for early-onset sepsis evaluations, ampicillin in combination with an aminoglycoside is the preferred choice. Similarly, for

TABLE 11.1 Cerebrospinal Fluid Indices in Neonates[13,14]

PRETERM NEONATE

Birth Weight (g)	Age (days)	No. of Samples	Red Blood Cells (mm³) Mean ± SD (range)	White Blood Cells (mm³) Mean ± SD (range)	Polymorphonuclear Leukocytes (%) Mean ± SD (range)	Glucose (mg/dL) Mean ± SD (range)	Protein (mg/dL) Mean ± SD (range)
≤1000	0–7	6	335 ± 709 (0–1780)	3 ± 3 (1–8)	11 ± 20 (0–50)	70 ± 17 (41–89)	162 ± 37 (115–222)
	8–28	17	1465 ± 4062 (0–19,050)	4 ± 4 (0–14)	8 ± 17 (0–66)	68 ± 48 (41–89)	159 ± 77 (95–370)
	29–84	15	808 ± 1843 (0–6850)	4 ± 3 (0–11)	2 ± 9 (0–36)	49 ± 22 (41–89)	137 ± 61 (76–260)
1001–1500	0–7	8	407 ± 853 (0–2450)	4 ± 4 (1–10)	4 ± 10 (0–28)	74 ± 19 (41–89)	136 ± 35 (85–176)
	8–28	14	1101 ± 2643 (0–9750)	7 ± 11 (0–44)	10 ± 19 (0–60)	59 ± 23 (41–89)	137 ± 46 (54–227)
	29–84	11	661 ± 1198 (0–3800)	8 ± 8 (0–23)	11 ± 19 (0–48)	47 ± 13 (41–89)	122 ± 47 (45–187)

FULL-TERM NEONATE

Age (days)	No. of Patients	Red Blood Cells (mm³)	White Blood Cells (mm³) Mean ± SD (range)	Polymorphonuclear Leukocytes Mean ± SD (range)	Glucose (mg/dL) Mean ± SD	Protein (mg/dL) Mean ± SD
0–30	108	≤1000/mm³	7.3 ± 13.9 (0–130) median 4	0.8 ± 6.2 (0–65) median 0	51.2 ± 12.9 (62% of serum glucose)	64.2 ± 24.2

late-onset sepsis evaluations, a penicillinase-resistant, semisynthetic penicillin such as oxacillin or nafcillin in combination with an aminoglycoside is the preferred choice.

Continuation of Case History

The infant was extubated and continuous positive airway pressure therapy was started on the first day of age. Trophic feedings were initiated on the second day of age, and a percutaneous intravenous central venous catheter was placed for parenteral nutrition. She achieved full enteral feedings on the 20th day. Over the subsequent 2 days, she developed lethargy, hyperglycemia, and increased episodes of apnea that resulted in reinitiation of mechanical ventilation. Blood cultures were obtained, and antimicrobial therapy with nafcillin and gentamicin was initiated.

Question 3: What Is the Optimal Evaluation for Possible Late-Onset Sepsis in Preterm Infants in the NICU-When Should a Lumbar Puncture Be Included?

Infants suspected of having late-onset sepsis in the NICU should have a complete evaluation that consists of a complete blood cell (CBC) count, blood and urine cultures. In critically ill hospitalized neonates, it is very difficult to distinguish infection from noninfectious clinical deteriorations; however, there should be a low threshold for also performing a lumbar puncture. Unfortunately, there are no laboratory or clinical findings that have a high sensitivity for the diagnosis of neonatal sepsis or meningitis.[18,19] Such laboratory tools as C-reactive protein; interleukin (IL)-6, IL-8, IL-10; and procalcitonin have suboptimal sensitivity and specificity to replace a blood or CSF culture as the gold standard. These biomarkers do not aid in the decision to initiate an evaluation for infection and whether or not to start antibiotics. In addition, their use has been associated with increased antibiotics and hospital days with no benefit of reduced morbidity or mortality.[20–25] These noninfectious biomarkers are really host markers and may better trend host response to complex infections but are not diagnostic.[25,26] PCR for detection of bacterial, viral and fungal DNA/RNA ultimately may lead to

an earlier diagnosis as well as detect CSF pathogens during a short window of about 24 hours after antibiotics and antivirals have been started.[17]

It is important to obtain a CBC count with platelets for reasons other than diagnosis. Neonatal sepsis may result in neutropenia, which is associated with a high mortality rate. The finding of a persistent absolute neutrophil count of 500/mm^3 or less after 48 hours of antimicrobial treatment may prompt consideration of adjuvant therapies such as recombinant granulocyte or granulocyte-macrophage colony-stimulating factors by some experts.[27,28] Routine use of IVIG infusions for suspected sepsis is not recommended, as studies have not demonstrated benefit in early or late morbidity or mortality but there may be special situations where it should be considered such as patient with a primary or secondary hypogammaglobinemia (e.g., chylothorax or sepsis with capillary leak syndrome).

Another reason for performance of a CBC is many infections may be complicated by thrombocytopenia and/or disseminated intravascular coagulation. Thrombocytopenia is common with many neonatal infections and is most severe with gram-negative and fungal infections.[29] The degree of thrombocytopenia should be factored into timing of safely performing the lumbar puncture. While controversial, the benefit of platelet transfusion prior to performing a lumbar puncture should be discussed. If severe thrombocytopenia is present and a lumbar puncture is indicated, administering a platelet infusion prior to procedure if counts <100,000/microliter in preterm infants and <50,000 in term infants are reasonable transfusion thresholds.[30] Significant thrombocytopenia could increase the risk of a local hematoma which can cause medullary compression and in rare cases lead to paralysis.[29]

A lumbar puncture should generally be performed in infants evaluated for possible late-onset sepsis for reasons stated in answer to Question 2. Risk factors for meningitis in preterm infants include low gestational age and prior bloodstream infection.[15] In VLBW infants, the average age of late-onset meningitis is 26 days (median 19 days; range 4–102 days).[15] Therapeutic decisions with regard to antibiotic choices can be made only if one knows whether the CNS is involved.

Question 4: What Factors Can Make a Lumbar Puncture Be Most Successful?

Early stylet removal and local anesthetic improve success of obtaining CSF and having a nontraumatic tap. Studies have found this more than doubles the success rate of both obtaining CSF and having a nontraumatic lumbar puncture.[31] Once just a few millimeters through the skin (epidermis and dermis), the stylet can be safely removed. The stylet is needed during skin penetration to reduce introduction of epidermoid cells in the CSF that can subsequently lead to an intraspinal epidermoid tumor. The needle is then slowly advanced until CSF is obtained. After CSF is obtained, replace stylet into the needle and remove it from the patient.

Question 5: What Is the Empirical Antimicrobial Choice for Possible Late-Onset Sepsis in the NICU?

In general, antimicrobial therapy for neonatal sepsis is dependent on the agents commonly seen in a particular nursery and their susceptibility pattern. For early-onset sepsis, ampicillin combined with an aminoglycoside, usually gentamicin, has been the empiric therapy of choice since group B *Streptococcus*, other streptococcal species, *Listeria monocytogenes*, and gram-negative bacilli predominate.[11]

For late-onset sepsis, a penicillinase-resistant, semisynthetic penicillin such as oxacillin or nafcillin in combination with an aminoglycoside is the preferred choice. For CNS infections, nafcillin is preferred because of improved penetration. Empiric vancomycin should not be used unless there is a prior history of colonization with methicillin-resistant *Staphylococcus aureus* (MRSA) or the infant has not been screened for MRSA and >10% of the infants in the NICU are colonized with MRSA to decrease the risk for emergence of vancomycin-resistant organisms.[32,33] Empiric vancomycin is not needed when there is a suspicion of a CoNS infection because outcomes are similar when initially treated with nafcillin and then changed to vancomycin when culture results are known.

The use of a penicillinase-resistant penicillin antibiotic such as nafcillin to treat a possible staphylococcal infection in this infant is based on the goal of reducing vancomycin use in NICUs. Clinical experience and intervention trials suggest that such a practice is safe.[32,33] Bloodstream infections caused by CoNS are rarely fulminant or fatal, and they are not associated with an increased case-fatality rate over that seen among uninfected VLBW infants.[34,35] The clinical outcome of CoNS bacteremia is similar whether the initial antibiotic therapy is vancomycin or another agent that does not reliably treat CoNS infections. In addition, only one of five evaluations for sepsis yields a causative organism. The observation that more than 80% of blood cultures that yield CoNS are positive by 24 hours of incubation makes it possible for the clinician to change antibiotic therapy in a timely fashion if needed. An additional concern of vancomycin therapy has been the association of prior vancomycin use with subsequent development of gram-negative bacteremia among hospitalized pediatric patients.[36]

Aminoglycosides have been the time-honored choice for empiric treatment of infections caused by gram-negative bacilli. They effectively cover the most common and severe gram-negative organisms including pseudomonas, *E. coli*, *Klebsiella*, *Serratia*, *Citrobacter*, and *Enterobacter* as well as other gram-negative pathogens. With extended-interval dosing, higher peak concentrations are achieved which increase concentration-dependent microbial killing in addition to a post antibiotic effect. Once-daily or extended dosing of gentamicin is based on sound pharmacodynamic and pharmacokinetic considerations and should be used for both full-term and preterm infants to achieve optimal peak concentrations for gram-negative pathogens and is associated with reduced toxicity and cost.[37] Extended-interval dosing maximizes the bactericidal activity of the aminoglycoside while minimizing its potential toxicity.

Aminoglycosides have the distinct advantage of exerting less selective pressure for development of resistance in closed units like the NICU, thus minimizing the risk of emergence of resistant bacteria.[38] This is in contrast to the rapid emergence of cephalosporin resistance when these agents are provided routinely for possible late-onset sepsis.[39] When used for empirical therapy of early-onset infection, cefotaxime has been associated with increased neonatal mortality.[40] However, because CSF penetration of aminoglycosides is poor, their use in meningitis is problematic. If a lumbar puncture is not performed as part of the initial evaluation for possible sepsis, and only an aminoglycoside is used, then effective therapy for gram-negative meningitis may not be provided. Delay in the determination of whether a neonate has meningitis will delay optimal therapy for this condition. Targeting the primary use of third- and fourth-generation cephalosporins and carbapenems for suspected meningitis and confirmed pathogens is important in preventing and controlling the emergence of resistance against these antimicrobials.

Once meningitis is confirmed or ruled out and susceptibilities are known, antibiotics should be narrowed and broad-spectrum antibiotics reserved for when they are needed.

Continuation of Case History

At 18 hours after collection, the blood cultures yielded gram-negative rods. Cefotaxime was added to the antibiotic regimen. E. coli was subsequently identified from the blood cultures. A lumbar puncture was then performed that demonstrated 4160 white blood cells/mm^3 (90% polymorphonuclear cells, 10% mononuclear cells); 8320 red blood cells/mm^3; protein of 433 mg/dL; and glucose of 84 mg/dL (serum glucose of 180 mg/dL). Culture of CSF yielded E. coli.

Question 6: What Is the Treatment of Meningitis in Neonates, Particularly That Caused by Gram-Negative Bacilli?

Table 11.1 provides the normal CSF values and we can see from our case the number of white blood cells with a predominance of polymorphonuclear cells and relatively low red blood cell count is consistent with meningitis even if CSF culture did not grow E. coli. The recommended antimicrobial treatment for neonatal meningitis based on causative organism and dosing for the antibiotics.[41] The treatment of gram-negative meningitis initially includes the addition of a third- or fourth-generation cephalosporin such as cefotaxime or cefepime, or a carbapenem antibiotic such as meropenem.[42–47] Meningitis caused by gram-negative enteric bacilli is challenging because eradication of the organism from CSF is often delayed. Moreover,

many of these pathogens are now resistant to ampicillin, and aminoglycoside concentrations in CSF may not be high enough to kill the organism. Cefotaxime has superior in vitro and CSF bactericidal activity and is the agent of choice for early-onset meningitis. Recently there has been a shortage of cefotaxime in the United States; ceftazidime or cefepime are suitable alternative agents and are preferred for late-onset meningitis pending identification and susceptibility testing as cefotaxime does not cover pseudomonas infections. The cephalosporin agent is often combined with an aminoglycoside at least until sterilization of CSF has been achieved. There is no experience or studies using extended-interval dosing of aminoglycosides for neonatal meningitis, although from a pharmacodynamic standpoint, such a dosing schedule should achieve higher CSF concentrations.[48] Continued treatment of gram-negative bacillary meningitis is based on in vitro susceptibility tests. Ampicillin may be used in infrequent cases when the organism is susceptible.

Of concern is the production by gram-negative bacteria of both chromosomally determined β-lactamases and plasmid-determined extended-spectrum β-lactamases (ESBLs), both of which can result in resistance to the third-generation cephalosporin antibiotics, even during therapy.[49–51] Chromosomally determined β-lactamases are seen in Enterobacter spp., Serratia spp., Pseudomonas aeruginosa, Citrobacter spp., and indole-positive Proteus, whereas ESBLs are present in the Enterobacteriaceae, especially Klebsiella pneumoniae and E. coli. Susceptibility testing is critical and if there is ESBL resistance to cephalosporins, treatment of such infections should include a carbapenem antibiotic (meropenem or imipenem), possibly in combination with an aminoglycoside.[52] Recently, carabapenem resistance has emerged among gram-negative bacilli.[50,53] Surveillance and studies on the impact of these organisms in NICUs and the appropriate antimicrobial therapy of neonatal infections with these organisms are ongoing.[54]

The treatment of GBS meningitis is ampicillin or penicillin G. The American Academy of Pediatrics recommends 14 days for uncomplicated GBS meningitis and a minimum of 4 weeks if complicated with ventriculitis, cerebritis, or abscess.[55] No GBS resistance to penicillin G in the United States has been documented despite its extensive use in mothers and neonates. Despite the in vitro resistance of GBS to aminoglycosides, the addition of gentamicin to a penicillin agent will provide synergy.

Similar considerations are applicable in the preterm infant in whom meningitis develops while in the NICU. Potential pathogens include *S. aureus*, CoNS, enterococci, and multiply resistant pathogens such as methicillin-resistant *S. aureus* and gentamicin-or cephalosporin-resistant gram-negative enteric bacilli. If blood or CSF culture yields a gram-positive organism for early-onset infection, ampicillin can be continued (assuming it is GBS), but for late-onset infection, one should modify treatment pending susceptibilities to vancomycin or a combination of ampicillin and/or vancomycin. If the blood or CSF culture yields a gram-negative organism, an aminoglycoside with the addition of cefotaxime for early-onset infection (since the most likely pathogens are *E. coli* or *Klebsiella*) and cefepime or ceftazidime for late-onset infections (since *P. aeruginosa* may be the responsible pathogen) should be administered pending susceptibilities. Local stewardship can vary, but reserving carbapenems for those infections resistant to cephalosporins should be included in antibiotic stewardship plans. *Chryseobacterium* (formerly *Flavobacterium*) *meningosepticum*, a multiply resistant gram-negative bacilli, is a rare cause of meningitis that requires treatment with vancomycin and rifampin, or even ciprofloxacin.

Meningitis caused by anaerobic bacteria is infrequent and is usually caused by *Bacteroides fragilis* and *Clostridium* spp., mostly *C. perfringens*. The mortality rate is high. Penicillin, ampicillin, cephalosporins, and vancomycin are active against many gram-positive anaerobes. They have little if any activity against most anaerobic gram-negative bacilli; metronidazole is the agent of choice for meningitis secondary to these organisms. Carbapenem antibiotics such as meropenem and imipenem have excellent anaerobic activity against both gram-positive and negative organisms and can also be used.

The treatment of neonatal infections caused by *Ureaplasma urealyticum* and *Mycoplasma* spp. is complicated by the susceptibility patterns of these organisms as they usually are resistant to most antibiotics commonly used in neonates.[56] For infections caused by *U. urealyticum* and *M. pneumoniae*, azithromycin is the preferred agent unless resistance is present and doxycycline can be used as an alternative. For *M. hominis*, which is usually resistant to macrolides, clindamycin or doxycycline is preferred, with ciprofloxacin as an alternative. Although the exact duration of therapy for meningitis for *Ureaplasma* and *Mycoplasma* infections is not known, a 10- to 14-day course seems reasonable when there is associated clinical improvement and microbiologic eradication during that period.

Neonatal fungal infection of the CNS is usually caused by *Candida* species.[57,58] Amphotericin deoxycholate remains the treatment of choice, and it has been used successfully as monotherapy. Amphotericin B lipid formulations may be used if renal toxicity occurs while the infant is receiving the deoxycholate preparation. Fluconazole has excellent CNS penetration and is frequently added to amphotericin therapy for meningitis and in cases of persistent fungemia or poor clinical response when the organism is susceptible. Voriconazole or an echinocandin is recommended for *Aspergillus* infections. Echinocandins such as micafungin and caspofungin penetrate into the brain tissue well and can be used to treat meningitis.[59–64]

Continuation of Case History

A lumbar puncture was repeated 72 hours after diagnosis of meningitis and the CSF showed 6900 white blood cells/mm^3 (90% polymorphonuclear cells, 10% mononuclear cells); 2400 red blood cells/mm^3; protein of 550 mg/dL; and glucose of 21 mg/dL. Culture of CSF again yielded *E. coli* that was resistant to ampicillin but susceptible to cefotaxime, ceftazidime, and gentamicin with minimum inhibitory concentrations of 2 μg/mL.

Question 7: Do Intrathecal or Intraventricular Antibiotic Treatment Have a Role?

Meningitis secondary to gram-negative bacilli is associated with persistently positive CSF cultures despite appropriate therapy. The median duration of positive CSF cultures is 3 days, and the duration of positivity is correlated with long-term prognosis. In addition, the duration of positive CSF culture will have an impact on the total length of therapy. For these reasons, it is recommended that a repeat lumbar puncture be performed to determine both occurrence

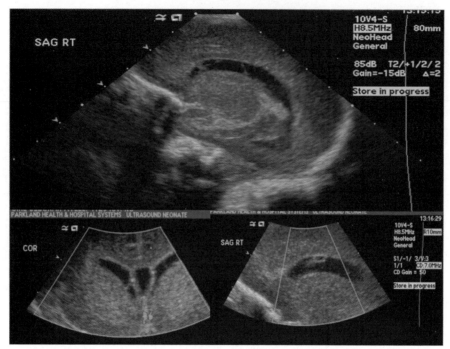

Fig. 11.1 Cranial ultrasound performed on a 2-week-old extremely low-birth-weight infant with meningitis caused by *Escherichia coli.* There are echogenic debris and septation consistent with purulent material within the dilated lateral ventricle.

and timing of CSF sterilization. The timing of the repeat lumbar puncture will be determined in part by the clinical findings and initial spinal fluid analysis.

Ventriculitis occurs in at least 70% of cases; however, ventricular fluid is poorly accessible to systemically administered antibiotics. Therefore both lumbar intrathecal and intraventricular gentamicin have been used for the treatment of gram-negative meningitis.[65,66] Among infants who received parenteral drug alone or parenteral plus intrathecal therapy (1 mg/ day for at least 3 days), no differences in either the case-fatality rate or neurologic residua were observed by the Neonatal Meningitis Cooperative Study Group.[65] These investigators subsequently studied the use of intraventricular gentamicin (2.5 mg); there was higher mortality among infants who received intraventricular gentamicin (43%) in combination with ampicillin and gentamicin than in those who received systemic antibiotics alone (13%). Subsequent evaluation of ventricular fluid from infants who received intraventricular gentamicin showed significantly greater concentrations of tumor necrosis factor and IL-1β in their CSFs, indicating that greater inflammatory injury

may result from this form of therapy.[67] In general, intraventricular therapy is not recommended, although it remains an option in those infants who already have a ventricular drain in place and persistently positive CSF cultures.

Continuation of Case History

A cranial ultrasound performed on days 2 and 7 after presentation did not demonstrate abscess formation or new intracranial hemorrhage, but it did show mild ventricular dilatation, and echogenic debris and septations were visualized within the ventricular system (Fig. 11.1). The infant continued to receive cefotaxime and was nearing 21 days of therapy.

Question 8: What Is the Duration of Treatment for Meningitis in Neonates?

Unfortunately, there are no randomized studies of duration of antibiotic therapy for neonatal meningitis.

In general, duration of therapy is dependent on the causative organism, site(s) of infection, clinical severity, and course. This is usually 7 days for uncomplicated bacteremia, 7 to 10 days for sepsis and pneumonia, and 14 to 21 days for meningitis, depending on the causative agent. Normalization of C-reactive protein or other inflammatory markers such as IL-8 or IL-10 has been used to discontinue antibiotic therapy in infants with sepsis. Although this approach seems reasonable, more studies involving high-risk neonates with serious infections such as meningitis are needed before such a strategy can be recommended routinely.

For meningitis caused by gram-negative bacilli, the duration of antimicrobial therapy is a minimum of 21 days or 2 weeks after the first sterile CSF culture, whichever is longest. Earlier discontinuation of antimicrobial therapy may result in bacterial relapse. Some experts recommend performance of another lumbar puncture after 21 days of treatment in infants with gram-negative enteric meningitis and before discontinuation of antibiotic therapy as it may be useful to determine the adequacy of therapy. Markedly abnormal CSF findings, such as glucose concentration less than 25 mg/dL, protein content higher than 300 mg/dL, or more than 50% polymorphonuclear cells, without other explanation warrant continued antimicrobial therapy to prevent relapse.

For meningitis caused by group B streptococcus, a minimum of 14 days of antimicrobial therapy is recommended. The decision of whether to perform an "end of therapy" lumbar puncture in these neonates can be based on clinical course. If the infant has experienced complications such as seizures, significant hypotension, or prolonged positive CSF cultures, or if the neuroimaging is abnormal, then it probably is prudent to do it.

The optimal duration of therapy for meningitis caused by other microorganisms is not known. Meningitis secondary to *S. aureus* should be treated with at least 3 weeks of antibiotic therapy. In general, cerebral abscess requires more prolonged therapy of 4 to 6 weeks, depending on whether it is surgically drained or there is persistence of abnormalities on neuroimaging. Similarly, ventriculitis, cerebritis, or any parenchymal brain disease diagnosed with imaging should be treated for a minimum of 4 weeks.

Question 9: When Should Neuroimaging Be Considered, and What Type of Examination Is Recommended?

The timing and the reason for performing neuroimaging studies are important considerations in the decision of which type of study should be performed. Cranial ultrasonography is safe, convenient, and readily available; it can be done at the bedside and does not require sedation. It provides rapid and reliable information on ventricular size and whether there is development of hydrocephalus. It is therefore useful to perform an ultrasound early in the course when the infant is too critical to transport to radiology. Cranial ultrasonography also will provide information on periventricular white matter injury; initially, ischemia may be manifested by increased periventricular echogenicity, which may progress to cystic periventricular leukomalacia in later studies (Fig. 11.2). Ultrasonography, however, does not allow for optimal evaluation of parenchymal abnormalities such as infarct, cerebritis, and abscess nor of presence of subdural empyema, all known complications of neonatal meningitis.

Computed tomography will provide information on whether the course of meningitis has been complicated by a cerebral abscess, hydrocephalus, or subdural collections if magnetic resonance imaging (MRI) is not available. In general, however, computed tomography scans should be avoided except when neuroimaging is required on an emergent basis as its use has been associated with subsequent neurodevelopmental impairment and increased risk for cancer.[68]

MRI is the best currently available modality for evaluation of the neonatal brain. It provides excellent information on the status of the white matter, cortex, subdural and epidural spaces, and even the posterior fossa in cases of tuberculous meningitis (Fig. 11.3). In addition, it has been used in preterm infants to predict neurodevelopmental outcome. For these reasons, infants with suspected cerebral injury either because of abnormalities on ultrasonography, seizures, persistent CSF abnormalities, or meningitis caused by *Citrobacter, Serratia*, or fungi that are associated with abscess formation should have brain MRI performed. Cerebral abscess formation can complicate up to 70% of cases of *C. koseri* meningitis (Fig. 11.4). Microabscesses are also common with neonatal fungal meningitis. For these reasons, many experts recommend that at least one brain MRI be performed for every infant with

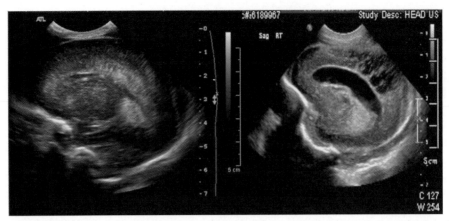

Fig. 11.2 Cranial ultrasound performed on an extremely low-birth-weight infant with meningitis that demonstrates echogenic periventricular white matter *(left)* with subsequent progression to cystic periventricular leukomalacia *(right)*.

neonatal meningitis. In addition, all infants with meningitis require hearing evaluation.

Question 10: Should Other Adjunctive Therapies Be Provided to an Infant With Meningitis?

Dexamethasone has been shown in some studies to decrease neurologic morbidity in older infants and children with meningitis. No studies are available in neonates, and its use is not recommended.[69] In a rabbit model of *E. coli* meningitis, the addition of dexamethasone to standard antibiotic therapy was associated with an increase in hippocampal neuronal apoptosis.[70]

The prolonged use of broad-spectrum antimicrobial agents, especially third-generation cephalosporins and carbapenems, has been associated with development of systemic candidiasis in preterm infants with birth weight less than 1000 g.[71] Prophylactic fluconazole has been shown to decrease the incidence of candidiasis in these infants, and its use should be considered in infants with meningitis who require prolonged broad-spectrum antimicrobial therapy with cephalosporins, carbapenems, or other broadly acting antibiotics.[72,73]

Question 11: What If the Infant's CSF Is Abnormal but Routine Bacterial Cultures of CSF and Blood Are Sterile?

The most frequent reason for a sterile CSF culture despite CSF changes indicative of meningitis is previous antimicrobial therapy. However, intraventricular hemorrhage can result in inflammatory changes such as pleocytosis with predominance of polymorphonuclear cells, elevated protein concentration, and hypoglycorrhachia in the absence of an infectious process, making the performance of a lumbar puncture before initiation of antimicrobial therapy important (Table 11.1).

When an infant in whom sepsis and meningitis are suspected has abnormal CSF indices but routine bacterial cultures are sterile, a repeat lumbar puncture should be performed. Pathogens that can result in an aseptic meningitis should be excluded (see Box 11.1), especially because specific therapy is available for some of them. To detect these pathogens, CSF should be tested for the presence of anaerobic bacteria, *M. hominis*, *Ureaplasma* spp., fungi (*Candida* grows in aerobic cultures, but other fungi need special culture methods), and viruses such as herpes simplex, cytomegalovirus, enteroviruses, and parechoviruses by culture or PCR as appropriate.[17]

Continuation of Case History

The infant's CSF evaluation was markedly improved after 21 days of cefotaxime, and MRI examination revealed only mild ventriculomegaly. At discharge to home at 3 months of age, he passed an automated auditory brainstem response test. At 22 months corrected gestational age, he had mild impairment in both mental and psychomotor development indexes by Bayley Scales of Infant Development.

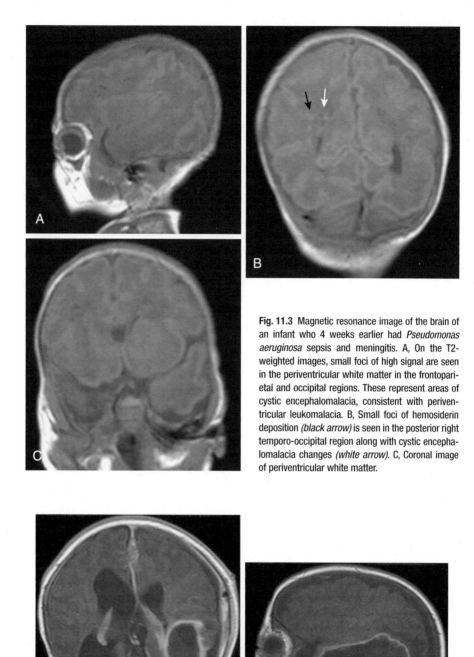

Fig. 11.3 Magnetic resonance image of the brain of an infant who 4 weeks earlier had *Pseudomonas aeruginosa* sepsis and meningitis. A, On the T2-weighted images, small foci of high signal are seen in the periventricular white matter in the frontoparietal and occipital regions. These represent areas of cystic encephalomalacia, consistent with periventricular leukomalacia. B, Small foci of hemosiderin deposition *(black arrow)* is seen in the posterior right temporo-occipital region along with cystic encephalomalacia changes *(white arrow)*. C, Coronal image of periventricular white matter.

Fig. 11.4 Magnetic resonance image of the brain of a 3-week-old full-term infant with meningitis and cerebral abscess caused by *Serratia marcescens*. Following gadolinium administration, (A) a large ring-enhancing lesion is seen that (B) extends from the posterior aspect of the temporal lobe into the adjacent parietal and occipital white matter.

Question 12: What Is the Outcome of Meningitis in Neonates?

Despite improvements in neonatal care and antibiotic therapy, significant morbidity and mortality persist[74] Among preterm infants with birth weights 1000 g, infants with meningitis are more likely to have low (<70) mental and psychomotor indices, cerebral palsy, vision impairment, and head circumference below the 10th percentile than uninfected infants of similar birth weight and gestation.[35]

Among infants with early or late-onset meningitis, the case-fatality rate and morbidity remain high. Survival outcomes have improved when comparing data from before and after 1990. Mortality has decreased from around 25% to 10% and has since remained stable. Despite improved survival, neurologic sequelae are found in approximately 50% of survivors. Risk factors for neurological sequelae include seizures as well as time to sterilization but are not related to the kind of pathogen. Adverse neurological sequelae include postinfectious hydrocephalus, seizure disorder, developmental delay, cerebral palsy, cognitive impairment, behavioral problems, hearing loss, and speech and visual impairment. Major neurologic sequelae include spastic quadriplegia, profound intellectual disability, hemiparesis, deafness, or cortical blindness. Prediction of late morbidity can be aided by the use of brain MRI performed toward the end of therapy.

On the other hand, children not identified early as having major sequelae performed intellectually, socially, and academically in a manner similar to other family members.

Conclusion

Meningitis is a serious infection for which early therapy is mandatory to improve both short- and long-term outcomes. This is possible only by the timely recognition of its occurrence, thus making performance of a lumbar puncture for CSF analysis and culture the key to rapid institution of effective antimicrobial therapy. Rapid PCR panels may also help identify pathogens before antibiotics are administered or if obtained within 12 to 24 hours of presentation if lumbar puncture needed to be deferred.[17] Ultimately, however, its prevention will be achieved when neonatal sepsis is controlled, an elusive but not impossible goal in neonatal medicine.[75]

REFERENCES

1. Kaufman D, Fairchild KD. Clinical microbiology of bacterial and fungal sepsis in very-low-birth-weight infants. *Clin Microbiol Rev*. 2004;17(3):638-680, table of contents. Available at: doi:org/10.1128/CMR.17.3.638-680.2004.
2. Cantey JB, Milstone AM. Bloodstream infections: epidemiology and resistance. *Clin Perinatol*. 2015;42(1):1-16, vii. Available at: doi:org/10.1016/j.clp.2014.10.002.
3. Cantey JB, Farris AC, McCormick SM. Bacteremia in early infancy: etiology and management. *Curr Infect Dis Rep*. 2016;18(1):1. Available at: doi:org/10.1007/s11908-015-0508-3.
4. Puopolo KM, Benitz WE, Zaoutis TE, Committee on Fetus and Newborn, Committee on Infectious Diseases. Management of neonates born at ≤34 6/7 weeks' gestation with suspected or proven early-onset bacterial sepsis. *Pediatrics*. 2018;142(6). Available at: doi:org/10.1542/peds.2018-2896.
5. Puopolo KM, Benitz WE, Zaoutis TE, Committee on Fetus and Newborn, Committee on Infectious Diseases. Management of neonates born at ≥35 0/7 weeks' gestation with suspected or proven early-onset bacterial sepsis. *Pediatrics*. 2018;142(6). Available at: doi:org/10.1542/peds.2018-2894.
6. Puopolo KM, Lynfield R, Cummings JJ, Committee on Fetus and Newborn, Committee on Infectious Diseases. Management of infants at risk for group B streptococcal disease. *Pediatrics*. 2019;144(2). Available at: doi:org/10.1542/peds.2019-1881.
7. Cetinkaya M, Cekmez F, Buyukkale G, et al. Lower vitamin D levels are associated with increased risk of early-onset neonatal sepsis in term infants. *J Perinatol*. 2015;35(1):39-45. Available at: doi:org/10.1038/jp.2014.146.
8. Schrag SJ, Verani JR. Intrapartum antibiotic prophylaxis for the prevention of perinatal group B streptococcal disease: experience in the United States and implications for a potential group B streptococcal vaccine. *Vaccine*. 2013;31(suppl 4):D20-D26. Available at: doi:org/10.1016/j.vaccine.2012.11.056.
9. Stoll BJ, Hansen N, Fanaroff AA, et al. Changes in pathogens causing early-onset sepsis in very-low-birth-weight infants. *N Engl J Med*. 2002;347(4):240-247. Available at: doi:org/10.1056/NEJMoa012657.
10. Stoll BJ, Hansen NI, Sánchez PJ, et al. Early onset neonatal sepsis: the burden of group B Streptococcal and E. coli disease continues. *Pediatrics*. 2011;127(5):817-826. Available at: doi:org/10.1542/peds.2010-2217.
11. Stoll BJ, Puopolo KM, Hansen NI, et al. Early-onset neonatal sepsis 2015 to 2017, the rise of *Escherichia coli*, and the need for novel prevention strategies. *JAMA Pediatr*. 2020;174(7):e200593. Available at: doi:org/10.1001/jamapediatrics.2020.0593.
12. Flannery DD, Akinboyo IC, Mukhopadhyay S, et al. Antibiotic susceptibility of *Escherichia coli* among infants admitted to neonatal intensive care units across the US from 2009 to 2017. *JAMA Pediatr*. 2021;175(2):168-175. Available at: doi:org/10.1001/jamapediatrics.2020.4719.
13. Rodriguez AF, Kaplan SL, Mason EO. Cerebrospinal fluid values in the very low birth weight infant. *J Pediatr*. 1990;116(6):971-974. Available at: doi:org/10.1016/s0022-3476(05)80663-8.
14. Ahmed A, Hickey SM, Ehrett S, et al. Cerebrospinal fluid values in the term neonate. *Pediatr Infect Dis J*. 1996;15(4):298-303. Available at: doi:org/10.1097/00006454-199604000-00004.
15. Stoll BJ, Hansen N, Fanaroff AA, et al. To tap or not to tap: high likelihood of meningitis without sepsis among very low birth weight infants. *Pediatrics*. 2004;113(5):1181-1186.
16. Bergin SP, Thaden JT, Ericson JE, et al. Neonatal *Escherichia coli* bloodstream infections: clinical outcomes and impact of initial antibiotic therapy. *Pediatr Infect Dis J*. 2015;34(9):933-936. Available at: doi:org/10.1097/INF.0000000000000769.

17. Arora HS, Asmar BI, Salimnia H, Agarwal P, Chawla S, Abdel-Haq N. Enhanced identification of group B *Streptococcus* and *Escherichia coli* in young infants with meningitis using the Bio-fire Filmarray meningitis/encephalitis panel. *Pediatr Infect Dis J.* 2017;36(7):685-687. Available at: doi:org/10.1097/INF.0000000000001551.

18. Laborada G, Rego M, Jain A, et al. Diagnostic value of cytokines and C-reactive protein in the first 24 hours of neonatal sepsis. *Am J Perinatol.* 2003;20(8):491-501. Available at: doi:org/10.1055/s-2003-45382.

19. Verboon-Maciolek MA, Thijsen SFT, Hemels MAC, et al. Inflammatory mediators for the diagnosis and treatment of sepsis in early infancy. *Pediatr Res.* 2006;59(3):457-461. Available at: doi:org/10.1203/01.pdr.0000200808.35368.57.

20. Sturgeon JP, Zanetti B, Lindo D. C-reactive Protein (CRP) levels in neonatal meningitis in England: an analysis of national variations in CRP cut-offs for lumbar puncture. *BMC Pediatr.* 2018;18(1):380. Available at: doi:org/10.1186/s12887-018-1354-x.

21. Goldfinch CD, Korman T, Kotsanas D, Burgner DP, Tan K. C-reactive protein and immature-to-total neutrophil ratio have no utility in guiding lumbar puncture in suspected neonatal sepsis. *J Paediatr Child Health.* 2018;54(8):848-854. Available at: doi:org/10.1111/jpc.13890.

22. Dhudasia MB, Benitz WE, Flannery DD, Christ L, Rub D, Remaschi G, et al. Diagnostic Performance and Patient Outcomes With C-Reactive Protein Use in Early-Onset Sepsis Evaluations. *J Pediatr.* 2022. https://doi.org/10.1016/j.jpeds.2022.12.007.

23. Brown JVE, Meader N, Wright K, Cleminson J, McGuire W. Assessment of C-reactive protein diagnostic test accuracy for late-onset infection in newborn infants: a systematic review and meta-analysis. *JAMA Pediatr.* 2020;174(3):260-268. Available at: doi:org/10.1001/jamapediatrics.2019.5669.

24. Mukherjee A, Davidson L, Anguvaa L, Duffy DA, Kennea N. NICE neonatal early onset sepsis guidance: greater consistency, but more investigations, and greater length of stay. *Arch Dis Child Fetal Neonatal Ed.* 2015;100(3):F248-F249. Available at: doi:org/10.1136/archdischild-2014-306349.

25. Tiozzo C, Mukhopadhyay S. Noninfectious influencers of early-onset sepsis biomarkers. *Pediatr Res.* 2022;91(2):425-431. Available at: doi:org/10.1038/s41390-021-01861-4.

26. Cantey JB, Lee JH. Biomarkers for the diagnosis of neonatal sepsis. *Clin Perinatol.* 2021;48(2):215-227. Available at: doi:org/10.1016/j.clp.2021.03.012.

27. Carr R, Modi N, Doré C. G-CSF and GM-CSF for treating or preventing neonatal infections. *Cochrane Database Syst Rev.* 2003;(3):CD003066. Available at: doi:org/10.1002/14651858.CD003066.

28. Chaudhuri J, Mitra S, Mukhopadhyay D, Chakraborty S, Chatterjee S. Granulocyte colony-stimulating factor for preterms with sepsis and neutropenia: a randomized controlled trial. *J Clin Neonatol.* 2012;1(4):202-206. Available at: doi:org/10.4103/2249-4847.105993.

29. Guida JD, Kunig AM, Leef KH, McKenzie SE, Paul DA. Platelet count and sepsis in very low birth weight neonates: is there an organism-specific response? *Pediatrics.* 2003;111(6 Pt 1):1411-1415.

30. Kusulas MP, Eutsler EP, DePiero AD. Bedside ultrasound for the evaluation of epidural hematoma after infant lumbar puncture. *Pediatr Emerg Care.* January 2018. Available at: doi:org/10.1097/PEC.0000000000001383.

31. Baxter AL, Fisher RG, Burke BL, Goldblatt SS, Isaacman DJ, Lawson ML. Local anesthetic and stylet styles: factors associated with resident lumbar puncture success. *Pediatrics.* 2006;117(3):876-881. Available at: doi:org/10.1542/peds.2005-0519.

32. Chiu CH, Michelow IC, Cronin J, Ringer SA, Ferris TG, Puopolo KM. Effectiveness of a guideline to reduce vancomycin use in the neonatal intensive care unit. *Pediatr Infect Dis J.* 2011;30(4):273-278. Available at: doi:org/10.1097/INF.0b013e3182011d12.

33. Hamdy RF, Bhattarai S, Basu SK, et al. Reducing vancomycin use in a level IV NICU. *Pediatrics.* 2020;146(2). Available at: doi:org/10.1542/peds.2019-2963.

34. Stoll BJ, Hansen N, Fanaroff AA, et al. Late-onset sepsis in very low birth weight neonates: the experience of the NICHD Neonatal Research Network. *Pediatrics.* 2002;110(2 Pt 1):285-291. Available at: doi:org/10.1542/peds.110.2.285.

35. Stoll BJ, Hansen NI, Adams-Chapman I, et al. Neurodevelopmental and growth impairment among extremely low-birth-weight infants with neonatal infection. *JAMA.* 2004;292(19):2357-2365. Available at: doi:org/10.1001/jama.292.19.2357.

36. Van Houten MA, Uiterwaal CS, Heesen GJ, Arends JP, Kimpen JL. Does the empiric use of vancomycin in pediatrics increase the risk for gram-negative bacteremia? *Pediatr Infect Dis J.* 2001;20(2):171-177. Available at: doi:org/10.1097/00006454-200102000-00011.

37. Mohamed AF, Nielsen EI, Cars O, Friberg LE. Pharmacokinetic-pharmacodynamic model for gentamicin and its adaptive resistance with predictions of dosing schedules in newborn infants. *Antimicrob Agents Chemother.* 2012;56(1):179-188. Available at: doi:org/10.1128/AAC.00694-11.

38. de Man P, Verhoeven BA, Verbrugh HA, Vos MC, van den Anker JN. An antibiotic policy to prevent emergence of resistant bacilli. *Lancet.* 2000;355(9208):973-978. Available at: doi:org/10.1016/s0140-6736(00)90015-1.

39. Saporito L, Graziano G, Mescolo F, et al. Efficacy of a coordinated strategy for containment of multidrug-resistant Gram-negative bacteria carriage in a neonatal intensive care unit in the context of an active surveillance program. *Antimicrob Resist Infect Control.* 2021;10(1):30. Available at: doi:org/10.1186/s13756-021-00902-1.

40. Clark RH, Bloom BT, Spitzer AR, Gerstmann DR. Empiric use of ampicillin and cefotaxime, compared with ampicillin and gentamicin, for neonates at risk for sepsis is associated with an increased risk of neonatal death. *Pediatrics.* 2006;117(1):67-74. Available at: doi:org/10.1542/peds.2005-0179.

41. Nelson B. *Nelson's Pediatric Antimicrobial Therapy.* 21st ed. Elk Grove Village, IL: American Academy of Pediatrics; 2015.

42. Sullins AK, Abdel-Rahman SM. Pharmacokinetics of antibacterial agents in the CSF of children and adolescents. *Paediatr Drugs.* 2013;15(2):93-117. Available at: doi:org/10.1007/s40272-013-0017-5.

43. Nau R, Sörgel F, Eiffert H. Penetration of drugs through the blood-cerebrospinal fluid/blood-brain barrier for treatment of central nervous system infections. *Clin Microbiol Rev.* 2010;23(4):858-883. Available at: doi:org/10.1128/CMR.00007-10.

44. Arnold CJ, Ericson J, Cho N, et al. Cefepime and ceftazidime safety in hospitalized infants. *Pediatr Infect Dis J.* 2015;34(9):964-968. Available at: doi:org/10.1097/INF.0000000000000778.

45. Capparelli E, Hochwald C, Rasmussen M, Parham A, Bradley J, Moya F. Population pharmacokinetics of cefepime in the neonate. *Antimicrob Agents Chemother.* 2005;49(7):2760-2766. Available at: doi:org/10.1128/AAC.49.7.2760-2766.2005.

46. Ellis JM, Rivera L, Reyes G, et al. Cefepime cerebrospinal fluid concentrations in neonatal bacterial meningitis. *Ann Pharmacother.* 2007;41(5):900-901. Available at: doi:org/10.1345/aph.1H585.

47. Patel SJ, Green N, Clock SA, et al. Gram-negative bacilli in infants hospitalized in the neonatal intensive care unit. *J Pediatric Infect Dis Soc.* 2017;6(3):227-230. Available at: doi:org/10.1093/jpids/piw032.

48. de Hoog M, Mouton JW, van den Anker JN. New dosing strategies for antibacterial agents in the neonate. *Semin Fetal Neonatal Med.* 2005;10(2):185-194. Available at: doi:org/10.1016/j.siny.2004.10.004.

49. Wong-Beringer A, Hindler J, Loeloff M, et al. Molecular correlation for the treatment outcomes in bloodstream infections caused by *Escherichia coli* and *Klebsiella pneumoniae* with reduced susceptibility to ceftazidime. *Clin Infect Dis.* 2002;34(2):135-146. Available at: doi:org/10.1086/324742.

50. Zerr DM, Weissman SJ, Zhou C, et al. The molecular and clinical epidemiology of extended-spectrum cephalosporin- and carbapenem-resistant *Enterobacteriaceae* at 4 US pediatric hospitals. *J Pediatric Infect Dis Soc.* 2017;6(4):366-375. Available at: doi:org/10.1093/jpids/piw076.

51. Abdel-Hady H, Hawas S, El-Daker M, El-Kady R. Extended-spectrum beta-lactamase producing *Klebsiella pneumoniae* in neonatal intensive care unit. *J Perinatol.* 2008;28(10):685-690. Available at: doi:org/10.1038/jp.2008.73.

52. Patterson JE. Extended spectrum beta-lactamases: a therapeutic dilemma. *Pediatr Infect Dis J.* 2002;21(10):957-959. Available at: doi:org/10.1097/00006454-200210000-00014.

53. Datta S, Roy S, Chatterjee S, et al. A five-year experience of carbapenem resistance in *Enterobacteriaceae* causing neonatal septicaemia: predominance of NDM-1. *PLoS One.* 2014;9(11):e112101. Available at: doi:org/10.1371/journal.pone.0112101.

54. Folgori L, Bielicki J, Heath PT, Sharland M. Antimicrobial-resistant Gram-negative infections in neonates: burden of disease and challenges in treatment. *Curr Opin Infect Dis.* 2017;30(3):281-288. Available at: doi:org/10.1097/QCO.0000000000000371.

55. Kimberlain DW, Barnett ED, Lynfield R, Sawyer MH, eds. Group B streptococcal infections. In: *Red Book: 2021–2024 Report of the Committee on Infectious Diseases.* Elk Grove Village, IL: American Academy of Pediatrics; 32nd ed. 2021:707-713.

56. Kimberlain DW, Barnett ED, Lynfield R, Sawyer MH, eds. *Mycoplasma pneumoniae* and other mycoplasma species infections. In: *Red Book: 2021–2024 Report of the Committee on Infectious Diseases.* Elk Grove Village, IL: American Academy of Pediatrics; 32nd ed. 2021.

57. Kimberlain DW, Barnett ED, Lynfield R, Sawyer MH, eds. Candidiasis. In: *Red Book: 2021–2024 Report of the Committee on Infectious Diseases.* Elk Grove Village, IL: American Academy of Pediatrics; 32nd ed. 2021.

58. Benjamin DK, Stoll BJ, Gantz MG, et al. Neonatal candidiasis: epidemiology, risk factors, and clinical judgment. *Pediatrics.* 2010;126(4):e865-e873. Available at: doi:org/10.1542/peds.2009-3412.

59. Benjamin DK, Kaufman DA, Hope WW, et al. A phase 3 study of micafungin versus amphotericin B deoxycholate in infants with invasive candidiasis. *Pediatr Infect Dis J.* 2018;37(10):992-998. Available at: doi:org/10.1097/INF0000000000001996.

60. Kovanda LL, Walsh TJ, Benjamin DK, et al. Exposure-response analysis of micafungin in neonatal candidiasis: pooled analysis of two clinical trials. *Pediatr Infect Dis J.* 2018;37(6):580-585. Available at: doi:org/10.1097/INF.0000000000001957.

61. Auriti C, Goffredo BM, Ronchetti MP, et al. High-dose micafungin in neonates and young infants with invasive candidiasis: results of a phase 2 study. *Antimicrob Agents Chemother.* 2021;65(4). Available at: doi:org/10.1128/AAC.02494-20.

62. Leroux S, Jacqz-Aigrain E, Elie V, et al. Pharmacokinetics and safety of fluconazole and micafungin in neonates with systemic candidiasis: a randomized, open-label clinical trial. *Br J Clin Pharmacol.* 2018;84(9):1989-1999. Available at: doi:org/10.1111/bcp.13628.

63. Auriti C, Falcone M, Ronchetti MP, et al. High-dose micafungin for preterm neonates and infants with invasive and central nervous system candidiasis. *Antimicrob Agents Chemother.* 2016;60(12):7333-7339. Available at: doi:org/10.1128/AAC.01172-16.

64. Hope WW, Mickiene D, Petraitis V, et al. The pharmacokinetics and pharmacodynamics of micafungin in experimental hematogenous Candida meningoencephalitis: implications for echinocandin therapy in neonates. *J Infect Dis.* 2008;197(1):163-171. Available at: doi:org/10.1086/524063.

65. McCracken GH, Mize SG. A controlled study of intrathecal antibiotic therapy in gram-negative enteric meningitis of infancy. Report of the neonatal meningitis cooperative study group. *J Pediatr.* 1976;89(1):66-72. Available at: doi:org/10.1016/s0022-3476(76)80929-8.

66. McCracken GH, Mize SG, Threlkeld N. Intraventricular gentamicin therapy in gram-negative bacillary meningitis of infancy. Report of the Second Neonatal Meningitis Cooperative Study Group. *Lancet.* 1980;1(8172):787-791.

67. Ramilo O, Sáez-Llorens X, Mertsola J, et al. Tumor necrosis factor alpha/cachectin and interleukin 1 beta initiate meningeal inflammation. *J Exp Med.* 1990;172(2):497-507. Available at: doi:org/10.1084/jem.172.2.497.

68. Frush DP, Donnelly LF, Rosen NS. Computed tomography and radiation risks: what pediatric health care providers should know. *Pediatrics.* 2003;112(4):951-957.

69. *Bacterial Meningitis in Children: Dexamethasone and Other Measures to Prevent Neurologic Complications.* UpToDate. Available at: https://www.uptodate.com/contents/bacterial-meningitis-in-children-dexamethasone-and-other-measures-to-prevent-neurologic-complications?search=bacterial%20meningitis%20children%20dexamethasone&source=search_result&selectedTitle=1~150&usage_type=default&display_rank=1. Accessed March 10, 2022.

70. Spreer A, Gerber J, Hanssen M, et al. Dexamethasone increases hippocampal neuronal apoptosis in a rabbit model of *Escherichia coli* meningitis. *Pediatr Res.* 2006;60(2):210-215. Available at: doi:org/10.1203/01.pdr.0000227553.47378.9f.

71. Cotten CM, McDonald S, Stoll B, et al. The association of third-generation cephalosporin use and invasive candidiasis in extremely low birth-weight infants. *Pediatrics.* 2006;118(2):717-722. Available at: doi:org/10.1542/peds.2005-2677.

72. Kaufman D, Boyle R, Hazen KC, Patrie JT, Robinson M, Donowitz LG. Fluconazole prophylaxis against fungal colonization and infection in preterm infants. *N Engl J Med.* 2001;345(23):1660-1666. Available at: doi:org/10.1056/NEJMoa010494.

73. Uko S, Soghier LM, Vega M, et al. Targeted short-term fluconazole prophylaxis among very low birth weight and extremely low birth weight infants. *Pediatrics.* 2006;117(4):1243-1252. Available at: doi:org/10.1542/peds.2005-1969.

74. Sewell E, Roberts J, Mukhopadhyay S. Association of infection in neonates and long-term neurodevelopmental outcome. *Clin Perinatol.* 2021;48(2):251-261. Available at: doi:org/10.1016/j.clp.2021.03.001.

75. Cantey JB, Ronchi A, Sánchez PJ. Spreading the benefits of infection prevention in the neonatal intensive care unit. *JAMA Pediatr.* 2015;169(12):1089. Available at: doi:org/10.1001/jamapediatrics.2015.2980.

Chapter 12

Neonatal Herpes Simplex Virus, Congenital Cytomegalovirus, Congenital Zika, and Congenital and Neonatal SARS-CoV-2 Virus Infections

Nazia Kabani and David W. Kimberlin

Chapter Outline

Key Points

- After reading this chapter, readers will be familiar with the epidemiology of congenital infections such as CMV, HSV, Zika, and SARS-CoV-2 virus.
- Risk factors for acquiring these infections are discussed.
- Clinical manifestations, diagnosis, treatment, and clinical outcomes are also discussed in detail.

Among the numerous viral pathogens that cause central nervous system (CNS) infections in the neonatal period, herpes simplex virus (HSV) and cytomegalovirus (CMV) are unique in their management. Both have commercially available antiviral drugs that treat the virus, as well as evidence-based data documenting the benefit of antiviral therapy. Neonatal HSV infection primarily is acquired in the peripartum period, whereas congenital CMV infection is the most common viral infection acquired in utero. Utilization of antiviral therapy to improve disease outcomes is influenced by these differences, with antiviral therapy of neonatal HSV disease aimed primarily at improving mortality and antiviral therapy of congenital CMV infections targeting improvement in longer-term audiologic outcomes. Additionally, the extent of data and clinical experience differs between the two viruses, with antiviral treatment of neonatal HSV disease required in all cases, but antiviral management of congenital CMV infection is an option rather than a requirement.

The studies conducted by the National Institute of Allergy and Infectious Diseases (NIAID) Collaborative Antiviral Study Group (CASG) over the past 30 years have defined the benefits and toxicities of antiviral treatment of neonatal HSV and congenital CMV. In conducting controlled investigations of these rare infections, the CASG also has characterized the natural history of infection with these viruses in neonates. These advances in our understanding of neonatal HSV and congenital CMV disease not only provide the foundation for advances in the management of these infections but also establish the scope through which newly recognized congenital and perinatal infections such as Zika and SARS-CoV-2 are appreciated.

Unlike HSV and CMV, which are transmitted person to person, Zika virus is unique among the viruses that cause congenital infections by being mosquito-borne. When a pregnant mother acquires a primary Zika infection, the virus can cross the placenta to infect the developing fetus with devastating consequences, including microcephaly, tremendous brain abnormalities, and even fetal loss. While much about congenital Zika virus infection remains to be elucidated, what we know already draws heavily from existing knowledge of congenital CMV and even rubella disease.

Novel coronavirus disease 2019 (COVID-19) is caused by severe acute respiratory syndrome coronavirus 2 (SARS-CoV-2).[1] It emerged in China in late 2019, and has caused over 200 million infections worldwide, with greater than 4 million deaths.[2] Cases of vertical transmission have been described but are rare, and most infected neonates tend to have no adverse outcomes.[3] Neonatal SARS-CoV-2 infection also can be acquired via horizontal transmission, from direct contact when feeding or via respiratory droplets of symptomatic mothers.[4] There is much still to be learned about SARS-CoV-2 infection, in neonates in particular.

Question 1: When Does Infection Occur?

NEONATAL HSV DISEASE

HSV disease of the newborn is acquired during one of three distinct times: intrauterine (in utero), peripartum (perinatal), and postpartum (postnatal). Among infected infants, the time of transmission for the majority (~85%) of neonates is in the peripartum period.[5] An additional 10% of infected neonates acquire the virus postnatally, and the final 5% are infected with HSV in utero.[5]

CONGENITAL CMV INFECTION

CMV infection also can occur at any of these three distinct times (intrauterine, peripartum, and postpartum). Congenital infection, though, is synonymous with in utero acquisition, and is clearly associated with long-term morbidity. In contrast, peripartum transmission can produce acute illness, but rarely if ever results in long-term sequelae. Infection of women both immediately before and during pregnancy puts the fetus at risk for congenital CMV infection.[6,7] In utero transmission occurs after primary maternal infection, as is the case with toxoplasmosis, rubella, and Zika (see later text), and also in recurrent infections, including reinfection with a different strain of the virus[8] or reactivation of latent virus.[9]

CONGENITAL ZIKA INFECTION

Zika virus infection in the Americas peaked in 2016, and then declined substantially through 2017 and 2018. Zika virus transmission has been found in all countries in the Region of the Americas except mainland Chile, Uruguay, and Canada, and is also found in Africa and parts of Asia and the Pacific Islands. Congenital Zika, like congenital CMV, is acquired most often in utero.[10] This happens when a pregnant woman acquires Zika for the first time from the bite of an infected mosquito. The resulting primary infection can cross the placenta and infect the developing fetus.[10]

Congenital SARS-CoV-2 or Neonatal SARS-CoV-2 Infection

SARS-CoV-2 infection spread throughout the world, starting initially in Wuhan, China at the end of 2019.[1] A global pandemic was declared by WHO on March 11, 2020, and continues at the time of the writing of this chapter. There have been numerous reviews, meta-analyses, and national registries that have collectively evaluated thousands of infected pregnant women with SARS-CoV-2, and in totality found that less than 5% result in congenital SARS-CoV-2 infection.[2,3,11–18] Currently, it is unclear what the exact timing of SARS-CoV-2 vertical transmission is.[19,20] Congenital SARS-CoV-2 infection can be acquired via vertical transmission (in utero) from an infected symptomatic or asymptomatic pregnant woman to neonate. Neonatal SARS-CoV-2 infection can also be acquired through intrapartum transmission, although it is quite rare. Finally, postpartum transmission seems to be the most common way of acquiring SARS-CoV-2.[19,20]

Question 2: What Are the Risk Factors for Neonatal Infection?

NEONATAL HSV DISEASE

The following five factors are known to influence transmission of HSV from mother to neonate:
1. Type of maternal infection (primary vs. recurrent)[21–25]
2. Maternal antibody status[25–28]
3. Duration of rupture of membranes[24]
4. Integrity of mucocutaneous barriers (e.g., use of fetal scalp electrodes)[11,29,30]
5. Mode of delivery (cesarean section vs. vaginal)[25]

Infants born to mothers who have a first episode of genital HSV infection near term are at much greater risk of developing neonatal herpes than are those whose mothers have recurrent genital herpes.[21–25] This increased risk is due both to lower concentrations of transplacentally passaged HSV-specific antibodies (which also are less reactive to expressed polypeptides) in women with primary infection,[27] and to the higher quantities of HSV that are shed for longer periods of time in the maternal genital tract when compared with women with recurrent genital HSV infection.[31]

The largest assessment of the influence of type of maternal infection on likelihood of neonatal transmission is a landmark study involving almost 6 women in labor who did not have clinical evidence of genital HSV infection, ~40,000 of whom had cultures performed within 48 hours of delivery (Fig. 12.1). Of these, 121 women were identified who both were asymptomatically shedding HSV and for whom sera were available for serologic analysis. In this large trial, 57% of infants delivered to women with first-episode primary infection developed neonatal HSV disease, compared with 25% of infants delivered to women with first-episode nonprimary infection and 2% of infants delivered to women with recurrent HSV disease (see Fig. 12.1).[25]

The duration of rupture of membranes and mode of delivery also appear to affect the risk for acquisition of neonatal infection. A small study published in 1971 demonstrated that cesarean delivery in a woman with active genital lesions can reduce the infant's risk of acquiring HSV if performed within 4 hours of rupture of membrane.[24] Based on this observation, it has been recommended for more than four decades that women with active genital lesions at the time of onset of labor be delivered by cesarean section.[32] It was not until 2003, however, that cesarean delivery was definitively proven to be effective in the prevention of HSV transmission to the neonate from a mother actively shedding virus from the genital tract.[25] Importantly, neonatal infection has occurred despite cesarean delivery performed before rupture of membranes.[33,34]

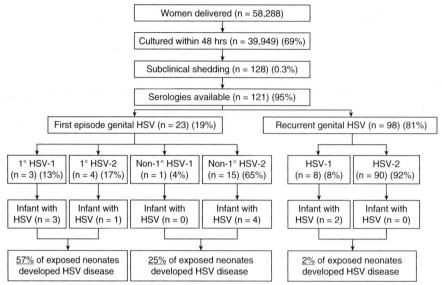

Fig. 12.1 Risk of neonatal herpes simplex virus *(HSV)* disease as a function of the type of maternal infection. *1°*, Primary infection. Data from Brown ZA, Wald A, Morrow RA, et al. Effect of serologic status and cesarean delivery on transmission rates of herpes simplex virus from mother to infant. *JAMA*. 2003;289(2):203-209.

CONGENITAL CMV INFECTION

Intrauterine infection usually is the result of a susceptible woman acquiring infection from a child in the family or from day care exposure early during her gestation.[35–37] Multiple studies in Sweden and the United States have shown that the rate of CMV infection is much higher in children who attend day care than those who do not.[36,38–40] Many initially seronegative children become infected with CMV from their day care peers. CMV infection then is transmitted horizontally from child to child, most likely through saliva on hands and toys.[41,42] Infected children excrete large amounts of CMV for extended periods of time, exposing parents and other caregivers who may become pregnant.

Maternal shedding of virus directly correlates with the risk of perinatal infection. Infected breast milk and exposure to CMV in the genital tract lead to high rates of peripartum and postnatal CMV transmission.[43] Infants who breastfeed from CMV-seropositive women have an estimated rate of infection between 39% and 59%. The risk is greater when the maternal viral load is higher than 7×10^3 genome equivalents/mL. Excretion of the virus in breast milk is greatest between 2 weeks and 2 months after birth. Infected

infants usually begin to excrete CMV between 3 weeks and 3 months after birth. Many of these infants excrete CMV chronically (for years), providing an opportunity to infect caretakers or others in contact with these children.

CONGENITAL ZIKA INFECTION

Zika virus is acquired by a pregnant woman in one of three ways:

1. The bite of an infected mosquito to a nonimmune pregnant woman
2. Sexual transmission from a carrier to a pregnant woman
3. Transfusion of an infected blood product[44]

The prevalence of Zika virus is related to the prevalence of the *Aedes aegypti* mosquito[44] and the proportion of seronegative hosts. The greatest risk of serious sequelae for the fetus occurs in the first or second trimester but has also been reported in the third trimester.[45] In a case series from Brazil, Zika virus caused adverse outcomes in 55% of infants when maternal infection occurred in the first trimester, in 52% of infants with maternal infection in the second trimester, and in 29% of infants with maternal infection in the third trimester.[19]

Congenital SARS-CoV-2 or Neonatal SARS-CoV-2

SARS-CoV-2 acquisition is possible via in utero transmission, peripartum transmission, or via postpartum transmission. Current data are insufficient to elucidate the effects of SARS-CoV-2 on the fetus in first-, second-, or third-trimester infections. Thus far, reports have been overwhelmingly from pregnant women infected in their third trimester and their fetal and neonatal outcomes in third trimester.[3,46] One retrospective cohort study with 882 infected pregnant women showed that a subset of women infected in first and second trimesters had an increased risk for preterm birth and stillbirth, but that a second subset was completely unaffected despite early gestation infection.[47] However, this study did not look at neonatal infections or maternal-to-fetal transmissions.[47] Another retrospective cohort study including 17 hospitals in the United States found that pregnant women with SARS-CoV-2 infection prior to 28 weeks of gestation had an increased risk of fetal or neonatal death or preterm birth at <37 weeks of gestation.[48] A systematic review including 936 neonates born to mothers with SARS-CoV-2 found only 3.2% rate of maternal-to-fetal transmission.[3] This rate was similar to positivity transmission rates in China (2%) where there were stringent precautions for babies born to infected mothers, and in studies done outside of China (3.5%).[49] Interestingly, in a national cohort study from Sweden which included 2323 neonates of infected mothers had only a 0.9% positivity rate, despite allowing rooming in of infant with mom, breastfeeding, and skin-to-skin.[12]

Question 3: What Are the Clinical Manifestations of Neonatal Infection and Disease?

NEONATAL HSV DISEASE

HSV infections acquired either peripartum or postpartum can be classified as (1) disseminated disease involving multiple visceral organs, including lung, liver, adrenal glands, skin, eye, and the brain (disseminated disease); (2) CNS disease, with or without skin lesions (CNS disease); and (3) disease limited to the skin, eyes, and/or mouth (SEM disease). This classification system is predictive of both morbidity and mortality.[50–54]

Neonatal HSV disseminated disease is manifest by hepatitis that can be very severe, disseminated intravascular coagulopathy, and pneumonitis. The mean age at presentation (±standard error [SE]) is 11.4 ± 0.8 days.[51] CNS involvement is a common component of this category of infection, occurring in about 60% to 75% of infants with disseminated disease.[55] Although the presence of a vesicular rash can greatly facilitate the diagnosis of HSV infection, more than 40% of neonates with disseminated HSV disease will not have cutaneous vesicles at the time of illness presentation.[33,51,56,57] Events associated with disseminated neonatal HSV infection that can result in death relate primarily to the severe coagulopathy, liver dysfunction, and pulmonary involvement of the disease.

Clinical manifestations of neonatal HSV CNS disease include seizures (both focal and generalized), lethargy, irritability, tremors, poor feeding, temperature instability, and bulging fontanelle. The mean age at presentation (±SE) is 19.7 ± 1.6 days.[51] Between 60% and 70% of infants classified as having CNS disease have associated skin vesicles at any point in the disease course.[51,56] With CNS neonatal HSV disease, mortality is usually the product of devastating brain destruction, with resulting acute neurologic and autonomic dysfunction.

SEM disease is the most favorable of the presenting categories of neonatal HSV infection. By definition, infection in infants with SEM disease has not progressed to multiorgan, visceral involvement and does not involve the CNS. Presenting signs and symptoms can include skin vesicles in approximately 80% of patients, fever, lethargy, and/or conjunctivitis.[51] The mean age at presentation (±SE) is 12.0 ± 2.2 days.[51] There is a high degree of likelihood that, in the absence of antiviral therapy, SEM disease will progress to one of the more severe categories of neonatal HSV infection.[33]

CONGENITAL CMV INFECTION

Congenital CMV infection is the most frequent known viral cause of mental retardation,[58] and is the leading nongenetic cause of neurosensory hearing loss in many countries including the United States.[59–61] It also is the most common congenital infection in humans, with approximately 0.5% of all live births in the United States involving CMV infection

(~20,000 infants per year).[62] CMV can be acquired in utero during any trimester of pregnancy.

Of the fetuses infected, approximately 10% will be symptomatic at birth, and ~20% of these patients will die in the neonatal period; of the survivors, 90% will have significant neurologic sequelae.[63–68] The majority of these infants will have sensorineural hearing loss (SNHL), mental retardation, microcephaly, seizures, and/or paresis/paralysis.[60,69–72] These impairments frequently result in spastic quadriplegia requiring lifelong dependence on a wheelchair, along with cognitive and speech impairments that dramatically limit their ability to interact with and function in the world. Between 25% and 40% of all childhood, SNHL is caused by intrauterine CMV infection.[73] Fetuses can be infected with CMV at any point throughout gestation. However, infections occurring earlier in gestation (first or early second trimesters) are more likely to result in severe forms of encephaloclastic injury.

Most infants (~90%) with congenital CMV infection have no detectable clinical abnormalities at birth (asymptomatic infection), and SNHL develops in about 10% of these children. Because most infants with congenital CMV have asymptomatic infection, approximately 70% of CMV-associated SNHL occurs in this group, even though the likelihood of sequelae in any given asymptomatically infected child is much lower than in a symptomatically infected child (Table 12.1).

CMV-associated SNHL is extremely variable with respect to the age of onset, laterality, degree of the deficit, and continued deterioration of the loss (progression) during early childhood.[59,70,72] About half of all children with CMV-associated SNHL have normal hearing at birth (delayed-onset SNHL) and therefore will not be detected by newborn hearing screening.[59] Delayed-onset SNHL, threshold fluctuations, and/or progressive loss of hearing are observed in both symptomatic and asymptomatic infections. The age of onset of delayed-onset SNHL can range from 6 to 197 months. However, the median age is 33 and 44 months for symptomatic and asymptomatic children, respectively.[59,70] Therefore, neither routine physical examination in the nursery nor newborn hearing screening will identify the majority of children with CMV-associated SNHL at birth.

TABLE 12.1   U.S. Public Health Impact of Congenital Cytomegalovirus Infection

	Estimated Number
No. of live births per year	4,000,000
Rate of congenital cytomegalovirus infection	1%
No. of infected infants	40,000
No. of infants symptomatic at birth (5%–7%)	2800
No. with fatal disease (±12%)	336
No. with sequelae (90% of survivors)	2160
No. of infants asymptomatic at birth (93%–95%)	37,200
No. with late sequelae (15%)	5580
Total no. with sequelae or fatal outcome	8076

From Dobbins JG, Stewart JA, Demmler GJ. Surveillance of congenital cytomegalovirus disease, 1990–1991. Collaborating Registry Group. *MMWR CDC Surveill Summ.* 1992;41(2):35-39.

The natural history of congenitally acquired CMV infection is well described.[59,63,70,74–77] In contrast, outcomes of perinatally and postnatally acquired CMV infections are less well characterized. It is generally agreed that postnatal acquisition of CMV in term infants does not lead to symptomatology or disease.[78] In preterm infants, initial case reports suggested that perinatally and postnatally acquired CMV infections could produce severe disease.[79–84] Larger series and case-controlled trials more recently suggest that symptomatic disease in preterm infants is less common than asymptomatic infection, and long-term sequelae are rare.[85–89] Nevertheless, severe disseminated CMV disease can occur in premature infants, including life-threatening pneumonitis, hepatitis, and thrombocytopenia.[90]

CONGENITAL ZIKA INFECTION

As with congenital CMV, congenital Zika infection can result in microcephaly, brain anomalies, and developmental delay.[91] In a review of 14 studies with radiologic assessment, the major findings in fetuses infected by Zika virus were ventriculomegaly in 33%, microcephaly in 24%, and intracranial calcifications in

27%.[91] There are multiple features of the congenital Zika virus syndrome, but the full spectrum of the syndrome is still under investigation.[92]

The principal clinical features of congenital Zika virus syndrome include microcephaly, facial dispro-portion, hypertonia/spasticity, hyperreflexia, and seizures.[92] Microcephaly is often a consequence of primary maternal infection in the first or second tri-mester. Microcephaly is defined by both the World Health Organization and the Centers for Disease Control and Prevention as an occipitofrontal circum-ference below the third percentile.[44] CNS abnormali-ties, positional abnormalities such as arthrogryposis, hearing loss, and ocular abnormalities are also pos-sible with congenital Zika infection. Finally, fetal loss, impaired fetal growth, and hydrops fetalis have also been reported in congenital Zika infection.[44]

Congenital SARS-CoV-2 or Neonatal SARS-CoV-2 Infection

Overall, neonates born to mothers with SARS-CoV-2 infection have fared well in most studies.[17,93] Some neonates are asymptomatic or present with mild symptoms such as cough, rhinorrhea, or fever.[4] Other symptoms have included respiratory distress, diar-rhea, lethargy, poor feeding, or even multiorgan failure requiring extracorporeal membrane oxygenation (ECMO). Lab findings range from leukocytosis, neu-tropenia, and thrombocytopenia, to nonspecific elevated inflammatory markers.[94] One retrospective cohort study found only 0.8% of neonates born to SARS-CoV-2-positive mothers tested positive after birth, but all were completely asymptomatic.[95] A large nationwide prospective cohort study in Sweden com-pared neonatal outcomes in 2323 neonates born to mothers with SARS-CoV2 with 9275 unexposed case-matched neonates, and found that maternal SARS-CoV-2 infection was associated with some poor neonatal outcomes.[12] These included respiratory dis-orders, NICU stays, preterm deliveries, and hyperbili-rubinemia. However, they were not associated with mortality or length of stay in NICU.[12] Several other studies also found significantly increased rates of pre-term deliveries.[11,13,14,17] One prospective web-based registry found that 9.3% of babies born to women

with SARS-CoV-2 infection during pregnancy were small for gestation age.[18] Additionally, it also found that 4.4% of all SARS-CoV-2-infected pregnancies were complicated by fetal growth restriction.[18] A review that included 52 studies looking at symptom-atic neonates with possible or confirmed vertical transmission of SARS-CoV-2 reported cases of pneumonia, encephalitic symptoms, hematologic abnormalities, prematurity, neurologic abnormalities including feeding difficulties, hypotonia, and leth-argy.[96] Another review looked at all possible neurode-velopmental sequelae of neonates born to mothers with SARS-CoV-2 infection during pregnancy and found a range of possible neurological findings, but no clear significant pattern of neurodevelopmental impairment.[97] As such, long-term follow-up studies will be needed to discern if SARS-CoV-2 during preg-nancy has an adverse effect on neurodevelopment of infants.[98]

Question 4: What Are the Treatments and Outcomes for HSV, CMV, Zika, and SARS-CoV-2 Virus Infections in Neonates?

NEONATAL HSV DISEASE

In the pre-antiviral era, 85% of patients with dissemi-nated neonatal HSV disease died by 1 year of age, as did 50% of patients with CNS neonatal HSV disease (Table 12.2).[54] Evaluations of two different doses of vidarabine and of a lower dose of acyclovir (30 mg/kg per day for 10 days) documented that both of these antiviral drugs reduce mortality to comparable de-grees,[52,54,99] with mortality rates at 1 year from dis-seminated disease decreasing to 54% and from CNS disease decreasing to 14% (see Table 12.2).[52] Despite its lack of therapeutic superiority, the lower dose of acyclovir quickly supplanted vidarabine as the treat-ment of choice for neonatal HSV disease because of its favorable safety profile and its ease of administration. Unlike acyclovir, vidarabine had to be administered over prolonged infusion times and in large volumes of fluid.

With utilization of a higher dose of acyclovir (60 mg/kg per day for 21 days), 12-month mortality is further reduced to 29% for disseminated neonatal HSV

TABLE 12.2   Mortality and Morbidity Outcomes Among 295 Infants With Neonatal HSV Infection, Evaluated by the National Institutes of Allergy and Infectious Diseases Collaborative Antiviral Study Group Between 1974 and 1997

	TREATMENT			
Extent of Disease	Placebo[39]	Vidarabine[37]	Acyclovir[37] (30 mg/kg per day)	Acyclovir[35] (60 mg/kg per day)
Disseminated disease	n = 13	n = 28	n = 18	n = 34
Dead	11 (85%)	14 (50%)	11 (61%)	10 (29%)
Alive	2 (15%)	14 (50%)	7 (39%)	24 (71%)
Normal	1 (50%)	7 (50%)	3 (43%)	15 (63%)
Abnormal	1 (50%)	5 (36%)	2 (29%)	3 (13%)
Unknown	0 (0%)	2 (14%)	2 (29%)	6 (25%)
Central nervous system infection	n = 6	n = 36	n = 35	n = 23
Dead	3 (50%)	5 (14%)	5 (14%)	1 (4%)
Alive	3 (50%)	31 (86%)	30 (86%)	22 (96%)
Normal	1 (33%)	13 (42%)	8 (27%)	4 (18%)
Abnormal	2 (67%)	17 (55%)	20 (67%)	9 (41%)
Unknown	0 (0%)	1 (3%)	2 (7%)	9 (41%)
Skin, eye, or mouth infection	n = 8	n = 31	n = 54	n = 9
Dead	0 (0%)	0 (0%)	0 (0%)	0 (0%)
Alive	8 (100%)	31 (100%)	54 (100%)	9 (100%)
Normal	5 (62%)	22 (71%)	45 (83%)	2 (22%)
Abnormal	3 (38%)	3 (10%)	1 (2%)	0 (0%)
Unknown	0 (0%)	6 (19%)	8 (15%)	7 (78%)

Adapted from Kimberlin DW. Advances in the treatment of neonatal herpes simplex infections. *Rev Med Virol.* 2001;11(3):157-163.

disease and to 4% for CNS HSV disease (Figs. 12.2 and 12.3, respectively).[50] Differences in mortality at 24 months among patients treated with the higher dose of acyclovir and the lower dose of acyclovir are statistically significant after stratification for disease category (CNS vs. disseminated; P = .0035; odds ratio = 3.3 with 95% confidence interval [CI] of 1.5–7.3).[50] Lethargy and severe hepatitis are associated with mortality among patients with disseminated disease, as are prematurity and seizures in patients with CNS disease.[51]

For neonates with disseminated or CNS neonatal HSV disease, improvements in morbidity rates with antiviral therapies have not been as dramatic as with mortality. In the pre-antiviral era, 50% of survivors of disseminated neonatal HSV infections were developing normally at 12 months of age (see Table 12.2).[54] With utilization of the higher dose of acyclovir for 21 days, this percentage has increased to 83% (Fig. 12.4).[50] In the case of CNS neonatal HSV disease, 33% of patients in the pre-antiviral era were developing normally at 12 months of age (see Table 12.2), whereas 31% of the recipients of the higher dose of acyclovir who develop normally at 12 months today (see Fig. 12.4).[50,54] A significant advance in outcomes from neonatal HSV CNS disease occurred with the determination by the CASG that oral acyclovir suppressive therapy for 6 months following acute parenteral treatment improves neurodevelopmental outcomes.[100] In

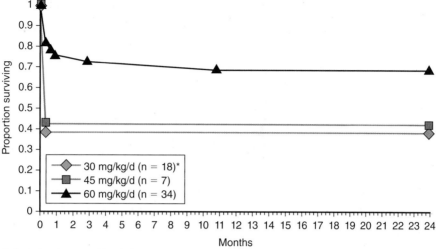

*indicate that these were historical controls

Fig. 12.2 Mortality in patients with disseminated neonatal herpes simplex virus disease. From Kimberlin DW, Lin CY, Jacobs RF, et al. Safety and efficacy of high-dose intravenous acyclovir in the management of neonatal herpes simplex virus infections. *Pediatrics.* 2001;108(2):230-238.

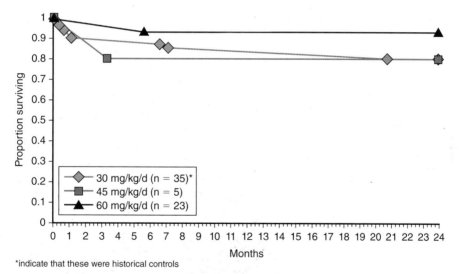

*indicate that these were historical controls

Fig. 12.3 Mortality in patients with central nervous system neonatal herpes simplex virus disease. From Kimberlin DW, Lin CY, Jacobs RF, et al. Safety and efficacy of high-dose intravenous acyclovir in the management of neonatal herpes simplex virus infections. *Pediatrics.* 2001;108(2):230-238.

this study involving infants with neonatal HSV with CNS involvement, Bayley developmental scores at 1 year of age were assessed in infants receiving 6 months of suppressive acyclovir therapy versus those receiving placebo. The acyclovir group had a significantly higher mean Bayley score than the placebo group (88.24 vs. 68.12, P = .046),[101] indicating

improved developmental outcomes in the suppression group (see Fig. 12.4). Suppressive acyclovir therapy also prevents skin recurrences in any classification of HSV disease.[101] Seizures at or before the time of initiation of antiviral therapy are associated with increased risk of morbidity both in patients with CNS disease and in patients with disseminated infection.[51]

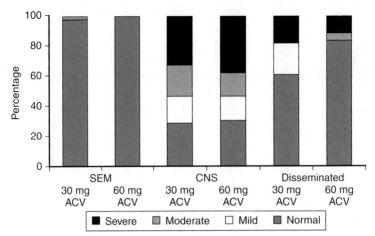

Fig. 12.4 Morbidity among patients with known outcomes after 12 months of life. *CNS*, Central nervous system; *SEM*, skin, eyes, and/or mouth. Adapted from Kimberlin DW, Whitley RJ, Wan W, et al. Oral acyclovir suppression and neurodevelopment after neonatal herpes. *N Engl J Med.* 2011;365(14):1284-1292.

Unlike disseminated or CNS neonatal HSV disease, morbidity following SEM disease has dramatically improved during the antiviral era. Before the use of antiviral therapies, 38% of SEM patients experienced developmental difficulties at 12 months of age (see Table 12.2).[54] With vidarabine and lower-dose acyclovir, these percentages were reduced to 12% and 2%, respectively.[52] In the high-dose acyclovir study, no SEM patients developed neurologic sequelae at 12 months of life (see Fig. 12.4).[50]

Infants with neonatal HSV disease should be treated with intravenous (IV) acyclovir at a dose of 60 mg/kg per day delivered intravenously in 3 divided daily doses.[35,102] The dosing interval of intravenous acyclovir may need to be increased in premature infants based on their creatinine clearance.[103] Duration of therapy is 21 days for patients with disseminated or CNS neonatal HSV disease and 14 days for patients with HSV infection limited to the SEM.[102] All patients with CNS HSV involvement should have a repeat lumbar puncture at the end of intravenous acyclovir therapy to determine that the CSF specimen is polymerase chain reaction (PCR)-negative in a reliable laboratory and to document the end-of-therapy CSF indices.[51] Those persons who remain PCR-positive should continue to receive intravenous antiviral therapy until PCR negativity is achieved.[51,104] Following treatment of the acute infection, all infants with any disease classification of neonatal HSV should receive oral acyclovir at 300 mg/m^2 per dose three times daily as suppressive therapy for 6 months.[89]

The primary apparent toxicity associated with the use of intravenous acyclovir administered at 60 mg/kg per day is neutropenia, with approximately one-fifth of patients developing an absolute neutrophil count (ANC) of 1000/μL or lower.[50] Although the neutropenia resolves either during continuation of intravenous acyclovir or following its cessation, it is prudent to monitor neutrophil counts at least twice weekly throughout the course of intravenous acyclovir therapy, with consideration given to decreasing the dose of acyclovir or administering granulocyte colony-stimulating factor if the ANC remains below 500/μL for a prolonged period.[50] Absolute neutrophil counts should be monitored at 2 and 4 weeks after starting oral suppressive therapy and then monthly thereafter while oral acyclovir is administered.[89]

CONGENITAL CMV INFECTION

Administration of antiviral therapy with parenteral ganciclovir or oral valganciclovir beginning within the first month of life improves audiologic and developmental outcomes among patients with symptomatic congenital CMV disease.[100,105] From 1991 through 1999, 100 patients with symptomatic congenital CMV disease involving the CNS were enrolled in a pivotal CASG study. Patients were randomly assigned to ganciclovir treatment (6 mg/kg per dose administered intravenously every 12 hours for 6 weeks) or to no treatment.[105] Infants in the no-treatment arm were managed in a fashion identical to those receiving active drug. This study demonstrated that a relatively short duration of therapy of 6 weeks provides benefit in protection against worsening of hearing during the first 2 years of life. Denver developmental assessments were performed during the conduct of the ganciclovir study, and post hoc blinded analysis of the results demonstrated that patients receiving 6 weeks of intravenous ganciclovir experienced fewer developmental delays at 6 months and 12 months of age,[106] suggesting there may be a neurodevelopmental benefit to antiviral therapy as well.

Following this pivotal trial, the CASG conducted a phase I/II pharmacokinetic/pharmacodynamic investigation of oral valganciclovir in infants with symptomatic congenital CMV disease.[107] This study identified the oral dose of valganciclovir of 16 mg/kg per dose administered twice daily as that which reliably achieves the same ganciclovir blood concentrations as the previously studied intravenous ganciclovir dose of 6 mg/kg per dose administered every 12 hours. It was this dose that then was taken into a large phase III trial of 6 weeks versus 6 months of oral valganciclovir for the treatment of infants with symptomatic congenital CMV disease.[100] Best-ear hearing outcomes at 6 months were similar for the groups ($P = .41$). Total-ear hearing was more likely to be improved or remain normal at 12 months in the 6-month group (73.4%) versus the 6-week group (57.1%) ($P = .01$). Benefit in total-ear hearing was maintained at 24 months (77.1% vs. 63.8%, respectively; $P = .04$). The 6-month group had higher Bayley-III Language Composite (84.6 ± 2.9 vs. 72.5 ± 2.9, $P < .01$) and Receptive Communication Scale (7.3 ± 0.5 vs. 5.2 ± 0.5, $P < .01$) neurodevelopmental scores at 24 months. Grade 3 or 4 neutropenia occurred in 19.3% during the first 6 weeks, and 21.3% (6-month group) versus 26.5% (6-week group) during the next 4.5 months of treatment ($P = .64$). As a consequence of this study, the standard duration of treatment of infants with symptomatic congenital CMV disease now is 6 months.[108] Antiviral therapy must be started within the first month of life when used to affect hearing and developmental outcomes in this population. Antiviral therapy now is being studied in the asymptomatic congenital CMV population as well, but there currently are no data to justify its use in that group.

CONGENITAL ZIKA INFECTION

There currently are no antiviral therapeutic options for congenital Zika infection. All management is supportive.[109] Medical management of seizures, spasticity, and hearing loss are all routine parts of newborn follow-ups of infants affected by congenital Zika infection.[109] Further studies and investigations are currently underway to look for potential vaccines or treatments.

CONGENITAL SARS-COV-2 OR NEONATAL SARS-COV-2 INFECTION

Currently, neonates infected with COVID-19 are mostly managed with supportive care, including supplemental oxygen, respiratory support, temperature control, and fluid resuscitation.[4] Currently, evidence for the use of antiviral medications and steroids in neonatal COVID-19 is lacking but have been used in a few emergency cases.[110,111] Remdesivir is an inhibitor of the viral RNA-dependent RNA polymerase, and inhibits viral replication by terminating RNA transcription.[112] It has in vitro inhibitory activity against SARS-CoV-1 and the Middle East respiratory syndrome (MERS-CoV), which has been used in adults and older children requiring oxygen.[112] Remdesevir use has been reported in several newborns, and it is currently being studied in a pharmacokinetic and safety study sponsored by its manufacturer, Gilead. A recent study by Tavakoli et al. found that neonates whose mothers did not receive remdesivir had a higher rate of positive PCR for SARS-CoV-2 after delivery, indicating a higher risk of vertical transmission in babies of SARS-CoV-2-positive mothers without remdesivir treatment.[113] Vaccines are not currently available for neonates, but are able to be given to infants 6 months and older. Of note, after COVID-19 vaccines became available for pregnant women, studies found that vaccinated pregnant women had decreased rates of maternal SARS-CoV-2 infection and had decreased severity of illness, when infected.[114] Studies have also reported no adverse outcomes for neonates of vaccinated mothers.[114] Additionally, babies born to vaccinated mothers can be protected from COVID-19 due to the passage of antibodies against

SARS-CoV-2 from the mother to the fetus via the umbilical cord, in utero.[114]

Question 5: Do All Infants With HSV, CMV, Zika, and SARS-CoV-2 Infections Have to Be Treated?

NEONATAL HSV DISEASE

Yes. Neonatal HSV disease has significant mortality and morbidity, and all affected infants require parenteral acyclovir therapy.

CONGENITAL CMV INFECTION

No. Antiviral therapy administered for 6 months improves audiologic and developmental outcomes for infants with symptomatic congenital CMV disease with or without CNS involvement. However, the toxicities from the therapy are not inconsequential, and the degree of benefit is modest. Therefore antiviral therapy should be considered for the management of symptomatic congenital CMV disease,[108] but managing physicians and families could opt to not treat in some cases.[108]

CONGENITAL ZIKA INFECTION

Not applicable. With no current treatment, antiviral therapy of congenital Zika infection is not feasible at this time. However, multiple follow-up visits and medical management of sequelae are necessary parts of the syndrome management and treatment.[109]

CONGENITAL SARS-COV-2

Not applicable, since there is no FDA approved or authorized treatment currently available for congenital SARS-CoV-2 infection. Currently, treatment is supportive, with studies underway of remdesivir antiviral treatment.

Question 6: What Is the Appropriate Diagnostic Approach to an Infant in Whom HSV, CMV, Congenital Zika, or Congenital SARS-CoV-2 Infection Is Suspected?

NEONATAL HSV DISEASE

For diagnosis of neonatal HSV infection, the following specimens should be obtained: (1) swabs of the mouth, nasopharynx, conjunctivae, and rectum ("surface cultures") for HSV PCR and culture; (2) specimens of skin vesicles and CSF for HSV PCR and culture; (3) whole blood for HSV PCR; and (4) whole blood for alanine aminotransferase.[102] Positive cultures obtained from any of the surface sites more than 12 to 24 hours after birth indicate viral replication, and therefore are suggestive of infant infection rather than merely contamination after intrapartum exposure. As with any PCR assay, false-negative and false-positive results can occur. The presence of red blood cells in spinal fluid historically has been associated with HSV CNS infections. The data suggesting this association are older and reflect a time when the hemorrhagic encephalitis produced by HSV was more advanced at the time of diagnosis. As a consequence of enhanced appreciation for HSV CNS infections and of rapid diagnostic testing such as PCR, most CNS HSV infections today do not have a significant amount of blood in the CSF. Whole blood PCR may be of benefit in the diagnosis of neonatal HSV disease, but its use should not supplant the standard workup of such patients (which includes surface cultures and CSF PCR); no data exist to support use of serial blood PCR assay to monitor response to therapy. Rapid diagnostic techniques also are available, such as direct fluorescent antibody staining of vesicle scrapings or enzyme immunoassay detection of HSV antigens. These techniques are as specific but slightly less sensitive than culture. Typing HSV strains differentiates between HSV-1 and HSV-2 isolates. Radiographs and clinical manifestations can suggest HSV pneumonitis, and elevated transaminase values can suggest HSV hepatitis; both are seen commonly in neonatal HSV disseminated disease. Histologic examination of lesions for the presence of multinucleated giant cells and eosinophilic intranuclear inclusions typical of HSV (e.g., with Tzanck test) has low sensitivity and should not be performed.

Serologic diagnosis of neonatal HSV infection is not of clinical value. The presence of transplacentally acquired maternal IgG confounds the assessment of the neonatal antibody status during acute infection, especially given the large proportions of the adult American population who are HSV-1- and HSV-2-seropositive. Serial antibody assessment may be useful in the very specific circumstance of a mother who has a primary infection late in gestation and transfers very little or no antibody to the fetus. In general, however, serologic studies play no role in the diagnosis of neonatal HSV disease.

CONGENITAL CMV INFECTION

Proof of congenital infection requires detection of CMV from urine, stool, respiratory tract secretions, or CSF obtained within 2 to 4 weeks of birth.[108] The sensitivity of CMV DNA detection by PCR of dried blood spots is low,[115] limiting use of this type of specimen for widespread screening for congenital CMV. A positive PCR result from a neonatal dried blood spot confirms congenital infection, but a negative result does not rule out congenital infection. Saliva PCR is emerging as the gold standard approach to the diagnosis of congenital CMV infection.[116] Differentiation between intrauterine and perinatal infection is difficult later than 2 to 4 weeks of age unless clinical manifestations of the former, such as chorioretinitis or intracranial calcifications, are present.

CONGENITAL ZIKA INFECTION

Proof of congenital Zika virus infection requires suspicion for Zika clinically as well as knowledge of confirmed Zika infection in the mother. Confirmation by laboratory evidence of maternal infection is accomplished by positive real-time reverse transcription (rRT)-PCR findings in any clinical specimen or positive Zika virus IgM with confirmatory neutralizing antibody titers from the mother.[109]

An infant suspected of having Zika should have samples collected within 2 days of birth. These samples include serum and urine for Zika virus ribonucleic acid (RNA) via PCR and serum Zika virus IgM enzyme-linked immunosorbent assay. CSF testing can be done for these as well but are not required for the diagnosis of Zika.[109] A false-positive IgM test result can be ruled out by performing the plaque reduction neutralization test (PRNT). This test measures virus-specific neutralizing antibodies. A false-negative PCR result is possible and does not exclude infection because viremia can be transient.[117] A positive IgM test rest with a negative PCR result would suggest Zika infection. However, if both are negative congenital infection can be excluded.

CONGENITAL SARS-COV-2 OR NEONATAL SARS-COV-2 INFECTION

In order to diagnose an infant with SARS-CoV-2, first a mother must be diagnosed with a positive SAR-CoV-2 RNA virologically (by nucleic acid amplification, antigen detection, etc.).[118] Sample for of SARS-CoV-2 RNA can be collected using nasopharynx, oropharynx, or nasal swab samples. Per CDC guidelines, symptomatic and asymptomatic neonates born to mothers with suspected or confirmed COVID-19 should have testing performed at approximately 24 hours of age. If initial test results are negative, or not available, testing should be repeated at 48 hours of age. If a neonate is asymptomatic and expected to be discharged at less than 48 hours of age, a test can be performed prior to discharge, between 24 and 48 hours of age.[118]

Question 7: How Should You Monitor the Response to Treatment?

NEONATAL HSV DISEASE

The primary measure of responsiveness to therapy is clinical improvement in the patient. All patients with CNS HSV involvement should have a repeat lumbar puncture at the end of intravenous acyclovir therapy to determine that the CSF specimen is PCR-negative in a reliable laboratory, and to document the end-of-therapy CSF indices.[51] Those persons who remain PCR-positive should continue to receive intravenous antiviral therapy until PCR negativity is achieved.[51,104] There are no data correlating clearance or persistence of HSV DNA in blood with clinical outcomes. Therefore serial blood PCR measurements of HSV DNA in blood are not recommended to establish response to antiviral therapy or to guide determinations regarding the appropriate time to discontinue therapy.

CONGENITAL CMV INFECTION

Although great deal of work is being performed in this area, at the current time there are no biomarkers that are clearly established for predicting audiologic outcomes in infants with congenital CMV infection.[76,77,119–122] Therefore, treatment duration should be based on the period established in the most recent controlled study (6 months) rather than on other measures of possible response to therapy such as serial blood PCR measurements of CMV DNA.

CONGENITAL ZIKA INFECTION

Because there is no current treatment for Zika virus, management of patients with Zika infection is purely supportive through medical management of individual symptoms.

CONGENITAL SARS-COV-2 INFECTION

Management of neonates with SARS-CoV-2 infection is mainly supportive and through medical management, as no approved treatment is yet available.

Question 8: What Are the Biggest Gaps in Our Current Understanding of the Natural History, Diagnosis, and Management of These Infections?

NEONATAL HSV DISEASE

The duration of parenteral therapy for neonatal HSV disease is well established at 14 (SEM disease) or 21 (CNS or disseminated disease) days. The CASG's randomized controlled trial of oral acyclovir suppression following parenteral therapy proved that such additional treatment improves outcomes further, suggesting that subclinical viral reactivation is occurring in the brain of affected infants. Understanding the full scope of this treatment is a major unmet need at this time. Additional gaps in our knowledge of neonatal HSV disease relate to detection of HSV DNA in whole blood, both for diagnosis of infection and for assessment of treatment efficacy over time.

CONGENITAL CMV INFECTION

There is a tremendous unmet need in the identification of biomarkers (either host or virus) that will predict who is at highest risk of sequelae from congenital CMV infection, especially asymptomatic infection. These will allow more targeted therapeutic approaches in patients with the highest risks of detrimental outcomes.

CONGENITAL ZIKA INFECTION

Unlike CMV and HSV, there is a tremendous amount of information currently unknown about Zika. This lack is likely due to the relatively recent nature of the Zika epidemic in the Americas, the lack of large clinical studies or case studies on the topic, the geographic areas affected by Zika transmission, and the (fortunate) decline in Zika cases following 2016. Even the exact definition of congenital Zika virus syndrome is still under development as more cases with different manifestations continue to be recognized.

CONGENITAL SARS-COV-2 OR NEONATAL SARS-COV-2 INFECTION

As with Zika, there is a very large information gap regarding SARS-CoV-2 infections in neonates, as well as its effects in utero from infection in a pregnant woman. As with Zika, there is no true definition or disease form yet of a congenital SARS-CoV-2 syndrome. Finally, as new variants continue to emerge during this pandemic, new information is likely to be reported.

Conclusions

An impressive amount of knowledge has been amassed over the past three decades about the pathogenesis, diagnosis, and treatment of congenital CMV infection and neonatal HSV disease. Management recommendations have been standardized and broadly implemented. The degree of distance traveled in our knowledge of neonatal HSV and congenital CMV infections can be seen in the Zika virus epidemic. The SARS-CoV-2 pandemic has been especially novel, though, particularly since a respiratory pathogen previously had not been known to cause congenital infections. Over time, we undoubtedly will increase our understanding of the extent and pathogenesis of congenital Zika and congenital and perinatal SARS-CoV-2 infections, and hopefully we will have a therapeutic drug or effective vaccine to manage and prevent infections from affecting the most vulnerable among us—namely neonates and infants. Frontiers will continue to be advanced as new therapeutic options and modalities are identified.

REFERENCES

1. American Academy of Pediatrics. Coronaviruses, including SARS-CoV-2 and MERS-CoV. In: Kimberlin DW, Barnett ED, Lynfield R, Sawyer MH, eds. *Red Book: 2021–2024 Report of the Committee on Infectious Diseases*. 32nd ed. Itasca, IL: American Academy of Pediatrics; 2021:281-285.

2. Kyle MH, Hussain M, Saltz V, Mollicone I, Bence M, Dumitriu D. Vertical transmission and neonatal outcomes following maternal SARS-CoV-2 infection during pregnancy. *Clin Obstet Gynecol*. 2022;65(1):195-202.
3. Kotlyar AM, Grechukhina O, Chen A, et al. Vertical transmission of coronavirus disease 2019: a systematic review and meta-analysis. *Am J Obstet Gynecol*. 2021;224:35.e3-53.e3.
4. Sankaran D, Nakra N, Cheema R, Blumberg D, Lakshminrusimha S. Perinatal SARS-CoV-2 infection and neonatal COVID-19: a 2021 update. *Neoreviews*. 2021;22(5):e284-e295.
5. Whitley RJ, Roizman B. Herpes simplex virus infections. *Lancet*. 2001;357:1513-1518.
6. Schopfer K, Lauber E, Krech U. Congenital cytomegalovirus infection in newborn infants of mothers infected before pregnancy. *Arch Dis Child*. 1978;53:536-539.
7. Stagno S, Reynolds DW, Huang ES, et al. Congenital cytomegalovirus infection. *N Engl J Med*. 1977;296:1254-1258.
8. Boppana SB, Rivera LB, Fowler KB, et al. Intrauterine transmission of cytomegalovirus to infants of women with preconceptional immunity. *N Engl J Med*. 2001;344:1366-1371.
9. Stagno S, Pass RF, Dworsky ME, et al. Maternal cytomegalovirus infection and perinatal transmission. *Clin Obstet Gynecol*. 1982;25:563-576.
10. Brasil P, Pereira Jr JP, Moreira ME, et al. Zika virus infection in pregnant women in Rio de Janeiro. *N Engl J Med*. 2016;375:2321-2334.
11. Mullins E, Hudak ML, Banerjee J, et al. Pregnancy and neonatal outcomes of COVID-19: coreporting of common outcomes from PAN-COVID and AAP-SONPM registries. *Ultrasound Obstet Gynecol*. 2021;57:573-581.
12. Norman M, Navér L, Söderling J, et al. Association of maternal SARS-CoV-2 infection in pregnancy with neonatal outcomes. *JAMA*. 2021;325:2076-2086.
13. Dhir SK, Kumar J, Meena J, et al. Clinical features and outcome of SARS-CoV-2 infection in neonates: a systematic review. *J Trop Pediatr*. 2021;67:fmaa059.
14. Jafari M, Pormohammad A, Sheikh Neshin SA, et al. Clinical characteristics and outcomes of pregnant women with COVID-19 and comparison with control patients: a systematic review and meta-analysis. *Rev Med Virol*. 2021;31:e2208.
15. Dumitriu D, Emeruwa UN, Hanft E, et al. Outcomes of neonates born to mothers with severe acute respiratory syndrome coronavirus 2 infection at a large medical center in New York City. *JAMA Pediatr*. 2021;175:157-167.
16. Kyle MH, Glassman ME, Khan A, et al. A review of newborn outcomes during the COVID-19 pandemic. *Semin Perinatol*. 2020;44:151286.
17. Masoumeh S, Nazarpour S, Sheidaie A. Evaluation of pregnancy outcomes in mothers with COVID-19 infection: a systematic review and meta-analysis. *J Obstet Gynaecol*. 2023;43(1):2162867. doi:10.1080/01443615.2022.2162867.
18. Mullins E, Perry A, Banerjee J, et al. PAN-COVID Investigators. Pregnancy and neonatal outcomes of COVID-19: The PAN-COVID study. *Eur J Obstet Gynecol Reprod Biol*. 2022;276:161-167. doi:10.1016/j.ejogrb.2022.07.010.
19. WHO Team (Sexual and Reproductive Health and Research, WHO Headquarters). *Definition and Categorisation of the Timing of Mother-to-Child Transmission of SARS-CoV-2*. WHO Scientific Brief. 2021;1. Available at: https://apps.who.int/iris/handle/10665/339422.
20. Grünebaum A, Dudenhausen J, Chervenak FA. Covid and pregnancy in the United States—an update as of August 2022. *J Perinat Med*. 2023;51(1):34-38. doi:10.1515/jpm-2022-0361.
21. Brown ZA, Benedetti J, Ashley R, et al. Neonatal herpes simplex virus infection in relation to asymptomatic maternal infection at the time of labor. *N Engl J Med*. 1991;324:1247-1252.
22. Brown ZA, Vontver LA, Benedetti J, et al. Effects on infants of a first episode of genital herpes during pregnancy. *N Engl J Med*. 1987;317:1246-1251.
23. Corey L, Wald A. Genital herpes. In: Holmes KK, Sparling PF, Mardh PA, et al., eds. *Sex Transm Dis*. 3rd ed. New York: McGraw-Hill; 1999:285-312.
24. Nahmias AJ, Josey WE, Naib ZM, et al. Perinatal risk associated with maternal genital herpes simplex virus infection. *Am J Obstet Gynecol*. 1971;110:825-837.
25. Brown ZA, Wald A, Morrow RA, et al. Effect of serologic status and cesarean delivery on transmission rates of herpes simplex virus from mother to infant. *JAMA*. 2003;289:203-209.
26. Yeager AS, Arvin AM. Reasons for the absence of a history of recurrent genital infections in mothers of neonates infected with herpes simplex virus. *Pediatrics*. 1984;73:188-193.
27. Prober CG, Sullender WM, Yasukawa LL, et al. Low risk of herpes simplex virus infections in neonates exposed to the virus at the time of vaginal delivery to mothers with recurrent genital herpes simplex virus infections. *N Engl J Med*. 1987;316:240-244.
28. Yeager AS, Arvin AM, Urbani LJ, et al. Relationship of antibody to outcome in neonatal herpes simplex virus infections. *Infect Immun*. 1980;29:532-538.
29. Parvey LS, Ch'ien LT. Neonatal herpes simplex virus infection introduced by fetal-monitor scalp electrodes. *Pediatrics*. 1980;65:1150-1153.
30. Kaye EM, Dooling EC. Neonatal herpes simplex meningoencephalitis associated with fetal monitor scalp electrodes. *Neurology*. 1981;31:1045-1047.
31. Whitley RJ. Herpes simplex viruses. In: Fields BN, Knipe DM, Howley PM, et al., eds. *Fields Virology*. 3rd ed. Philadelphia: Lippincott-Raven Publishers; 1996:2297-2342.
32. Anonymous. ACOG practice bulletin. Management of herpes in pregnancy. Number 8 October 1999. Clinical management guidelines for obstetrician-gynecologists. *Int J Gynaecol Obstet*. 2000;68:165-173.
33. Whitley RJ, Corey L, Arvin A, et al. Changing presentation of herpes simplex virus infection in neonates. *J Infect Dis*. 1988;158:109-116.
34. Peng J, Krause PJ, Kresch M. Neonatal herpes simplex virus infection after cesarean section with intact amniotic membranes. *J Perinatol*. 1996;16:397-399.
35. Taber LH, Frank AL, Yow MD, et al. Acquisition of cytomegaloviral infections in families with young children: a serological study. *J Infect Dis*. 1985;151:948-952.
36. Pass RF, August AM, Dworsky M, et al. Cytomegalovirus infection in day-care center. *N Engl J Med*. 1982;307:477-479.
37. Pass RF, Hutto C, Ricks R, et al. Increased rate of cytomegalovirus infection among parents of children attending day-care centers. *N Engl J Med*. 1986;314:1414-1418.
38. Adler SP. The molecular epidemiology of cytomegalovirus transmission among children attending a day care center. *J Infect Dis*. 1985;152:760-768.
39. Hutto C, Ricks R, Garvie M, et al. Epidemiology of cytomegalovirus infections in young children: day care vs. home care. *Pediatr Infect Dis*. 1985;4:149-152.
40. Pass RF, Little EA, Stagno S, et al. Young children as a probable source of maternal and congenital cytomegalovirus infection. *N Engl J Med*. 1987;316:1366-1370.

41. Hutto C, Little EA, Ricks R, et al. Isolation of cytomegalovirus from toys and hands in a day care center. *J Infect Dis.* 1986;154: 527-530.

42. Faix RG. Survival of cytomegalovirus on environmental surfaces. *J Pediatr.* 1985;106:649-652.

43. Stagno S, Reynolds DW, Pass RF, et al. Breast milk and the risk of cytomegalovirus infection. *N Engl J Med.* 1980;302:1073-1076.

44. Rasmussen SA, Jamieson DJ, Honein MA, et al. Zika virus and birth defects—reviewing the evidence for causality. *N Engl J Med.* 2016;374:1981-1987.

45. Pacheco O, Beltran M, Nelson CA, et al. Zika virus disease in Colombia—preliminary report. *N Engl J Med.* 2016;383: e44(1–10).

46. Sturrock S, Ali S, Gale C, et al. Neonatal outcomes and indirect consequences following maternal SARS-CoV-2 infection in pregnancy: a systematic review. *BMJ Open.* 2023;13(3):e063052. doi:10.1136/bmjopen-2022-063052.

47. Piekos SN, Roper RT, Hwang YM, et al. The effect of maternal SARS-CoV-2 infection timing on birth outcomes: a retrospective multicentre cohort study. *Lancet Digit Health.* 2022;4(2): e95-e104.

48. Hughes BL, Sandoval GJ, Metz TD, et al. First- or second-trimester SARS-CoV-2 infection and subsequent pregnancy outcomes. *Am J Obstet Gynecol.* 2023;228(2):226.e1-226.e9. doi:10.1016/j.ajog.2022.08.009.

49. Fang F, Chen Y, Zhao D, et al. Recommendations for the diagnosis, prevention, and control of coronavirus disease-19 in children—the Chinese perspectives. *Front Pediatr.* 2020;8:553394.

50. Kimberlin DW, Lin CY, Jacobs RF, et al. Safety and efficacy of high-dose intravenous acyclovir in the management of neonatal herpes simplex virus infections. *Pediatrics.* 2001;108:230-238.

51. Kimberlin DW, Lin CY, Jacobs RF, et al. Natural history of neonatal herpes simplex virus infections in the acyclovir era. *Pediatrics.* 2001;108:223-229.

52. Whitley R, Arvin A, Prober C, et al. A controlled trial comparing vidarabine with acyclovir in neonatal herpes simplex virus infection. *N Engl J Med.* 1991;324:444-449.

53. Whitley R, Arvin A, Prober C, et al. Predictors of morbidity and mortality in neonates with herpes simplex virus infections. *N Engl J Med.* 1991;324:450-454.

54. Whitley RJ, Nahmias AJ, Soong SJ, et al. Vidarabine therapy of neonatal herpes simplex virus infection. *Pediatrics.* 1980;66: 495-501.

55. Whitley RJ. Herpes simplex virus infections. In: Remington JS, Klein JO, eds. *Infectious Diseases of the Fetus and Newborn Infants.* 3rd ed. Philadelphia: WB Saunders Company; 1990:282-305.

56. Sullivan-Bolyai JZ, Hull HF, Wilson C, et al. Presentation of neonatal herpes simplex virus infections: implications for a change in therapeutic strategy. *Pediatr Infect Dis.* 1986;5:309-314.

57. Arvin AM, Yeager AS, Bruhn FW, et al. Neonatal herpes simplex infection in the absence of mucocutaneous lesions. *J Pediatr.* 1982;100:715-721.

58. Elek SD, Stern H. Development of a vaccine against mental retardation caused by cytomegalovirus infection in utero. *Lancet.* 1974;1:1-5.

59. Fowler KB, McCollister FP, Dahle AJ, et al. Progressive and fluctuating sensorineural hearing loss in children with asymptomatic congenital cytomegalovirus infection. *J Pediatr.* 1997;130:624-630.

60. Harris S, Ahlfors K, Ivarsson S, et al. Congenital cytomegalovirus infection and sensorineural hearing loss. *Ear Hear.* 1984; 5:352-355.

61. Fowler KB, Dahle AJ, Boppana SB, et al. Newborn hearing screening: will children with hearing loss caused by congenital cytomegalovirus infection be missed? *J Pediatr.* 1999;135:60-64.

62. Demmler GJ. Infectious Diseases Society of America and Centers for Disease Control. Summary of a workshop on surveillance for congenital cytomegalovirus disease. *Rev Infect Dis.* 1991;13:315-329.

63. Stagno S, Whitley RJ. Herpesvirus infections of pregnancy. Part I: cytomegalovirus and Epstein-Barr virus infections. *N Engl J Med.* 1985;313:1270-1274.

64. McCracken Jr GH, Shinefield HM, Cobb K, et al. Congenital cytomegalic inclusion disease. A longitudinal study of 20 patients. *Am J Dis Child.* 1969;117:522-539.

65. Pass RF, Stagno S, Myers GJ, et al. Outcome of symptomatic congenital cytomegalovirus infection: results of long-term longitudinal follow-up. *Pediatrics.* 1980;66:758-762.

66. Weller TH. The cytomegaloviruses: ubiquitous agents with protean clinical manifestations. I. *N Engl J Med.* 1971;285: 203-214.

67. Weller TH, Hanshaw JB. Virologic and clinical observations on cytomegalic inclusion disease. *N Engl J Med.* 1962;266: 1233-1244.

68. Conboy TJ, Pass RF, Stagno S, et al. Early clinical manifestations and intellectual outcome in children with symptomatic congenital cytomegalovirus infection. *J Pediatr.* 1987;111:343-348.

69. Ahlfors K, Ivarsson SA, Harris S. Report on a long-term study of maternal and congenital cytomegalovirus infection in Sweden. Review of prospective studies available in the literature. *Scand J Infect Dis.* 1999;31:443-457.

70. Dahle AJ, Fowler KB, Wright JD, et al. Longitudinal investigation of hearing disorders in children with congenital cytomegalovirus. *J Am Acad Audiol.* 2000;11:283-290.

71. Williamson WD, Desmond MM, LaFevers N, et al. Symptomatic congenital cytomegalovirus. Disorders of language, learning, and hearing. *Am J Dis Child.* 1982;136:902-905.

72. Williamson WD, Percy AK, Yow MD, et al. Asymptomatic congenital cytomegalovirus infection. Audiologic, neuroradiologic, and neurodevelopmental abnormalities during the first year. *Am J Dis Child.* 1990;144:1365-1368.

73. Morton CC, Nance WE. Newborn hearing screening—a silent revolution. *N Engl J Med.* 2006;354:2151-2164.

74. Boppana SB, Fowler KB, Vaid Y, et al. Neuroradiographic findings in the newborn period and long-term outcome in children with symptomatic congenital cytomegalovirus infection. *Pediatrics.* 1997;99:409-414.

75. Boppana SB, Pass RF, Britt WJ, et al. Symptomatic congenital cytomegalovirus infection: neonatal morbidity and mortality. *Pediatr Infect Dis J.* 1992;11:93-99.

76. Fowler KB, Boppana SB. Congenital cytomegalovirus (CMV) infection and hearing deficit. *J Clin Virol.* 2006;35:226-231.

77. Rivera LB, Boppana SB, Fowler KB, et al. Predictors of hearing loss in children with symptomatic congenital cytomegalovirus infection. *Pediatrics.* 2002;110:762-767.

78. Stronati M, Lombardi G, Di Comite A, et al. Breastfeeding and cytomegalovirus infections. *J Chemother.* 2007;19(suppl 2): 49-51.

79. Vochem M, Hamprecht K, Jahn G, et al. Transmission of cytomegalovirus to preterm infants through breast milk. *Pediatr Infect Dis J.* 1998;17:53-58.

80. Maschmann J, Hamprecht K, Dietz K, et al. Cytomegalovirus infection of extremely low-birth weight infants via breast milk. *Clin Infect Dis.* 2001;33:1998-2003.

81. Takahashi R, Tagawa M, Sanjo M, et al. Severe postnatal cytomegalovirus infection in a very premature infant. *Neonatology.* 2007;92:236-239.

82. Vancikova Z, Kucerova T, Pelikan L, et al. Perinatal cytomegalovirus hepatitis: to treat or not to treat with ganciclovir. *J Paediatr Child Health.* 2004;40:444-448.

83. Bradshaw JH, Moore PP. Perinatal cytomegalovirus infection associated with lung cysts. *J Paediatr Child Health.* 2003;39:563-566.

84. Hsu ML, Cheng SN, Huang CF, et al. Perinatal cytomegalovirus infection complicated with pneumonitis and adrenalitis in a premature infant. *J Microbiol Immunol Infect.* 2001;34:297-300.

85. Neuberger P, Hamprecht K, Vochem M, et al. Case-control study of symptoms and neonatal outcome of human milk-transmitted cytomegalovirus infection in premature infants. *J Pediatr.* 2006;148:326-331.

86. Kothari A, Ramachandran VG, Gupta P. Cytomegalovirus infection in neonates following exchange transfusion. *Indian J Pediatr.* 2006;73:519-521.

87. Mussi-Pinhata MM, Yamamoto AY, do Carmo Rego MA, et al. Perinatal or early-postnatal cytomegalovirus infection in preterm infants under 34 weeks gestation born to CMV-seropositive mothers within a high-seroprevalence population. *J Pediatr.* 2004;145:685-688.

88. Yasuda A, Kimura H, Hayakawa M, et al. Evaluation of cytomegalovirus infections transmitted via breast milk in preterm infants with a real-time polymerase chain reaction assay. *Pediatrics.* 2003;111:1333-1336.

89. Vollmer B, Seibold-Weiger K, Schmitz-Salue C, et al. Postnatally acquired cytomegalovirus infection via breast milk: effects on hearing and development in preterm infants. *Pediatr Infect Dis J.* 2004;23:322-327.

90. Hamprecht K, Maschmann J, Jahn G, et al. Cytomegalovirus transmission to preterm infants during lactation. *J Clin Virol.* 2008;41:198-205.

91. Vouga M, Baud D. Imaging of congenital Zika virus infection: the route to identification of prognostic factors. *Prenat Diagn.* 2016;36:799-811.

92. Costello A, Dua T, Duran P, et al. Defining the syndrome associated with congenital Zika virus infection. *Bull World Health Organ.* 2016;94:406-406A.

93. Ryan L, Plötz FB, van den Hoogen A, et al. Neonates and COVID-19: state of the art. *Pediatr Res.* 2022;91:432-439.

94. Zeng L, Xia S, Yuan W, et al. Neonatal early-onset infection with SARS-CoV-2 in 33 neonates born to mothers with COVID-19 in Wuhan, China. *JAMA Pediatr.* 2020;174(7):722-725.

95. Getahun D, Peltier MR, Lurvey LD, et al. Association between SARS-CoV-2 infection and adverse perinatal outcomes in a large health maintenance organization. *Am J Perinatol.* 2022. doi:10.1055/s-0042-1749666.

96. Moza A, Duica F, Anotniadis P, et al. Outcome of newborns with confirmed or possible SARS-CoV-2 vertical infection-A scoping review. *Diagnostics (Basel).* 2023;13(2):245. doi:10.3390/diagnostics13020245.

97. Brum AC, Vain NE. Impact of perinatal COVID on fetal and neonatal brain and neurodevelopmental outcomes. *Semin Fetal Neonatal Med.* 2023;28(2):101427. doi:10.1016/j.siny.2023.101427.

98. McClymont E, Albert AY, Alton GD, et al. CANCOVID-Preg Team. Association of SARS-CoV-2 infection during pregnancy with maternal and perinatal outcomes. *JAMA.* 2022;327(20):1983-1991. doi:10.1001/jama.2022.5906.

99. Whitley RJ, Yeager A, Kartus P, et al. Neonatal herpes simplex virus infection: follow-up evaluation of vidarabine therapy. *Pediatrics.* 1983;72:778-785.

100. Kimberlin DW, Jester PM, Sanchez PJ, et al. Valganciclovir for symptomatic congenital cytomegalovirus disease. *N Engl J Med.* 2015;372:933-943.

101. Kimberlin DW, Whitley RJ, Wan W, et al. Oral acyclovir suppression and neurodevelopment after neonatal herpes. *N Engl J Med.* 2011;365:1284-1292.

102. American Academy of Pediatrics. Herpes simplex. In: Kimberlin DW, Barnett ED, Lynfield R, Sawyer MH, eds. *Red Book: 2021–2024 Report of the Committee on Infectious Diseases.* 32nd ed. Itasca, IL: American Academy of Pediatrics; 2021: 407-417.

103. Englund JA, Fletcher CV, Balfour Jr HH. Acyclovir therapy in neonates. *J Pediatr.* 1991;119:129-135.

104. Kimberlin DW, Lakeman FD, Arvin AM, et al. Application of the polymerase chain reaction to the diagnosis and management of neonatal herpes simplex virus disease. *J Infect Dis.* 1996;174:1162-1167.

105. Kimberlin DW, Lin CY, Sanchez PJ, et al. Effect of ganciclovir therapy on hearing in symptomatic congenital cytomegalovirus disease involving the central nervous system: a randomized, controlled trial. *J Pediatr.* 2003;143:16-25.

106. Oliver SE, Cloud GA, Sanchez PJ, et al. Neurodevelopmental outcomes following ganciclovir therapy in symptomatic congenital cytomegalovirus infections involving the central nervous system. *J Clin Virol.* 2009;46(suppl 4):S22-S26.

107. Kimberlin DW, Acosta EP, Sanchez PJ, et al. Pharmacokinetic and pharmacodynamic assessment of oral valganciclovir in the treatment of symptomatic congenital cytomegalovirus disease. *J Infect Dis.* 2008;197:836-845.

108. American Academy of Pediatrics. Cytomegalovirus infection. In: Kimberlin DW, Barnett ED, Lynfield R, Sawyer MH, eds. *Red Book: 2021–2024 Report of the Committee on Infectious Diseases.* 32nd ed. Itasca, IL: American Academy of Pediatrics; 2021:294-300.

109. Russell K, Oliver SE, Lewis L, et al. Update: Interim guidance for the evaluation and management of infants with possible congenital zika virus infection—United States. *MMWR Morb Mortal Wkly Rep.* 2016;65:870-878.

110. Wardell H, Campbell JI, VanderPluym C, Dixit A. Severe acute respiratory syndrome coronavirus 2 infection in febrile neonates. *J Pediatric Infect Dis Soc.* 2020;9(5):630-635. doi:10.1093/jpids/piaa084.

111. Hopwood AJ, Jordan-Villegas A, Gutierrez LD, et al. Severe acute respiratory syndrome coronavirus-2 pneumonia in a newborn treated with remdesivir and coronavirus disease 2019 convalescent plasma [published online ahead of print December 11, 2020]. *J Pediatr Infect Dis Soc.* doi:10.1093/jpids/piaa165.

112. Beigel JH, Tomashek KM, Dodd LE, et al. Remdesivir for the treatment of Covid-19—final report. *N Engl J Med.* 2020;383:1813-1826.

113. Tavakoli N, Chaichian S, Sadraie JS, et al. Is it possible to reduce the rate of vertical transmission and improve perinatal outcomes by inclusion of remdesivir in treatment regimen of pregnant women with COVID-19? *BMC Pregnancy Childbirth.* 2023;23(1):110. doi:10.1186/s12884-023-05405-y.

114. Piekos SN, Price ND, Hood L, Hadlock JJ. The impact of maternal SARS-CoV-2 infection and COVID-19 vaccination on maternal-fetal outcomes. *Reprod Toxicol.* 2022;114:33-43. doi:10.1016/j.reprotox.2022.10.003.

115. Boppana SB, Ross SA, Novak Z, et al. Dried blood spot real-time polymerase chain reaction assays to screen newborns for congenital cytomegalovirus infection. *JAMA*. 2010;303:1375-1382.
116. Boppana SB, Ross SA, Shimamura M, et al. Saliva polymerase-chain-reaction assay for cytomegalovirus screening in newborns. *N Engl J Med*. 2011;364:2111-2118.
117. Rabe IB, Staples JE, Villanueva J, et al. Interim guidance for interpretation of Zika virus antibody test results. *MMWR Morb Mortal Wkly Rep*. 2016;65:543-546.
118. Centers for Disease Control and Prevention. *Evaluation and Management Considerations for Neonates at Risk for COVID-19*. Available at: https://www.cdc.gov/coronavirus/2019-ncov/hcp/caring-for-newborns.html.
119. Noyola DE, Demmler GJ, Williamson WD, et al. Cytomegalovirus urinary excretion and long term outcome in children with congenital cytomegalovirus infection. Congenital CMV Longitudinal Study Group. *Pediatr Infect Dis J*. 2000;19:505-510.
120. Rosenthal LS, Fowler KB, Boppana SB, et al. Cytomegalovirus shedding and delayed sensorineural hearing loss: results from longitudinal follow-up of children with congenital infection. *Pediatr Infect Dis J*. 2009;28:515-520.
121. Boppana SB, Fowler KB, Pass RF, et al. Congenital cytomegalovirus infection: association between virus burden in infancy and hearing loss. *J Pediatr*. 2005;146:817-823.
122. Ross SA, Novak Z, Fowler KB, et al. Cytomegalovirus blood viral load and hearing loss in young children with congenital infection. *Pediatr Infect Dis J*. 2009;28:588-592.

Chapter 13

Neonatal Hypotonia and Neuromuscular Disorders

Crystal Jing Jing Yeo, Jahannaz Dastgir, and Basil T. Darras

Chapter Outline

Gaps in Knowledge

1. The severe hypotonia and hyporeflexia in Prader-Willi syndrome (PWS) may lead to unnecessary invasive tests such as electromyography, muscle biopsy, and/or genetic testing for spinal muscular atrophy (SMA). Genetic testing for PWS is not well understood by most clinicians and, if ordered incorrectly, may lead to false normal results.

2. It is important for clinicians to know that normal creatine phosphokinase (CPK) and electromyography do not exclude a congenital myopathy.

3. Correct ordering of genetic testing, and interpretation of results, are not common knowledge among clinicians caring for newborn infants with hypotonia. For example, ordering a motor neuron disease gene panel instead of single gene *SMN* testing to exclude or confirm the diagnosis of SMA will lead to delays in diagnosis and treatment.

4. Aminoglycoside antibiotics must be used with caution in hypotonic small preterm infants with hypermagnesemia because they increase neuromuscular blockade and thus worsen the hypotonia.

Introduction

Neonatal hypotonia, often referred to as the "floppy infant," is the main presenting clinical feature of most neuromuscular diseases of early life.[1] However, disorders of the central nervous system (CNS) may also manifest

213

with hypotonia. In this chapter, we will attempt to (1) define hypotonia, (2) discuss the physical examination and assessment of the hypotonic infant, (3) discuss the differential anatomic diagnosis of hypotonia, (4) summarize the most common neuromuscular disorders presenting principally with hypotonia, and (5) present our stepwise diagnostic approach to the investigation of neonatal hypotonia.

Definition of Hypotonia

Two types of muscle tone can be assessed clinically: postural and phasic. *Postural* (antigravity) tone is a sustained, low-intensity muscle contraction in response to gravity. It is mediated by both gamma and alpha motor neuron systems in the spinal cord, and it is assessed clinically by passive manipulation of the limbs. *Phasic* tone is a brief contraction in response to a high-intensity stretch. It is mediated by the alpha motor neuron system only and is examined clinically by eliciting the muscle stretch reflexes. *Hypotonia* is defined as reduction in postural tone, with or without a change in phasic tone. When postural tone is depressed, the trunk and limbs cannot overcome gravity and the child appears hypotonic or floppy.

An approximate caudal-rostral progression in the development of muscle tone has been described by Sainte-Anne Dargassies.[2] At postconceptional age of 28 weeks, there is minimal resistance to passive manipulation in all limbs; by 32 weeks, flexor tone can be appreciated in the lower extremities; and by 36 weeks, flexor tone is also present in the upper limbs. By term, strong flexor tone in all four limbs can be demonstrated by passive movements.

Physical Examination and Assessment of a Hypotonic Child

Volpe[3] describes the physical examination of a hypotonic infant in detail. Following a careful general physical examination, the neurological assessment should include an evaluation of primary neonatal reflexes, a sensory examination, and most importantly, a motor examination (Box 13.1). *General physical examination* may reveal organomegaly, skin changes, dysmorphic features, contractures, abnormalities of the genitalia, respiratory rate or pattern irregularities,

BOX 13.1 HYPOTONIA: PHYSICAL EXAMINATION

- General physical examination
- Appearance/posture (flaccid)
- Passive manipulation of the limbs
- Mobility and muscle power
- Muscle stretch reflexes
- Primary neonatal reflexes
- Sensation
- Traction response ("head lag")
- Vertical suspension ("slips through")
- Horizontal suspension ("drapes over")
- "Scarf sign," "Heel to ear or chin"

or evidence of traumatic injury (e.g., bruising, petechiae). The general examination may also be normal. Abnormal *primary neonatal reflexes* refer to their persistence. In normal infants, the Moro reflex disappears by 6 months of age,[4,5] the palmar grasp becomes less obvious after 2 months of age, and the tonic neck response should diminish by 6 to 7 months of age.[4–6] *Sensation* can be tested by withdrawal from a stimulus (e.g., touching the infant with a small brush), and abnormalities in sensation may suggest the presence of a congenital neuropathy (e.g., hereditary motor-sensory or sensory-autonomic neuropathies), but, admittedly, this is difficult to assess in infants.

The motor examination includes assessment of posture, muscle tone, mobility, muscle power, and muscle stretch reflexes. When assessing muscle tone, the infant's head should be placed in the midline in order to eliminate the effect of the tonic neck response. Minimal resistance to passive manipulation of arms or legs is an important clinical feature of hypotonia. Weak cry, poor suck, and poor respiratory effort may be noted in an otherwise very alert infant. Pectus excavatum or carinatum is sometimes seen, reflecting long-standing weakness of chest wall musculature. Most hypotonic infants demonstrate a classic "frog-like" posture: full abduction and external rotation of the legs as well as a flaccid extension or flexion of the arms. Congenital dislocation of the hips may be noted because poor muscle tone in utero failed to maintain the femoral head in the acetabulum. Another sign of intrauterine hypotonia and limited fetal movements is arthrogryposis (i.e., contractures of multiple joints). Spontaneous antigravity movements of limbs may be absent or decreased. In a full-term newborn or older infant, passive movement of the infant's elbow across the midline produces a positive "scarf sign." Similarly, a positive heel-to-ear test is readily demonstrated by opposing the heel to the ear. Finally, muscle stretch reflexes may be normal, brisk or hypoactive (i.e., absent or decreased).

Muscle tone can be evaluated further by performing the traction response, vertical suspension, and horizontal suspension maneuvers.[7]

TRACTION RESPONSE

To elicit the traction response, the examiner grasps the infant's hands and wrists and slowly raises the infant from the supine to a seated position. The normal infant's head is maintained at midline or at least for a few seconds when the seated position is reached. However, the hypotonic infant tends to have significant head lag when pulled to the seated position and will not maintain his/her head erect when sitting.

VERTICAL SUSPENSION

The examiner places both hands beneath the infant's armpits and lifts the infant straight up. In a normal infant, the shoulder muscles press down against the examiner's hands and enable him/her to suspend vertically without falling. When the normal infant is in vertical suspension, the head is maintained in the midline and hips, knees, and ankles are in flexion. When this maneuver is performed in the hypotonic infant, the infant slips through the examiner's hands with both legs usually extended.

HORIZONTAL SUSPENSION

The examiner uses one hand to support the infant's trunk in a prone position and observes the resulting posture. A normal infant flexes or fully extends the limbs, straightens the back, and maintains the head in the midline position for at least a few seconds. The hypotonic infant's head and limbs hang loosely and the trunk "drapes over" the examiner's hand.

Some clinicians use signs borrowed from the premature infant examination (described above), such as the "scarf sign" (i.e., approximation of elbow to opposite shoulder) or "heel to ear or chin," in an effort to quantitate muscle tone. We do not use these routinely in the assessment of tone but have found them useful in the diagnosis of congenital laxity of ligaments.

Differential Anatomic Diagnosis of Hypotonia

Neonatal hypotonia may be the manifestation of pathology involving the CNS, the peripheral nervous system (i.e., lower motor unit), or both (Box 13.2). In infants with *cerebral or central hypotonia,* nearly two-thirds of cases, the perinatal or prenatal history may suggest a CNS insult. There may also be associated global (rather than an isolated gross-motor) developmental delay, occasionally seizures, microcephaly, dysmorphic features, and/or malformation of the brain and/or other organs. Central hypotonia may be associated with brisk and/or persistent primitive reflexes and normal-brisk muscle stretch reflexes. The degree of weakness noted in these infants is usually less than the degree of hypotonia (*"nonparalytic" hypotonia*) (Table 13.1). In *lower motor unit hypotonia or peripheral hypotonia,* developmental delay is primarily gross-motor and is associated with absent or depressed muscle stretch reflexes and/or muscle atrophy and fasciculations of the tongue. In general, antigravity limb movements are decreased and cannot be elicited via postural reflexes. In these infants, the degree of weakness is proportional or in excess of the degree of hypotonia (*"paralytic" hypotonia*) (Table 13.1). Trauma to the high cervical cord due to traction in breech or cervical presentation may also initially manifest itself as flaccid paralysis, which may be asymmetric, and absent muscle stretch reflexes; later on, however, upper motor neuron signs develop.

Because muscle tone is also determined by the visco-elastic properties of muscle and joints, connective tissue disorders such as *Marfan, Ehlers-Danlos* syndromes, osteogenesis imperfecta and also benign laxity of the ligaments can present with hypotonia. In

BOX 13.2 HYPOTONIA: DIFFERENTIAL ANATOMIC DIAGNOSIS

- Brain
- Spinal cord
- Anterior horn cell
- Peripheral nerve
- Neuromuscular junction
- Muscle

TABLE 13.1   Cerebral (Central) Versus Lower Motor Unit (Peripheral) Hypotonia

	Cerebral (Central)	Lower Motor Unit (Peripheral)
History	Consistent with CNS insult; seizures	
Developmental delay	Decreased level of alertness; global developmental delay	Alert look; no global delay; delayed gross motor development
General physical examination	Microcephaly, dysmorphic features	Muscle atrophy, fasciculations, joint contractures, weak cry, weak suck
Other organ involvement	Malformation of other organs	No abnormalities of other organs besides musculoskeletal
Weakness	Weakness less than degree of hypotonia (nonparalytic hypotonia)	Weakness in proportion/excess to degree of hypotonia (paralytic hypotonia)
Postural reflexes	Movement through postural reflexes (e.g., tonic neck reflex)	Failure of movement with postural reflexes
Muscle stretch reflexes	Normal or brisk, clonus, Babinski sign	Absent or depressed
Other	Brisk and/or persistent infantile reflexes (e.g., Moro, palmar grasp)	Decreased antigravity limb movements

BOX 13.3 COMBINED CEREBRAL AND MOTOR UNIT HYPOTONIA

- Congenital myotonic dystrophy
- Congenital muscular dystrophies
- Peroxisomal disorders
- Leukodystrophies
- Mitochondrial encephalomyopathies
- Neuroaxonal dystrophy
- Familial dysautonomia
- Asphyxia secondary to motor unit disease

addition, there is *combined cerebral and lower motor unit hypotonia* seen in infants and older children with congenital myotonic dystrophy, some congenital muscular dystrophies (CMD), peroxisomal disorders, mitochondrial encephalomyopathies, neuroaxonal dystrophy, leukodystrophies (e.g., globoid cell leukodystrophy), familial dysautonomia, and asphyxia secondary to motor unit disease (Box 13.3). Further, hypotonia without significant weakness may be a feature of systemic diseases such as sepsis, congenital heart disease, hypothyroidism, rickets, renal tubular acidosis, and others.

Neuromuscular diseases in infancy present primarily with *hypotonia* and *weakness*; however, infants with severe hypotonia but only marginal weakness usually do not have a disorder of the lower motor unit (anterior horn cell, peripheral and cranial nerves, neuromuscular junction, and muscle). These infants may have genetic conditions, metabolic disturbances, or systemic disorders (e.g., congenital heart disease, renal failure). Early on, neonates with CNS pathology may present with profound hypotonia, decreased reflexes, and moderate to severe but transient weakness; however, they also tend to have seizures, obtundation, cranial nerve abnormalities, and/or history of perinatal asphyxia. With recovery, they gradually develop better strength, increased muscle stretch reflexes and muscle tone. This is in contrast to the asphyxiated infants with disorders of the lower motor unit, in whom the weakness, hypotonia, and hyporeflexia persist. Alternatively, profound weakness and hypotonia without signs of CNS involvement occur in newborn infants with isolated neuromuscular disease and no history of perinatal asphyxia. Muscle stretch reflexes vary depending on the anatomical level of pathology along the motor unit (i.e., prominent hyporeflexia or total areflexia in anterior horn cell disorders and neuropathies, reduced reflexes in proportion to the degree of weakness in myopathies, and often normal reflexes in disorders of the neuromuscular junction). Again, approximately two-thirds of patients with neonatal hypotonia have cerebral etiologies and one-third have lower motor unit diseases.[8]

Box 13.4 lists the most common causes of cerebral (central) hypotonia. Prasad and Prasad[9] review the metabolic and genetic disorders presenting with hypotonia and suggest a diagnostic algorithm.

BOX 13.4 CEREBRAL (CENTRAL) HYPOTONIA

- Chromosomal disorders
- Other genetic defects
- Acute hemorrhagic and other brain injury
- Hypoxic/ischemic encephalopathy
- Chronic nonprogressive encephalopathies
- Peroxisomal disorders (Zellweger syndrome, neonatal ALD, etc.)
- Metabolic defects
- Drug intoxication
- "Benign" congenital hypotonia

Common Neuromuscular Disorders Presenting Principally With Hypotonia

This chapter will review the most frequent genetic and acquired disorders of the lower motor unit (Table 13.2). Most of these conditions present with hypotonia.

ANTERIOR HORN CELL/PERIPHERAL NERVE DISORDERS

Spinal Muscular Atrophies

Three clinical variants have been described based on the rate of progression and age at onset of the disease: (1) SMA Type I, or Werdnig-Hoffmann disease, (2) intermediate SMA, or SMA Type II, and (3) SMA Type III, or Kugelberg-Welander disease.[10,11] Here, we will discuss primarily SMA Type I, which may be seen clinically during infancy.

SMA Type I, Werdnig-Hoffmann Disease

Generalized hypotonia and *weakness* may be noted during the first 6 months of life, and in 95% of the cases before the age of 4 months. *Prenatal* onset has been described and it is experienced by the mother as weakening of fetal movements during the last trimester of the pregnancy. At birth or in the first 6 months of life, weak sucking, difficulty with swallowing, labored breathing, extreme hypotonia, severe weakness, and hyperabduction of the hips ("*frog legs*") become apparent. *Arthrogryposis* multiplex congenita is uncommon in SMA Type I but, nonetheless, has been observed rarely in infants who are symptomatic at birth; this is known as SMA Type 0 or Type Ia. Type I SMA patients never sit unsupported.[10,12] Examination shows hypotonia, areflexia, and weakness typically affecting the lower extremities earlier and more severely than the upper extremities and the proximal muscles more often than the distal ones. The anterior/posterior diameter of the thorax is decreased and there may be pectus excavatum with paradoxical respirations. As the disease advances, there is paralysis of the bulbar muscles, loss of the cough reflex, and an inaudible cry. Wasting and fasciculations of the tongue may be observed, but they can be easily confused with simple tongue tremors. Without disease-modifying treatments, death usually occurs in the first year or less often in the second year of life, most commonly related to aspiration pneumonia. An unusual genetically distinct variety of SMA related to diaphragmatic paralysis (spinal muscular atrophy

TABLE 13.2 Neuromuscular Diseases in the Hypotonic Infant and Child

Anterior Horn Cell/Peripheral Nerve	Neuromuscular Junction	Muscle
Spinal muscular atrophies	Transient neonatal MG	Congenital muscular dystrophies
Hypoxic-ischemic myelopathy	Congenital myasthenic syndromes	Congenital myotonic dystrophy
Traumatic myelopathy	Hypermagnesemia	Infantile FSHD
Neurogenic arthrogryposis	Aminoglycoside toxicity	Congenital myopathies
Congenital neuropathies	Infantile botulism	Metabolic myopathies
Axonal		Mitochondrial myopathies
Hypomyelinating		
Dejerine-Sottas		
HSAN		
Giant axonal neuropathy		
Metabolic		
Inflammatory		

FSHD, Facioscapulohumeral muscular dystrophy; *HSAN,* hereditary sensory and autonomic neuropathy; *MG,* myasthenia gravis.

with respiratory distress Type I, SMARD1) has been described, presenting primarily with respiratory distress in the first 2 months of life before any skeletal muscle involvement. In classic SMA Type I, the respiratory insufficiency is due to intercostal rather than diaphragmatic paralysis.[13]

Although used rarely, the electromyogram (EMG) may reveal excessive spontaneous activity during the first 3 months of life consisting of multiple discharges at a frequency 5 to 15 Hz in relaxed muscles, which persist during sleep. Fibrillation potentials may also appear later on. Motor unit potentials are increased in duration, and many are polyphasic and poorly recruited by voluntary activation. *Muscle biopsy* examination demonstrates small and large-group atrophy, with intermixed groups of hypertrophic fibers. The *hypertrophic* fibers are histochemically Type I fibers while the atrophic fibers are *Type I* and *Type II*.[10] Postmortem histologic examination of the spinal cord shows loss of anterior horn cells. CPK can be mildly to moderately elevated, usually up to 5 times the upper limit of normal. Given the availability of genetic diagnosis, EMG and, in particular, muscle biopsy are used only rarely in the diagnosis of SMA.

In 1990, all three types of autosomal recessive SMA were mapped to a single locus on chromosome 5q11.2-13.3.[14] Subsequently, in 1995, two groups reported the preferential deletion of two genes, the survival motor neuron (*SMN*)[15,16] and the neuronal apoptosis inhibitory protein gene (*NAIP*)[17] in SMA patients. Homozygous deletions of exon 7 or exons 7 and 8 of the telomeric copy of the *SMN* gene (*SMN1*) can be detected in 90% to 95% of patients with SMA, regardless of severity (Types I, II, and III).[15] Most of the remaining patients have deletion of *SMN1* in one allele and a point mutation in the other; a very small fraction of the deletion-negative patients has rare non-chromosome 5 types of SMA. Commercially available assays for the homozygous loss of exon 7 or exons 7 and 8 of the *SMN1* gene thus provide a highly correlated marker for the prenatal and postnatal diagnosis of SMA Type I. *NAIP* deletions are seen in over 45% of SMA Type I and less than 20% of Type II and Type III SMA patients.[17] Despite the occurrence of *NAIP* deletions, *NAIP* has not been proven to be important in the pathogenesis of SMA.

Since 2017, three SMN protein augmenting therapies, nusinersen, onasemnogene abeparvovec-xioi, and risdiplam, have become available for SMA patients and can substantially improve clinical outcomes with early treatment.[18] Testing for deletion of *SMN1* exon 7/8 is now included in routine newborn screening in 39 states across the United States and internationally.[19,20] This allows 91% of SMA infants to be diagnosed in the United States in the first week of life for the early initiation of treatment.

SMA Type II, SMA Type III

Most patients with SMA Type II and III are normal at birth. In a series of 19 infants who were later classified as SMA Type II, all of them were found to be normal at birth.[21] The onset of the disease, however, is before the age of 18 months and typically after the age of 6 months.[22] Patients can sit unsupported but never stand. Survival to ages 5 and 25 years is 98.5% and 68.5%, respectively, was reported in patients with disease-modifying treatments. Many patients with SMA Type III achieve normal gross motor milestones early on and often into later childhood. The onset of symptoms is usually after the age of 18 months (either before the age of 3 years [Type IIIa] or after [Type IIIb]) and patients can stand alone; lifespan is almost normal. The SMA phenotype is determined, at least in part, by the number of copies of the centromeric copy of the *SMN* gene, known as *SMN2* (which produces a small amount (~10%) of full-length SMN protein); patients with milder phenotypes tend to have more copies of *SMN2*. Most SMA Type I patients have one to two copies of *SMN2* (80%), while most SMA Type II patients have two or three copies (82% have three copies), and the vast majority (96%) of SMA Type III patients have three or four copies of *SMN2*.[23] Treatment with SMN augmenting therapy is recommended in SMA patients with up to four copies of *SMN2*.[24]

Congenital Neuropathies

Congenital Hypomyelinating and Axonal Neuropathies

Fourteen infants with neuropathy were reviewed by Sladky.[25] He described nine infants with demyelinating neuropathy, including four with hypomyelination, three with steroid-responsive chronic inflammatory demyelinating polyneuropathy (CIDP), and two with a leukodystrophy. *Four* of five axonal neuropathies in the same sibship were X-linked and one was a sporadic case. Neonates with congenital neuropathies usually present with severe hypotonia, weakness, and hyporeflexia or areflexia closely resembling SMA Type I. However, cerebrospinal fluid protein is elevated in most infants with congenital neuropathies, not a finding in SMA Type I. *EMG* and *nerve conduction* studies (NCS) are not only important for confirming the diagnosis and distinguishing between neuropathies and SMA Type I, but they can also help identify whether demyelinating or axonal features. Nevertheless, electrophysiological studies may be unable to differentiate between inherited noninflammatory and acquired inflammatory neuropathies. Though sural nerve biopsy may help establish the diagnosis, it may not exclude CIDP. A number of infants with congenital neuropathies may also have the early onset of hereditary motor and sensory neuropathies (HMSN) such as Charcot-Marie-Tooth (CMT)1A and CMT1B (known as *Dejerine-Sottas disease*), CMT 4E (neonatal hypotonia and arthrogryposis), a metabolic disease such as mitochondrial cytopathy or a leukodystrophy, hereditary sensory and autonomic neuropathy (e.g., Riley-Day syndrome), or giant axonal neuropathy.

DISTURBANCES OF NEUROMUSCULAR TRANSMISSION

Transient Neonatal Myasthenia Gravis

This syndrome results from the transplacental transfer of circulating anti-acetylcholine receptor (AChR) antibodies from a myasthenic mother. It develops in about 10% to 20% of infants born to myasthenic mothers. The syndrome usually presents within hours of birth but may be delayed for up to 3 days; the main features are feeding difficulties (87%), generalized weakness (69%), respiratory difficulties (65%), weak cry (60%), facial diplegia (54%), ptosis (50%), and sometimes external ophthalmoplegia. Respiratory failure is uncommon, but it may occur. The presence of arthrogryposis, pulmonary hypoplasia, polyhydramnios, weak fetal movements, or stillbirth signifies onset in utero. The severity of the disease in infants correlates poorly with clinical severity in mothers

and with maternal antibody titer; however, falling antibody titers correlate with clinical improvement. Infants with transient neonatal myasthenia gravis (TNMG) are born to mothers with a relatively high ratio of antibodies directed against the fetal versus the adult AChR. TNMG may rarely occur in infants born to seronegative mothers and may rarely be secondary to anti-MuSK antibodies.[26] The mean duration of symptoms is 18 days, with a range of 5 days to 3 months. The diagnosis is confirmed by demonstrating high serum concentration of AChR antibody in newborn infants. Though less frequently utilized, diagnosis may also be confirmed via reversal of the symptoms with edrophonium chloride (Tensilon), given either as an intramuscular or subcutaneous injection of 0.04 to 0.15 mg/kg or 0.1 mg/kg body weight intravenously delivered in fractional amounts over a number of minutes after a test dose of 0.01 mg/kg. Clinical improvement becomes apparent in a few minutes after the intravenous administration of edrophonium chloride and may last for 10 to 15 minutes. Given the possibility of cardiac bradyarrhythmias subsequent to the intravenous use of edrophonium chloride, however, the intramuscular and subcutaneous routes are preferable in newborn infants. In severely compromised neonates, an exchange transfusion should be attempted. For infants with only feeding and swallowing problems, a longer-lasting effect (1–3 hours) may be achieved by the intramuscular or subcutaneous injection of about 0.05 mg/kg per dose neostigmine methyl sulfate 15 to 30 minutes before each feeding, though this may induce increased tracheal secretions. The same medication can also be administered through a nasogastric tube at ten times the parenteral dose (0.5 mg/kg/dose) 45 to 60 minutes prior to feeding.

Acquired Autoimmune Myasthenia Gravis

Only minor differences exist between acquired autoimmune myasthenia gravis in children and adults, but the onset of symptoms is always after age 6 months and in most cases after 2 years.

Congenital Myasthenic Syndromes

Congenital myasthenic syndromes can be classified according to the site of the defect, that is, presynaptic, postsynaptic, synaptic, and mixed.[27] These are defects of neuromuscular transmission, and the classification and main features of the most common forms are shown in Table 13.3. Congenital myasthenic syndromes usually present in infancy with generalized hypotonia and fluctuating weakness, weak cry and suck, respiratory distress, apnea, and feeding difficulties. Fluctuating ptosis, ophthalmoparesis, and fatigability on exertion may also be present during infancy and childhood. Later on, delayed motor milestones may be noted and will, in some cases, progress during adolescence and adulthood. Testing for anti-AChR antibodies is negative. The diagnosis is based on clinical history and examination, family history (if present), EMG findings, and the clinical response to acetylcholinesterase inhibitors and confirmed with genetic testing. Tensilon (edrophonium chloride) chloride testing, though less frequently in use today,

is positive in most types of congenital myasthenic syndromes, except in the classic slow channel syndrome and in congenital end-plate acetylcholinesterase deficiency (see Table 13.3). If clinical response to edrophonium chloride occurs, long-term treatment with neostigmine or pyridostigmine may be needed. In most cases, however, detailed EMG studies, in vitro microphysiologic, ultrastructural, and histochemical studies of intercostal muscle biopsies have been used to establish the diagnosis. Nevertheless, currently genetic testing may be the first step in the work-up of individuals suspected of the diagnosis. Treatments may also be tailored to the specific mutation with medications such as albuterol or ephedrine.

Infantile Botulism

Patients developing botulism in infancy are normal at birth but between the age of 10 days and 12 months

TABLE 13.3   Main Congenital Myasthenic Syndromes

Defect	Inheritance	Clinical Features	Tensilon Test	Treatment
Presynaptic				
Familial infantile myasthenia with episodic apnea (ChAT mutations)	AR	Hypotonia Ptosis, apnea No ophthalmoparesis Generalized weakness	+	AChE inhibitors
Postsynaptic Or Synaptic				
Congenital end-plate AChE deficiency (COLQ mutations)	AR	Asymmetric ptosis Ophthalmoparesis Distal weakness Delayed pupillary constriction to light	–	No response to AChE inhibitors
Classic slow channel syndrome (AChR A1, AChR B1, AChR D, AChr E mutations)	AD	Ophthalmoparesis Fluctuating ptosis Head and wrist extensor weakness	–	No response to AChE inhibitors
Congenital AChR deficiency (rapsyn or ε-subunit mutations)	AR	Hypotonia, ptosis Ophthalmoplegia (ε-subunit) Strabismus (rapsyn) Respiratory failure (rapsyn) Feeding difficulties Arthrogryposis (rapsyn)	+	AChE inhibitors
Dok-7 myasthenia (*DOK-7* mutations)	AR	Proximal weakness Ptosis Facial weakness Respiratory failure	–	Poor response to AchE inhibitors

AChE, acetylcholinesterase; *AChR,* Acetylcholine receptor; *AD,* autosomal dominant; *AR,* autosomal recessive; *ChAT,* choline acetyltransferase.

(median age at presentation is 10 weeks) develop acutely severe weakness, dysphagia, constipation, weak cry, severe hypotonia, and respiratory insufficiency.[28] On examination, there is diffuse hypotonia and weakness, ptosis, ophthalmoplegia with pupillary involvement (mydriasis) in some cases, reduced gag reflex, and usually preservation of muscle stretch reflexes.[29] The history of presentation is suggestive of a descending pattern of paralysis. Affected infants tend to deteriorate if given aminoglycosides or other neuromuscular blocking agents. On EMG examination, the compound motor unit potential amplitude is low at rest; repetitive stimulation at 2 to 5 Hz typically produces decrement, but with 20 to 50 Hz stimulation, facilitation of 125% to 3000% is seen in almost all cases. To demonstrate the increment, however, a prolonged period of stimulation (10–20 seconds) may be required.[30] During infancy, the pathogenesis of botulism is different. The *Clostridium botulinum* (*C. botulinum*) is ingested, colonizes the intestinal tract, and produces toxin in situ. This is in contrast to older children and adults in whom the disease is related to ingestion of food contaminated by preformed exotoxin.[31] The diagnosis in infants is confirmed by isolation of the organism in stool. Infantile botulism is a self-limited disease, but the period of profound hypotonia can last from 2 to 6 weeks, so the infant should be observed in the intensive care unit and be supported, if respiratory failure occurs. Botulinum immune globulin (BIG) seems to be safe and reduces the duration of the disease, the cost of hospitalization, and the severity of illness.[32]

Magnesium Intoxication

Generalized weakness, hypotonia and mental status changes may be seen in infants born to mothers treated with high doses of magnesium sulfate for eclampsia. Because this is a self-limited condition brought about by elevated magnesium levels that impair neuromuscular transmission, specialized testing (e.g., EMG/NCS) is not necessary. These infants may have depressed deep tendon reflexes, abdominal distension secondary to ileus, and irregularities of cardiac rhythm. Aminoglycoside antibiotics may worsen the hypotonia in small preterm infants with hypermagnesemia because of increased neuromuscular blockade and, therefore they should be used with caution.

Muscle Disorders

The muscle disorders reviewed in this chapter usually present with hypotonia and weakness during infancy; however, a later onset may occur. They are listed in Box 13.5.

CONGENITAL MUSCULAR DYSTROPHIES

In CMDs, the muscle biopsy is abnormal (it shows features often seen in the major muscular dystrophies of later onset); however, there are no unique identifying features and thus the need for genetic confirmation.

CMDs can be classified into two major groups depending on the association with structural brain abnormalities on neuroimaging studies or autopsy examination.[33] The CMDs without structural CNS anomalies, also known as "Classical" CMD, form a heterogenous group of disorders. In the second group, i.e., those with associated structural CNS abnormalities, concomitant eye involvement, and clinical evidence of significant neurological dysfunction may be evident. The latter group includes *Fukuyama muscular dystrophy* (FMD), *Walker-Warburg* syndrome (WWS), and *muscle-eye-brain* disease (MEBD) (Box 13.6; Table 13.4). A biochemical classification has been proposed as well (Table 13.5).

BOX 13.5 MUSCLE DISORDERS IN THE HYPOTONIC INFANT

Congenital muscular dystrophies
Congenital myotonic dystrophy
Infantile facioscapulohumeral muscular dystrophy
Congenital myopathies
    Nemaline myopathy
    Central core disease
    Centronuclear/myotubular myopathy
    Congenital fiber type disproportion
    Minicore disease
    Other congenital myopathies
Metabolic myopathies
    Acid maltase deficiency
    Mitochondrial myopathies
        Cytochrome c oxidase deficiency
        Fatty acid oxidation defects
Nonlysosomal glycogenoses

BOX 13.6 CLASSIFICATION OF CONGENITAL MUSCULAR DYSTROPHY

CLASSICAL CMD
  Merosin-Deficient CMD
    Primary merosin deficiency (MDC1A)
    Secondary merosin deficiency (MDC1B, MDC1C)
  Merosin-positive CMD
    Rigid spine syndrome
    CMD with distal hyperextensibility (Ullrich type)
    Other merosin-positive CMDs
CMD WITH CENTRAL NERVOUS SYSTEM ABNORMALITIES AND/OR MENTAL RETARDATION
  Fukuyama CMD
  Muscle-eye-brain disease
  Walker-Warburg syndrome
  LARGE-related CMD (MDC1D)

CMD, Congenital muscular dystrophy. Modified from Darras BT. Oculopharyngeal, distal, and congenital muscular dystrophies. In: Dashe JF, ed. *UpToDate* Waltham, MA; 2022.
From Nordli DR, Shefner JM, section eds. Dashe JF, deputy ed. Post TW, ed. UpToDate. Waltham, MA: UpToDate Inc. http://www.uptodate.com.

Congenital Muscular Dystrophies Without Structural CNS Anomalies

The CMDs without structural CNS anomalies can be subclassified now on the basis of merosin (laminin α2-chain gene mutation) staining results of their muscle biopsies into merosin-deficient and merosin-positive CMDs (Boxes 13.5 and 13.6). Both subgroups can present in early infancy with hypotonia, weakness, elevated serum CPK, and joint contractures. Children may exhibit respiratory muscle weakness or difficulty with feeding. The diagnosis in this group of CMDs rests on head MRI imaging, EMG/NCS, CPK testing and muscle biopsy histology, histochemistry, and merosin immunostaining but confirmation is achieved with genetic analysis.

Merosin Deficient Classic Congenital Muscular Dystrophy (MDC1A)

All merosin-deficient patients studied with cranial MRI have abnormalities of the white matter on T2-weighted images that were not seen in the merosin-positive group.[33] Given the expression of merosin in peripheral nerve and brain, slowing of motor nerve conduction velocities[34] and delayed somatosensory evoked potentials have been found. Of interest, both the peripheral and the CNS involvement become more pronounced with age and may be only minimal early in the course of the disease. The *merosin-negative subgroup* is quite unique because of the associated hypomyelination of brain white matter detected by head MRI, the involvement of peripheral nerves[34] and the somewhat severe clinical involvement.[35,36] Despite the white matter changes, most of these patients do not exhibit major neurological deficits on standard evaluation; nonetheless, patients with seizures have been described. *In general,* the merosin-deficient subgroup comprises a more severe neuromuscular phenotype with relatively high-serum CPKs.[37] Most patients are unable to stand or walk, in contrast to the merosin-positive patients, most of whom will walk independently.[38] The phenotype of merosin-deficient CMD seems to be broadening, however. On the one hand, there are patients with mild phenotype who function well into adulthood, but on the other hand, a few patients have also demonstrated evidence of focal cortical dysgenesis (10% occipital agyria) or cerebellar hypoplasia (20%) on brain imaging. An *intermediate phenotype,* with incomplete deficiency and later onset in achievement of ambulation, has also been described. Further, two siblings from a consanguineous family with an internally deleted laminin α2-chain gene, as a result of a splice site mutation in the LAMA2 gene, were reported recently; interestingly, these patients appear mildly affected compared to others who completely lack this protein.[39] Secondary merosin-deficient CMDs such as FKRP-related CMD (MDC1C) are listed in Table 13.5.

Merosin Positive Classic Congenital Muscular Dystrophy

This group of patients with classic CMD, who are merosin positive, may well be quite heterogeneous genetically. As alluded to earlier in the comparative studies with the merosin-deficient patients, it has become apparent that the prognosis for ambulation, for the most part, appears to be much better in the merosin-positive patients.[37,40–42] However, delayed deterioration has been described in a large study from Japan.[43] This would indicate that the underlying dystrophic process is progressive, albeit so slowly that initial motor development outpaces this deterioration. Various merosin-positive CMDs such as rigid-spine syndrome and Ullrich muscular dystrophy are listed in Box 13.6.

TABLE 13.4 Genetic Loci for Congenital Muscular Dystrophy Identified to Date

Disease	Mode of Inheritance	Gene Location	Symbol (Gene Product)	Alternative Disease Symbol
Classical CMD*				
Primary merosin deficiency (MDC1A)	AR	6q22-q23	*LAMA2* (laminin α2 chain of merosin)	
Secondary merosin deficiency (MDC1B)	AR	1q42	?	
Secondary merosin deficiency (MDC1C)	AR	19q13.3	*FKRP* (fukutin-related protein)	MDDGB5
Rigid spine syndrome (RSMD)	AR	1p35-p36	*RSMD1* (selenoprotein N)	
Ullrich muscular dystrophy (UCMD)	AR	21q22.3	*COL6A1* (collagen VI α1 chain)	
Bethlem myopathy	AD			
	AD	21q22.3	*COL6A2* (collagen VI α2 chain)	
	AR			
	AD	2q37	*COL6A3* (collagen VI α3 chain)	
	AR			
Lamin A-related congenital muscular dystrophy (L-CMD)	AD	1q21.2	*LMNA*	
Integrin α7 deficiency	AR	12q13	Integrin α7	
CMD-dystroglycanopathy with CNS abnormalities and/or mental retardation				
Fukuyama CMD	AR	9q31-33	*FCMD* (fukutin)	MDDGA4
Muscle-eye-brain disease (MEB) or Walker-Warburg syndrome (WWS)	AR	1p33-p34	*POMGnT1* (glycosyl-transferase)	MDDGA3
	AR	9q34.1	*POMT1* (O-mannosyl-transferase)	MDDGA1
	AR	9q31-q33	*FCMD* (fukutin)	MDDGA4
	AR	19q13.3	*FKRP* (fukutin-related protein)	MDDGA5
	AR	14q24.3	*POMT2* (mannosyl-transferase)	MDDGA2
LARGE-related CMDs (MDC1D) (WWS-MEB)	AR	22q12.3	*LARGE* (putative glycosyl-transferase)	MDDGA6 MDDGB6

*Structural CNS abnormalities have been described in some patients with classical CMD.

AR, Autosomal recessive; *CMD*, congenital muscular dystrophy; *CNS*, central nervous system; *MDDG*, muscular dystrophy-dystroglycanopathy. Adapted with permission from Jones, K, North, K. The congenital muscular dystrophies. In: Jones HR, De Vivo DC, Darras BT, eds. *Neuromuscular Disorders of Infancy, Childhood, and Adolescence: A Clinician's Approach.* Philadelphia, PA: Butterworth Heinemann; 2003:633. Also from Online Mendelian Inheritance in Man (OMIM).

Congenital Muscular Dystrophies With Structural CNS Anomalies and/or Mental Retardation

Fukuyama Muscular Dystrophy

Of the CMDs with structural CNS anomalies, FMD is a major representative.[44] Described in 1960, FMD is the second most prevalent form of muscular dystrophy in Japan with a DMD/FMD prevalence ratio of 2.1/1 after Duchenne muscular dystrophy (DMD). FMD has been described in non-Japanese Americans and Europeans but, overall, is rare outside Japan. The *FMD gene locus* has been mapped to chromosome 9q31-33;[45,46] it appears to be inherited as an autosomal recessive

TABLE 13.5 Biochemical Classification of Congenital Muscular Dystrophies

Conditions affecting the endoplasmic reticulum	SEPN1 (RSMD1)
Conditions involving the extracellular matrix	Laminin α-2 (MDC1A) Integrin α-7 (CMD) Integrin α-9 (CMD) Collagen VI (Ullrich syndrome)
Conditions affecting the glycosylation of proteins	Fukutin (FCMD) FKRP (MDC1C) *Large* (MDC1D) POMT1 (WWS) POMT2 (WWS) POMGnT1 (MEB) CDG Type I (N-glycosylation disorder)*
Other	Conditions affecting nuclear envelope proteins: severe laminopathies

CDG, Congenital disorder of glycosylation; *CMD,* congenital muscular dystrophy; *FCMD,* Fukuyama congenital muscular dystrophy; *FKRP,* fukutin-related protein; *MDC,* muscular dystrophy, congenital; *MEB,* muscle-eye-brain disease; *RSMD1,* rigid spine syndrome, 1; *SEPN1,* selenoprotein N1; *WWS,* Walker-Warburg syndrome.

*Lefeber DJ, Schonberger J, Morava E, et al. Deficiency of Dol-P-Man synthase subunit DPM3 bridges the congenital disorders of glycosylation with the dystroglycanopathies. *Am J Hum Genet.* 2009;85:76.

trait; the defective gene has been isolated and the respective protein product has been named fukutin.[43]

FMD presents with generalized weakness and hypotonia at birth, joint contractures, and depressed muscle stretch reflexes. Other clinical features include microcephaly and delayed psychomotor development. Convulsions occur in 50% of cases. CPK is usually significantly elevated (10–50 times the upper limit of normal). *Muscle biopsy* shows myopathic changes consisting of endomysial and perimysial fibrosis, rounded muscle fibers with involvement of both *Type I and II fibers* and increased number of Type IIC fibers. Head MRI and autopsy studies usually show diffuse cerebral pachygyria, cerebral and cerebellar polymicrogyria, hydrocephalus ex vacuo, subpial gliosis, and heterotopias. Polymicrogyria is found consistently in the cerebellum. Death usually occurs by 10 years of age.

Walker–Warburg Syndrome

The WWS also seems to be inherited as an autosomal recessive trait. Although a case of WWS has been described in a family with FMD, linkage to the FMD locus on 9q31-33 has been excluded in at least a number of families. The major features are a severe neonatal phenotype with weakness, hypotonia, hydrocephalus, macrocephaly, and eye abnormalities.[47] The muscle biopsy findings are indistinguishable from other disorders in this group; there are major myopathic changes, albeit nonspecific. Deficient laminin α2-chain and α-dystroglycan staining has been described.[48]

The *neuropathologic* features detected by head MRI imaging and autopsy examination vary little from case to case and include hydrocephalus (communicating or ex vacuo), Type II (cobblestone) lissencephaly[49] with or without polymicrogyria, cerebellar hypoplasia, *Dandy-Walker* malformation, small optic nerves and olfactory tracts, absent corpus callosum, colpocephaly, encephalocele(s), and heterotopias. The cortex is composed of two layers separated by an irregular plain layer containing glial fibers and axons. All cerebellar cortical layers can be seen, however. The pathologic changes affecting the eye include optic nerve hypoplasia, retinal detachment and dysplasia, microphthalmia, anterior segment abnormalities, cataract formation, corneal opacities, and shallow anterior chamber. Most WWS patients die in early infancy. A fraction of patients (20%) with WWS have mutations in the gene coding for POMT1 (mannosyltransferase) on chromosome 9q34.1 (Table 13.4) but also in fukutin, fukutin-related protein, POMT2, POMGnT1, and LARGE genes.[48,50–52]

Muscle-Eye-Brain Disease (Santavuori Congenital Muscular Dystrophy)

The *clinical features* of this disorder have been described in a number of Finnish families,[53] some with a history of consanguinity, suggesting autosomal recessive inheritance. Again, the 9q31-q33 locus of FMD has been excluded in a number of Finnish pedigrees, and although the muscle, eye, and brain findings resemble WWS, the phenotype is much milder. Affected patients can usually sit, stand and walk, but subsequent development of spasticity (usually by age 5 years) leads to loss of gross-motor skills.

There is *hypotonia* early in life, slow gross-motor development, hydrocephalus, seizures probably related to cortical dysplasia (pachygyria and polymicrogyria)[54] and, of course, eye involvement with optic atrophy, retinal dysplasia, high myopia, progressive failure of vision and abnormal electroretinogram (ERG), and visual evoked potentials (VEPs). In the Santavuori variety of CMD, eye involvement is usually not obvious in the newborn period. In fact, the ERG may remain normal until 7 years of age. VEPs become delayed and increased in amplitude. Patients survive beyond age 3 years, but death usually occurs between 6 and 16 years. Haltia et al.[54] reported weak immunostaining for merosin with normal laminin β2-chain staining in muscle from patients with MEB. α-dystroglycan immunostaining is reduced in MEB disease. The gene mutated in MEB disease is a glycosyltransferase (POMGnT1) gene and has been mapped at 1p32-p34.[55] Fukutin, LARGE, POMT1, POMT2, and POMGnT1 are putative glycosyltransferases involved in the glycosylation of α-dystroglycan (Table 13.4); mutations in these genes can also result in an MEB phenotype.

CONGENITAL MYOTONIC DYSTROPHY

Myotonic dystrophy, a multisystem disease originally described by Steinert in 1909, is the most prevalent form of muscular dystrophy. The congenital form of the disease occurs in 15% to 25% of infants born to affected mothers. The pregnancy is usually complicated by poor fetal movements and polyhydramnios. Clinical features include hypotonia at birth, respiratory distress, club feet, poor suck and swallow, and myopathic facies. Contractures may be present and may reflect weakness in utero. The weakness of facial and jaw muscles produces a "tented upper lip." At birth, respiratory distress is a common occurrence, but myotonia is not present during the neonatal period. In fact, myotonia may not be present until the age of 5 to 8 years. As the child gets older, mental retardation becomes apparent in most cases. Congenital myotonic dystrophy is always transmitted through an affected mother, who may be asymptomatic or only mildly symptomatic.

In *congenital myotonic dystrophy*, the *CPK* is usually normal. While the infant's EMG may fail to show myotonia, the maternal EMG is always abnormal. *Muscle biopsy* shows nonspecific abnormalities consisting of increased variability in fiber size with Type I fiber atrophy in some cases. The *genetic defect* in myotonic dystrophy has been identified as an expansion of a trinucleotide CTG repeat located in the 3′ untranslated region of a gene, which codes for a serine-threonine protein kinase, also known as myotonin protein kinase.[56,57] Normal individuals contain between 4 and 49 copies of the CTG repeat; normal individuals with 38 to 49 copies of the repeat are classified as a borderline category (premutation) because of the small possibility of expansion of the CTG repeat in their offspring.[58] Mildly affected individuals, or asymptomatic mutation "*carriers*," have 50 to 80 CTG repeats, whereas affected subjects have between 100 and 2000 or more copies (*full mutation*). Infants with congenital myotonic dystrophy usually have more than 750 copies. The CTG copy number increases during successive generations, which explains the phenomenon of genetic anticipation (increasing severity of the disease phenotype and/or earlier onset in successive generations) in myotonic dystrophy families.[59] Although for a given number of repeats (above 100), a wide range in disease severity may be observed, infants with severe congenital myotonic dystrophy and their mothers tend to have a greater number of CTG repeats. The greater the CTG repeat expansion in the mother, the higher the probability of her offspring being affected with the congenital form of illness. Unfortunately, these findings do not explain the exclusive maternal inheritance in cases of congenital myotonic dystrophy. Genomic imprinting or the presence of a maternal intrauterine factor have been proposed as possible mechanisms.

If *myotonic dystrophy* is suspected in a hypotonic neonate, the mother should be examined, even if she is thought to be asymptomatic, the examiner should look closely for evidence of myotonia or weakness of distal muscles and also neck flexors. Currently, the most sensitive way to confirm the diagnosis in an infant is blood testing for the CTG repeat expansion utilizing PCR and/or Southern blot.[60] If the diagnosis of myotonic dystrophy cannot be established in the mother on the basis of clinical presentation and physical examination, EMG sampling of multiple muscles may be necessary to identify myotonia.

INFANTILE FACIOSCAPULOHUMERAL MUSCULAR DYSTROPHY

Facioscapulohumeral dystrophy (FSHD) is an autosomal dominant dystrophy with a distinct phenotype.[61,62] The diagnosis in FSH dystrophy can be suspected and/or easily made clinically in most patients with this disorder. Typically, these children have prominent facial as well as scapulohumeral muscle weakness; Striking asymmetry of muscle involvement is a typical feature of FSH muscular dystrophy.

The infantile variety of FSHD, which is often sporadic in inheritance, has a very early onset (usually within the first few years of life) and is rapidly progressive, with wheelchair confinement by the age of 9 to 10 years in most cases.[62] There is profound facial weakness, with an inability to close the eyes in sleep, to smile, and to show any evidence of facial expression. The weakness rapidly involves the shoulder and hip girdles with lumbar lordosis, resulting in pronounced forward pelvic tilt, and hyperextension of the knees and the head upon walking. Marked weakness of the wrist extensors may result in a wrist drop. Young children with early onset FSHD1 and a very small number of chromosome 4q35 repeats often have epilepsy, mental retardation, and severe sensorineural hearing loss.[63]

A commercial DNA test is available for FSH muscular dystrophy;[64] most patients with classic FSHD1, for whom detailed molecular studies have been done, carry a chromosomal rearrangement within the subtelomere of chromosome 4q (4q35).[65] A tandem array of 3.3 kb repeated DNA elements (D4Z4) is deleted in patients with FSHD1.[66] In the general population, the number of repeat units varies from 11 to >100; in FSHD1 patients, an allele of 1 to 10 residual units is observed because of the deletion of an integral number of these units.[67] Most infants with FSHD1 have only one to three copies of the repeat unit. This diagnostic test is positive in 95% of typical FSH cases.[68] FSHD2, which phenotypically is very similar to FSHD1, is caused by heterozygous mutations in the *SMCHD1* gene on chromosome 18p11 in patients with a permissive haplotype on chromosome 4 that allows the inappropriate expression of the *DUX4* gene; the DUX4 product has a toxic effect on skeletal muscle fibers.[69]

CONGENITAL MYOPATHIES

Shy and Magee introduced the term "*congenital myopathy*" to describe central core disease (CCD) and any myopathy present at birth excluding muscular dystrophy.[70] Unfortunately, inclusion of conditions like nemaline and centronuclear myopathies, which may be progressive and in some cases lethal, blurred the clinical distinction from the muscular dystrophies. These conditions are, however, distinct at a pathological level. In CMDs, the muscle biopsy findings are dystrophic and nonspecific, whereas in congenital myopathies, there are distinct myopathological features without significant fibrosis, muscle fiber degeneration, or replacement with adipose tissue. In *congenital myopathies*, the specificity of distinguishing pathological features has declined recently with the inclusion of conditions with similar but not identical histological features, such as multicore or minicore disease.

Hypotonia and *weakness* are the major clinical features. However, other characteristic features of congenital myopathy like scoliosis, ptosis, and ophthalmoplegia may not be apparent at birth. Therefore, despite the frequent history of infantile hypotonia, diagnosis may be delayed until gross-motor developmental delay and associated weakness develop in late infancy or early childhood. In the congenital myopathies, the EMG may be normal or myopathic with small polyphasic motor unit potentials, normal NCS, normal repetitive nerve stimulation, and absence of abnormal spontaneous activity. The *CPK level* is usually normal or slightly elevated. This is a helpful distinction from CMDs, in which CPK levels are usually moderately to markedly elevated. The diagnosis of congenital myopathies is heavily dependent on the muscle biopsy, which reveals the characteristic features for which the disorder has been named.[71] Table 13.6 summarizes the genetics and main clinical features of congenital myopathies.

Nemaline Myopathy

The term nemaline has been used to characterize the presence of rods or thread-like structures (Greek *nema*, thread) seen in the muscle biopsies of patients with this type of congenital myopathy.[72,73] Of the three different types (neonatal, late infantile/early childhood, late childhood/adult), the neonatal type is the most

TABLE 13.6 Congenital Myopathies

Disease	Genes	Proteins	Onset	Weakness	Cardiac	Respiratory	Facial	Oculo-motor	Prognosis
Myotubular myopathy (centronuclear myopathy, X-linked)	MTM1	Myotubularin	Prenatal to congenital	+++	-	++	+++	+++	Death during infancy, some survive to adulthood
Centronuclear myopathy, classic	BIN-1	Amphiphysin 2	Late infancy to early childhood	+	-	++	++	++	Ambulation until adolescence
Centronuclear myopathy, adult	DMM2 BIN1 RYR1 TTN	Dynamin 2 Amphiphysin 2 Ryanodine receptor 1 Titin	Infancy, childhood, 2nd-3rd decade	+	-	-	+	+/-	Slowly progressive
Nemaline myopathy, severe (congenital)	ACTA1 NEB TPM3 TNNT1 LMOD3	α-actin Nebulin Tropomyosin 3 Troponin T Type I Leiomodin 3	Birth	+++	-	++	+++	-	Death in neonatal period
Nemaline myopathy, typical (congenital)	ACTA1 NEB TPM3 TPM2 CFL2 KBTD13 KLHL40 KLHL41	α-actin Nebulin Tropomyosin 3 Tropomyosin 2 Cofilin 2	1st year	++	+/-	+	+++	-	Many survive to adulthood
Nemaline myopathy, childhood	ACTA1 NEB TPM3	α-actin Nebulin Tropomyosin 3	Pre-pubertal	+	-	-	-	-	Many survive to adulthood
Nemaline myopathy, adult	ACTA1 NEB	α-actin Nebulin	3rd-6th decade	+	+	+/-	++	-	Adulthood
Central core, classical	RYR1	Ryanodine receptor	Infancy	+	Rare	-	+	-	Adulthood?
Multi-minicore disease	SEPN1	Selenoprotein N1	Infancy to early childhood	++	Rare	++	++	Rare	Variable

Continued

TABLE 13.6 Congenital Myopathies—cont'd

Disease	Genes	Proteins	Onset	Weakness	Cardiac	Respiratory	Facial	Oculo-motor	Prognosis
Congenital myopathy and fatal cardiomyopathy	*TTN*	Titin	Infancy to childhood	+ to +++	+++	?	−	−	?
Congenital fiber-type disproportion	*ACTA1* SEPN1 TPM3 RYR1 MYH7 TPM2 XLCFTD	α-actin Selenoprotein N1 Tropomyosin 3 Ryanodine receptor 1 Myosin heavy chain 7 Tropomyosin 2	1st year		Rare	+ to +++ (30%)	+	+/−	Variable
Actin myopathy (non-nemaline)	*ACTA1*	α-actin	Congenital	+++	+	+++	++	?	High mortality
Hyaline body myopathy	*MYH7*	Slow β-cardiac myosin heavy chain	Congenital to adult						
Reducing body myopathy	*FHL-1*	Four and a half LIM domain-1 protein	Congenital to adult	+++ to +	+			+; ptosis	

+++, severe; ++, moderate; +, mild; +/−, mild or absent; −, not reported; ?, not reported so far. Courtesy Dr. Peter Kang, University of Minnesota Medical School.

severe, presenting with hypotonia, diminished spontaneous activity, history of poor fetal movements, and early respiratory distress.[74] More commonly, presentation is delayed until after the newborn period when gross-motor delay with proximal weakness develops.

Serum CPK is usually normal or slightly elevated and the EMG may be normal, myopathic, neuropathic, or mixed. The diagnosis is made by the characteristic nemaline bodies on muscle biopsy. These bodies originate from the Z disks and tend to cluster under the sarcolemma. Frequently Type I fiber predominance is present. Histochemically, α-actinin, myosin, and actin have been detected in nemaline bodies.[75] In a large Australian family characterized by relatively late onset and predominantly distal muscle involvement, close linkage to the 1q22-q23 region[76] was found with subsequent detection of mutations in tropomyosin-3 gene.[77] In this family, the inheritance was autosomal dominant. This form has been named NEM1. A second type of the autosomal recessive form of the disease (NEM2) has been linked to a locus on chromosome 2q21.2-q22, where the nebulin gene has been mapped; recently, mutations in this gene have been identified in patients with nemaline myopathy. In the autosomal dominant families, there is a curious female predominance.[78] To date, more than ten genes have been involved in the pathogenesis of nemaline myopathy (the most common are α-tropomyosin, nebulin, α-actin, β-tropomyosin, troponin T Type I, and cofilin 2). Cardiac involvement may also be present in individuals with *ACTA1* or *MYPN* (myopalladin) mutations.

Central Core Disease

The vast majority of patients with CCD present with hypotonia in early infancy and childhood and a subsequent delay in motor milestones.[79] Rarely, severe hypotonia and marked contractures are present at birth. More commonly, skeletal abnormalities are present, particularly congenital dislocation of the hips, flat feet, pes cavus, club feet, and kyphoscoliosis. The clinical course varies from nonprogressive to slowly progressive. An association between CCD and malignant hyperthermia has been observed even in individuals without evidence of weakness.[80] The diagnosis is based primarily on the histologic finding of central cores on muscle biopsy. The cores appear to be packed with myofiber material and depleted of organelles.

CCD is transmitted by autosomal dominant inheritance.[81] Linkage analysis in four families with CCD has resulted in mapping of the locus to chromosome 19q12-13.2 and more specifically to the 19q13.1[82] segment where the ryanodine receptor-1 gene (*RYR1*) is located. Autosomal dominant and recessive mutations of the ryanodine receptor-1 have been detected in families susceptible to malignant hyperthermia and patients with CCD.[83] Therefore, it appears that at least some forms of CCD and malignant hyperthermia are allelic disorders of the same genetic defect. Therefore the expression of CCD may be related to some additional as yet unidentified factor.

Centronuclear/Myotubular Myopathy

The mode of inheritance of the centronuclear/myotubular myopathy has been debated. Two major forms of inheritance have emerged, i.e., an X-linked form seen primarily in congenital, severely affected cases, and an autosomal dominant late-onset form. In some early-onset cases, the inheritance appears to be autosomal recessive. Early-onset cases are the most common form of *centronuclear/myotubular* myopathy and present with severe hypotonia, weakness, and respiratory distress. Affected infants are very weak and have major feeding difficulties, facial diplegia, bilateral ptosis, and limitation of eye movements (*external ophthalmoplegia*). Frequently, dysmorphic features are evident, such as pectus carinatum, micrognathia, simian creases, high-arched palate, and talipes equinovarus.[84] Chest X-ray always shows slender ribs. Despite intensive respiratory support, infants rarely survive and improve their motor function. Survivors have a marfanoid appearance. Focal or generalized seizures, albeit uncommon, have been reported. The muscle biopsy shows central nuclei present in many muscle fibers and Type I fiber predominance.[85] A radial pattern of staining is noted with oxidative enzyme stains. The gene defect in the X-linked recessive variety (*MTM1*) was mapped to Xq28[86] and subsequently isolated. The protein product was designated myotubularin.[87] The *myotubularin gene* is highly conserved in evolution (expressed in yeast) and is ubiquitously expressed in human tissue despite the fact that the disease shows muscle specificity. No specific treatment is available and most patients with the neonatal form require intensive respiratory support and gastric feeding. Although some improvement is usually noted with maturation, most neonates remain ventilator dependent. Dynamin 2, Amphiphysin 2 (*B1N1*), titin, and also *RYR1* (Table 13.6) mutations have also been described in patients with centronuclear myopathy.[88]

Congenital Fiber Type Disproportion

Congenital fiber type disproportion (CFTD) typically presents with hypotonia and weakness at birth or in the neonatal period.[89] Contractures of the hands and feet and skeletal abnormalities are common. There is delay in acquisition of motor milestones.[90] CPK is normal and EMG may be normal or myopathic. The muscle biopsy shows Type I fiber atrophy, which is a nonspecific finding, noted in other clinically diverse conditions. Therefore, the existence of the CFTD as an entity has been debated. A group of patients with hypotonia and Type I fiber predominance has been described in whom a decrease in the size of Type I fibers is not observed. Type I fiber predominance is another nonspecific feature of many myopathies. Despite the debate over the specificity of CFTD, it is not unusual to find Type I fiber atrophy and Type I fiber predominance in muscle biopsies of hypotonic infants. Although these findings do not reliably predict an improving course, many of these infants will have a good outcome and, as such, deserve supportive measures. α-Actin (*ACTA1*), *RYR1*, α-tropomyosin, b-tropomyosin, *MYH7*, and selenoprotein N (*SEPN1*) mutations have been described in patients with CFTD.[91,92]

Minicore Myopathy

Minicore myopathy (multi-minicore disease [MmD]) is a recessive congenital myopathy characterized by multiple areas of loss of oxidative activity on muscle biopsy. Its onset is usually at birth or during infancy and sometimes in childhood. It presents with predominantly axial and proximal weakness, hypotonia, and arthrogryposis. Two-thirds of affected children develop scoliosis and respiratory difficulties. The presence of minicores has been linked to four clinical phenotypes: (1) classic phenotype with significant axial weakness, early respiratory impairment, and severe scoliosis; (2) predominantly hip girdle weakness sometimes associated with arthrogryposis at birth; (3) classic phenotype with associated external

ophthalmoplegia; and (4) marked distal atrophy and weakness affecting primarily the upper extremities.

Patients with the classic axial presentation of MmD have recessive mutations in the selenoprotein N (*SEPN1*) gene, also causing CMD with rigidity of the spine (*RSMD1*). MmD with predominant hip girdle weakness and the one with distal atrophy and weakness have been linked to mutations in the skeletal muscle ryanodine receptor (*RYR1*) gene. Recently, *RYR1*, titin, and *MYH7* gene recessive mutations were also identified in the subset of patients with MmD and external ophthalmoplegia or cardiomyopathy.[93]

Other Congenital Myopathies

In addition to the four most common congenital myopathies described above, there are uncommon types of congenital myopathies characterized by hypotonia, weakness, delay in motor milestones, and a less well-defined pattern of inheritance. Their names reflect their myopathological features and include: (1) actin myopathy (non-nemaline), (2) fingerprint body myopathy, (3) sarcotubular myopathy, (4) hyaline body myopathy, (5) reducing body myopathy, (6) cytoplasmic body myopathy, (7) myopathy with myotubular aggregates, (8) zebra body myopathy, and (9) trilaminar myopathy. Although the mutated genes are known in some of them (Table 13.6), in all of these conditions, the diagnosis is made by muscle biopsy, which underscores the significance of this procedure in the evaluation of newborns with weakness and hypotonia unrelated to CNS dysfunction or systemic disease.

METABOLIC MYOPATHIES

Acid Maltase Deficiency (Glycogen Storage Disease II)

Acid maltase is a lysosomal α-1,4-glucosidase which releases glucose from glycogen, oligosaccharides, and maltose. Acid maltase deficiency (AMD) is divided into three major groups: infantile, childhood, and adult AMD. All types are transmitted by autosomal recessive inheritance.

Infantile Acid Maltase Deficiency (Pompe Disease)

Infantile AMD may present in the newborn period, but the onset is usually during the second or third month of life. The presentation is usually that of rapidly progressive weakness, hypotonia, and enlargement of the heart, tongue, and liver. Storage of glycogen in the brain and spinal cord results in CNS dysfunction with diminished alertness and hyporeflexia. Respiratory and feeding difficulties are common and death, usually from cardiorespiratory failure, commonly occurs before the age of 2 years. The *electrocardiogram* (EKG) shows a short PR interval, high QRS amplitude, and left ventricular hypertrophy.[94] In one infant, a *Wolff-Parkinson-White* syndrome was noted. The diagnosis is supported by an increased CPK, generally less than ten times the upper limit of normal, and a myopathic EMG, with abundant myotonic discharges and occasionally with fibrillation potentials and positive waves. Acid maltase activity is deficient in muscle, liver, heart, leukocytes, and cultured fibroblasts. To confirm the diagnosis, the enzyme is usually assayed in lymphocytes and/or muscle tissue and sometimes in urine.[95] The *muscle biopsy* shows large vacuoles with a high glycogen content (PAS-positive) and strong reactivity for acid phosphatase, identifying them as secondary lysosomes. Despite the detection of numerous mutations in the acid α-1,4-glucosidase gene on chromosome 17q23,[96] DNA testing is not yet routinely available. In the past, aside from supportive management of cardiorespiratory insufficiency, there was no effective treatment for infantile AMD. Enzyme replacement therapy has become available with good results.[97]

MITOCHONDRIAL MYOPATHIES

Cytochrome c Oxidase (COX) Deficiency

Fatal Infantile Myopathy

This condition presents soon after birth with severe *lactic acidosis*, profound *hypotonia* and *weakness*, feeding difficulties, and respiratory insufficiency. In some cases, myopathy with or without an associated cardiomyopathy may be the only manifestation. More commonly, however, there is an associated renal *deToni-Fanconi-Debre* syndrome. Most of these infants die from cardiorespiratory insufficiency before 1 year of age. The muscle biopsy shows ragged-red fibers with accumulation of glycogen and lipid in most but not all cases. *Histochemical* staining for COX activity is undetectable, and biochemical analysis of skeletal muscle tissue shows virtual absence of COX activity.[98]

Recently, a severe depletion of mitochondrial DNA (mtDNA) has been detected in patients with fatal infantile myopathy.

Benign Infantile Myopathy

The benign variety presents at or soon after birth with generalized weakness and hypotonia, respiratory and feeding difficulties, and severe lactic acidosis.[99] Unlike the fatal form, this condition is confined to the skeletal muscle. These infants tend to improve spontaneously during the first year of life and are normal by the age of 3 years. Muscle histochemistry and/or standard biochemical assays show almost undetectable COX activity. With age, this enzyme activity recovers. Ragged-red fibers have been observed in early muscle biopsies but disappear during childhood. The benign variety is distinguished from the fatal form by the immunological detection (*immunotitration by ELISA*) of the enzyme in muscle tissue.[100] In the fatal type of COX deficiency, the enzyme protein is undetectable by ELISA.[101] Most cases have been sporadic. This condition is thought to result from mutations in a tissue-specific and developmentally regulated fetal COX isoform. Since the enzymatic deficiency is reversible, aggressive support is advised in infants with COX deficiency.

FATTY ACID OXIDATION DEFECTS

This *group* of disorders *includes*: (1) the carnitine deficiency syndromes, (2) defects in carnitine palmitoyltransferases, CPT I, CPT II, and translocase, and (3) defects of fatty acid β-oxidation enzymes. Most of these conditions present in infancy with hypotonia, generalized weakness, and in some cases cardiomegaly and/or hepatic failure. There may be associated nonketotic or hypoketotic hypoglycemia, hyperammonemia, reduced total and/or free carnitine (rarely, increased free and total carnitine), elevated serum acylcarnitines, and abnormal urine dicarboxylic acids and acylglycines. Serum CPK may be normal or highly elevated. Affected newborns may be lethargic and/or comatose. Muscle biopsy may reveal accumulation of lipid, primarily in Type I fibers. The *diagnosis* requires detection of the enzymatic deficiency in cultured skin fibroblasts and/or muscle tissue. In cases of true primary muscle carnitine deficiency, the clinical response to carnitine supplementation may be dramatic.

Therefore a trial of carnitine supplementation is warranted in infants with carnitine transport defects. *Organic acidurias* may also present with weakness, hypotonia, cardiomyopathy, and liver enlargement, probably due to secondary carnitine deficiency. In the secondary syndromes, the muscle biopsy shows lipid but not glycogen accumulation. Abnormal organic acids and acylcarnitines can be demonstrated by the appropriate testing of urine and serum.

NONLYSOSOMAL GLYCOGENOSES

Phosphorylase Deficiency

Phosphorylase deficiency may present in early infancy with severe generalized weakness and hypotonia, feeding difficulties, and respiratory insufficiency.[102] Areflexia or hyporeflexia is usually present but the child remains alert without evidence of encephalopathy.[103] Serum CPK concentration is elevated and the muscle biopsy is diagnostic, showing myopathic changes with subsarcolemmal and intermyofibrillar deposits of glycogen. Phosphorylase activity is undetectable in muscle tissue by either histochemistry or enzymatic methods.

Phosphofructokinase Deficiency

A neonatal variety of phosphofructokinase (PFK) deficiency has been described, presenting with congenital weakness, hypotonia, swollen joints, multiple contractures, and, in some cases, seizures, cortical blindness, and corneal opacifications.[104] There may be evidence of cardiomyopathy, but none of the infantile cases develop hemolysis. *CPK values* and uric acid are increased in most patients. The muscle biopsy shows accumulation of glycogen under the sarcolemma and between myofibrils. The *diagnosis* is confirmed by the *immunohistochemical* demonstration of absent PFK staining in muscle, and diminished muscle PFK activity by enzymatic assay. In infants with PFK deficiency, the enzyme is present in red blood cells in normal amounts. The biochemical basis of the infantile variety of PFK deficiency is unclear and probably heterogenous.

Approach to Hypotonia

The following describes our stepwise approach to the diagnostic investigation of infantile hypotonia (Fig. 13.1).

- Conduct a detailed history (h/o polyhydramnios, intrauterine growth retardation, reduced fetal movement) and physical examination (as described above) including tests of muscle stretch reflexes, antigravity limb movements, and contractures.[105]
- Exclude systemic illness and congenital laxity of ligaments.
  - If *central hypotonia* is suspected, conduct genetic testing for Prader-Willi (deletion of 15q11-13) and Down (trisomy 21) syndrome using chromosomal microarray and/or methylation array. In centers where rapid genomic or exon sequencing are available, consider clinical genetics consultation for likelihood of a monogenetic disorder and rapid genome-wide testing for infants as the first-line diagnostic test. If molecular diagnosis is unavailable, consider further phenotyping with MRI/MRS studies, metabolic studies, and tests for very long-chain fatty acids and/or other peroxisomal tests. Consider lumbar puncture for CSF lactate, glucose, and protein; and, if indicated, CSF neurotransmitter testing.
- If *peripheral hypotonia* is suspected, first examine the mother. If she has signs of myotonic dystrophy, perform a DNA test for 19qCTG repeat expansion in the child. Elicit any history of autoimmune myasthenia gravis in the mother. If SMA has not been tested as part of newborn screening and clinical suspicion is high, perform targeted testing for *SMN1* exon 7/8 deletion.
  - Consider clinical genetics consultation for likelihood of a monogenetic disorder and rapid genome-wide testing for infants as the first line diagnostic test, after gold standard testing for Prader-Willi, SMA, and myotonic dystrophy if clinical suspicion of these disorders is high. Both parents' sequences can be compared with the infant's sequence to prioritize variants of interests and establish inheritance patterns. Rapid genome-wide testing can mitigate prolonged and invasive diagnostic testing, such as electromyography and muscle biopsy, and optimize medical management. If a molecular diagnosis is identified,

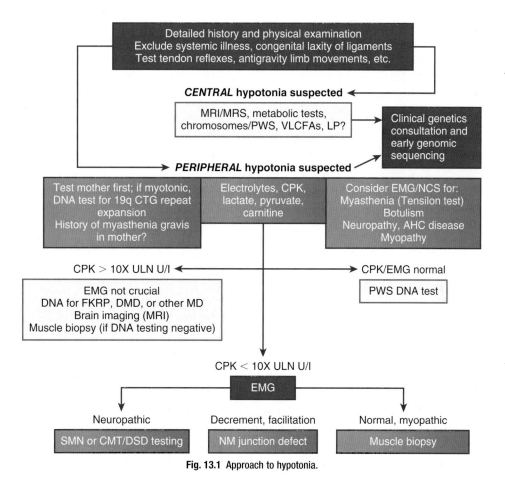

Fig. 13.1 Approach to hypotonia.

evaluate for targeted treatment options and provide prognostic information to guide medical decisions and goals of care.
- If no molecular diagnosis is made, consider mitochondrial genome analysis and additional phenotyping as follows:
- Consider electromyography and NCS to evaluate for myasthenia, botulism, neuropathy or anterior horn cell disease, and myopathy. Consider performing a Tensilon test if myasthenic syndrome is suspected.
- Test the child's electrolytes, CPK, lactate, pyruvate, carnitine, and/or other biochemical tests.
  - If CPK/EMG are normal, conduct a DNA test for Prader-Willi syndrome.

- If CPK is greater than ten times the upper limit of normal, electromyography is not crucial. Perform DNA tests for *FKRP* (fukutin-related protein) gene mutations and/or other muscular dystrophies. Targeted gene testing can circumvent the limitations of genome-wide sequencing in detecting large deletions, inversions, and repeat expansions. Consider brain imaging (MRI). If DNA testing is negative, conduct a muscle biopsy.
- If CPK is elevated less than ten times the upper limit of normal, conduct electromyography. If the EMG is neuropathic, order genetic testing for *SMN* gene or Charcot-Marie-Tooth/Dejerine-Sottas disease. An

EMG showing decrement/facilitation indicates a neuromuscular junction defect. If the EMG is normal or myopathic, conduct a muscle biopsy (electromyography may be normal in certain myopathies).

The future of the field leaves several further gaps including the timing and type of genomic testing in all infants with hypotonia, in addition to the genetic therapies that may be targeted to improve neurological outcomes.

REFERENCES

1. Volpe JJ, Inder TE, Darras BT, et al., eds. *Volpe's Neurology of the Newborn*. 6th ed. Philadelphia: Elsevier; 2018.
2. Sainte-Anne Dargassies S. *Neurological Development in the Full-Term and Premature Neonate*. New York: Elsevier North Holland; 1979.
3. Volpe JJ. Neonatal hypotonia. In: Jones HR Jr, De Vivo DC, Darras BT, eds. *Neuromuscular Disorders of Infancy, Childhood, and Adolescence: A Clinician's Approach*. Philadelphia: Butterworth Heinemann; 2003:113-122.
4. Gingold MK, Jaynes ME, Bodensteiner JB, et al. The rise and fall of the plantar response in infancy. *J Pediatr*. 1998;133:568.
5. Paine RS, Brazelton TB, Donovan DE, et al. Evolution of postural reflexes in normal infants and in the presence of chronic brain syndromes. *Neurology*. 1964;14:1036.
6. Futagi Y, Tagawa T, Otani K. Primitive reflex profiles in infants: differences based on categories of neurological abnormality. *Brain Dev*. 1992;14:294.
7. Fenichel GM. The hypotonic infant. In: *Clinical Pediatric Neurology, a Signs and Symptoms Approach*. 5th ed. Philadelphia: Elsevier Saunders; 2005:149-169.
8. Richer LP, Shevell MI, Miller SP. Diagnostic profile of neonatal hypotonia: an 11-year study. *Pediatr Neurol*. 2001;25:32.
9. Prasad AN, Prasad C. Genetic evaluation of the floppy infant. *Semin Fetal Neonatal Med*. 2011;16:99.
10. Dubowitz V. Disorders of the lower motor neurone: the spinal muscular atrophies. In: Dubowitz V, ed. *Muscle Disorders in Childhood*. London: Saunders; 1995:325-369.
11. Morrison KE, Harding AE. Disorders of the motor neuron. In: Harding AE, ed. *Genetics and Neurology*. London: Bailliere Tindall; 1994:431-445.
12. Bundey S. Spinal muscular atrophies (SMAs). In: Bundey S, ed. *Genetics and Neurology*. Edinburgh: Churchill Livingstone; 1985: 172-193.
13. Grohmann K, Varon R, Stolz P, et al. Infantile spinal muscular atrophy with respiratory distress type I (SMARD1). *Ann Neurol*. 2003;54:719.
14. Gilliam TC, Brzustowicz LM. The molecular basis of the spinal muscular atrophies. In: Rosenberg RN, Pruisner SB, DiMauro S, et al., eds. *The Molecular and Genetic Basis of Neurological Disease*. Philadelphia: Butterworth Heinemann; 1993:883-887.
15. Hahnen E, Forkert R, Marke C, et al. Molecular analysis of candidate genes on 5q13 in autosomal recessive spinal muscular atrophy: evidence of homozygous deletions of the SMN gene in unaffected individuals. *Hum Mol Genet*. 1995;4: 1927.
16. Lefebvre S, Burglen L, Reboullet S, et al. Identification and characterization of a spinal muscular atrophy-determining gene. *Cell*. 1995;80:155.
17. Roy N, Mahadevan MS, McLean M. The gene for neuronal apoptosis inhibitor protein (NAIP), a novel protein with homology to baculoviral inhibitors of apoptosis is partially deleted in individuals with type I, II, and III spinal muscular atrophy (SMA). *Cell*. 1995;80:167.
18. Yeo CJJ, Simmons Z, De Vivo DC, et al. Ethical perspectives on treatment options with spinal muscular atrophy patients. *Ann Neurol*. 2022;91:305.
19. Cure SMA. *What is Newborn Screening?* Available at: http://www.curesma.org/newborn-screening-for-sma/. Accessed September 19, 2021.
20. SMA NBS Alliance. *Status of Newborn Screening for Spinal Muscular Atrophy*. Available at: http://www.sma-screening-alliance.org/map/. Accessed September 19, 2021.
21. Byers RK, Banker BQ. Infantile muscular atrophy. *Arch Neurol*. 1961;5:140.
22. Munsat TL. Workshop report. International SMA collaboration. *Neuromusc Disord*. 1991;1:81.
23. Feldkotter M, Schwarzer V, Wirth R, et al. Quantitative analyses of SMN1 and SMN2 based on real-time light cycler PCR: fast and highly reliable carrier testing and prediction of severity of spinal muscular atrophy. *Am J Hum Genet*. 2002;70:358.
24. Glascock J, Sampson J, Connolly AM, et al. Revised recommendations for the treatment of infants diagnosed with spinal muscular atrophy via newborn screening who have 4 copies of SMN2. *J Neuromuscul Dis*. 2020;7:97.
25. Sladky JT. Chronic sensory-motor neuropathies in children. Paper presented at Annual Meeting of the American Association of Electrodiagnostic Medicine Course A, 1993; New Orleans, LA.
26. Behin A, Mayer M, Kassis-Makhoul B, et al. Severe neonatal myasthenia due to maternal anti-MuSK antibodies. *Neuromuscul Disord*. 2008;18:443.
27. Engel AG, Ohno K, Harper CM. Congenital myasthenic syndromes. In: Jones Jr HR, De Vivo DC, Darras BT, eds. *Neuromuscular Disorders of Infancy, Childhood, and Adolescence: A Clinician's Approach*. Philadelphia: Butterworth Heinemann; 2003:555-574.
28. Gutmann L, Pratt L. Pathophysiologic aspects of human botulism. *Arch Neurol*. 1976;33:175.
29. Cherington M. Botulism: clinical, electrical and therapeutic considerations. In: Lewis GE, ed. *Biomedical Aspects of Botulism*. New York: Academic; 1981:327-330.
30. Cornblath DR, Sladky JT, Sumner AJ. Clinical electrophysiology of infantile botulism. *Muscle Nerve*. 1983;6:448.
31. Sunada Y, Bernier SM, Utani A, et al. Identification of a novel mutant transcript of laminin alpha 2 chain gene responsible for muscular dystrophy and dysmyelination in dy2J mice. *Hum Mol Genet*. 1995;4:1055.
32. Arnon SS, Schechter R, Maslanka SE, et al. Human botulism immune globulin for the treatment of infant botulism. *N Engl J Med*. 2006;354:462.
33. Dubowitz V. 41st ENMC international workshop on congenital muscular dystrophy. *Neuromusc Disord*. 1996;6:295.
34. Shorer Z, Philpot J, Muntoni F, et al. Demyelinating peripheral neuropathy in merosin-deficient congenital muscular dystrophy. *J Child Neurol*. 1995;10:472.
35. Helbling-Leclerc A, Zhang X, Topaloglu H, et al. Mutations in the laminin alpha 2-chain gene (LAMA2) cause merosin-deficient congenital muscular dystrophy. *Nat Genet*. 1995;11:216.

36. Tome FM, Evangelista T, Leclerc A, et al. Congenital muscular dystrophy with merosin deficiency. *C R Acad Sci III*. 1994; 317:351.
37. Philpot J, Sewry C, Pennock J, et al. Clinical phenotype in congenital muscular dystrophy: correlation with expression of merosin in skeletal muscle. *Neuromusc Disord*. 1995;5:301.
38. Kobayashi O, Hayashi Y, Arahata K, et al. Congenital muscular dystrophy: clinical and pathologic study of 50 patients with the classical (occidental) merosin-positive form. *Neurology*. 1996; 46:815.
39. Allamand V, Sunada Y, Salih MAM, et al. Mild congenital muscular dystrophy in two patients with an internally deleted laminin α2-chain. *Hum Mol Genet*. 1997;6:747.
40. Vainzof M, Marie SKN, Reed UC, et al. Deficiency of merosin (laminin M or α2) in congenital muscular dystrophy associated with cerebral white matter alterations. *Neuropediatrics*. 1995; 26:293.
41. Connolly AM, Pestronk A, Planer GJ, et al. Congenital muscular dystrophy syndromes distinguished by alkaline and acid phosphatase, merosin, and dystrophin staining. *Neurology*. 1996;46:810.
42. North KN, Specht LA, Sethi RK, et al. Congenital muscular dystrophy associated with merosin deficiency. *Neurology*. 1996;11:291.
43. Kobayashi K, Nakahori Y, Miyake M, et al. An ancient retrotransposal insertion causes Fukuyama-type congenital muscular dystrophy. *Nature*. 1998;394:388.
44. Fukuyama Y, Osawa M, Suzuki H. Congenital progressive muscular dystrophy of the Fukuyama type: clinical, genetic and pathological considerations. *Brain Dev*. 1981;3:1.
45. Toda T, Segawa M, Nomura Y, et al. Localization of a gene for Fukuyama type congenital muscular dystrophy to chromosome 9q31−33. *Nat Genet*. 1993;5:283.
46. Yoshioka M, Kuroki S. Clinical spectrum and genetic studies of Fukuyama congenital muscular dystrophy. *Am J Med Genet*. 1994;53:245.
47. Dobyns WB, Pagon RA, Armstrong D, et al. Diagnostic criteria for Walker-Warburg syndrome. *Am J Med Genet*. 1989;32:195.
48. Beltran-Valero de Bernabe D, Currier S, Steinbrecher A, et al. Mutations in the O-mannosyltransferase gene POMT1 give rise to the severe neuronal migration disorder Walker-Warburg syndrome. *Am J Hum Genet*. 2002;71:1033.
49. Dobyns WB, Truwit CL. Lissencephaly and other malformations of cortical development: 1995 update. *Neuropediatrics*. 1995;26:132.
50. de Bernabe DB, van Bokhoven H, van Beusekom E, et al. A homozygous nonsense mutation in the fukutin gene causes a Walker-Warburg syndrome phenotype. *J Med Genet*. 2003;40:845.
51. Beltran-Valero de Bernabe D, Voit T, Longman C, et al. Mutations in the FKRP gene can cause muscle-eye-brain disease and Walker-Warburg syndrome. *J Med Genet*. 2004;41:e61.
52. van Reeuwijk J, Janssen M, van den Elzen C, et al. POMT2 mutations cause alpha-dystroglycan hypoglycosylation and Walker-Warburg syndrome. *J Med Genet*. 2005;42:907.
53. Santavuori P, Somer H, Sainio K, et al. Muscle-eye brain disease (MEB). *Brain Dev*. 1989;11:147.
54. Haltia M, Leivo I, Sorne RH, et al. Muscle-eye-brain disease: a neuropathological study. *Ann Neurol*. 1997;41:173.
55. Yoshida A, Kobayashi K, Manya H, et al. Muscular dystrophy and neuronal migration disorder caused by mutations in a glycosyltransferase, POMGnT1. *Dev Cell*. 2001;1:717.
56. Aslanidis C, Jansen G, Amemiya C, et al. Cloning of the essential myotonic dystrophy region and mapping of the putative defect. *Nature*. 1992;355:548.
57. Brook JD, McCurrach ME, Harley HG, et al. Molecular basis of myotonic dystrophy: expansion of a trinucleotide (CTG) repeat at the 3′ end of a transcript encoding a protein kinase family member. *Cell*. 1992;68:799.
58. Harley HG, Rundle SA, Reardon W. Unstable DNA sequence in myotonic dystrophy. *Lancet*. 1992;339:1125.
59. Suthers GK, Huson SM, Davies KE. Instability versus predictability: the molecular diagnosis of myotonic dystrophy. *J Med Genet*. 1992;29:761.
60. Brunner HG, Nillesen W, van Oost BA. Presymptomatic diagnosis of myotonic dystrophy. *J Med Genet*. 1992;29:780.
61. Munsat TL, Piper D, Cancilla P, et al. Inflammatory myopathy with facioscapulohumeral distribution. *Neurology*. 1972;22:335.
62. Taylor DA, Carroll JE, Smith ME, et al. Facioscapulohumeral dystrophy associated with hearing loss and Coats syndrome. *Ann Neurol*. 1982;12:395.
63. Funakoshi M, Goto K, Arahata K. Epilepsy and mental retardation in a subset of early onset 4q35-facioscapulohumeral muscular dystrophy. *Neurology*. 1998;50:1791.
64. Kohler J, Rohrig D, Bathke KD, et al. Evaluation of the facioscapulohumeral muscular dystrophy (FSHD1) phenotype in correlation to the concurrence of 4q35 and 10q26 fragments. *Clin Genet*. 1999;55:88.
65. Griggs RC, Tawil R, Storvick D, et al. Genetics of facioscapulohumeral muscular dystrophy: new mutations in sporadic cases. *Neurology*. 1993;43:2369.
66. Hewitt JE, Lyle R, Clark LN, et al. Analysis of the tandem repeat locus D4Z4 associated with facioscapulohumeral muscular dystrophy. *Hum Mol Genet*. 1994;3:1287.
67. Tawil R, Figlewicz DA, Griggs RC, et al. Facioscapulohumeral dystrophy: a distinct regional myopathy with a novel molecular pathogenesis. FSH Consortium. *Ann Neurol*. 1998;43:279.
68. Ricci E, Galluzzi G, Deidda G, et al. Progress in the molecular diagnosis of facioscapulohumeral muscular dystrophy and correlation between the number of KpnI repeats at the 4q35 locus and clinical phenotype. *Ann Neurol*. 1999;45:751.
69. Lemmers RJ, Tawil R, Petek LM, et al. Digenic inheritance of an SMCHD1 mutation and an FSHD-permissive D4Z4 allele causes facioscapulohumeral muscular dystrophy type 2. *Nat Genet*. 2012;44:1370.
70. Shy GM, Magee KR. A new congenital non-progressive myopathy. *Brain*. 1956;79:610.
71. Sewry CA. Pathological defects in congenital myopathies. *J Muscle Res Cell Motil*. 2008;29:231.
72. Shy GM, Engel WK, Somers JE, et al. Nemaline myopathy: a new congenital myopathy. *Brain*. 1963;86:793.
73. Sewry CA, Laitila JM, Wallgren-Pettersson C. Nemaline myopathies: a current view. *J Muscle Res Cell Motil*. 2019;40:111.
74. Shafiq SA, Dubowitz V, Peterson H, et al. Nemaline myopathy: report of a fatal case with histochemical and electron microscopic studies. *Brain*. 1967;90:817.
75. Wallgren-Pettersson C, Arjomaa P, Holmberg C. Alpha-actinin and myosin light chains in congenital nemaline myopathy. *Pediatr Neurol*. 1990;6:171.
76. Laing NG, Majda BT, Akkari PA, et al. Assignment of a gene (NEMI) for autosomal dominant nemaline myopathy to chromosome I. *Am J Hum Genet*. 1992;50:576.
77. Laing NG, Wilton SD, Akkari PA, et al. A mutation in the alpha tropomyosin gene TPM3 associated with autosomal dominant nemaline myopathy. *Nat Genet*. 1995;9:75.
78. Scarlato G, Pellegrini G, Moggio M. Familial nemaline myopathy. *Neuropediatrics*. 1982;13:211.

79. Engel WK, Foster JB, Hughes BP. Central core disease-an investigation of a rare muscle cell abnormality. *Brain.* 1961;84:167.
80. Denborough MA, Dennett XK, Anderson RM. Central core disease and malignant hyperthermia. *Br Med J.* 1973;1:272.
81. Byrne E, Blumbergs PC, Hallpike JF. Central core disease. Study of a family with five affected generations. *J Neurol Sci.* 1982;53:77.
82. Haan EA, Freemantle CJ, McCure JA, et al. Assignment of the gene for central core disease to chromosome 19. *Hum Genet.* 1990;86:187.
83. Zhang Y, Chen HS, Khanna VK. A mutation in the human ryanodine receptor gene associated with central core disease. *Nature Genet.* 1993;5:46.
84. Kinoshita M, Cadman TE. Myotubular myopathy. *Arch Neurol.* 1968;18:265.
85. Spiro AJ, Shy GM, Gonatas NK. Myotubular myopathy: persistence of fetal muscle in an adolescent boy. *Arch Neurol.* 1966;14:1.
86. Thomas NST, Sarfarazi M, Roberts K, et al. X-linked myotubular myopathy (MTM1) evidence for linkage to Xq28 DNA marker loci. *J Med Genet.* 1990;27:284.
87. Laporte J, Hu LJ, Kretz C, et al. A gene mutated in X-linked myotubular myopathy defines a new putative tyrosine phosphatase family conserved in yeast. *Nature Genet.* 1996;13:175.
88. Bitoun M, Maugenre S, Jeannet PY, et al. Mutations in dynamin 2 cause dominant centronuclear myopathy. *Nat Genet.* 2005;37:1207.
89. Brooke MH. Congenital fiber type disproportion. In: Kakulas BA, ed. *Clinical Studies in Myology.* Vol. 295. Amsterdam: Excerpta Medica ICS; 1973:147.
90. Lenard HG, Goebel HH. Congenital fibre type disproportion. *Neuropediatrics.* 1975;6:220.
91. Laing NG, Clarke NF, Dye DE, et al. Actin mutations are one cause of congenital fibre type disproportion. *Ann Neurol.* 2004;56:689.
92. Clarke NF, Kidson W, Quijano-Roy S, et al. SEPN1: associated with congenital fiber-type disproportion and insulin resistance. *Ann Neurol.* 2006;59:546.
93. Jungbluth H, Zhou H, Hartley L, et al. Minicore myopathy with ophthalmoplegia caused by mutations in the ryanodine receptor type I gene. *Neurology.* 2005;65:1930.
94. Bulkley BH, Hutchins GM. Pompe's disease presenting as hypertrophic myocardiopathy with Wolff-Parkinson-White syndrome. *Am Heart J.* 1978;92:246.
95. Salafsky IS, Nadler HL. Deficiency of acid alpha glucosidase in the urine of patients with Pompe disease. *J Pediatr.* 1973;82:294.
96. Zhong N, Martiniuk F, Tzall S, et al. Identification of a missense mutation in one allele of a patient with Pompe disease, and use of endonuclease digestion of PCR-amplified RNA to demonstrate lack of mRNA expression from the second allele. *Am J Hum Genet.* 1991;49:635.
97. Kishnani PS, Nicolino M, Voit T, et al. Chinese hamster ovary cell-derived recombinant human acid alpha-glucosidase in infantile-onset Pompe disease. *J Pediatr.* 2006;149:89.
98. Rimoldi M, Bottacchi E, Rossi L. Cytochrome-c-oxidase deficiency in muscle of a floppy infant without mitochondrial myopathy. *J Neurol.* 1982;227:201.
99. Zeviani M, Peterson P, Servidei S. Benign reversible muscle cytochrome c oxidase deficiency: a second case. *Neurology.* 1987;37:64.
100. Tritschler HJ, Bonilla E, Lombes A, et al. Differential diagnosis of fatal and benign cytochrome c oxidase-deficient myopathies of infancy: an immunohistochemical approach. *Neurology.* 1991;41:300.
101. Bresolin N, Zeviani M, Bonilla E. Molecular defects in cytochrome c oxidase deficiency: decrease of immunologically detectable enzyme in muscle. *Neurology.* 1985;35:802.
102. DiMauro S, Hartlage P. Fatal infantile form of muscle phosphorylase deficiency. *Neurology.* 1978;28:1124.
103. Milstein J, Herron T, Haas J. Fatal infantile muscle phosphorylase deficiency. *J Child Neurol.* 1989;4:186.
104. Servidei S, Bonilla E, Diedrich RG. Fatal infantile form of muscle phosphofructokinase deficiency. *Neurology.* 1986;36:1465.
105. Vasta I, Kinali M, Messina S, et al. Can clinical signs identify newborns with neuromuscular disorders? *J Pediatr.* 2005;146:73.

Chapter 14

Amplitude-Integrated EEG and Its Potential Role in Improving Neonatal Care Within the NICU

Lauren C. Weeke, Maria Luisa Tataranno, and Mohamed El-Dib

Chapter Outline

Case Description (Fig. 14.1)

The patient was born at 40 weeks' gestation and weighed 3150 g at birth. An emergency cesarean section was performed for suspected fetal compromise with bradycardia on the cardiotocogram because of a nuchal cord. Apgar scores were 1, 0, 0 at 1, 5, and 10 minutes, respectively. The infant was resuscitated for 15 minutes with intravenous adrenalin given once. The umbilical cord pH was 7.25, and base excess was −3.5. The first arterial lactate concentration was 26.4 mmol/L. The infant was cooled for 72 hours at 33.5°C. Seizures were treated with phenobarbital, midazolam, and lidocaine. Magnetic resonance imaging (MRI) on day 4 showed severe abnormalities in the basal ganglia and thalami. The infant died on day 5 after redirection of care.

Key Points

- aEEG is easy to apply and interpret at the cotside.
- The aEEG background pattern is a reliable marker for encephalopathy in full-term infants and for brain maturation in preterm infants and can guide prognostication.
- Electrographic seizures detected with the aEEG compressed tracing should always be confirmed on the raw EEG, with two channels having greater reliability than single channel.
- Factors influencing the aEEG such as interelectrode spacing, medications, and common artifacts should be considered when interpreting the aEEG.

Introduction

Interest in the neonatal brain has increased considerably throughout the past decades. Imaging techniques such as ultrasound and magnetic resonance imaging (MRI) can evaluate the presence and extent of structural lesions of the brain. Near-infrared spectroscopy (NIRS) allows noninvasive monitoring of

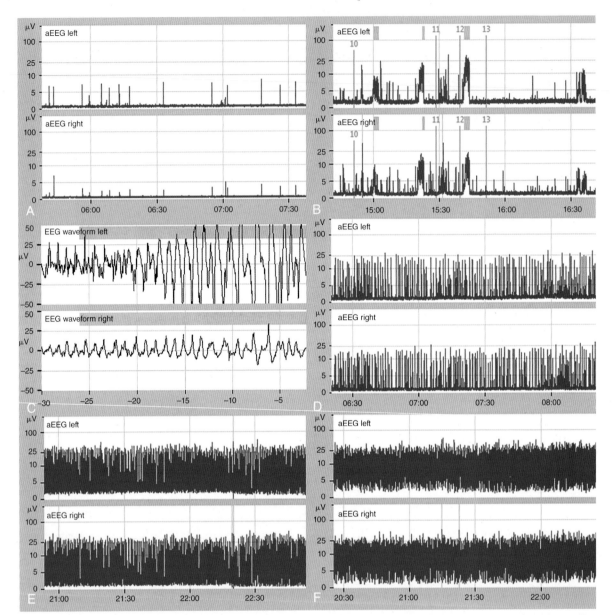

Fig. 14.1 A, Cooling was started at 3 hours after birth. B, Amplitude-integrated electroencephalogram (aEEG) at 18 hours after birth during cooling shows a flat trace pattern with seizures (indicated by the *pink bars*). *10*, care; *11*, x-ray; *12+13*, midazolam is given. C, The raw EEG showing a typical ictal discharge with evolution in amplitude and frequency. D, A sparse burst suppression pattern is seen 36 hours after birth (during cooling). E, A dense burst suppression is seen 48 hours after birth. F, A discontinuous normal voltage pattern is seen 72 hours after birth.

brain oxygenation and cerebral hemodynamics. Conventional multichannel electroencephalography (will be referred to as cEEG) and amplitude-integrated EEG (aEEG) provide information about brain function. EEG may detect epileptic discharges, reflect encephalopathy, from common etiologies such as hypoxic-ischemic encephalopathy (HIE, as illustrated in Fig. 14.1), and may give valuable information on brain maturation. Today, aEEG is used routinely in an increasing number of neonatal intensive care units (NICUs) due to its ease of use at the cotside. The extent of EEG monitoring in the NICU has been evaluated by analyzing 210 surveys (124 from Europe and 54 from the United States). Ninety percent of respondents had access to either cEEG or aEEG monitoring; 51% had both. The cEEG was mainly interpreted by neurophysiologists (72%), whereas aEEG was usually interpreted by the neonatologist (80%). However, as many as 31% of the respondents reported that they were not confident in their ability to interpret aEEG/cEEG.[1]

Amplitude-Integrated EEG

Maynard originally constructed the cerebral function monitor (CFM) in the late 1960s for continuous brain monitoring. Prior developed the clinical application for monitoring adult patients during anesthesia and intensive care, after cardiac arrest, during status epilepticus, or after heart surgery.[2]

The term aEEG is currently preferred to denote a method for encephalographic monitoring, whereas CFM refers to a specific type of equipment. The EEG signal for the single-channel aEEG is usually recorded from a pair of electrodes placed over the parietal lobes (corresponding to P3 and P4 according to the international EEG 10–20 classification, ground Fz, Fig. 14.2A). Two-channel EEG places frontal-parietal or central-parietal leads (F3-P3 and F4-P4 or C3-P3 and C4-P4, ground Fz according to the international EEG 10–20 classification, Fig. 14.2B and C) and is now predominantly used. This provides additional information about hemispheric asymmetry, which may be especially helpful in children with unilateral brain lesions.[3] In the two-channel recording, the F3-P3 and F4-P4

position is preferred for assessment of the background pattern. This arrangement is in opposition to the short electrode distance of the C3-P3 and C4-P4 positions, which is better for seizure detection but may alter the background pattern.[4]

For aEEG processing, the raw EEG signal is amplified and passed through an asymmetric band-pass filter that prefers higher frequencies over lower ones and suppresses activity below two Hz and above 15 Hz to minimize artifacts from sweating, movement, muscle activity, and electrical interference. Additional processing includes rectification (negative waves become positive), smoothing, and considerable time compression. The signal is displayed on a semilogarithmic scale at slow speed (6 cm/hr) at the cotside. A second tracing continuously displays the original or raw EEG from either one or two channels. The electrode impedance is continuously recorded but not necessarily displayed; there is an alarm when the impedance is high, often as a result of a loose electrode. The bandwidth (BW) in the output reflects variations in minimum and maximum EEG amplitude, both of which depend on the maturity and severity of illness of the newborn. Because the semilogarithmic scale is used to plot the output, changes in background activity of very low amplitude (<5 μV) are enhanced.[5]

The aEEG traces are assessed visually based on pattern recognition and are classified into the following five categories in full-term infants[6]:

1. *The continuous normal voltage (CNV)* pattern is a continuous trace with a voltage between 10 and 25 (–50) μV (Fig. 14.3A).
2. *The discontinuous normal voltage (DNV)* pattern in which the lower margin is predominantly below 5 μV (no burst suppression [BS]) (Fig. 14.3B).
3. *The BS pattern* with periods of low amplitude (inactivity) intermixed with bursts of higher amplitude (usually >25 μV). According to spacing between bursts, tracing can be classified either as sparse or dense BS pattern (Fig. 14.3C and D).
4. *The continuous low voltage pattern (CLV)* of very low voltage (around or below 5 μV) (Fig. 14.3E).

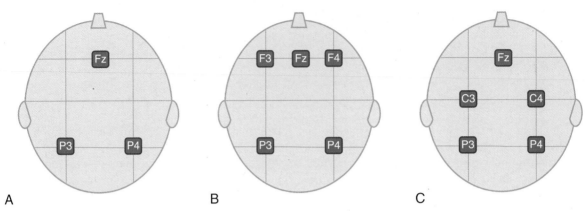

Fig. 14.2 Examples of electrode position in single channel aEEG using P3 and P4 (A) atypical two channel with F3-P3/F4-P4 (B) and more commonly used two channel with C3-P3/C4-P4 (C)

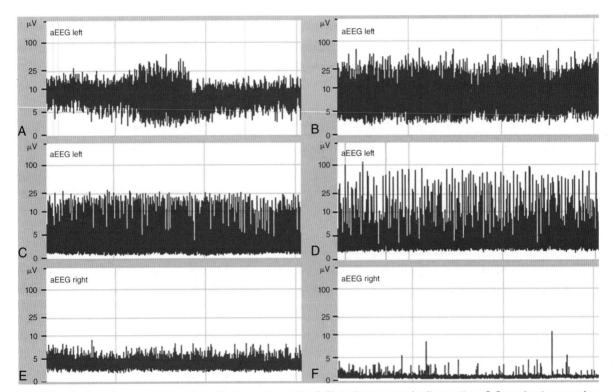

Fig. 14.3 A, Continuous normal voltage pattern with sleep-wake cycling. B, Discontinuous normal voltage pattern. C, Dense burst suppression. D, Sparse burst suppression pattern. E, Continuous low-voltage pattern. F, Flat trace pattern. *aEEG*, Amplitude-integrated electroencephalogram.

5. *The flat tracing (FT)* which has very low voltage, mainly inactive tracing with activity below 5 μV (Fig. 14.3F).

Another classification according to al Naqeeb[7] uses absolute values for background patterns in term infants:

- Normal: upper margin greater than 10 μV; lower margin above 5 μV.
- Moderately abnormal: upper margin greater than 10 μV; lower margin less than 5 μV.
- Severely abnormal: upper margin less than 10 μV; lower margin less than 5 μV.

We prefer the pattern recognition criteria because the background pattern may be influenced by a baseline drift (Fig. 14.4). This drift is especially common in infants with very poor background activity where the lower margin is lifted upward by a high-frequency external signal, such as the ECG signal.[8] When these two aEEG scoring systems were compared in the same dataset containing comparable normothermia and hypothermia-treated infants,[9] it was noted that the pattern recognition method was superior for early outcome prediction in a subgroup of patients with HIE. Interobserver agreement was slightly higher using the voltage criteria compared with the pattern recognition method. However, both methods are equally good in determining the background pattern compared with the use of cEEG.[10] The voltage classification system is easier to use for clinicians with little

experience in reading aEEG, but one should always try to assess the underlying pattern. It has been shown that a BS pattern may be read as a normal voltage pattern when a drift of the baseline is bringing the lower margin above 5 μV.[11] When this artifact is not recognized, the background pattern may be misclassified and consequently hypothermia may not be offered to eligible infants (see Fig. 14.4).

Comparison With cEEG

Several studies investigating simultaneous use of aEEG and cEEG have been performed to compare the two techniques for background pattern recognition. A good correlation between the aEEG background pattern and cEEG background activity was seen in full-term infants with moderate to severe neonatal encephalopathy.[12–15]

PROGNOSTIC VALUE OF aEEG IN HIE PRIOR TO THE ERA OF THERAPEUTIC HYPOTHERMIA

The value of the background pattern in the prediction of neurodevelopmental outcome in term infants with HIE has been well established with the use of the cEEG. A poor background pattern, which persists beyond the first 12 to 24 hours after birth (BS, low voltage, and FT), is well known to carry a poor prognosis. The best predictive ability was seen at 6 hours

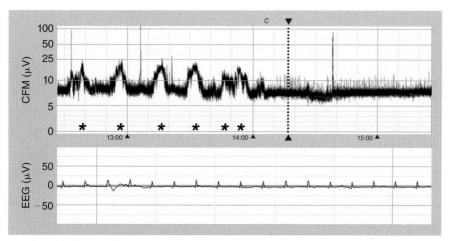

Fig. 14.4 The patient was born at full-term via an emergency cesarean section. Sinusoidal cardiotocography was seen. Arterial umbilical pH was 6.70, and the first arterial lactate level was 30 mmol/L. Upper panel, drift of the baseline with seizures (indicated by *). Lower panel, raw EEG shows electrocardiogram artifact. The loading dose of lidocaine was given at point *C*. *CFM*, Cerebral function monitor; *EEG*, electroencephalogram. (Figure from first book publication by Mona Toet and Linda de Vries. Fig. 2 in the previous version from 2016.)

of age. cEEG features associated with an abnormal outcome included a background amplitude less than 30 μV, interburst intervals (IBIs) of more than 30 seconds, electrographic seizures, and absence of sleep-wake cycling (SWC) at 48 hours after birth.

The prognostic value of early aEEG in HIE is described in the meta-analysis of eight studies by Spitzmiller et al.[16] A minimum amplitude of less than 4 μV was useful in predicting severe MRI abnormalities.[17] Both positive and negative predictive values were slightly lower when aEEG was assessed at three instead of 6 hours after birth, but they were still considered sufficiently high to use this technique for early selection in hypothermia or other intervention studies. Combining a neurologic examination with aEEG performed less than 12 hours after birth further increased predictive accuracy from 75% to 85%.[18] A significant correlation was described between clinical examination, by using the Thompson score, and the aEEG background pattern. They have similar predictive values for adverse outcome. However, the aEEG has several advantages over the Thompson score as it is a continuous measurement which can identify deteriorations in neurological status, identify electrographic-only seizures, and can be sent out for expert review.[19]

In one study, recovery of poor background activity (BS, FT, and CLV) within 24 hours after perinatal asphyxia has been reported in 20% of the cases.[20] Of these infants, 60% survived with a mild disability or were normal at follow-up. The patients who did not recover either died in the neonatal period or survived with a severe disability.

Another way of looking at recovery of the background pattern is to assess the presence, quality, and time of onset of SWC (see also Figs. 14.3A, and 14.10C). The time of onset of SWC was shown to predict neurodevelopmental outcome in infants with HIE based on whether SWC returns before 36 hours (good outcome) or after 36 hours (poor outcome).[21]

PROGNOSTIC VALUE OF aEEG IN HIE IN THE ERA OF THERAPEUTIC HYPOTHERMIA

Del Rio and colleagues[22] performed a systematic review investigating and comparing the prognostic value of aEEG in cooled and noncooled infants with HIE. Seven studies have reported on the predictive value of

aEEG in cooled infants (Table 14.1).[9,23–28] All found the predictive value, especially the specificity, of aEEG to be poor at 6 to 24 hours after birth. However, from 36 hours onward, both the sensitivity and specificity were above 80% and comparable to the predictive value of aEEG in the normothermic situation.

The positive predictive value (PPV) of aEEG changes over the course of hypothermia. It is well known that the aEEG background may gradually improve over the first 48 to 72 hours of cooling.[9,23,29] The PPV of an abnormal aEEG in cooled infants increases from 66% at 24 hours to 85% at 48 hours and 89% at 72 hours.[30] These findings along with the findings of Sewell et al.,[31] who showed a better predictive value using a background evolution pattern compared to defining the background at specific timepoints, highlight the importance of monitoring infants throughout the duration of cooling and rewarming to inform the trajectory of recovery, or absence of recovery, over time.

The appearance of SWC in cooled infants with HIE has been addressed in several studies.[9,27,32] Researchers found that the onset of SWC may be markedly delayed in term infants with moderate to severe HIE treated with hypothermia, but when SWC returns within 36 hours, the majority of infants will have a normal outcome.[27,32] However, when SWC is never achieved, this predicts a poor outcome with a PPV of 0.73.[9,27] Therefore, SWC is an important additional tool for assessing recovery in term infants with moderate to severe HIE treated with hypothermia.

Care should be taken when antiseizure medication (ASM) is given in infants who have not recovered their background pattern within 24 to 48 hours. High blood levels of ASM, as a result of altered metabolism and accumulation under hypothermia, may influence the background pattern of the aEEG.

New quantitative EEG measures of delta power and discontinuity are being developed which can aid real-time prognostication in infants with HIE as well.[33,34]

aEEG AND SEIZURES
Seizure Detection

A multichannel video cEEG study by Murray et al.[35] showed that only one-third of neonatal EEG seizures display clinical signs on simultaneous video recordings. Two-thirds of these clinical manifestations were

TABLE 14.1 Studies Investigating the Predictive Value of aEEG in Hypothermia-Treated Infants

Study (Year of Publication)	Normothermia (n)	Hypothermia (n)	Follow-Up (mo)	6 hours		24 hours		36 hours		48 hours	
				Sensitivity,% (95% CI)	Specificity,% (95% CI)	Sensitivity,% (95% CI)	Specificity,% (95% CI)	Sensitivity,% (95% CI)	Specificity,% (95% CI)	Sensitivity,% (95% CI)	Specificity,% (95% CI)
Hallberg et al.[22] (2010)	0	23	12	100 (54–100)	31 (11–59)	100 (54–100)	76 (50–93)	100 (54–100)	82 (57–96)	80 (28–99)	100 (80–100)
Thoresen et al.[8] (2010)	31	43	18	100 (80–100)	62 (41–80)	94 (71–100)	73 (52–88)	88 (64–99)	96 (80–100)	82 (57–96)	100 (87–100)
Ancora et al.[23] (2013)	0	12	≥12	100 (40–100)	50 (16–84)	75 (19–99)	25 (3–65)	NR	NR	NR	NR
Shankaran et al.[24] (2011)	51	57	18	100 (86–100)	30 (16–49)	NR	NR	NR	NR	NR	NR
Gucuyener et al.[25] (2012)	0	10	8–24	100 (16–100)	38 (9–76)	NR	NR	NR	NR	NR	NR
Cseko et al.[26] (2013)	0	70	18–24	100 (87–100)	40 (25–56)	95 (76–100)	74 (50–93)	95 (74–100)	83 (68–93)	82 (57–96)	93 (80–98)
Azzopardi[27] (2014)	158	156	18	97 (89–100)	31 (21–42)	NR	NR	NR	NR	NR	NR

aEEG, Amplitude-integrated electroencephalogram; CI, confidence interval; HT, hypothermia; NR, not reported; NT, normothermia.

not recognized or were misinterpreted by experienced neonatal staff with very low interobserver agreement.[36] These findings show that clinical diagnosis is not sufficient for the recognition and management of neonatal seizures and underline the importance of EEG monitoring in infants at risk of developing seizures.

A rapid rise of both the lower and the upper margins of the aEEG tracing is suggestive of an ictal discharge (Fig. 14.1B). Seizures can be recognized as single seizures, repetitive seizures, and status epilepticus (see also Fig. 14.11C). The latter usually resembles a sawtooth pattern. Correct interpretation of aEEG is greatly improved by simultaneous reading of the raw EEG, which is now available on all modern digital aEEG monitors (see Fig. 14.10A).

Multichannel video cEEG is the gold standard for neonatal seizure detection,[37] but it is not always readily available or feasible in the NICU. The advantages of limited channel aEEG compared with cEEG are the easy application and interpretation that can be done in real time by NICU personnel. This can significantly reduce the time to diagnosis and treatment of seizures.[38] However, owing to the nature of the aEEG technique, it is not surprising that very brief seizure activity and focal seizures may be missed.[39] Thus, cEEG remains the gold standard for quantification of seizure burden. Infants with focal seizures, however, usually develop more widespread ictal discharges, which will be identified by limited channel aEEG. In addition, 81% of the neonatal seizures originate from central temporal or midline vertex electrodes, which can potentially be picked up by the aEEG electrodes.[12] A recent systematic review by Falsaperla et al. investigating the sensitivity of aEEG in neonatal seizure detection (14 studies included) showed an overall sensitivity varying between 31% and 90% (median 56.8%). When stratified for aEEG technique, the sensitivity for single-channel aEEG was 52.3% (range 29.7%–78%), for two-channel aEEG, it was 58.5% (range 37.5%–90%) and when two-channel aEEG was combined with analysis of the raw EEG, the sensitivity was 80.8% (range 76%–85.6%).[40] This underlines the importance of using at least two channels in combination with the raw EEG, especially in infants with suspected unilateral brain lesions.[3]

It has been noted that the aEEG can show a pattern consistent with a seizure, but the two-channel raw EEG is inconclusive. This could be due to multifocal epileptiform activity, which can only be confirmed on a cEEG (Fig. 14.5).

Since the increased use of continuous monitoring, it has become clear that electrographic-only seizures are common and occur especially following administration of the first ASM. This so-called uncoupling or electroclinical dissociation has been reported by several groups and was found in 50% to 60% of the children studied. The aEEG may play an important role in the detection of these electrographic-only seizures.[41,42]

Importantly it has been recognized that status epilepticus is not uncommon occurring in 18% of 56 full-term infants admitted with neonatal seizures recorded with aEEG.[43,44] The background pattern at the onset of status epilepticus appears to be the main predictor of outcome in all infants with status epilepticus. The background pattern also proved to be an independent predictor of seizures in infants with HIE treated with therapeutic hypothermia.[45] The incidence of seizures did not change after the introduction of therapeutic hypothermia, but the overall seizure burden was reduced.[46] However, status epilepticus is not uncommon in infants with HIE treated with hypothermia (10%–23%).[47–49] A high seizure burden and status epilepticus have been related to more severe brain injury on MRI and postneonatal epilepsy in hypothermia-treated infants.[47,48,50–54] While it is highly recommended to monitor infants with HIE throughout cooling and rewarming, a recent study by Benedetti et al. showed that infants with normal or mildly abnormal background pattern developed seizures during the first 24 hours or not at all, while infants who developed seizures after 24 hours had markedly abnormal background patterns. In limited resource settings, this could guide tailored duration of monitoring.[55]

Should We Treat Electrographic-Only Seizures?

There is no consensus on whether clinical events without an EEG correlate should be treated or how aggressively to treat electrographic-only seizures.[56,57] Although human data are scarce, several studies do suggest an adverse effect of both clinical and electrographic-only seizures on neurodevelopmental outcome. Neonatal seizures have been reported to predispose patients to later problems with regard to

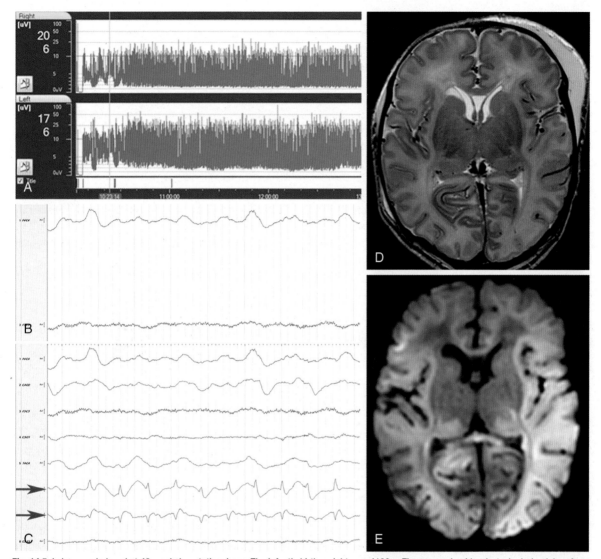

Fig. 14.5 Labor was induced at 42 weeks' gestational age. The infant's birth weight was 4100 g. There was shoulder dystocia during labor. Apgar scores were 2 and 5 after 1 and 5 minutes, respectively. The infant was resuscitated for 4 minutes. Umbilical pH was 6.98 and base excess was −18. The infant was not cooled but started to have seizures within 12 hours after birth. He was treated initially with phenobarbital and was transferred to the neonatal intensive care unit. He subsequently needed ventilatory support and was treated with phenobarbital, lidocaine, and midazolam. Cranial ultrasound performed within 24 hours after birth showed diffuse echogenicities in the subcortical white matter and basal ganglia. Magnetic resonance imaging showed extensive cortical gray matter and subcortical white matter abnormalities in the entire left hemisphere and in large areas of the right hemisphere together with the thalami. A, Amplitude-integrated electroencephalogram at 25 hours after birth was performed for suspected seizures, but findings from the two-channel aEEG and raw electroencephalogram (B) were not conclusive. C, Multichannel electroencephalogram showed epileptic activity over the vertex *(red arrows)*. D, Axial T2-weighted image. E, Axial diffusion-weighted image.

cognition, behavior, and development of postneonatal epilepsy.[58-60] Two previous aEEG studies have shown that infants treated for both clinical and electrographic-only seizures had a lower incidence of postneonatal epilepsy (8%–9%) compared with those treated only for clinical seizures (20%–50%).[61-64] Prolonged seizures can increase brain temperature and thus increase metabolic demands.[65] Moreover, prolonged seizures cause progressive cerebral hypoxia, increase local cerebral blood flow, and may steal perfusion from injured brain regions.[66] In a study by Miller et al. on term newborns with HIE, brain injury was independently associated with the severity of seizures.[59] They performed MRI and proton magnetic resonance spectroscopy (MRS) in 90 full-term infants. Seizure severity was associated with increased lactate/choline in both the intervascular boundary zone ($P < .001$) and the basal nuclei ($P = .011$) when controlling for potential confounders of MRI abnormalities and the extent of resuscitation at birth. Seizure severity was independently associated with diminished N-acetylaspartate/choline in the intervascular boundary zone ($P = .034$).

In the randomized controlled trial of van Rooij et al.,[67] the seizure burden was very high in both groups (treated for electrographic-only seizures vs. clinical seizures only), but the burden was higher in the treatment of the clinical seizures only group. It was interesting to see that there was a significant correlation between the duration of seizure patterns and the severity of brain injury on MRI in the blinded group, which was not present in the nonblinded group. Another randomized controlled trial showed that infants treated for electrographic-only seizures had fewer seizures, a lower seizure burden, and a shorter time to treatment than infants treated for clinical seizures only. These authors also confirmed that seizure burden was associated with more severe brain injury and showed that high seizure burden was associated with poorer outcome at 18 to 24 months.[50] Recently, a study by Hunt et al. showed no difference in outcome, seizure burden, MRI injury, death, or disability between electrographic-only and clinically treated seizures in a heterogenous group of infants. Moreover, there was a concern about cognitive outcomes for those treated for electrographic seizures. Limitations of this study include the heterogenicity of

its population, possible difference in seizure burden (though not statistically different), unclear use of raw EEG or seizure detection algorithms, and that both groups received equal ASMs. This study, as in previous studies, was underpowered, making it difficult to draw conclusions.[68]

Adequate and fast detection of electrographic seizures is important to reduce seizure burden. However, it is difficult to constantly monitor real-time EEG. On some digital aEEG machines, seizure detection algorithms are available, which may help in detecting seizures.[69] More recently, a neonatal seizure detection algorithm for cEEG was tested in a multicenter randomized controlled trial.[70,71] Although the algorithm did not enhance identification of individual infants with seizures, the percentage of correctly identified seizure hours was higher in the algorithm group. The authors concluded that the benefit of the algorithm might be greater in less experienced centers.

aEEG IN PRETERM INFANTS

In parallel with cEEG, aEEG background activity is more discontinuous in preterm infants. In relatively healthy and stable premature infants, the maturation of the aEEG background pattern is dependent on both gestational age (GA) and postmenstrual age (PMA). The greater the GA, the more mature the aEEG background pattern is at birth, and subsequently the higher the maturation rate will be.[72] Moreover, preterm infants of lower GA display a relatively faster aEEG maturation compared with others of higher GA at the same PMA.[73] Normative values for aEEG background activity at different GA have been published.[74] A scoring system for evaluation of brain maturation in preterm infants has also been developed.[75] Zhang et al. described reference values for aEEG amplitude obtained for 274 infants with a wide range of PMA (30–55 weeks).[76]

The normative amplitudes of aEEG margins, especially of the lower margin in quiet sleep, were recommended as a source of reference data for the identification of potentially abnormal aEEG results. The upper and lower margins of the aEEG in both active and quiet sleep clearly rose after the neonatal period. The BW decreased almost monotonically throughout the PMA range from 30 to 55 weeks. The lower margin of the aEEG was positively correlated with PMA, with a larger rank correlation coefficient during quiet sleep (r = 0.89) than during active sleep (r = 0.49).

The aEEG in preterm infants develops with three major trends through to full-term age: increase in continuity, with defined decreasing periods of normal EEG suppression for specific GA, appearance of several normal and specific transient waveforms of prematurity, and the appearance of SWC. Interpretation of background pattern and SWC maturational patterns may give useful information on brain maturity and eventually also the severity of brain injury, thus it may be useful also for prognosis.[77–79] Currently, non-expert readers still struggle to interpret the patterns produced and to distinguish abnormal from normal aEEG/EEG pattern. For this reason, in the last years, there has been an attempt to use quantitative measures for the analysis of neonatal EEG in order to assess neonatal brain function.[80] New aEEG/EEG devices already implemented some real-time quantitative algorithms such as the IBI, which indicates the grade of EEG suppression, helping the clinical interpretation at the cotside.

Niemarkt et al. described a method where the upper margin amplitude (UMA), lower margin amplitude (LMA), and BW were quantitatively calculated using a special software system.[81] In addition, the relative duration of discontinuous background pattern (discontinuous background defined as activity with LMA <5 μV, expressed as a percentage) was calculated. They found that GA and postnatal age both contributed independently and equally to LMA and the percentage of discontinuous pattern. Both GA and PMA correlated positively with LMA and negatively with percentage of discontinuous pattern. They concluded that LMA and percentage of discontinuous pattern are simple quantitative measures of neurophysiologic development and may be used to evaluate neurodevelopment in infants.

Other groups studied IBI duration or burst duration as a measure of discontinuity (or maturation). Palmu et al. described the characteristics of activity bursts in the early preterm EEG to assess interrater agreement of burst detection by visual inspection, and to determine the performance of an automated burst detector that uses a nonlinear energy operator (NLEO).[82] They concluded that visual detection of bursts from the early preterm EEG is comparable, albeit not identical, between raters. The original automated detector underestimates the amount of burst occurrence but can be readily improved to yield results comparable to visual detection. More recently, Koolen et al. developed an automated burst detection method based on line length, which had a sensitivity and specificity above 0.84 and even performed well with a limited number of channels.[83] The same group also developed a quantitative measure of discontinuity called the suppression curve, which proved to be a reliable measure of preterm brain maturation.[84] Further clinical studies are warranted to assess the optimal descriptors of burst detection for monitoring and prognostication. Validation of a burst detector may offer an evidence-based platform for further development of brain monitors in very preterm babies.

SWC can be clearly identified in the aEEG from around 30 weeks GA or postnatal age (PNA), but a cyclical pattern resembling immature SWC can also be seen in stable infants born as early as 25 to 26 weeks GA. As expected, SWC matures with GA and with PNA; using an SWC scoring system, a more mature SWC at 34 weeks PMA was associated with improved neurodevelopmental outcome in preterm infants.[85]

Effects from common medications (e.g., surfactant, morphine, and diazepam) and elevated carbon dioxide blood levels can be readily seen as a deterioration of the aEEG background pattern in preterm infants.[86–90]

Early prediction of outcome based on aEEG is a more complicated issue in preterm infants than in full-term infants. A predominantly discontinuous background pattern can be considered normal in most infants younger than 30 weeks GA. In the most immature infants, factors other than initial brain function may influence long-term neurodevelopmental outcome (e.g., bronchopulmonary dysplasia and late-onset sepsis), which makes prediction of outcome from the early EEG less certain. Several studies have investigated the prognostic value of early aEEG in preterm infants. Klebermass et al. showed that an aEEG-pattern score (evaluating the background pattern, SWC, and presence of seizure activity) was highly predictive of adverse outcome at 3 years (defined as death, Bayley-II <85, CP, and neurosensory impairment).[79] A recent study investigated whether there was an association between early postnatal EEG and neurocognitive outcomes at 10 to 12 years of age in extremely preterm born infants. They found a significantly lower absolute band power in all frequency bands in infants with unfavorable outcome on the full intelligence quotient, adaptive behavior composite score, and global executive composite score ($P < .05$).[91] However, West et al. showed that the neurophysiologist's assessment of two-channel EEG in infants <29 weeks GA within 48 hours after delivery was a better predictor of adverse outcome than quantitative continuity measures defined as percentage of time above 25 μV. Moreover, all infants with definite seizures identified by the neurophysiologist had poor outcomes.[92]

Several cEEG and aEEG studies have shown correlation between early background depression and the severity of a periventricular-intraventricular hemorrhage.[93] aEEG is a useful tool for the evaluation of preterm infants with progressive posthemorrhagic ventricular dilatation (PHVD). In a study by Klebermass-Schrehof and colleagues, the aEEG background pattern of 17 preterm infants with PHVD showed increased suppression in 13 patients (76%) with increasing ventricular dilatation. The changes in aEEG background patterns were detected before clinical signs of elevated intracranial pressure occurred and aEEG showed normalization within a week of successful therapeutic intervention.[94]

aEEG has also been related to illness severity (using the Score for Neonatal Acute Physiology II [SNAP-II]) in preterm infants.[95] They found that severity of illness as measured by the SNAP-II and low blood pressure had a negative effect on the aEEGs of preterm infants (n = 38, mean GA 29+7 weeks [range 26+0–31+8 weeks]). These findings were confirmed by two recent studies relating the SNAP-II and hemodynamic parameters to the Burdjalov score and aEEG amplitudes.[77,96]

Epileptic seizure activity in preterm infants can be identified in a manner similar to that used in full-term infants. Identifying seizure activity on a discontinuous background pattern can be very difficult. With access to the raw EEG on the digital devices, this problem can be handled more easily, especially with the seizure detection algorithm available on some devices (Fig. 14.6). However, care should be taken to distinguish ictal discharges from artifacts.[97]

Pitfalls and Artifacts

The simultaneous recording of the raw EEG, present on digital devices, helps in the identification of artifacts that are quite common during long-term recordings.[98] Hagmann et al. have shown that 12% of their 200 hours of recordings were affected by artifacts.[11] This was due to electrical interference in 55% of cases, which could be either ECG artifact (39%) or fast activity (>50 Hz, 61%), and to movement artifact in the remaining 45%. They state that the dual facility (aEEG with simultaneous raw EEG) is crucial for the correct interpretation of the aEEG.

Inappropriate electrode position can also lead to aEEG recordings with artifact or drift of the baseline as noted earlier in this chapter. Some apparently normal aEEGs in infants with severe encephalopathy have electrocardiographic artifacts that could explain a drift of a severely depressed baseline to a baseline within the normal voltage range (see Fig. 14.4). It is very important to recognize this so-called drift of the baseline because the interpretation of aEEG background patterns is used for selection for therapeutic hypothermia.

Medication can also affect the background pattern. ASMs can lead to a temporary decrease in amplitude on the aEEG recording, although this decrease does not influence prognosis.[18,99] Other drugs, such as morphine, can have a similar effect.[89] (Fig. 14.7) We therefore recommend the use of pattern recognition, taking the values of upper and lower margins into account as well.

Any movement or handling of the infant, such as a ventilation artifact resulting in a sudden increase of the baseline of the aEEG recording, can mimic seizure activity on the aEEG (Fig. 14.8). The simultaneously recorded raw EEG signal can help to interpret aEEG traces more accurately.[98,100] In addition, marking events on the aEEG recording by nursing staff is extremely important.

aEEG IN OTHER CLINICAL CONDITIONS

Continuous monitoring of EEG is also useful in infants with congenital heart disease (CHD). A few studies describe the role of the aEEG in this condition, some in combination with NIRS.[101–104] A study by Claessens et al. describes the perioperative use of aEEG in CHD. Preoperatively, none of the infants had an abnormal

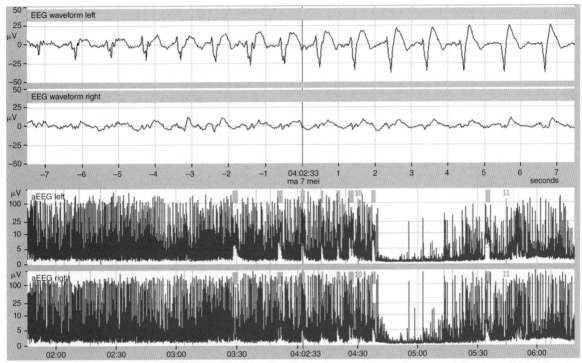

Fig. 14.6 Preterm infant born at 28+5 weeks gestational age with a birth weight of 1065 g, unexplained preterm delivery. Apgar scores were 5 and 9 after 1 and 5 minutes, respectively. Cranial ultrasound revealed a bilateral IVH grade 2 with parenchymal involvement on the left. Therefore a two-channel aEEG recording was obtained. No clinical seizures were observed. The aEEG at 52 hours after birth showed electrographic-only seizures, which were picked up by the seizure detection algorithm and visible in the aEEG. There was no posthemorrhagic ventricular dilatation. Three loading doses (10 mg/kg) of phenobarbital, lidocaine, and clonazepam were given. The infant died on day 6 after redirection of care. A discontinuous pattern without cycling at 29 weeks postmenstrual age with a sudden depression of the aEEG after administration of clonazepam. On day 3, electrographic-only seizures picked up by the seizure detection algorithm *(orange squares)* and the aEEG (abrupt, transient rise of the lower border).

background pattern or ictal discharges. Postoperatively, abnormal background pattern was seen in 24% (95% CI, 14%–33%) and ictal discharges were seen in 17% (95% CI, 8%–26%). Abnormal background pattern and ictal discharges were more frequent in infants with new postoperative brain injury ($P = .08$ and .01, respectively). Abnormal brain activity (i.e., abnormal background pattern or ictal discharges) was the single risk factor associated with new postoperative brain injury in multivariable logistic regression analysis (OR, 4.0; 95% CI, 1.3–12.3; $P = .02$).[104]

Another group studied aEEG during neonatal sepsis with or without meningitis in infants 34 to 42 weeks GA.[105] They found that low-voltage background pattern, SWC, and epileptiform activity on the aEEG are helpful to predict neurologic outcome in infants with

neonatal sepsis or meningitis. Others looked at the effect of sepsis on the aEEG in extremely premature infants.[106] They found that sepsis was associated with acute aEEG changes, as indicated by a BS pattern, but was not associated with a decrease in aEEG maturation score.

The use of aEEG in monitoring the depth of anesthesia has also been described in infants with noncardiac congenital anomalies.[107] aEEG showed a variable reduction of brain activity in response to anesthesia in infants with noncardiac congenital anomalies, with fast recovery—mostly within 24 hours—after cessation of anesthesia. The degree of reduction in brain activity was related to GA and the dose of sevoflurane.

A sudden rise of arterial partial pressure of carbon dioxide ($PaCO_2$) levels can result in a sudden drop in

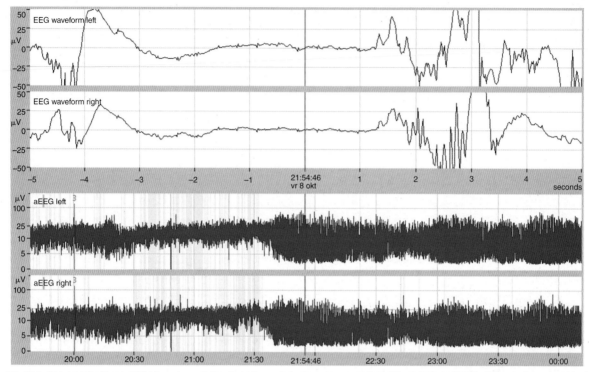

Fig. 14.7 Preterm infant born at 33+2 weeks gestational age from a twin pregnancy, complicated by preeclampsia. The baby was born via vaginal delivery and was diagnosed with bilateral choanal atresia after birth. Thus she needed oral intubation and was administered a bolus of morphine followed by continuous infusion. Afterward, she needed surgical correction of the choanal atresia. She was suspected to be affected by 22q11 deletion; however, the genetic test resulted normal. The aEEG shows a sudden change in the BGP from CNV to DNV after the start of morphine.

aEEG amplitude (Fig. 14.9).[90] An observational study describing 25 infants (21 preterm, 4 full-term) comprising 32 episodes of acute severe hypercapnia showed that 27 episodes were accompanied by a transient aEEG depression.[90]

Severe hyperbilirubinemia (Fig. 14.10) may also lead to aEEG background depression with or without seizures. aEEG can be used in congenital metabolic disorders, resulting in hyperammonemia and seizures (Fig. 14.11).[108] Deterioration of background patterns, abnormal SWC patterns, and seizures have been described and can be recognized in various metabolic diseases.[109]

Finally, aEEG can be of use in genetic disorders associated with neonatal epilepsy as well. For example, neonatal seizures associated with mutations in the KCNQ2 gene result in a specific aEEG pattern (Fig. 14.12).[110] The interictal background activity in infants with genetic disorders and neonatal seizures

may be normal (as seen in Fig. 14.12 and as was described in infants with neonatal seizures and mutations in the SLC13A5 gene).[111]

Gaps in Knowledge

As with all (new) techniques, there is a learning curve for aEEG. From the paper by Boylan et al.,[1] we know that the aEEG is mainly assessed by neonatologists, 30% of whom are not confident in their ability to interpret it. Because of this lack of confidence in reading aEEGs, proper training is essential. As cEEG remains the gold standard, a cEEG should be performed if one is unsure about the assessment of the aEEG. To provide the best care, neonatologists must collaborate with neurophysiologists. Furthermore, if an aEEG recording lasts several days, we recommend performing a cEEG at least once. Several centers are now using continuous multichannel recording that allows for

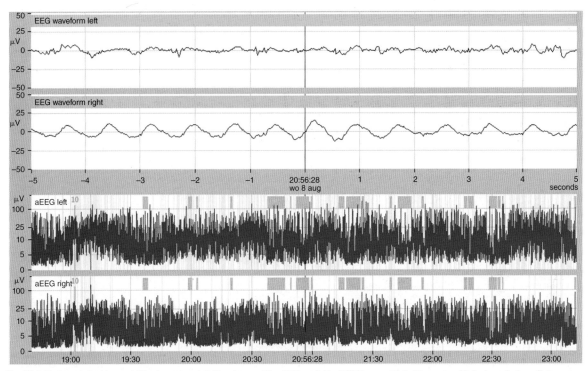

Fig. 14.8 Preterm infant born at 27 + 1 weeks gestational age with a birth weight of 1020 g, ventilated because of infant respiratory distress syndrome. This patient had a normal cranial ultrasound examination. At 2 years of age, the infant had a cognition composite score of 115 and a motor composite score of 127 on the Bayley-III. Two-channel recording showing several seizure detection alerts because of a rhythmic pattern. This turned out to be an artifact as the waveform pattern on the raw EEG form the right hemisphere synchronizes with the ventilator settings while the infant was lying on its right side.

remote access to all channels for the neurophysiologist, but that also offers a two-channel display for the neonatologist.

The aEEG assessment of the preterm infant is different and more difficult to interpret than the aEEG assessment of a term infant. With digital equipment and advanced techniques increasingly available, quantitative assessment of IBI and the use of automated burst detectors will be performed more often.

Conclusion

aEEG monitoring is increasingly considered the standard of care in the neonatal unit, not only in infants with HIE or those with seizures, but also in infants who are seriously ill with CHD, sepsis with or without meningitis, and metabolic diseases and in preterm born infants. We should therefore be aware not only of the advantages of aEEG monitoring, but also of its pitfalls.

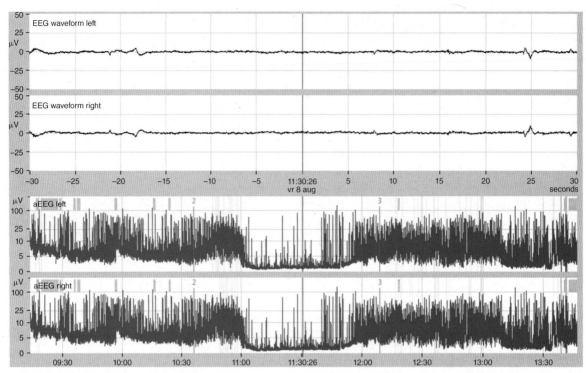

Fig. 14.9 Full-term infant who was discharged home after a normal vaginal delivery with good Apgar scores. The infant was admitted to the neonatal intensive care unit on the second day after birth because of a group B streptococcal septicemia. The patient needed high-frequency oscillation because of pulmonary hypertension and required inotropes to maintain a normal blood pressure. On day 7, there was a sudden drop in amplitude to an almost flat trace. During this period of low amplitude, there was a sudden rise in $Paco_2$ up to 130 mm Hg caused by an obstructed endotracheal tube. The amplitude-integrated electroencephalogram pattern normalized again when the $Paco_2$ normalized. *CFM*, Cerebral function monitor; *EEG*, electroencephalogram. (Figure from the second book publication; Fig. 8 in the previous version from 2016)

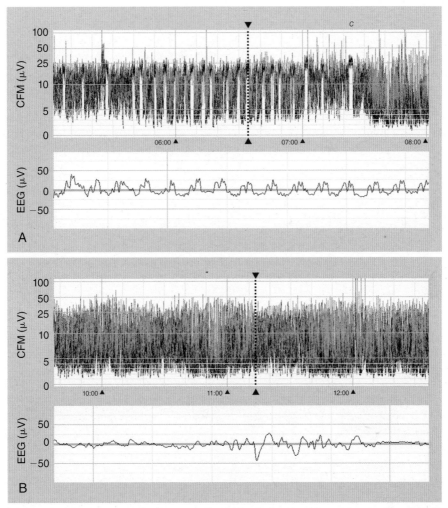

Fig. 14.10 Full-term infant of Chinese nationality, born at 37 + 2 weeks gestational age. The infant developed severe hyperbilirubinemia with a blood level of 588 μmol/L on day 5. He developed seizures at a referring hospital where they started aEEG monitoring. Following a loading dose of phenobarbital (20 mg/kg), he was referred to the neonatal intensive care unit. Brainstem auditory evoked potentials were abnormal, and magnetic resonance imaging showed clear signal intensity changes in the globus pallidus. Exchange transfusion and phototherapy were performed. Further evaluation revealed a G6PD deficiency. The infant developed an auditory neuropathy, but motor and cognitive function were in the normal range at the age of 7 years. A, Epileptiform activity at the referring hospital on an aEEG *(top panel).* The lower panel shows epileptiform activity on the raw aEEG. A loading dose of phenobarbital was given at point *C.* B, Day 5 aEEG on admission (after phenobarbital). A discontinuous normal voltage pattern without seizures was seen.

Continued

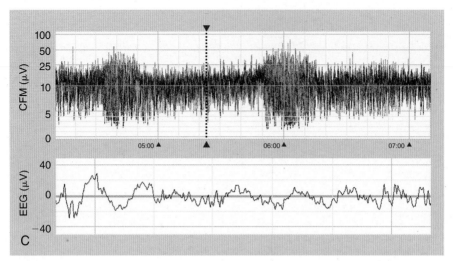

Fig. 14.10, cont'd C, Day 6 aEEG (1 day after admission) shows continuous normal voltage pattern with sleep-wake cycling. *CFM*, Cerebral function monitor; *EEG*, electroencephalogram. (Figure from first publication by Mona Toet and Linda de Vries; Fig. 9 in previous version from 2016.)

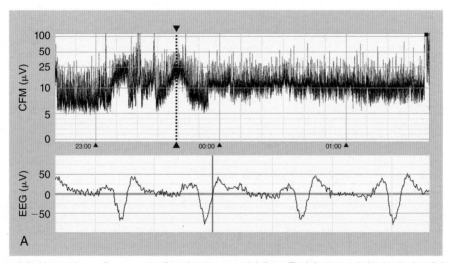

Fig. 14.11 Full-term infant born at home after an uncomplicated pregnancy and delivery. The infant was admitted to the hospital on day 2 because of a low body temperature and an incident after oral feeding. The infant developed seizures with apneas, needed ventilation, and was referred to a neonatal intensive care unit. He was treated with phenobarbital, midazolam, lidocaine, and pyridoxine because of refractory seizures. Serum ammonia level was elevated on admission and increased linearly (1245—3293—3293—8700—4719 μmol/L). He was subsequently diagnosed to have a urea cycle defect (ornithine transcarbamylase deficiency) and died on day 4. A, Seizures were noted on admission.

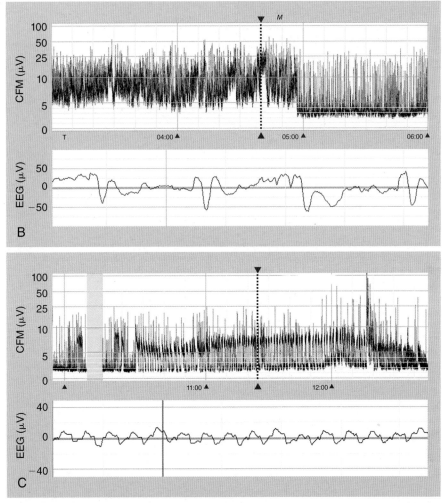

Fig. 14.11, cont'd B, Repetitive seizures were observed the day after admission. After a loading dose of midazolam (at *M*), a sparse burst suppression pattern was seen. C, Several hours after the repetitive seizures shown in B, status epilepticus on a flat background pattern is seen. *CFM*, Cerebral function monitor; *EEG*, electroencephalogram.

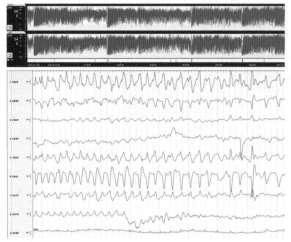

Fig. 14.12 Full-term infant born after an uncomplicated pregnancy and delivery. On day 2, the infant developed clinical seizures. On day 3, the infant was admitted to the neonatal intensive care unit where seizures were confirmed on amplitude-integrated electroencephalogram (aEEG). Seizures were treated with phenobarbital, midazolam, lidocaine, levetiracetam, and carbamazepine. Only lidocaine and carbamazepine were effective. Magnetic resonance imaging showed no structural abnormalities, but on proton MR spectroscopy, a low *N*-acetyl aspartate peak was noted. The infant was diagnosed with a mutation in the *KCNQ2* gene. The aEEG on admission shows four seizures with a typical pattern: a short, transient rise followed by a short, transient decrease of the upper and lower margin *(upper panel)*. This corresponds to seizures in the real EEG *(lower panel)*. Afterward, the background pattern is suppressed (discontinuous normal voltage) but returns rapidly to normal (continuous normal voltage).

REFERENCES

1. Boylan G, Burgoyne L, Moore C, O'Flaherty B, Rennie J. An international survey of EEG use in the neonatal intensive care unit. *Acta Paediatr (Oslo, Norway: 1992)*. 2010;99(8):1150-1155. doi:10.1111/j.1651-2227.2010.01809.x.
2. Prior P, Maynard D, Sheaff P, et al. Monitoring cerebral function: clinical experience with new device for continuous recording of electrical activity of brain. *Br Med J*. 1971;2(5764): 736-738. doi:10.1136/bmj.2.5764.736.
3. van Rooij LG, de Vries LS, van Huffelen AC, Toet MC. Additional value of two-channel amplitude integrated EEG recording in full-term infants with unilateral brain injury. *Arch Dis Child Fetal Neonatal Ed*. 2010;95(3):F160-F168. doi:10.1136/adc.2008.156711.
4. Quigg M, Leiner D. Engineering aspects of the quantified amplitude-integrated electroencephalogram in neonatal cerebral monitoring. *J Clin Neurophysiol*. 2009;26(3):145-149. doi:10.1097/WNP.0b013e3181a18711.
5. El-Dib M, Chang T, Tsuchida TN, Clancy RR. Amplitude-integrated electroencephalography in neonates. *Pediatr Neurol*. 2009;41(5):315-326. doi:10.1016/j.pediatrneurol.2009.05.002.

6. Hellstrom-Westas L, Rosen I, de Vries L, Greisen G. Amplitude-integrated EEG classification and interpretation in preterm and term infants. *NeoReviews*. 2006;7(2):e72-e87.
7. al Naqeeb N, Edwards A, Cowan F, Azzopardi D. Assessment of neonatal encephalopathy by amplitude-integrated electroencephalography. *Pediatrics*. 1999;103(6 Pt 1):1263-1271. doi:10.1542/peds.103.6.1263.
8. Toet MC, van Rooij LG, de Vries LS. The use of amplitude integrated electroencephalography for assessing neonatal neurologic injury. *Clin Perinatol*. 2008;35(4):665-678, v. doi:10.1016/j.clp.2008.07.017.
9. Thoresen M, Hellström-Westas L, Liu X, de Vries LS. Effect of hypothermia on amplitude-integrated electroencephalogram in infants with asphyxia. *Pediatrics*. 2010;126(1):e131-e139. doi:10.1542/peds.2009-2938.
10. Shellhaas RA, Gallagher PR, Clancy RR. Assessment of neonatal electroencephalography (EEG) background by conventional and two amplitude-integrated EEG classification systems. *J Pediatr*. 2008;153(3):369-374. doi:10.1016/j.jpeds.2008.03.004.
11. Hagmann CF, Robertson NJ, Azzopardi D. Artifacts on electroencephalograms may influence the amplitude-integrated EEG classification: a qualitative analysis in neonatal encephalopathy. *Pediatrics*. 2006;118(6):2552-2554. doi:10.1542/peds.2006-2519.
12. Toet MC, van der Meij W, de Vries LS, Uiterwaal CSPM, van Huffelen KC. Comparison between simultaneously recorded amplitude integrated electroencephalogram (cerebral function monitor) and standard electroencephalogram in neonates. *Pediatrics*. 2002;109(5):772-779. doi:10.1542/peds.109.5.772.
13. Evans E, Koh S, Lerner J, Sankar R, Garg M. Accuracy of amplitude integrated EEG in a neonatal cohort. *Arch Dis Child Fetal Neonatal Ed*. 2010;95(3):F169-F173. doi:10.1136/adc.2009.165969.
14. Bennet L, Fyfe KL, Yiallourou SR, Merk H, Wong FY, Horne RSC. Discrimination of sleep states using continuous cerebral bedside monitoring (amplitude-integrated electroencephalography) compared to polysomnography in infants. *Acta Paediatr*. 2016;105(12):e582-e587. doi:10.1111/apa.13602.
15. Meledin I, Abu Tailakh M, Gilat S, et al. Comparison of amplitude-integrated EEG and conventional EEG in a cohort of premature infants. *Clin EEG Neurosci*. 2017;48(2):146-154. doi:10.1177/1550059416648044.
16. Spitzmiller RE, Phillips T, Meinzen-Derr J, Hoath SB. Amplitude-integrated EEG is useful in predicting neurodevelopmental outcome in full-term infants with hypoxic-ischemic encephalopathy: a meta-analysis. *J Child Neurol*. 2007;22(9):1069-1078. doi:10.1177/0883073807306258.
17. Shah DK, Lavery S, Doyle LW, Wong C, McDougall P, Inder TE. Use of 2-channel bedside electroencephalogram monitoring in term-born encephalopathic infants related to cerebral injury defined by magnetic resonance imaging. *Pediatrics*. 2006; 118(1):47-55. doi:10.1542/peds.2005-1294.
18. Shalak LF, Laptook AR, Velaphi SC, Perlman JM. Amplitude-integrated electroencephalography coupled with an early neurologic examination enhances prediction of term infants at risk for persistent encephalopathy. *Pediatrics*. 2003;111(2): 351-357. doi:10.1542/peds.111.2.351.
19. Weeke LC, Vilan A, Toet MC, van Haastert IC, de Vries LS, Groenendaal F. A comparison of the Thompson encephalopathy score and amplitude-integrated electroencephalography in infants with perinatal asphyxia and therapeutic hypothermia. *Neonatology*. 2017;112(1):24-29. doi:10.1159/000455819.

20. van Rooij LGM, Toet MC, Osredkar D, van Huffelen AC, Groenendaal F, de Vries LS. Recovery of amplitude integrated electroencephalographic background patterns within 24 hours of perinatal asphyxia. *Arch Dis Child Fetal Neonatal Ed.* 2005; 90(3):F245-F251. doi:10.1136/adc.2004.064964.

21. Osredkar D, Derganc M, Paro-Panjan D, Neubauer D. Amplitude-integrated electroencephalography in full-term newborns without severe hypoxic-ischemic encephalopathy: case series. *Croat Med J.* 2006;47(2):285-291.

22. del Río R, Ochoa C, Alarcon A, Arnáez J, Blanco D, García-Alix A. Amplitude integrated electroencephalogram as a prognostic tool in neonates with hypoxic-ischemic encephalopathy: a systematic review. *PLoS One.* 2016;11(11):e0165744. doi:10.1371/journal.pone.0165744.

23. Hallberg B, Grossmann K, Bartocci M, Blennow M. The prognostic value of early aEEG in asphyxiated infants undergoing systemic hypothermia treatment. *Acta Paediatr.* 2010;99(4): 531-536. doi:10.1111/j.1651-2227.2009.01653.x.

24. Ancora G, Maranella E, Grandi S, et al. Early predictors of short term neurodevelopmental outcome in asphyxiated cooled infants. A combined brain amplitude integrated electroencephalography and near infrared spectroscopy study. *Brain Dev.* 2013;35(1):26-31. doi:10.1016/j.braindev.2011.09.008.

25. Shankaran S, Pappas A, McDonald SA, et al. Predictive value of an early amplitude integrated electroencephalogram and neurologic examination. *Pediatrics.* 2011;128(1):e112-e120. doi:10.1542/peds.2010-2036.

26. Gucuyener K, Beken S, Ergenekon E, et al. Use of amplitude-integrated electroencephalography (aEEG) and near infrared spectroscopy findings in neonates with asphyxia during selective head cooling. *Brain Dev.* 2012;34(4):280-286. doi:10.1016/j.braindev.2011.06.005.

27. Csekő A, Bangó M, Lakatos P, Kárdási J, Pusztai L, Szabó M. Accuracy of amplitude-integrated electroencephalography in the prediction of neurodevelopmental outcome in asphyxiated infants receiving hypothermia treatment. *Acta Paediatr.* 2013; 102(7):707-711. doi:10.1111/apa.12226.

28. Azzopardi D. Predictive value of the amplitude integrated EEG in infants with hypoxic ischaemic encephalopathy: data from a randomised trial of therapeutic hypothermia. *Arch Dis Child Fetal Neonatal Ed.* 2014;99(1):F80-F82. doi:10.1136/archdischild-2013-303710.

29. Massaro AN, Tsuchida T, Kadom N, et al. aEEG evolution during therapeutic hypothermia and prediction of NICU outcome in encephalopathic neonates. *Neonatology.* 2012;102(3): 197-202. doi:10.1159/000339570.

30. Chandrasekaran M, Chaban B, Montaldo P, Thayyil S. Predictive value of amplitude-integrated EEG (aEEG) after rescue hypothermic neuroprotection for hypoxic ischemic encephalopathy: a meta-analysis. *J Perinatol.* 2017;37(6):684-689. doi:10.1038/jp.2017.14.

31. Sewell EK, Vezina G, Chang T, et al. Evolution of amplitude-integrated electroencephalogram as a predictor of outcome in term encephalopathic neonates receiving therapeutic hypothermia. *Am J Perinatol.* 2018;35(3):277-285. doi:10.1055/s-0037-1607212.

32. Takenouchi T, Rubens EO, Yap VL, Ross G, Engel M, Perlman JM. Delayed onset of sleep-wake cycling with favorable outcome in hypothermic-treated neonates with encephalopathy. *J Pediatr.* 2011;159(2):232-237. doi:10.1016/j.jpeds.2011.01.006.

33. Korotchikova I, Stevenson NJ, Walsh BH, Murray DM, Boylan GB. Quantitative EEG analysis in neonatal hypoxic ischaemic

encephalopathy. *Clin Neurophysiol.* 2011;122(8):1671-1678. doi:10.1016/j.clinph.2010.12.059.

34. Kota S, Massaro AN, Chang T, et al. Prognostic value of continuous electroencephalogram delta power in neonates with hypoxic-ischemic encephalopathy. *J Child Neurol.* 2020; 35(8):517-525. doi:10.1177/0883073820915323.

35. Murray DM, Boylan GB, Ali I, Ryan CA, Murphy BP, Connolly S. Defining the gap between electrographic seizure burden, clinical expression and staff recognition of neonatal seizures. *Arch Dis Child Fetal Neonatal Ed.* 2008;93(3):F187-F191. doi:10.1136/adc.2005.086314.

36. Malone A, Anthony Ryan C, Fitzgerald A, Burgoyne L, Connolly S, Boylan GB. Interobserver agreement in neonatal seizure identification. *Epilepsia.* 2009;50(9):2097-2101. doi:10.1111/j.1528-1167.2009.02132.x.

37. Shellhaas RA, Chang T, Tsuchida T, et al. The American Clinical Neurophysiology Society's Guideline on continuous electroencephalography monitoring in neonates. *J Clin Neurophysiol.* 2011;28(6):611-617. doi:10.1097/WNP.0b013e31823e96d7.

38. Apers WMJ, de Vries LS, Groenendaal F, Toet MC, Weeke LC. Delay in treatment of neonatal seizures: a retrospective cohort study. *Neonatology.* 2020;117(5):599-605. doi:10.1159/000509282.

39. Shellhaas RA, Clancy RR. Characterization of neonatal seizures by conventional EEG and single-channel EEG. *Clin Neurophysiol.* 2007;118(10):2156-2161. doi:10.1016/j.clinph.2007.06.061.

40. Falsaperla R, Scalia B, Giaccone F, et al. aEEG vs cEEG's sensivity for seizure detection in the setting of neonatal intensive care units: a systematic review and meta-analysis. *Acta Paediatr (Oslo, Norway: 1992).* 2022;111(5):916-926. doi:10.1111/apa.16251.

41. Boylan GB, Rennie J, Pressler R, Wilson G, Morton M, Binnie C. Phenobarbitone, neonatal seizures, and video-EEG. *Arch Dis Child Fetal Neonatal Ed.* 2002;86(3):F165-F170. doi:10.1136/fn.86.3.F165.

42. Scher MS, Alvin J, Gaus L, Minnigh B, Painter MJ. Uncoupling of EEG-clinical neonatal seizures after antiepileptic drug use. *Pediatr Neurol.* 2003;28(4):277-280. doi:10.1016/S0887-8994(02)00621-5.

43. van Rooij LGM, de Vries LS, Handryastuti S, et al. Neurodevelopmental outcome in term infants with status epilepticus detected with amplitude-integrated electroencephalography. *Pediatrics.* 2007;120(2):e354-e363. doi:10.1542/peds.2006-3007.

44. Pisani F, Cerminara C, Fusco C, Sisti L. Neonatal status epilepticus vs recurrent neonatal seizures: clinical findings and outcome. *Neurology.* 2007;69(23):2177-2185. doi:10.1212/01.wnl.0000295674.34193.9e.

45. Rothman SM, Glass HC, Chang T, Sullivan JE, Bonifacio SL, Shellhaas RA. Risk factors for EEG seizures in neonates treated with hypothermia: a multicenter cohort study. *Neurology.* 2014;83(19):1773-1774. doi:10.1212/01.wnl.0000456637.05253.24.

46. Boylan GB, Kharoshankaya L, Wusthoff CJ. Seizures and hypothermia: importance of electroencephalographic monitoring and considerations for treatment. *Semin Fetal Neonatal Med.* 2015;20(2):103-108. doi:10.1016/j.siny.2015.01.001.

47. Glass HC, Nash KB, Bonifacio SL, et al. Seizures and magnetic resonance imaging–detected brain injury in newborns cooled for hypoxic-ischemic encephalopathy. *J Pediatr.* 2011;159(5): 731-735.e1. doi:10.1016/j.jpeds.2011.07.015.

48. Nash KB, Bonifacio SL, Glass HC, et al. Video-EEG monitoring in newborns with hypoxic-ischemic encephalopathy treated with hypothermia. *Neurology.* 2011;76(6):556-562. doi:10.1212/WNL.0b013e31820af91a.

49. Wusthoff CJ, Dlugos DJ, Gutierrez-Colina A, et al. Electrographic seizures during therapeutic hypothermia for neonatal hypoxic-ischemic encephalopathy. *J Child Neurol.* 2011;26(6): 724-728. doi:10.1177/0883073810390036.

50. Srinivasakumar P, Zempel J, Trivedi S, et al. Treating EEG seizures in hypoxic ischemic encephalopathy: a randomized controlled trial. *Pediatrics.* 2015;136(5):e1302-e1309. doi:10. 1542/peds.2014-3777.

51. Shah DK, Wusthoff CJ, Clarke P, et al. Electrographic seizures are associated with brain injury in newborns undergoing therapeutic hypothermia. *Arch Dis Child Fetal Neonatal Ed.* 2014;99(3): F219-F224. doi:10.1136/archdischild-2013-305206.

52. Chen YJ, Chiang MC, Lin JJ, et al. Seizures severity during rewarming can predict seizure outcomes of infants with neonatal hypoxic-ischemic encephalopathy following therapeutic hypothermia. *Biomed J.* 2020;43(3):285-292. doi:10.1016/j.bj.2020. 06.008.

53. Fitzgerald MP, Massey SL, Fung FW, Kessler SK, Abend NS. High electroencephalographic seizure exposure is associated with unfavorable outcomes in neonates with hypoxic-ischemic encephalopathy. *Seizure.* 2018;61:221-226. doi:10.1016/j. seizure.2018.09.003.

54. Kharoshankaya L, Stevenson NJ, Livingstone V, et al. Seizure burden and neurodevelopmental outcome in neonates with hypoxic-ischemic encephalopathy. *Dev Med Child Neurol.* 2016;58(12):1242-1248. doi:10.1111/dmcn.13215.

55. Benedetti GM, Vartanian RJ, McCaffery H, Shellhaas RA. Early electroencephalogram background could guide tailored duration of monitoring for neonatal encephalopathy treated with therapeutic hypothermia. *J Pediatr.* 2020;221:81-87.e1. doi:10.1016/j.jpeds.2020.01.066.

56. Sankar R, Painter MJ. Neonatal seizures. *Neurology.* 2005; 64(5):776-777. doi:10.1212/01.WNL.0000157320.78071.6D.

57. Silverstein FS, Jensen FE. Neonatal seizures. *Ann Neurol.* 2007;62(2):112-120. doi:10.1002/ana.21167.

58. McBride MC, Laroia N, Guillet R. Electrographic seizures in neonates correlate with poor neurodevelopmental outcome. *Neurology.* 2000;55(4):506-514. doi:10.1212/WNL.55.4.506.

59. Miller SP, Weiss J, Barnwell A, et al. Seizure-associated brain injury in term newborns with perinatal asphyxia. *Neurology.* 2002;58(4):542-548. doi:10.1212/WNL.58.4.542.

60. Brunquell PJ, Glennon CM, DiMario FJ, Lerer T, Eisenfeld L. Prediction of outcome based on clinical seizure type in newborn infants. *J Pediatr.* 2002;140(6):707-712. doi:10.1067/ mpd.2002.124773.

61. Hellstrom-Westas L, Blennow G, Lindroth M, Rosen I, Svenningsen NW. Low risk of seizure recurrence after early withdrawal of antiepileptic treatment in the neonatal period. *Arch Dis Child Fetal Neonatal Ed.* 1995;72(2):F97-F101. doi:10. 1136/fn.72.2.F97.

62. Toet MC, Groenendaal F, Osredkar D, van Huffelen AC, de Vries LS. Postneonatal epilepsy following amplitude-integrated EEG-detected neonatal seizures. *Pediatr Neurol.* 2005;32(4): 241-247. doi:10.1016/j.pediatrneurol.2004.11.005.

63. Clancy RR, Legido A. Postnatal epilepsy after EEG-confirmed neonatal seizures. *Epilepsia.* 1991;32(1):69-76. doi:10.1111/j. 1528-1157.1991.tb05614.x.

64. Ronen GM, Buckley D, Penney S, Streiner DL. Long-term prognosis in children with neonatal seizures: a population-based study. *Neurology.* 2007;69(19):1816-1822. doi:10.1212/01. wnl.0000279335.85797.2c.

65. Yager JY, Armstrong EA, Jaharus C, Saucier DM, Wirrell EC. Preventing hyperthermia decreases brain damage following neonatal hypoxic-ischemic seizures. *Brain Res.* 2004;1011(1): 48-57. doi:10.1016/j.brainres.2004.02.070.

66. Boylan GB, Panerai RB, Rennie JM, Evans DH, Rabe-Hesketh S, Binnie CD. Cerebral blood flow velocity during neonatal seizures. *Arch Dis Child Fetal Neonatal Ed.* 1999;80(2):F105-F110. doi:10.1136/fn.80.2.F105.

67. van Rooij LGM, Toet MC, van Huffelen AC, et al. Effect of treatment of subclinical neonatal seizures detected with aEEG: randomized, controlled trial. *Pediatrics.* 2010;125(2):e358-e366. doi:10.1542/peds.2009-0136.

68. Hunt RW, Liley HG, Wagh D, et al. Effect of treatment of clinical seizures vs electrographic seizures in full-term and near-term neonates. *JAMA Netw Open.* 2021;4(12):e2139604. doi:10. 1001/jamanetworkopen.2021.39604.

69. Navakatikyan MA, Colditz PB, Burke CJ, Inder TE, Richmond J, Williams CE. Seizure detection algorithm for neonates based on wave-sequence analysis. *Clin Neurophysiol.* 2006;117(6): 1190-1203. doi:10.1016/j.clinph.2006.02.016.

70. Mathieson SR, Stevenson NJ, Low E, et al. Validation of an automated seizure detection algorithm for term neonates. *Clin Neurophysiol.* 2016;127(1):156-168. doi:10.1016/j.clinph.2015.04.075.

71. Pavel AM, Rennie JM, de Vries LS, et al. A machine-learning algorithm for neonatal seizure recognition: a multicentre, randomised, controlled trial. *Lancet Child Adolesc Health.* 2020;4(10):740-749. doi:10.1016/S2352-4642(20)30239-X.

72. Klebermass K, Kuhle S, Olischar M, Rücklinger E, Pollak A, Weninger M. Intra- and extrauterine maturation of amplitude-integrated electroencephalographic activity in preterm infants younger than 30 weeks of gestation. *Neonatology.* 2006;89(2): 120-125. doi:10.1159/000088912.

73. O'Toole JM, Pavlidis E, Korotchikova I, Boylan GB, Stevenson NJ. Temporal evolution of quantitative EEG within 3 days of birth in early preterm infants. *Sci Rep.* 2019;9(1):4859. doi:10.1038/s41598-019-41227-9.

74. Olischar M, Klebermass K, Kuhle S, et al. Reference values for amplitude-integrated electroencephalographic activity in preterm infants younger than 30 weeks' gestational age. *Pediatrics.* 2004;113(1):e61-e66. doi:10.1542/peds.113.1.e61.

75. Burdjalov VF, Baumgart S, Spitzer AR. Cerebral function monitoring: a new scoring system for the evaluation of brain maturation in neonates. *Pediatrics.* 2003;112(4):855-861. doi:10.1542/peds. 112.4.855.

76. Zhang D, Liu Y, Hou X, et al. Reference values for amplitude-integrated EEGs in infants from preterm to 3.5 months of age. *Pediatrics.* 2011;127(5):e1280-e1287. doi:10.1542/peds. 2010-2833.

77. Bowen JR, Paradisis M, Shah D. Decreased aEEG continuity and baseline variability in the first 48 hours of life associated with poor short-term outcome in neonates born before 29 weeks gestation. *Pediatr Res.* 2010;67(5):538-544. doi:10.1203/PDR. 0b013e3181d4ecda.

78. Wikström S, Pupp IH, Rosén I, et al. Early single-channel aEEG/EEG predicts outcome in very preterm infants. *Acta Paediatr (Oslo, Norway: 1992).* 2012;101(7):719-726. doi:10.1111/ j.1651-2227.2012.02677.x.

79. Klebermass K, Olischar M, Waldhoer T, Fuiko R, Pollak A, Weninger M. Amplitude-integrated EEG pattern predicts further outcome in preterm infants. *Pediatr Res.* 2011;70(1): 102-108. doi:10.1203/PDR.0b013e31821ba200.

80. O'Toole JM, Boylan GB. Quantitative preterm EEG analysis: the need for caution in using modern data science techniques. *Front Pediatr.* 2019;7:174. doi:10.3389/fped.2019.00174.

81. Niemarkt HJ, Andriessen P, Peters CHL, et al. Quantitative analysis of amplitude-integrated electroencephalogram patterns in stable preterm infants, with normal neurological development at one year. *Neonatology.* 2010;97(2):175-182. doi:10.1159/000252969.

82. Palmu K, Wikström S, Hippeläinen E, Boylan G, Hellström-Westas L, Vanhatalo S. Detection of "EEG bursts" in the early preterm EEG: visual vs. automated detection. *Clin Neurophysiol.* 2010;121(7):1015-1022. doi:10.1016/j.clinph.2010.02.010.

83. Koolen N, Jansen K, Vervisch J, et al. Line length as a robust method to detect high-activity events: Automated burst detection in premature EEG recordings. *Clin Neurophysiol.* 2014;125(10):1985-1994. doi:10.1016/j.clinph.2014.02.015.

84. Dereymaeker A, Koolen N, Jansen K, et al. The suppression curve as a quantitative approach for measuring brain maturation in preterm infants. *Clin Neurophysiol.* 2016;127(8):2760-2765. doi:10.1016/j.clinph.2016.05.362.

85. El-Dib M, Massaro AN, Glass P, Aly H. Sleep wake cycling and neurodevelopmental outcome in very low birth weight infants. *J Matern-Fetal Neonatal Med.* 2014;27(9):892-897. doi:10.3109/14767058.2013.845160.

86. Shany E, Benzaquen O, Friger M, Richardson J, Golan A. Influence of antiepileptic drugs on amplitude-integrated electroencephalography. *Pediatr Neurol.* 2008;39(6):387-391. doi:10.1016/j.pediatrneurol.2008.08.005.

87. Hellström-Westas L, Bell AH, Skov L, Greisen G, Svenningsen NW. Cerebroelectrical depression following surfactant treatment in preterm neonates. *Pediatrics.* 1992;89(4 Pt 1):643-647.

88. Bell AH, Greisen G, Pryds O. Comparison of the effects of phenobarbitone and morphine administration on EEG activity in preterm babies. *Acta Paediatr.* 1993;82(1):35-39. doi:10.1111/j.1651-2227.1993.tb12511.x.

89. Young GB, da Silva OP. Effects of morphine on the electroencephalograms of neonates: a prospective, observational study. *Clin Neurophysiol.* 2000;111(11):1955-1960. doi:10.1016/S1388-2457(00)00433-8.

90. Weeke LC, Dix LML, Groenendaal F, et al. Severe hypercapnia causes reversible depression of aEEG background activity in neonates: an observational study. *Arch Dis Child Fetal Neonatal Ed.* 2017;102(5):F383-F388. doi:10.1136/archdischild-2016-311770.

91. Nordvik T, Schumacher EM, Larsson PG, Pripp AH, Løhaugen GC, Stiris T. Early spectral EEG in preterm infants correlates with neurocognitive outcomes in late childhood. *Pediatr Res.* 2022;92(4):1132-1139. doi:10.1038/s41390-021-01915-7.

92. West CR, Harding JE, Williams CE, Nolan M, Battin MR. Cot-side electroencephalography for outcome prediction in preterm infants: observational study. *Arch Dis Child Fetal Neonatal Ed.* 2011;96(2):F108-F113. doi:10.1136/adc.2009.180539.

93. Hellström-Westas L, Klette H, Thorngren-Jerneck K, Rosén I. Early prediction of outcome with aEEG in preterm infants with large intraventricular hemorrhages. *Neuropediatrics.* 2002;32(6):319-324. doi:10.1055/s-2001-20408.

94. Klebermass-Schrehof K, Rona Z, Waldhör T, et al. Can neurophysiological assessment improve timing of intervention in posthaemorrhagic ventricular dilatation? *Arch Dis Child Fetal Neonatal Ed.* 2013;98(4):F291-F297. doi:10.1136/archdischild-2012-302323.

95. ter Horst HJ, Jongbloed-Pereboom M, van Eykern LA, Bos AF. Amplitude-integrated electroencephalographic activity is suppressed in preterm infants with high scores on illness severity. *Early Hum Dev.* 2011;87(5):385-390. doi:10.1016/j.earlhumdev.2011.02.006.

96. Shibasaki J, Toyoshima K, Kishigami M. Blood pressure and aEEG in the 96h after birth and correlations with neurodevelopmental outcome in extremely preterm infants. *Early Hum Dev.* 2016;101:79-84. doi:10.1016/j.earlhumdev.2016.08.010.

97. Weeke LC, van Ooijen IM, Groenendaal F, et al. Rhythmic EEG patterns in extremely preterm infants: classification and association with brain injury and outcome. *Clin Neurophysiol.* 2017;128(12):2428-2435. doi:10.1016/j.clinph.2017.08.035.

98. de Vries NKS, ter Horst HJ, Bos AF. The added value of simultaneous EEG and amplitude-integrated EEG recordings in three newborn infants. *Neonatology.* 2007;91(3):212-216. doi:10.1159/000097456.

99. Murray DM, Boylan GB, Ryan CA, Connolly S. Early EEG Findings in hypoxic-ischemic encephalopathy predict outcomes at 2 years. *Pediatrics.* 2009;124(3):e459-e467. doi:10.1542/peds.2008-2190.

100. Weeke LC, van Ooijen IM, Groenendaal F, et al. Rhythmic EEG patterns in extremely preterm infants: classification and association with brain injury and outcome. *Clin Neurophysiol.* 2017;128(12):2428-2435. doi:10.1016/j.clinph.2017.08.035.

101. Toet MC, Flinterman A, Laar I van de, et al. Cerebral oxygen saturation and electrical brain activity before, during, and up to 36 hours after arterial switch procedure in neonates without pre-existing brain damage: its relationship to neurodevelopmental outcome. *Exp Brain Res.* 2005;165(3):343-350. doi:10.1007/s00221-005-2300-3.

102. Latal B, Wohlrab G, Brotschi B, Beck I, Knirsch W, Bernet V. Postoperative amplitude-integrated electroencephalography predicts four-year neurodevelopmental outcome in children with complex congenital heart disease. *J Pediatr.* 2016;178:55-60.e1. doi:10.1016/j.jpeds.2016.06.050.

103. Algra SO, Schouten ANJ, Jansen NJG, et al. Perioperative and bedside cerebral monitoring identifies cerebral injury after surgical correction of congenital aortic arch obstruction. *Intensive Care Med.* 2015;41(11):2011-2012. doi:10.1007/s00134-015-3996-6.

104. Claessens NHP, Noorlag L, Weeke LC, et al. Amplitude-integrated electroencephalography for early recognition of brain injury in neonates with critical congenital heart disease. *J Pediatr.* 2018;202:199-205.e1. doi:10.1016/j.jpeds.2018.06.048.

105. ter Horst H, van Olffen M, Remmelts H, de Vries H, Bos A. The prognostic value of amplitude integrated EEG in neonatal sepsis and/or meningitis. *Acta Paediatr.* 2010;99(2):194-200. doi:10.1111/j.1651-2227.2009.01567.x.

106. Helderman JB, Welch CD, Leng X, O'Shea TM. Sepsis-associated electroencephalographic changes in extremely low gestational age neonates. *Early Hum Dev.* 2010;86(8):509-513. doi:10.1016/j.earlhumdev.2010.06.006.

107. Stolwijk LJ, Weeke LC, de Vries LS, et al. Effect of general anesthesia on neonatal aEEG-A cohort study of patients with non-cardiac congenital anomalies. *PLoS One.* 2017;12(8):e0183581. doi:10.1371/journal.pone.0183581.

108. Olischar M, Shany E, Aygün C, et al. Amplitude-integrated electroencephalography in newborns with inborn errors of metabolism. *Neonatology.* 2012;102(3):203-211. doi:10.1159/000339567.

109. Theda C. Use of amplitude integrated electroencephalography (aEEG) in patients with inborn errors of metabolism—a new tool for the metabolic geneticist. *Mol Genet Metab.* 2010; 100:S42-S48. doi:10.1016/j.ymgme.2010.02.013.

110. Vilan A, Mendes Ribeiro J, Striano P, et al. A distinctive ictal amplitude-integrated electroencephalography pattern in newborns with neonatal epilepsy associated with KCNQ2 mutations. *Neonatology.* 2017;112(4):387-393. doi:10.1159/000478651.

111. Weeke LC, Brilstra E, Braun KP, et al. Punctate white matter lesions in full-term infants with neonatal seizures associated with SLC13A5 mutations. *Eur J Paediatr Neurol.* 2017;21(2): 396-403. doi:10.1016/j.ejpn.2016.11.002.

Chapter 15

Magnetic Resonance Imaging—Newer Techniques and Overall Value in Diagnosis and Predicting Long-Term Outcome

Gregory A. Lodygensky, Caroline Menache Starobinski, Linda S. de Vries and Petra S. Hüppi

Chapter Outline

Introduction

Despite marked improvements in antenatal and perinatal care, perinatal brain injury remains one of the most important medical complications in the newborn resulting in significant handicap later in life. Experimental advances have helped to understand many of the cellular and vascular mechanisms of perinatal brain damage, showing a correlation between the nature of the injury and the maturation of the brain, but effects on long-term circuit formation are just emerging.[1-3] Early identification of brain injury and appropriate prognostication though remain a major challenge to neonatal care. Different forms of imaging are diagnostic tools that have emerged to detect early brain injury and help predict outcome.

Magnetic resonance (MR) techniques are one of these relatively new diagnostic tools that allow the assessment of the developing brain in detail thanks to their resolving power and their noninvasiveness. Their capacity to provide detailed structural as well as metabolic and functional information without the use of ionizing radiation is unique.

Conventional MR imaging is therefore now widely used for identifying normal and pathologic brain morphology giving objective information about the structure of the neonatal brain during development.

Susceptibility-weighted imaging (SWI) with phase postprocessing[4] is particularly useful for detecting intravascular venous deoxygenated blood as well as extravascular blood products. Diffusion-weighted imaging (DWI),[5,6] spectroscopy[7,8] and functional MR imaging (blood-oxygenation-dependent [BOLD] imaging)[9] are newer MR techniques that complement conventional MR imaging and can indicate some of the pathophysiologic mechanisms occurring during brain injury in the newborn and the postinjury plasticity. This article will focus on the role of the different MR techniques in the study of perinatal brain injury. The specific patterns of brain injury identified by different imaging techniques will be illustrated by case presentations, followed by the discussion of pathophysiologic and neurodevelopmental outcome associated with the described brain lesion. This approach should allow the reader to make the right choice of imaging method at the right time to decide on intervention, withdrawal of care, and accurate prediction of a range of neurofunctional outcomes.

Brain injury in the Term Newborn

Neonatal brain injury in the term infant is most frequently related to cerebral hypoperfusion and/or hypoxemia followed by reperfusion as the infant is resuscitated, typically shortly after delivery. This is summarized in the term "asphyxia," progressive hypoxemia, and hypercapnia with significant metabolic acidosis occurring both in the antenatal, intrapartum, and neonatal period.[1,10] Perinatal asphyxia may lead to hypoxic-ischemic encephalopathy (HIE) which is the clinically defined condition of disturbed neurologic function in the newborn, characterized by insufficient respiration, depression of tone and reflexes, altered level of consciousness, and often seizures.[11] The subsequent neurological deficits of concern are grouped together under the term of cerebral palsy[10,12,13] but include different motor deficits, such as spasticity, choreoathetosis, dyskinesia, dystonia, and ataxia. Further cognitive deficits, behavior, memory problems, and seizures might also be the end result of neonatal HIE.

The major varieties of neuropathologies that are found in neonatal HIE are listed in Table 15.1.

Selective neuronal necrosis is the most common pathology observed in HIE and refers to necrosis of neurons in a characteristic, although often widespread, distribution. The four basic patterns of the topography of the neuronal injury depend on the severity and temporal characteristics of the insult, and on the gestational age. Thus pontosubicular necrosis[14] occurs more frequently in premature than in term infants and the basal ganglia neurons of the putamen are more likely to be affected in term infants,[15] whereas neurons from the globus pallidus are more frequently affected in premature infants.[16]

The reason why a term infant with hypoxia-ischemia may develop one of the various patterns of selective neuronal necrosis or primarily parasagittal cerebral injury is not entirely clear but might be related to brain stem and basal ganglia sparing reflex,[17] where the blood flow is redirected to basal ganglia, the brainstem, and the cerebellum in case of

TABLE 15.1   Major Varieties of Neonatal HIE

Major Neuropathological Varieties of Neonatal HIE in the Term Infant	Characteristics of the Usual Insult According to the Pattern of Injury or Pathogenesis of the Injury
Selective neuronal necrosis: • diffuse • cerebral cortex–deep nuclear • deep nuclear–brainstem • pontosubicular Parasagittal cerebral injury (watershed injury)	Characteristics of the insult: • very severe, very prolonged • moderate to severe, prolonged • severe, abrupt • unknown Pathogenesis: Disturbance in cerebral perfusion due to: • parasagittal anatomical factors (arterial border zones and end zones) • impaired cerebrovascular autoregulation (pressure-passive state due to cerebral ischemia)
Focal and multifocal ischemic necrosis	Pathogenesis: Generalized systemic circulatory insufficiency (pre- or postnatal) • intrauterine • neonatal

mild to moderate asphyxia that does not occur in case of severe abrupt hypoperfusion, i.e., in case of a sentinel event like uterine rupture or cord compression.[18]

Pre- or postnatal generalized systemic circulatory insufficiency can also generate focal or multifocal ischemic necrosis.

The occurrence of a neonatal neurological syndrome requires the search for brain injury either from ante-, intra-, or postpartum events. The neurological symptoms of severe HIE are described in Table 15.2. Important systemic abnormalities (renal, cardiac, hepatic, etc.) related to ischemia accompany the neurological manifestations in most cases but show no relation to outcome.[19]

Clinicopathological correlations can be made for the different neuropathological varieties of neonatal HIE in the term infant and are summarized in Table 15.3.

The following four cases of term perinatal asphyxia illustrate the clinical course, the neuroimaging characteristics, and the subsequent neurodevelopmental outcome and will illustrate the role and appropriate timing of MR imaging in the evaluation of the term newborn after perinatal asphyxia.

TABLE 15.2 Neurological Encephalopathic Syndrome of a Severe HIE

Birth to 12 hours	12–24 hours	24–72 hours	After 72 hours
Deep stupor or coma Periodic breathing or respiratory failure Intact pupillary and oculomotor response Hypotonia and minimal movements/occasionally hypertonia Seizures	Variable change in alertness More seizures Apneic spells Jitteriness Weakness (upper limbs in terms; lower limbs in preterms)	Stupor or coma Respiratory arrest Oculomotor and pupillary disturbance	Persistent but diminished stupor Disturbed sucking, swallowing, gag, and tongue movements Hypotonia >hypertonia Weakness (upper limbs in terms; lower limbs in preterms)

Modified from Volpe JJ. *Neurology of the Newborn.* 6th ed. Philadelphia: Elsevier; 2018.

TABLE 15.3 Neonatal and Long-Term Clinical Correlates of Brain Injury in the Term Infant With HIE

Topography of the Major Injury	Neonatal Correlates	Long-Term Correlates
Selective neuronal necrosis of the *diffuse* type	Stupor and coma (cortical injury) Seizures (cortical injury) often of the subtle type Hypotonia (cortical or anterior horn injury) Oculomotor disturbance (cranial nerve nuclei injury) Disturbed sucking, swallowing (brainstem involvement)	Intellectual retardation (cortical injury) Spastic quadriparesis (cortical injury) Seizure disorder (10%–30%) (cortical injury) Impairment of cortical visual function Precocious puberty (10%) (hypothalamus) Impairment of sucking, swallowing, drooling, fixed facial expression (bulbar or pseudobulbar palsy) Hearing deficits (cochlear neurons) Atonic cerebral palsy (rare) (anterior horn cells)
Selective neuronal necrosis of *cortical–deep nuclear* type	Same symptoms except that the tone is usually increased, especially with stimulation	Same symptoms Additionally delayed onset of dystonia (6–12 months and even as late as 7–14 years of age)
Selective neuronal necrosis of *deep nuclear–brainstem* type	Same symptoms as above Additionally: ptosis, facial diparesis, ventilatory disturbances	Prolonged difficulties with feeding Normal cognition in 50%
Parasagittal cortical cerebral injury	Proximal weakness predominant in the upper limbs Seizures (variable) Disturbed level of alertness (variable)	Rarely spastic quadriparesis in severe cases Intellectual deficits (often "specific") usually recognized at school age
Focal and multifocal brain necrosis (cortical and subcortical)	Seizures, usually focal Hemiparesis or quadriparesis if bilateral	Spastic hemiparesis or quadriparesis Cognitive deficits Seizure disorder

Case 1

History: Term pregnancy with signs of fetal distress, cesarean section, low Apgar score, perinatal acidosis (pH 6.99). On day 1, general hypotonia, tonic deviations of eyes, sucking, smacking "subtle seizures." Normal neurologic exam on day 10.

Neuroimaging studies (see Fig. 15.1): Neonatal head ultrasound performed on day 1 is normal. MRI on day 3 reveals no significant signal abnormalities on T2-weighted images and some signal hyperintensities on T1-weighted images especially in the central cortex. DWI shows abnormal signal intensities with reduced apparent diffusion coefficient (ADC) bilaterally in the thalamus and internal capsule. Some discrete areas of reduced ADC are seen in the cortex. A repeat follow-up study on day 10 (see Fig. 15.2) shows thalami appearing brighter than normal on T2-weighted images with central white matter of relatively high intensity, often difficult to judge as normal or abnormal and might require repeat scanning to detect gliosis in the white matter later.

Clinical correlates in the neonatal period: This child developed signs of moderately severe impairment of bilateral hemispheres which characteristically results in diffuse hypotonia. He also presented with neonatal seizures of the "subtle" type which are thought to result from diffuse cortical injury, and could be relation to the discrete areas or reduced ADC seen in the cortex. The normalization of the neurological examination at 10 days of life can be viewed as a positive prognostic sign but does not preclude developmental issues.

Long-term clinical correlates: Ultimately, he developed signs of moderate spasticity especially in the upper limbs, but was able to walk unaided at the age of 3 years with a certain degree of truncal hypotonia. His fine motor skills were delayed due to dystonic movements of the arms. The onset of dystonia started around the age of 12 months and became more prominent with time. He had no major cognitive deficits. The mild spasticity is explained by the involvement of the central white matter and perirolandic cortex (seen best on DWI and T1 at day 3) and the dystonia is the result of the thalamo-putaminal lesions. The relatively good functional outcome of this patient was in part predictable from the normalization of his neurological exam at 10 days of life. The diagnosis still is dystonic CP with a spastic component (GMFCS level II), so unaided walking but needs help for stairs.

Case 2

History: Term pregnancy with signs of fetal distress, emergency cesarean section for uterine rupture, meconium aspiration, low Apgar score (1/3/5), perinatal acidosis (pH 6.84). Initial general hypotonia, then hypertonicity, no seizures.

Neuroimaging studies: Neonatal head ultrasound performed on day 1 is normal. MRI on day 1 reveals no significant signal abnormalities on T2- and T1-weighted images and on DWI. Single voxel ^{1}H-MRS performed on basal ganglia reveals elevated lactate (Lac) resonance at 1.3 ppm with no loss of N-acetylaspartate (NAA) (see Fig. 15.3). Follow-up MRI at day 10 shows bilateral thalami and putamen appearing hyperintense on T2-weighted images with clear distinction on proton density images with no cortical signal abnormalities (see Fig. 15.3). On T1-weighted images hyperintensities in this region can be confounded with hyperintensities due to myelination (see Figs. 15.3 and 15.4). ^{1}H-MRS now shows normalization of lactate and reduction of NAA (Fig. 15.4)

Clinical correlates in the neonatal period: After a brief period of hypotonia, corresponding most likely to the bilateral involvement of the reticular activating system in the diencephalon, this child developed rapidly the characteristic hypertonia associated to basal ganglia lesions and due to the involvement of the extrapyramidal system. It is interesting to note that no seizures were observed, most likely in relation to the fact that there were no cortical lesions.

Long-term clinical correlates: This child developed striking truncal hypotonia and severe dystonic posturing of the upper extremities limiting severely her motor development, although there was no spasticity. She is unable to walk unaided. Her receptive language competence is normal but her expressive language is noninterpretable and she uses vocal synthesis device. Her cognitive functions are however preserved. The diagnosis is severe CP of the dystonic type with a GMFCS IV.

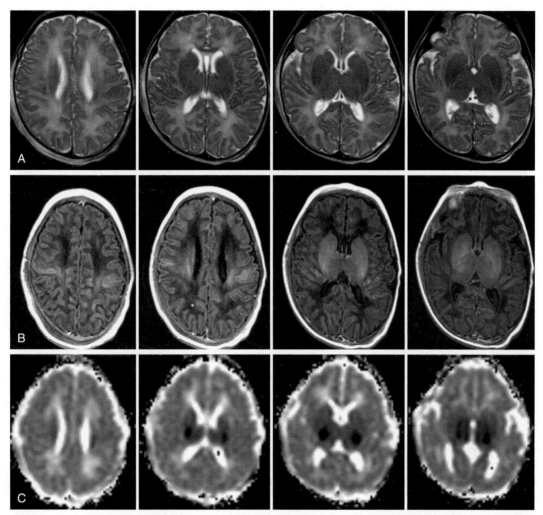

Fig. 15.1 Case 1 with perinatal asphyxia and MRI at day 3 of life. A, T2-weighted images with slight T2 hyperintensity of the thalami, no striking signal abnormalities. B, T1-weighted images show abnormal high signal intensities in several cortical areas, specifically in the depth of sulci. Thalamic area slightly hypointense. C, Diffusion-weighted imaging (DWI) shows striking lesions (*dark*) with apparent diffusion coefficient (ADC) reduction in bilateral thalami and in some discrete central cortical areas.

Case 3

History: Term pregnancy with intrauterine growth restriction, fetal distress, cesarean section, meconium aspiration perinatal acidosis, persistent pulmonary hypertension (pH 7.08).

Neuroimaging studies: Neonatal head ultrasound performed on day 1 is normal. MRI on day 1 reveals no significant signal abnormalities on T2- and T1-weighted images and standard DWIs reveal no striking signal abnormality ADC values measured in the left basal ganglia (ADC 0.8 mm^2/ms) and central white matter (ADC 0.8 mm^2/ms), respectively reveals markedly reduced ADC values compared to normal term neonates (1.0–1.2/1.4)[45] (see Fig. 15.5). ^{1}H-MRS performed on basal ganglia reveals elevated lactate resonance at 1.3 ppm with no loss of NAA. Follow-up MRI shows marked T2 signal

Continued on following page

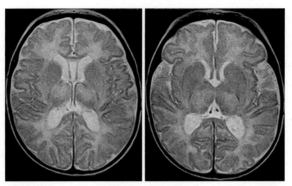

Fig. 15.2 Case 1: MRI 10 days after perinatal asphyxia. T2-weighted images show marked hyperintensities in bilateral thalami as well as the posterior limb of the internal capsule. Please note a mild ventricular dilatation as well.

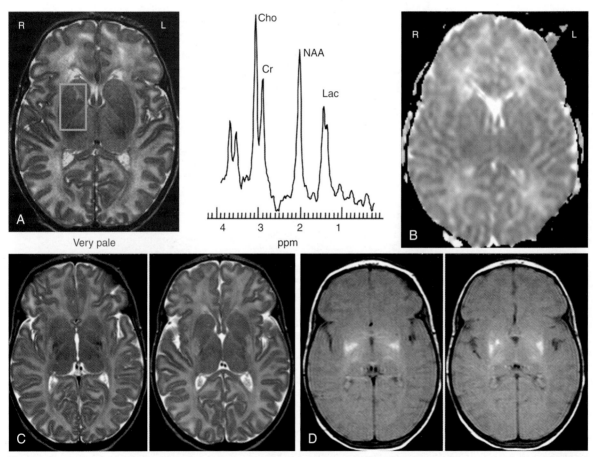

Fig. 15.3 Case 2: A, MR examination obtained at 12 hours after perinatal asphyxia. Axial T2-weighted image shows no signal abnormalities and single voxel ¹H-MRS performed over the right basal ganglia shows markedly increased lactate resonance with preserved *N*-acetylaspartate (NAA), Cr, and Cho resonances. B, Diffusion-weighted imaging (DWI) with axial apparent diffusion coefficient (ADC) map shows no diffusion abnormalities. C and D, MRI at 10 days after perinatal asphyxia. C, Axial T2-weighted images show areas of high signal intensity in the putamen and thalamus representing clear ischemic-lesions. D, Axial Proton density images with excellent detection of the lesion extension.

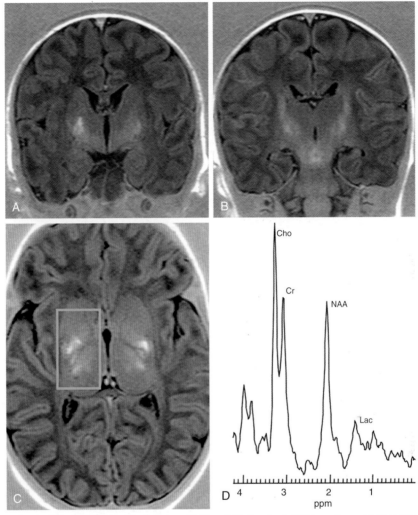

Fig. 15.4 Case 2: Coronal and axial inversion recovery sequences with T1-weighted contrast at 10 days after perinatal asphyxia. T1 hyperintensities appear irregular (A, C) (compare to regular distribution of beginning myelination in B). D, ^{1}H-MRS shows normalization of lactate and reduction of N-acetylaspartate (NAA) compared to ^{1}H-MRS at day 1.

Case 3 (Continued)

abnormalities in the basal ganglia with involvement of the left internal capsule with extension into the central white matter in a parasagittal distribution (see Fig. 15.6).

Clinical correlates in the neonatal period: This infant did not develop striking neurological abnormalities in the neonatal period. The only symptom was a moderate hypotonia and some weakness in the upper extremities.

Long-term clinical correlates: Development of marked right upper extremity palsy at the age of 6 months. The child did not reach for objects with the right hand and exhibited a spastic position of the right arm during leg movements. In the ventral position, she was unable to elevate her right arm. These impairments were in relation with the lesions of the left internal capsule. Later, at age 18 months, she showed signs of hyperreflexia in all four limbs as a result of the bilateral white matter lesions, but spasticity predominated on the right side, as a sequela of the unilateral left internal capsule lesion. Her cognitive performances were mildly delayed. She was able to walk unaided at the age of 2 years. The diagnosis is spastic CP GMFCS level II, predominating on the right side.

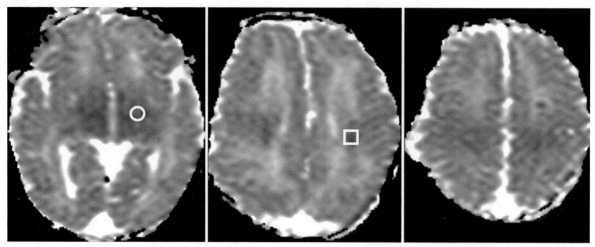

Fig. 15.5 Case 3. MRI on day 1 after perinatal asphyxia. Conventional MR Imaging reveals no signal abnormalities (not shown). DWI shows no overt lesions but ADC values measured in the left basal ganglia (ADC 0.8 mm^2/ms) (*circle*) and central white matter (ADC 0.8 mm^2/ms) (*square*), respectively, reveal markedly reduced ADC values compared to normal term neonates (around 1.6 mm^2/m). (Reference ADC values are from Rutherford M et al. Pediatrics. 2004 Oct;114(4):1004-14. doi: 10.1542/peds.2004-0222)

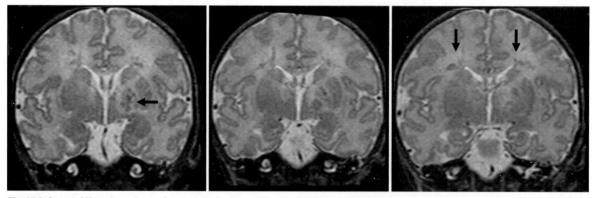

Fig. 15.6 Case 3: MRI 7 days after perinatal asphyxia. Coronal T2-weighted images showing T2 hypo- and hyperintensities in the central white matter with additional left-sided lesions in the internal capsule and lateral thalamus (*arrows*).

Case 4

History: Term pregnancy with uterine rupture at delivery. Perinatal resuscitation with Apgar scores at 0/0/3 and severe perinatal acidosis. On day 1, development of a moderate HIE with lethargy and hypotonia. Efforts in arousing the infant resulted in hypertonia and jitteriness. Spontaneous movements were diminished. Convulsions appeared rapidly.

Neuroimaging studies: Neonatal head ultrasound performed on day 1 is normal. MRI on day 2 reveals no significant signal abnormalities on T2- and T1-weighted images. DWIs reveal abnormally high signal corresponding to reduced ADC in ADC maps (not shown) bilaterally in putamen and thalami as well as in the perirolandic cortex (see Fig. 15.7). ^{1}H-MRS performed in basal ganglia reveals elevated lactate resonance at 1.3 ppm with no loss of NAA (not shown). Follow-up MRI at 17 days shows marked T2 signal abnormalities in the basal ganglia and alteration of the perirolandic cortex bilaterally visible both on proton density images as well as on T2-weighted images (see Fig. 15.7). At 2 months of age, additional atrophy and delay in myelination is present (see Fig. 15.8).

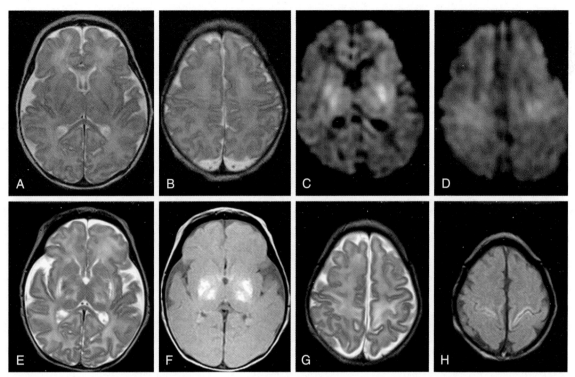

Fig. 15.7 Case 4: A–D, MRI at day 2 after perinatal asphyxia. A, B, Conventional T2-weighted images at the level of the basal ganglia and the centrum semiovale show no signal abnormalities. Diffusion-weighted imaging (DWI) shows striking hyperintensities in diffusion-weighted images in the bilateral putamen and thalamus in (C) and some high signal in the central cortex (D). MR imaging at 10 days after the insult confirms distribution of lesions with hyper- and hypointensities on T2-weighted images (E), typical high signal intensity with good lesion definition in proton density images (F), the perirolandic cortex shows typical T2 and PD hyperintensity (G, H).

Case 4 (Continued)

Clinical correlates in the neonatal period: The infant presented with neonatal seizures and a disturbed level of consciousness which reflected the bilateral cortical lesions.

Long-term clinical correlates: The child developed a severe spastic quadriplegia related to the injury in the perirolandic cortex. Additionally, dystonia started around the age of 12 to 18 months. This extrapyramidal syndrome was the result of the additional basal ganglia lesions. The child is thus severely disabled and unable to walk unaided (GMFCS level IV–V). However, the cognitive impairment is mild and she uses vocal synthesis for communication.

Case 5

History: Term pregnancy with persistent signs of fetal distress, cesarean section, low Apgar score with meconium aspiration, and cardiorespiratory resuscitation.

On day 1, general hypotonia, tonic deviations of eyes, sucking, smacking "subtle seizures," and electroencephalographic status epilepticus.

Neuroimaging studies: Neonatal head ultrasound performed on day 1 shows small ventricles and increased parenchymal echogenicity, suggestive of an insult prior to delivery. MRI performed on day 7 shows extensive signal intensity changes in the white matter with the cortex roughly isointense with white matter, especially posteriorly on

Continued on following page

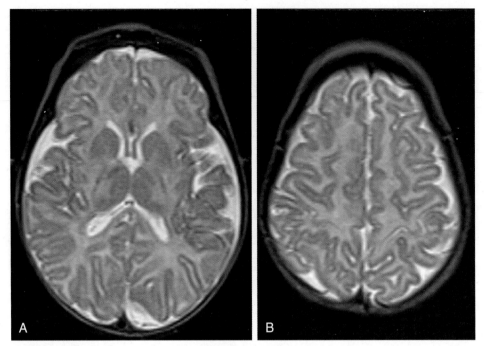

Fig. 15.8 Case 4: MR imaging at 2 months of age reveals the same lesions with marked atrophy and delay in myelination.

Case 5 (Continued)

T2- and T1-weighted images and apparent sparing of the thalami and basal ganglia, except for the pulvinar (see Fig. 15.9A, B). Also note the swollen mammillary bodies with increased signal intensity on T2 (see Fig. 15.9A). On DWI, markedly decreased ADC in both cortex, white matter (0.70), and basal ganglia (see Fig. 15.9C). Follow-up MRI 6 weeks later shows evolution into multicystic encephalomalacia with loss of both hemispheric gray and white matter and severe ex vacuo hydrocephaly (see Fig. 15.9D, E).

Clinical correlates in the neonatal period: the generalized hypotonia and the seizures reflect the bilateral extensive cortical injuries. The status epilepticus which is not uncommon in full-term asphyxia is the sign of the severity of the insult.

Long-term clinical correlates: The child developed a severe spastic quadriplegia with cognitive impairment and microcephaly. Spasticity was a major issue. The seizure disorder remained active during the first months of life. The EEG remained severely depressed indicating diffuse cortical necrosis. The diagnosis is severe spastic CP (GMFCS level V) and severe intellectual disability.

Cranial Ultrasonography in the Evaluation of Perinatal Asphyxia or HIE

Neonatal sonography is still the only bedside technique to image the neonatal brain. In term perinatal asphyxia and HIE, the most typical findings in the acute phase are represented by poor differentiation of cortical sulci and diffuse increase of parenchymal echogenicity and slit-like ventricles. These features can be primarily related to diffuse cerebral edema. Injury in the basal ganglia can lead to hyperechogenic basal ganglia, but these abnormalities take time to develop and are usually first seen 48 to 72 hours after birth. When echogenicity develops in the thalami as well as the basal ganglia, a "four column" pattern can be recognized.[20] This pattern has been shown to be predictive of poor outcome[21,22] and an echolucent line running between the thalami and basal ganglia corresponding to the posterior limb of the internal capsule has been shown to be predictive of poor outcome. But many early ultrasound

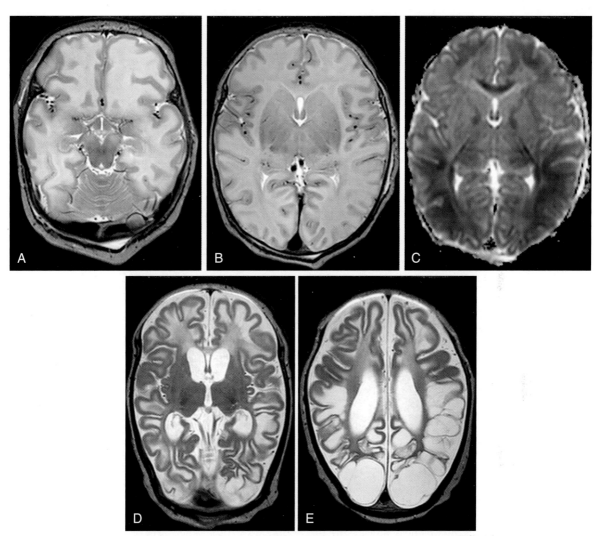

Fig. 15.9 Case 5: Neonatal head ultrasound performed on day 1 showed small ventricles and increased parenchymal echogenicity. A–C, MRI performed on day 7 demonstrated extensive signal intensity changes in the white matter and cortex with loss of gray/white matter differentiation, especially posteriorly and apparent sparing of thalami and basal ganglia except for the pulvinar. Also noted the swollen mammillary bodies with increased signal intensity on T2. On Diffusion-weighted imaging (DWI), markedly reduced apparent diffusion coefficients (ADCs) (0.70) were present in the occipital white matter, the corpus callosum but not in the thalami. D and E, Follow-up MRI 6 weeks later demonstrated evolution into multicystic encephalopathy with loss of both hemispheric gray and white matter and ex vacuo ventricular dilatation.

scans in neonates with HIE lesions are normal or nonspecific, as illustrated in the cases shown. Ultrasound examinations can be considered as a first-step technique that will exclude significant hemorrhage, periventricular calcifications, overt brain malformation, or signs of well-established injury dating the insult before birth. However, accurate assessment of brain injury should be done with an MRI study.

MR Techniques in the Evaluation of Perinatal Asphyxia or HIE

MR has become the technique of choice to evaluate the hypoxic-ischemic brain both in adults and in the newborn. Additional MR imaging techniques, such as the use of DWI, SWI, and MR spectroscopy, have further improved the MR capability to investigate the neonatal brain. Generally, to increase the signal-to-noise ratio, a higher field magnet (1.5–3 T) should be used, allowing for high-resolution imaging and increased sensitivity for spectroscopy.[23-25]

CONVENTIONAL MRI SEQUENCES AND FEATURES IN HIE

The basic information in conventional MR imaging is represented by T1- and T2-weighted images. Proton density and FLAIR images help illustrate brain lesions with slightly different contrast than T1- and T2-weighted images. A neonatal MR imaging protocol should provide good quality T1- and T2-weighted images with a maximum field of view of 16 to 18 cm and a slice thickness of 2 mm or less. Due to increased water content of the neonatal brain with longer T1 and T2 relaxation times, the repetition time (TR) should be increased in both T1-weighted and T2-weighted imaging sequences. Typically MR sequence parameters for T1-weighted images should include an increased TR to 800 ms and a TR above 5000 ms with an echo time (TE) of 125 to 150 ms for T2-weighted imaging.[23,26] To compensate for a long TR, the echo-train-length can be increased.

Selective Neuronal Necrosis After Perinatal Asphyxia

As shown in the three cases previously with a history of acute perinatal asphyxia, selective involvement of areas with advanced maturation and higher energy demands, i.e., the putamen, ventrolateral thalami, and perirolandic cortex, are particularly vulnerable. Characteristic changes representing selective neuronal necrosis in these areas on T1-weighted images are T1 hyperintensities, which become apparent 3 to 7 days after the insult. These T1 hyperintensities might represent cellular reaction of glial cells and macrophages containing lipid droplets and/or some mineralization of necrotic cells. Some difficulties in identifying these lesions arise from the fact that early myelination shows the same imaging characteristics. T1 hyperintensities in the internal capsule due to beginning myelination need to be differentiated from lateral thalamic lesions and lesions in the putamen. Often the posterior limb appears swollen and has lost its normal T1 hyperintensity/T2 hypointensity, which has a bad prognostic value and is associated with development of cerebral palsy.[27] These T1 changes are not apparent till the end

of the first week and most infants are now scanned on the day following rewarming, which is often too early to see these changes in the PLIC.[26] On T2-weighted images, thalami might appear slightly hyperintense in the acute phase (see Case 1) but these signal changes tend to be very difficult to detect. T2 hyperintensities become more apparent at a later stage, illustrated also by well-defined lesions on proton-density images (see Case 2). Evolution of these lesions is marked by progressive atrophy of the involved area (i.e., putamen, thalami, rolandic cortex) with persistent T2 hyperintensity and possible cavitation.[28]

Of note, similar lesions in the bilateral thalami, lentiform nucleus, and globus pallidum can be detected also in premature infants with documented severe anoxic insults, most frequently associated with the typical periventricular white matter injuries.[16]

Parasagittal Cerebral Injury

Isolated parasagittal injury refers to a lesion of the cerebral cortex and the subcortical white matter with a defined distribution, i.e., parasagittal, superomedial aspects of the cortical convexities, usually bilateral but often asymmetric in its extension.[29,30] During the acute phase, the cortex might show increased T1-weighted signal intensity or little abnormality on conventional MR imaging (see Fig. 15.10). On the T2-weighted sequence, loss of the cortical ribbon is best seen. Chronic changes involve cortical thinning and atrophy and less often subcortical cysts.

Multicystic Encephalomalacia

Case 5 shows another form of brain injury associated with HIE. Early on (<2 days), conventional MRI is characterized by a diffuse T1 hypointensity and T2 hyperintensity involving both the cortex and the subcortical white matter but sparing the cerebellum and the more basal structures of the medulla (see Fig. 15.9). Late intrauterine generalized prolonged systemic circulatory insufficiency is probably at the origin of these lesions, which evolve into severe cortical atrophy with cavitation and are invariably associated with a severe neurological syndrome.

Cerebellar Injury

There is still limited data about cerebellar injury on MRI in term neonates with HIE. Conventional T1- and

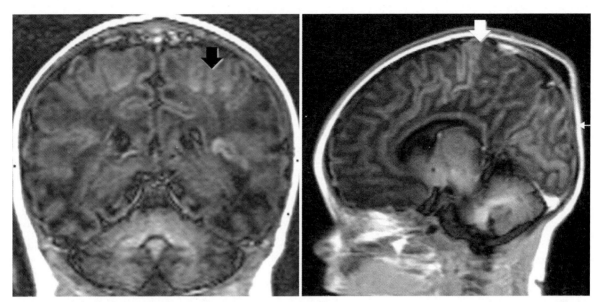

Fig. 15.10 Typical parasagittal distribution of T1 hyperintensities in cortical neuronal necrosis of deep sulcal cortex of another patient with acute perinatal asphyxia.

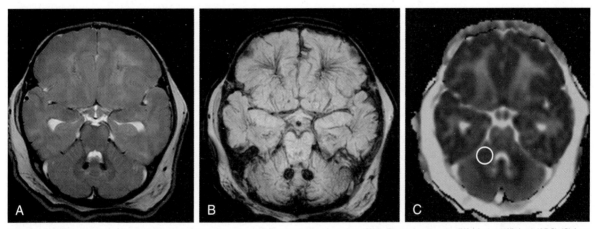

Fig. 15.11 MRI, axial plane, T2-weighted sequence (A), susceptibility-weighted imaging (SWI) (B), and apparent diffusion coefficient (ADC) (C) in a term infant with severe HIE Grade III and a near total pattern of injury on day 2. The brain is severely swollen and there is loss of gray-white matter differentiation. Blood is seen in the fourth ventricle on T2 and SWI. The ADC values in the cerebellar hemisphere were severely reduced (0.61). The infant died.

T2- weighted sequences do not often suggest cerebellar injury in neonates with HIE.[31] SWI will additionally identify the presence of hemorrhagic lesions (Fig. 15.11). Several studies measured ADC values in cerebellar hemispheres, vermis, and pons. One study looked at 28 infants with HIE and hypothermia, 8 with HIE and normothermia, and 9 controls and found ADC values to be significantly related to death and motor outcome.[32] In a recent study, ADC values were found to be significantly reduced in the vermis ($p = 0.021$) and dentate nucleus ($p < 0.001$) in infants with HIE compared to controls. ADC values in the vermis were significantly correlated with Purkinje cells injury.[33] Another study looked at 59 infants and noted combined pontine and dentate nucleus in eight of them and noted that these abnormalities were always associated with a more severe brain injury pattern as well as being predictive of major disability.[34] More advanced MRI studies have identified cerebellar injury in HIE using diffusion tensor imaging (DTI) in the first month after birth.[35]

DIFFUSION WEIGHTED IMAGING SEQUENCES AND FEATURES IN HIE

DWI measures the self-diffusion of water. The two primary pieces of information available from DWI studies—water apparent diffusion coefficient (ADC) and diffusion anisotropy measures—change dramatically during development, reflecting underlying changes in tissue water content and cytoarchitecture.[36] ADC being a quantitative measure (velocity) of overall water diffusion in tissue and anisotropy being a measure of directionality of water diffusion in a given tissue. The developing human brain presents several challenges for the application of DWI. Values for the water diffusion parameters differ markedly between neonatal brain and adult brain and vary with age. As a result, much of the knowledge regarding DWI derived from studies of mature, adult human brain is not directly applicable to the developing brain.

In order to perform DWI, the optimum b value required to make the measurement has to be optimized, as it differs between the newborn and adult brain. Generally, a b value corresponding to approximately 1.1/ADC provides the greatest contrast-to-noise ratio for such a measurement.[9] In neonatal brain, the high b value is typically on the order of 700 to 1000 mm²/s. EPI rather than SE[37]-like sequences are generally used, and the recent use of multiband acceleration techniques helps to reduce the acquisition time. Indeed "high angular resolution diffusion imaging" (HARDI) and multicompartmental diffusion techniques require the acquisition of multiple shells (data for several b values in the newborn up to 2600 ms) with multiple diffusion gradient directions to provide an accurate estimation of the diffusion model and the extraction of microstructural features of the developing brain.[38]

DWI parameters also change in response to brain injury. The decrease in water diffusion associated with injury was initially described for animals[39] and adult human stroke,[40] and was subsequently confirmed for

human infants.[41] Case 1 and Case 4 clearly show the marked reduction of ADC in the basal ganglia with only slight hyperintensities on T2-weighted images which can be easily missed. DWI in this case detects the lesion more reliably.

There is still debate on the precise mechanism for the decrease in the ADC associated with injury. Changes in ADC following injury are dynamic. ADC values are initially decreased, but subsequently increase so that they are greater than normal and remain so in the chronic phase of injury. During the transition between decreased and increased values, there is a brief period during which values are normal, a process referred to as "pseudo-normalization." Pseudo-normalization takes place roughly 2 days following stroke in a rat model[42] and at approximately 9 days following injury in adult human stroke.[43] Preliminary data indicate that the timing of pseudo-normalization in human newborns follows more closely that of adult humans than that of rodents, taking place at roughly 7 days following the injury.[44] Interpretation of ADC values to detect acute brain injury in the developing brain needs to be adjusted for the regional differences in ADC values according to age (see Fig. 15.5).[45] Case 3 illustrates that without numerical measurement of ADC, acute tissue alteration on diffusion maps can be missed.[46]

Case 2 illustrates that in the human newborns, very early (<24 hours) DWI might also miss detection of ischemic injury, which has been reported in several studies.[45,47,48]

From these studies, we can summarize the current role of DWI in the evaluation of the term newborn with HIE:

1. DWI obtained less than 24 hours after injury may demonstrate focal abnormalities when measuring ADC values and comparing them to regional age-corresponding values; however, the full extent of lesions might not be detected.
2. DWI with ADC measurement obtained between day 2 and 4 may detect lesions not detected by conventional MRI.
3. DWI at 7 to 10 days is less sensitive than conventional MRI due to the "pseudo-normalization."

MAGNETIC RESONANCE SPECTROSCOPY IN HIE

Proton magnetic resonance spectroscopy (¹H-MRS) has also entered the clinical arena of MR techniques routinely used for the evaluation of the brain and permits the noninvasive study of metabolic alterations in the brain tissue.[49]

The physiologist is usually interested in the intracellular concentration of a chemical species in a particular cell type. It must be noted, though, that the in vivo human MR measurement in single voxel MRS is an average (over the sensitive volume) of all tissue types. In the brain, therefore, we generally assess a combination of glial and neuronal cells with different extracellular space depending upon how much white matter, gray matter, or cerebrospinal fluid (CSF) the volume-of-interest contains.

When oxidative phosphorylation is impaired, energy metabolism follows the alternative route of anaerobic glycolysis and produces lactic acid. Lactate has a chemical shift of 1.3 ppm and presents as a doublet peak in the in vivo ^{1}H-MRS due to coupling effects. Groenendaal et al. first described markedly elevated lactate levels in five infants with severe perinatal asphyxia.[50] The five patients died within the neonatal period. ^{1}H-MRS data has been generated that demonstrates regional differences in lactate elevation after hypoxic-ischemic events in newborns. Single volume ^{1}H-MRS in these patients showed greater increase of the Lac/NAA ratio in the basal ganglia than in the occipito-parietal cerebrum.[51] This corresponds to the signal abnormalities observed with early DWI after term hypoxia-ischemia. Case 2 illustrates the typical changes in ^{1}H-MRS after term perinatal hypoxia-ischemia.

Early spectroscopy (<18 hours after event) and measurement of high Lac/creatine (Cr) ratio in ^{1}H-MRS correlated well with neurodevelopmental outcome at 1 year.[50] This acute phase lactic acidosis is followed by persistently elevated lactate levels not associated with acidosis 1 to 2 weeks after the event to several weeks after the hypoxic-ischemic event.[52,53] However, ^{1}H-MRS performed in the first 24 hours after the insult is sensitive to the presence of hypoxic-ischemic brain injury, and seems to be suitable for the detection of brain injury on the first day when conventional MR imaging and DWI might not yet detect the injury. Early MR spectroscopy, within a few hours of insult has been shown to predict outcome more accurately than very early DWI alone.[26,54-56]

As markers of cell integrity other metabolites visible on ^{1}H-MRS can be used for the assessment of HIE.

Ratios of NAA/Cho and NAA/Cr have been used to assess cellular metabolic integrity in neonatal brain injury.[57,58] Studies using ^{1}H-MRS at a distance (>1–2 weeks) to the hypoxic-ischemic event showed good correlation between reduced NAA ratios with adverse neurodevelopmental outcome[57] whereas in early (acute stage) ^{1}H-MRS Lac/NAA ratios are good predictors of outcome.

From these studies, we can summarize the current role of ^{1}H-MRS in the evaluation of the term newborn with HIE:

1. ^{1}H-MRS can play an important role in the assessment of encephalopathic term infants. Elevated lactate/NAA, lactate/creatine, and lactate/choline (Cho) ratios or elevated absolute concentrations of lactate at less than 24 hours reliably indicate cellular injury.
2. ^{1}H-MRS might therefore be more useful than DWI techniques in identifying infants who would benefit from early therapeutic interventions.

MRI in the Settings of Therapeutic Neonatal Hypothermia

Mild therapeutic hypothermia is now recognized as the only available treatment after hypoxia-ischemia. In such an acute context, thorough assessment of brain integrity is mandatory in order to manage the patient and help the family. Estimating the severity of neonatal resuscitation, the neurological status according to Sarnat classification and assessing the electroencephalographic trace are so far the only available bedside tools. Cerebral ultrasonography performed prior to starting hypothermia can be useful to identify injury of antenatal onset and abnormalities suggestive of HIE mimics. Abnormalities in central gray nuclei can be seen with ultrasound but only after 48 to 72 hours.[20] MRI in this setting requiring close collaboration between the neonatologists, nursing staff, and neuroradiologist will give a thorough assessment of brain integrity and map out the extent of injury following asphyxia and might guide neuro-interventions such as hypothermia.

To date, relatively few studies have addressed the question of how MRI can be used, when assessing newborns undergoing therapeutic hypothermia or after the completion of therapeutic hypothermia,[26,58-61] but generally, the MRI predictability of outcome is not changed by hypothermia when scanned after hypothermia.[59]

MRI DURING HYPOTHERMIA

The rational of performing an MRI during hypothermia is to answer whether there is massive brain injury questioning ongoing medical treatment with possible withdrawal of life-sustaining therapies and eventually whether this is significant well-established injury dating the time of insult before birth. It is possible also that it might be used in the future to monitor and tailor the length of hypothermia.

The question becomes: What do we know of the validity of neonatal cerebral MRI under hypothermia? What are the effects on proton spectroscopy? What are the effects on DWI?

The ADC has a biphasic evolution following HI in newborns in conditions of normothermia.[44] Animal data has shown that it corresponds to cytotoxic edema with ongoing cell death and that its measure correlates with caspase-3 activation.[62] The measurement of the ADC is directly influenced by temperature, with a calculated 6% reduction of the ADC at 33.5°C. Referring to normative data established by Rutherford et al.[45] in conditions of normothermia, the measurement of ADC in normal un-injured tissue might give falsely decreased measures, although the hypoxic-ischemic brain regions express generally a much higher reduction with 35% or more. Moreover, the direct effect of localized cortical cooling in rhesus monkeys has been shown to induce a measurable decrease in ADC only with temperatures as low as 20°C.[52] Bednarek et al.[60] compared serial ADC values in hypothermia patients compared to a historic control group and showed that indeed the ADC drop after hypoxia-ischemia was prolonged by hypothermia with pseudo-normalization after 10 days rather than between 6 and 8 days as shown without hypothermia. The question remains whether the ADC in this setting is a reliable biomarker of injury. In a small prospective cohort, qualitative analysis of MRI during hypothermia has been performed on day of life 1, 2, and 10.[63] Restricted ADC values could be identified in case of brain injury. Similarly, to normothermic condition, significant injury was better defined on ADC map on day 2 rather than within the first 24 hours of life.

Phosphorus spectroscopy has been studied during hypothermia in an animal model with a keystone article showing that therapeutic hypothermia reduced the degree of second energy failure after hypoxic-ischemic injury.[64] Temperature changes will induce minimal chemical shift of the water peak that can be used to quantify temperature when studied in relation to the temperature-independent shift of the neighboring metabolites[65,66] and should not affect the magnitude of metabolic peak of lactate or NAA. Clinical experience and data published by Wintermark and colleagues[63] show that spectroscopy remains a reliable tool to assess brain integrity during hypothermia. Interestingly, the repeat exam on day 2 showed greater increase in lactate than the exam done within a few hours of birth.

MRI PERFORMED AFTER HYPOTHERMIA

The rational of performing an MRI after the completion of therapeutic hypothermia is to establish the extent of brain injury. The question in this setting is when is the best time to perform the exam? Is the MRI valid?

Conventional T1- and T2-weighted after completion of hypothermia (8 days of life: 6–11) has been demonstrated to have the same predictive ability when compared to noncooled newborn infants.[61] Unfortunately, the TOBY trial didn't include early predetermined timing for MRI with the precise analysis of the ADC. Massaro and colleagues found that T2 hyperintensity quantification of the putamen and the thalamus when normalizing to the ocular vitreous signal intensity had superior predictive value compared to T1 or ADC analysis.[67] In this study, the MRI was performed during the second week of life, explaining why the ADC had limited value, as injury can produce an ADC value within the pseudo-normalization timeframe. Further studies are needed to define lesion evolution by MRI in neonatal HIE and hypothermia treatment. Recent large retrospective analysis of predictive value of MRI for outcome prognosis confirm the value of MRI equally in cohort with or without hypothermia.[59,61] Data from a metaanalysis showed a better predictive value of MRI performed during the first week than the second week of life, most likely due to improved recognition of central gray nuclei injury with DWI.[56]

Focal and Multifocal Ischemic Brain Necrosis Without Asphyxia

As mentioned previously, focal and multifocal ischemic brain necrosis can also occur without HIE and the sole presence of these brain lesions also puts the neonate in the "high-risk infant" category even if they have not suffered asphyxia. However, they do significantly more often have at least one or two intrapartum risk factors compared to controls.[68] These lesions occur within the distribution of single or multiple major blood vessels. Almost 90% of the infarcts are unilateral, and of these lesions nearly all involve the middle cerebral artery (MCA), 75% of them involving the distribution of the left MCA for a yet unexplained reason and most often (57%) the posterior branch of the left MCA.[69] The major etiologies of these infarcts occurring without significant asphyxia are presented in Table 15.4.

The neonatal and long-term clinical correlates are described in Table 15.3. Neonatal seizures occur in 80% to 85% of these patients and are in most cases focal, with clonic movements contralateral to the lesion. Regarding long-term correlates, hemiparesis occurs in 25% of the patients with unilateral lesion, but depends on the size and site of the lesion.[71] The likelihood of hemiparesis depends on the extent of the lesion and especially on the involvement, of the corticospinal tracts.[72] DWI performed a few days after the insult will be able to show restricted diffusion in the PLIC and/or cerebral peduncle. This is known as pre-Wallerian degeneration and will be seen as Wallerian degeneration on a repeat MRI at 6 to 12 weeks of age.[73] Thus, hemiparesis is almost certain if the distribution of the stem of the MCA is affected, or if there is corticospinal tract involvement. However, if only a cortical branch or lenticulostriate vessels are affected, the likelihood of hemiparesis is around 10%. This relatively good outcome in unilateral lesions is probably related to the ability of the opposite hemisphere to reestablish ipsilateral corticospinal tract innervation (brain plasticity). Seizure disorders occur in 10% to 50% of infants depending on size of the lesion.[71,74,75] Cognitive function is more likely to be impaired if lesions are bilateral. In unilateral lesions, only 20% to 25% of infants develop cognitive problems.

TABLE 15.4 Etiologies of Focal and Multifocal Ischemic Lesions

Idiopathic (majority of cases)
Vascular maldevelopment
Vasculopathy
Vasospasm (i.e., with cocaine use)
Vascular distortion (obstetrical trauma to head and neck)
Vascular manipulation-ligation (i.e., for extracorporeal membrane oxygenation)
Embolus:
- placental thrombosis or tissue fragments (twin pregnancy with death of co-twin)
- involuting fetal vessels (thrombi)
- catheterized vessels (thrombi or air)
- cardiac: myxoma or rhabdomyoma, right to left shunt, patent foramen ovale
Thrombus:
- meningitis with arteritis or phlebitis
- trauma
- disseminated intravascular coagulation
- polycythemia
- hypercoagulable state: prot C or prot S or antithrombin III deficiency, antiphospholipid antibodies, factor V Leiden mutation in only rare cases, as recent population studies do not confirm the association in childhood follow-up[70]
- hypernatremia–dehydration

Modified from Volpe JJ. *Neurology of the Newborn*. 6th ed. Philadelphia: Elsevier; 2018.

Case 6

History: The pregnancy was uneventful but marked for cocaine exposure. During spontaneous labor, the cardiotocogram showed variable decelerations with signs of fetal distress and emergency cesarean section was performed for acute fetal bradycardia. The Apgar score was noted 5/9/9 with rapid clinical recovery. The infant was transferred to the neonatal unit for surveillance. On day 3 of life, the infant developed apneic attacks and convulsions were noted with head deviation.

Neuroimaging studies: MRI on day 4 reveals significant signal abnormalities on ADC maps and DWIs during the acute phase. DWI showed a striking reduction of diffusivity and ADC in the left temporo-parieto-occipital region with involvement also of the basal ganglia and internal capsule, consistent with an acute infarction (see Fig. 15.12A–C). Thus the mean value for ADC in the intact right hemisphere was $1.68 \pm 0.12 \ \mu m^2/ms$, whereas in the corresponding left hemisphere, the ADC was $0.60 \pm 0.04 \ \mu m^2/ms$, reflecting the dramatic decline in ADC during acute ischemic injury. MR angiography showed permeable vessels on both sides (Fig. 15.12D). On day 8 of life, the ADC was $1.69 \pm 0.09 \ \mu m^2/ms$ in the right hemisphere and $0.93 \pm 0.19 \ \mu m^2/ms$ in the left hemisphere. The MRI at 6 weeks of age showed

tissue dissolution in the left posterior cerebral region with an increased ADC of $2.85 \pm 0.15 \ \mu m^2/ms$, compared to normal ADC of $1.44 \pm 0.16 \ \mu m^2/ms$ in the right hemisphere. T2-weighted images at 6 weeks of age showed that the lesion had evolved with cavitation (see Fig. 15.12E–G). At 13 weeks, diffusion tensor images showed loss of optic radiation fibers and loss of cortical visual response on fMRI (not shown). At 12 and 20 months of age, DTI with fiber tracking illustrates partial recovery of optic radiation fibers and preserved anterior cerebral activation upon visual stimulation in the lesioned hemisphere (see Fig. 15.13).

Clinical correlates in the neonatal period: This is a typical case of focal infarct where the seizure starts after 2 to 3 days of life, without other neurological signs. In particular, no hypotonia or lethargy was described. In this situation, the seizures are the result of a focal cortical lesion and not due to diffuse cortical impairment.

Long-term clinical correlates: This child-developed hemiplegia contralateral to the side of the lesion, which was expected due to the extent of the lesion. Alteration of the visual field in the area of the infarct also occurred but vision was normal at age 5. Some degree of intellectual impairment developed as well.

MR Techniques in the Evaluation of Focal Ischemic Infarction in the Term Newborn

MRI is the technique of choice for evaluating focal neonatal cerebral infarctions, as ultrasonography only shows the infarction after several days as a wedge shape echogenic lesion, if it is within the field of view (perforator, large MCA). However, smaller cortical infarcts or a posterior cerebral artery stroke may be missed.[76]

Conventional MRI shows loss of cortico-subcortical differentiation in both T1- and T2-weighted imaging due to the increase of T2 signal intensity in the edematous cortex, thus approaching the signal intensity of the unmyelinated white matter. This sign is also called the "disappeared cortex" sign. The best modality to identify a focal ischemic infarct is DWI, with striking reduction of ADC in the acute phase and tissue dissolution thereafter, which results in cavitation with T2 characteristics of CSF.

As outlined in the clinical description, focal ischemic infarction may have less severe neurological sequelae probably due to the brain's potential for plasticity.[71,72]

Advanced MR techniques such as *DTI* and *fMRI* have recently been shown to be of use in the study of postinjury plasticity.[73,77] The geometric nature of the

diffusion tensor can be used to display the architecture of the brain white matter fiber tracts illustrating them by vector images. fMRI can illustrate functional brain activation by measuring changes in local perfusion based on the BOLD contrast. In a case of perinatal MCA stroke (Case 5) at 20 months of age, event-related fMRI showed significant activation in the visual cortex of the injured left hemisphere that was not observed at 3 months of age.[77] DTI vector maps suggest recovery of the optic radiation in the vicinity of the lesion. Optic radiations in the injured hemisphere were more prominent in DTI at 20 months of age than in DTI at 12 months of age which indicates that functional cortical recovery is supported by structural modifications that concern major pathways of the visual system.

Traumatic Brain Lesions of the Posterior Fossa

Intracranial hemorrhage as such is another important brain lesion in the neonatal period, particularly affecting the preterm infant but also occurring in the full-term infant in certain situations. In particular, traumatic brain lesions of the posterior fossa in the term newborn

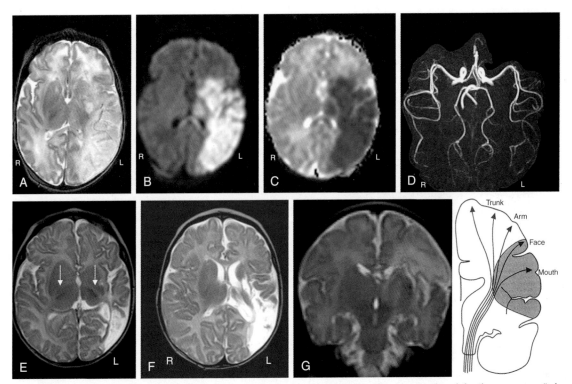

Fig. 15.12 Case 6: Acute left middle cerebral artery infarction in the newborn. A, Axial T2-weighted image where infarction appears as "missed cortex" with absence of cortical-subcortical differentiation due to acute edema. B, Diffusion-weighted image. C, Apparent diffusion coefficient (ADC) map with clear demarcation of ischemic zone. D, Shows reperfused middle cerebral artery on the left with MR angiography. E and F, Axial T2-weighted images in the chronic phase of infarction with cystic transformation of the initial ischemic zone and absence of left-sided myelination in the posterior limb of internal capsule (*arrows*). G, Coronal T2-weighted image corresponding to figure representing corticospinal tracts and innervation. (From Jeffrey J. Neil, Joseph J. Volpe, Chapter 16 - Encephalopathy of Prematurity: Clinical-Neurological Features, Diagnosis, Imaging, Prognosis, Therapy, Editor(s): Joseph J. Volpe, Terrie E. Inder, Basil T. Darras, Linda S. de Vries, Adré J. du Plessis, Jeffrey J. Neil, Jeffrey M. Perlman, Volpe's Neurology of the Newborn (Sixth Edition), Elsevier, 2018, Pages 425-457.e11. https://doi.org/10.1016/B978-0-323-42876-7.00016-8.)

associated with massive hemorrhage can cause serious neurological sequelae. The mechanism responsible for this lesion is occipital osteodiastasis. This consists of traumatic separation of the cartilaginous joint between the squamous and lateral portions of the occipital bone. In the most severe forms, the dura and the occipital sinus are torn resulting in massive subdural hemorrhage in the posterior fossa and cerebellar laceration. Risk factors are breech delivery, vacuum extraction, primiparity, and fetomaternal disproportion.

Clinical manifestations in the most severe cases are immediate signs of brainstem compression (stupor or coma, oculomotor and pupillary abnormalities, nuchal rigidity with opisthotonos, respiratory abnormalities, bradycardia, and then respiratory arrest) and this syndrome is rapidly lethal. In less severe forms, neurological signs can be absent in the first hours,

then symptoms of increased intracranial pressure develop due to ventricular dilatation (block of the CSF flow in the posterior fossa). The signs of brainstem compression due to the posterior fossa hematoma appear later. In addition, seizures occur in the majority of patients, most likely due to the accompanying subarachnoid blood. Long-term outcome is poor in severe occipital diastasis. If the posterior fossa hemorrhage is less pronounced, the outcome is more variable, depending on the rate of rapidity of diagnosis and intervention. With extension of the hemorrhage into the cerebellum, cerebellar deficits due to destruction of the cerebellar tissue are almost invariably present (intention tremor, dysmetria, truncal ataxia, and hypotonia). Hydrocephalus requiring ventriculoperitoneal shunts occur in 50% of cases. Cognitive deficits are also variably present.

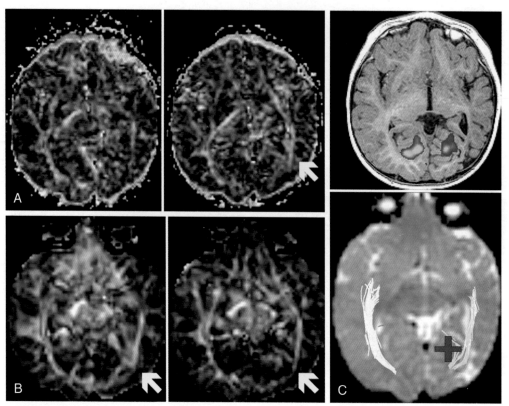

Fig. 15.13 Case 6: Diffusion tensor imaging with anisotropy maps at 12 months (A) and 20 months (B) arrows indicate recovery of optic radiation fibers visualized by diffusion tensor imaging (DTI). fMRI response to visual stimulation at 20 months of age shows recovery of cortical vision in the area of tract recovery. (Adapted from Seghier ML, Lazeyras F, Zimine S, Saudan-Frei S, Safran AB, Hüppi PS. Visual recovery after perinatal stroke evidenced by functional and diffusion MRI: case report. *BMC Neurol.* 2005;5:17.)

Case 7

History: Term pregnancy with vaginal delivery instrumented by vacuum for nonprogression, Apgar score (9/9/10), (pH 7.23). On day 1, appearance of general hypotonia, tonic-clonic seizure, subsequent tonic seizures.

Neuroimaging studies: Neonatal head ultrasound performed on day 2 shows posterior fossa hemorrhage with enlarged ventricles. MRI on day 2 reveals a large T2-hypointense lesion in the posterior fossa involving the cerebellar vermis with concomitant ventricular dilatation. On the sagittal images, the Vein of Galen can be identified. MR angiogram shows no arterial or venous malformation. Tonsillar herniation of the cerebellum is present. On follow-up, T2-weighted images marked cerebellar lesions are visualized (see Fig. 15.14).

Clinical correlates in the neonatal period: This child presented with hypotonia which could be due to brain stem compression and seizures due to cortical "irritation" by the subarachnoid blood. The brainstem compression signs which are common in these situations had not yet taken place when the diagnosis was made thanks to the occurrence of seizures which resulted in the emergency neuroimaging. Surgical removal of the hematoma was then realized. The child developed a cardiac arrest during surgery due to the massive blood loss and was immediately resuscitated with success.

Long-term clinical correlates: The patient presented with severe truncal hypotonia and truncal ataxia with delayed spontaneous walking. This child also developed mild spasticity in the lower extremities, most likely as a sequela of a mild cortical injury which happened during the short cardiac arrest during surgery. Her cognitive function is normal at the age of 5 years. However, the cerebellar deficits are still very important (intention tremor, dysmetria, and truncal ataxia).

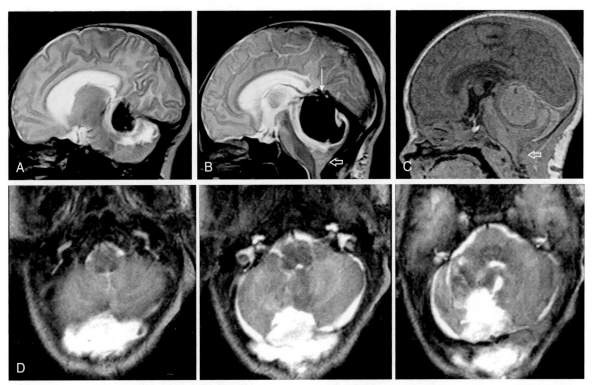

Fig. 15.14 Case 7: Sagittal T2-weighted images acquired on day 2 reveal a large T2-hypointense lesion in the posterior fossa involving the cerebellum with concomitant ventricular dilatation (A, B). On B, the vein of Galen can be identified (*small arrow*). Tonsillar herniation of the cerebellum is present (*large arrows*) (B, C). D shows axial T2-weighted images with residual cerebellar lesion.

MR Techniques in the Evaluation of Traumatic Brain Injury in the Term Newborn

As the posterior fossa is the primary site of subdural hemorrhage after traumatic birth, cranial ultrasound through the anterior fontanelle has limited capacity in detection of extent of posterior fossa lesions. The MRI appearance of blood is dependent on the oxidative state of hemoglobin and its environment. Acute hemorrhage (3 hours–10 days) therefore shows isointensity to slight hyperintensity on T1-weighted images (gradient-echo sequences preferred) and low signal intensity on T2-weighted images (see Fig. 15.14) with evolution to high signal intensity on T2-weighted images between 10 days and 3 weeks after the hemorrhage (Fig. 15.14). Sagittal image planes are necessary to look for cerebellar tonsillar herniation in the presence of posterior fossa hemorrhage. MR venography can exclude Vein of Galen malformations or sinus thrombosis, which is one of the major reasons for intracerebral hemorrhages in the term newborn[78] illustrated in Fig. 15.15.

Brain Injury in the Preterm Infant

Brain injury in the premature infant is composed of multiple lesions, principally described as germinal matrix (GM) intraventricular hemorrhage (IVH), venous hemorrhagic infarction, post hemorrhagic hydrocephalus, and periventricular leukomalacia (PVL) and many preterm infants show neurodevelopmental delay without having been diagnosed with any of these typical perinatal brain injuries.

The site of origin of IVH is the subependymal GM, which is a very cellular, gelatinous, highly vascularized region. Mechanisms underlying fragility of the

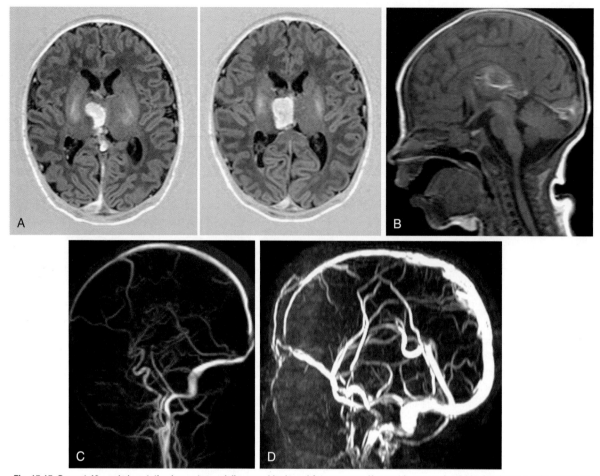

Fig. 15.15 Born at 40 weeks' gestation by ventouse delivery and had good Apgar scores. He went home on day 2 but developed hemiconvulsions on day 6. Ultrasound noted a thalamic hemorrhage and cerebral venous sinus thrombosis (CSVT) was suspected. An MRI confirmed the diagnosis with a thrombus in the straight sinus on the midsagittal T1-weighted image (A, axial, B sagittal, C, lack of flow on the MRV, D, normal MRV for comparison). He was treated for 3 months with low-molecular-weight heparin and a repeat MRV showed recanalization of the straight sinus. A normal MRV is shown for comparison. His outcome was good with good motor and cognitive skills at 7 years of age. He is left-handed and has a score on the movement-ABC on the 50th centile.

GM vasculature relate to the hypoxic GM which induces VEGF and angiopoietin-2 expression. These growth factors trigger angiogenesis. The nascent vessels of the GM exhibit paucity of pericytes and deficiency of fibronectin in immature basal lamina and are therefore fragile.[79] The exact site of the hemorrhage seems to be the capillary-venule or small venule level.[80] In 80% of cases, the blood subsequently enters the lateral ventricles and spread occurs through the ventricular system. The presence of blood may create an obliterative arachnoiditis over days to weeks with obstruction of CSF flow. The blood clot can also lead to impaired CSF circulation at the aqueduct of Sylvius and the arachnoid villi. One of the possible consequences of this phenomenon is the development of progressive ventricular dilation and hydrocephalus which may require neurosurgical intervention. Posthemorrhagic hydrocephalus may happen in an acute, subacute, or chronic way. Approximately, 15% of infants also develop a characteristic parenchymal

TABLE 15.5	White Matter Lesions in the Premature Infant			
Lesion	**Circulation Affected**	**Massive Hemorrhage**	**Unilateral in Most Cases**	**Long-Term Outcome in Most Cases**
PVHI	Venous	Yes	Yes	Spastic hemiparesis or asymmetrical spastic quadriparesis
PVL	Arterial/inflammatory	No	No	Spastic diplegia

PVHI, Periventricular hemorrhagic infarction; *PVL*, periventricular leukomalacia.
Modified from Cebeci B, Alderliesten T, Wijnen JP, et al. Brain proton magnetic resonance spectroscopy and neurodevelopment after preterm birth: a systematic review. *Pediatr Res* 2022;91(6):1322-1333. doi:10.1038/s41390-021-01539-x.

lesion, with a triangular shape, in the white matter situated dorsally and laterally to the external angle of the lateral ventricle. This lesion corresponds to a periventricular hemorrhagic infarction (PVHI).[81] The current prevailing hypothesis regarding its pathogenesis is that the GM hemorrhage creates an obstruction of the terminal vein and impaired blood flow in the medullary veins, resulting in hemorrhagic venous infarction which is usually unilateral. Indeed, the terminal vein draining the medullary veins runs essentially within the GM. The venous congestion creates a periventricular ischemia, leading to the PVHI which is a very different lesion from PVL (see Table 15.5). The time of onset of IVH is the first day of life in 50% of cases and the 3 first days of life in 90% of cases. The neonatal clinical correlates vary from a catastrophic neurological deterioration of the infant in minutes to hours if the IVH is massive, to a clinically silent syndrome. The long-term neurological prognosis is mostly dictated by the extent of the intraparenchymal lesion. Neurological sequelae mostly consist of spastic hemiparesis or asymmetrical quadriparesis with cognitive deficits. Posthemorrhagic ventricular dilatation (PHVD) occurs more likely if the IVH is severe and can contribute to the neurological sequelae in some cases.

PVL has classically been described as a disorder characterized by multifocal areas of necrosis, forming cysts in the deep periventricular cerebral white matter, which are often bilateral but not necessarily symmetrical and occur adjacent to the lateral ventricles. The earliest neuropathological changes are of *coagulation necrosis* of all cellular elements with loss of cytoarchitecture and tissue vacuolation.[82] *Axonal swelling* and intense activated *microglial reactivity* and proliferation are observed as early as 3 hours after the insult.[83,84] In addition, in the periphery of these focal lesions, a marked *astrocytic and vascular endothelial hyperplasia* characterizes the brain tissue reaction at the end of the first week. After 1 to 2 weeks, *macrophage activity with characteristic lipid-laden macrophages* is predominant over the astrocytic reactivity, with progressive cavitation of the tissue and cyst formation thereafter. During subacute and chronic stages of PVL, swollen axons calcify, accumulate iron, and degenerate particularly at the periphery of the injured zone. The deep focal necrotic lesions of PVL occur in areas that are considered arterial end zones. The state of development of the periventricular vessels is a function of gestational age and the degree of ischemia required to produce these focal lesions may vary upon the state of development of these vessels and thus upon gestational age.[85]

These *focal* necrotic lesions correlate well with the development of spastic cerebral palsy in VLBW infants (see Fig. 15.16), whereas the increasingly large number of VLBW infants with mild motor impairment and cognitive and behavioral deficits may relate to a more *diffuse* injury to the developing white matter which has more recently been recognized. Diffuse white matter damage is macroscopically characterized by a paucity of white matter, thinning of the corpus callosum and, in later stages, ventriculomegaly and delayed myelination.

The pathogenesis of the more diffuse lesions may relate in part to the development of the penetrating vessels, more peripherally. These diffuse lesions also seem to be related to less severe ischemia than the focal ones. In sick preterm infants, the cerebral circulation tends to become pressure passive, i.e., when blood pressure falls, so does the cerebral blood flow. This mechanism adds to ischemia in the pathogenesis of cerebral white matter injury. Neuropathological findings of the diffuse type of cerebral injury in the preterm infant further include preferential death of

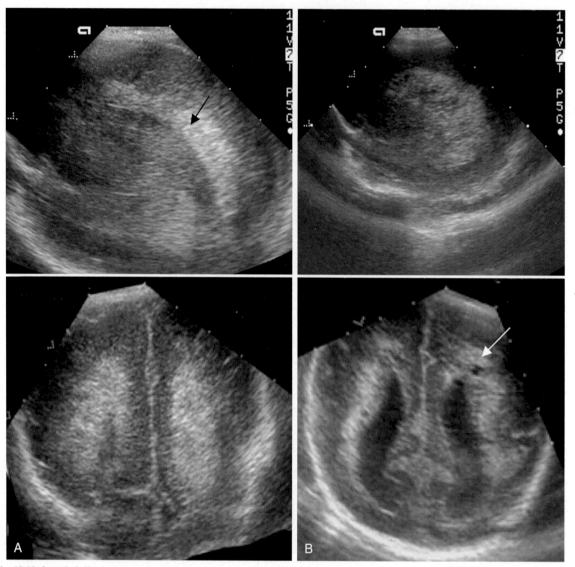

Fig. 15.16 Case 8: A, Head ultrasound examination on day 5 of life with increased slightly irregular periventricular hyperechogenicity (*arrows*). B, Head ultrasound at day 10 with persisting periventricular hyperechogenicity and appearance of echolucencies (*white arrow*). Typical ultrasound images of evolving periventricular leukomalacia.

preoligodendrocytes,[86,87] axonal damage,[84] and death of the transitory subplate neurons[88] through mechanisms of oxidative injury, glutamate toxicity, and presence of cytotoxic cytokines produced by infection and inflammation. The injury of the white matter secondary to cytotoxic cytokines has been shown to occur prenatally in the setting of chorioamnionitis[89,90] or postnatally in the setting of sepsis or necrotizing enterocolitis. These inflammatory factors are likely to be more important in the pathogenesis of the more diffuse type PVL. *Diffuse neuronal loss*, especially in lower cortical layers, the hippocampus, and in the cerebellar Purkinje cell layer, is described in preterm brain neuropathological studies.[91]

The clinical correlates of PVL are described in Table 15.6. At least some of the cognitive deficits associated to PVL may be due to subsequent disturbance of cortical neuronal organization, because of injury to subplate neurons, to late migrating astrocytes, or to axons with retrograde disturbances in dendritic development.[92]

The role of MRI in the diagnosis a nd prognosis of these lesions will be illustrated with four cases.

Case 8

History: Premature infant of 27 weeks gestational age, hyaline membrane disease, pneumothorax, neonatal sepsis.

Neuroimaging studies: Neonatal head ultrasound performed on day 5 shows bilaterally increased periventricular echodensities. At day 12, persistent periventricular echodensities with appearance of small echolucencies (Fig. 15.16). MRI at term shows periventricular cysts surrounded by hyperintense areas on T1-weighted images consistent with gliosis. The lateral ventricles are enlarged and irregularly shaped. There is overall volume reduction of the white matter especially posteriorly (Fig. 15.17).

Clinical correlates in the neonatal period: There was no definite neurological syndrome in the neonatal period.

Long-term clinical correlates: The child developed spastic diplegia as a sequela of the bilateral PVL. This is a good example of PVL occurring in the setting of hemodynamic alterations but also inflammation due to the neonatal sepsis. The spastic diplegia was severe (GMFCS level II), so walking with aids was reached at age 3 years. There was mild intellectual impairment. The child also presented with a strabismus.

Case 9

History: Preterm infant of 29 weeks gestation, emergency cesarean section for signs of placental abruption, primary resuscitation, perinatal acidosis, respiratory distress syndrome.

Neuroimaging studies: Neonatal head ultrasound performed on day 2 shows bilateral IVH with mild ventricular dilatation and local extension into frontal white matter indicative of periventricular venous infarction. MRI on day 2 confirms IVH with unilateral venous infarction with large T2 hypointense ventricles and T2 hypointensity adjacent to the ventricle with typical triangular shaped pattern. The rest of the white matter parenchyma shows no focal T2 abnormalities, but DWI measurements reveal abnormal low ADC (0.8 μm^2/ms) in the periventricular white matter (Fig. 15.18A, B). Follow-up MRI 3 weeks later shows tissue dissolution in the peripheral white matter with T2 signal similar to CSF, residual IVH illustrated by T2 hypointensities and hydrocephalus (Fig. 15.18C).

Clinical correlates in the neonatal period: There was no major neurological syndrome in the neonatal period.

Long-term clinical correlates: This child had a very poor outcome with severe spastic quadriplegia, epilepsy, and visual and cognitive impairment. All these sequelae are due to the severe bilateral cystic leukomalacia and not to the bilateral IVH or the unilateral PVHI. This is a good example of early leukomalacia detectable only by ADC measurements which clearly changes neurological prognosis early on. The hydrocephalus in this case is partly due to tissue loss surrounding the ventricles (ex vacuo hydrocephalus).

TABLE 15.6 Clinical Correlates of PVL		
Topography of the Injury	**Neonatal Correlates**	**Long-Term Correlates**
Periventricular white matter (descending motor fibers, optic radiations, and association fibers)	Lower limb weakness may be seen	• Spastic diplegia • Visual deficits • In the more severe forms: involvement of upper extremities and intellectual impairment • Epilepsy in 3% • Intellectual and visual deficits can also occur in infants without motor deficits in the more diffuse form of PVL

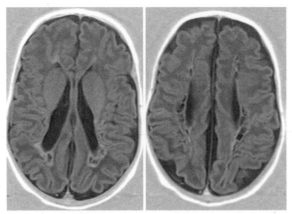

Fig. 15.17 Case 8: MRI examination at term age with inversion recovery (IR) sequence and T1-weighted contrast illustrating the periventricular cysts surrounded by hyperintense areas on T1-weighted images consistent with gliosis. The lateral ventricles are enlarged and irregularly shaped with squared-off posterior horns. There seems to be overall volume reduction of the white matter especially posteriorly. These findings are typical for late stage periventricular leukomalacia.

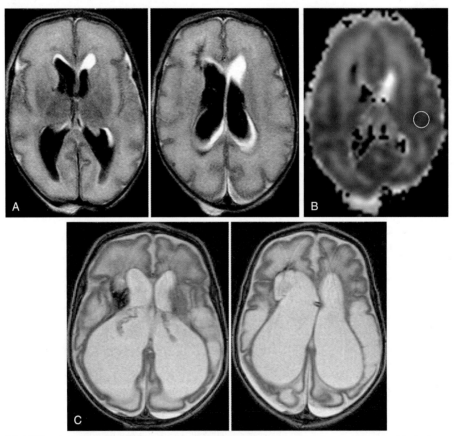

Fig. 15.18 Case 9: Axial T2-weighted images (A) with ventricles filled with blood (low intensity) of an acute intraventricular hemorrhage with periventricular hemorrhagic infarction into frontal parenchyma normal-appearing adjacent white matter. DWI in (B) shows reduced apparent diffusion coefficient (ADC) values (circle 0.8 mm^2/ms) in the parietal white matter. Evolution after 3 weeks shows multicystic encephalomalacia with marked hydrocephalus on axial T2-weighted images.

Case 10

History: Triplet pregnancy with moderate preterm labor at 24 to 26 weeks gestation and premature rupture of membranes at 30 weeks gestation. Reduced growth of one triplet and alteration of umbilical Doppler measurements leads to cesarean section at 33 weeks gestation. Triplet 1 small-for-gestational age, normal Apgar score.

Neuroimaging studies: Neonatal ultrasonography on day 2 describes bilateral periventricular hyperechogenicity (Fig. 15.19). Conventional MR imaging at term reveals multiple areas of diffuse T2 excessive high signal intensity (DEHSI) some T2 hypointensities/T1 hyperintensities in the white matter and subcortical white matter cysts as well as some T2 hyperintensities/T1 hyperintensities corresponding to gliotic changes in the periventricular white matter (Fig. 15.20).

Clinical correlates in the neonatal period: There was no major neurological syndrome in the neonatal period.

Long-term clinical correlates: This patient developed increased tone in the four limbs, predominating however in lower limbs with hyperreflexia and moderate spasticity of both legs, in relation with the white matter cysts visualized on neuroimaging. She was however able to walk without help at age 2 years. Her intellectual performances were markedly delayed, most likely as a sequela of the more diffuse white matter alterations. This case illustrates the fact that white matter injuries of both types (cystic and diffuse) can also happen prenatally in utero as a sequela of poor perfusion and/or inflammation.

Case 11

History: Preterm infant with gestational age at birth of 25 weeks, birth weight 650 g. Neonatal course significant for RDS with subsequent chronic lung disease, PDA ligation, necrotizing enterocolitis, and nosocomial sepsis.

Neuroimaging studies: Neonatal ultrasonography normal throughout neonatal period. Conventional MR imaging at term reveals diffuse T2 hyperintensities and T1 hypointensities in the white matter with poor cortical gyrification and on DWI markedly elevated ADC values (ADC > 1.8 mm^2/ms throughout the central white matter) (Fig. 15.21).

Clinical correlates in the neonatal period: There was no major neurological syndrome in the neonatal period.

Long-term clinical correlates: General neurodevelopmental delay noted on follow-up with increased tone in all four extremities and poor fine motor performance. Motor development of 16 months at 24 months corrected age. Marked delay in cognitive development with a developmental age of 15 months at the age of 24 months corrected and poor attention control. He receives special neurodevelopmental interventions since birth. This case is a good illustration of diffuse white matter alteration which was not visualized by cranial ultrasound.

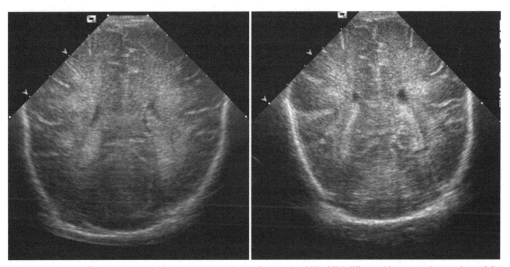

Fig. 15.19 Case 10: Cranial ultrasound images acquired in the first week of life. Mild diffuse white matter hyperechogenicity.

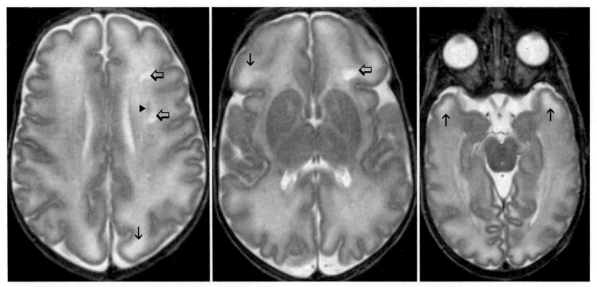

Fig. 15.20 Case 10: MRI examination at term. Axial T2-weighted images show diffuse excessive hyperintense white matter (DEHSI) (*small arrows*) with some small cystic lesions (*wide arrow*) in periventricular white matter. In the periventricular white matter small punctate hypointense lesions (*triangle*).

Cranial Ultrasonography in the Preterm Infant

Neonatal sonography is the one major bedside technique to image the neonatal brain. In preterm infants with severe IVH, serial ultrasound will allow early detection of PHVD and will help to guide intervention.[93] In those with a PVHI, assessment of the size and site of the lesion in a sagittal plane can predict development of a hemiparesis.[81] Leviton et al. postulated in 1990 that ultrasonographic white matter echodensities and echolucencies in low-birth-weight infants predicted later handicap more accurately than any other antecedent.[94] Unlike IVH, damage to the white matter can have different appearances and depending on the timing of the injury, the imaging characteristics can be nonspecific with generally an increase in echogenicity in the acute phase of the injury (Figs. 15.16 and 15.19). In clinical practice, at least in the older preterm infant, the condition of white matter is judged by its echogenic potential as compared to choroid plexus. Generally, the echogenicity found in early PVL is similar in intensity to choroid plexus, with a bilateral but slightly asymmetric appearance, can be sharply delineated and may have nodular components. This has to

be differentiated from normal peritrigonal flaring which is perfectly symmetric and with a radial appearance. Evolution of such hyperechogenicity can be twofold, either complete disappearance or evolution into cysts and/or ventricular dilatation. Cyst formation in analog to neuropathology is a process typical for the second week (10–40 days) after the insult. De Vries et al.[95] postulated an ultrasound-based classification for PVL of four grades, increasing grades being associated with increasing neurodevelopmental handicap. Grade I being the transient (>7 days) periventricular densities without cyst formation. If cysts develop and are few in numbers, localized primarily in frontal and frontoparietal white matter this is classified as Grade II. When they are widespread and extend into the parieto-occipital region they are referred to as Grade III, they may grow and gradually disappear leaving an irregularly dilated lateral ventricle. If cysts are present all the way into the subcortical area resembling porencephaly, this is referred to as Grade IV (Table 15.7).

Ultrasound can be viewed as the ideal mode of imaging to detect cystic PVL, especially when performed every week or every other week. Cysts are known to disappear after several weeks and may no

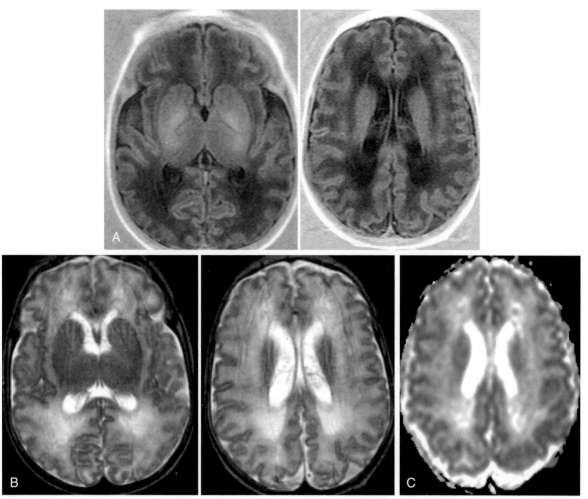

Fig. 15.21 Case 11: MRI examination at term of a 25-week gestation preterm infant. Normal cranial ultrasounds throughout perinatal period. Axial inversion recovery sequence with T1-weighted contrast shows low signal intensity in the white matter which corresponds in the T2-weighted images to high signal intensity throughout the white matter with moderately dilated ventricles and poor cortical folding (B). Apparent diffusion coefficient (ADC) values (C) of the central white matter is diffusely elevated with values >1.8 mm²/ms. Also note the poor cortical gyrification with simple gyri that most likely represent secondary rather than tertiary sulci.

TABLE 15.7	Ultrasound Classification of PVL[96]
Grade I	Transient periventricular echodensities (PVE) (>7 days)
Grade II	PVE evolving into localized fronto-parietal cystic lesions
Grade III	PVE evolving into extensive periventricular cystic lesions
Grade IV	Echodensities evolving into extensive periventricular and subcortical cysts

Classification needs longitudinal assessment with daily to weekly ultrasound evaluations.

longer be present at discharge or at term equivalent age.[97] Ultrasound has very limited value for detecting diffuse white matter injury as shown in studies comparing neonatal sonography with MRI.[13,98,99]

CONVENTIONAL MAGNETIC RESONANCE IMAGING IN THE PRETERM INFANT

Conventional MR imaging features of chronic white matter injury in the immature brain are characterized either by cysts similar to ultrasound but also and more importantly by a persistent high signal intensity of the white matter in T2-weighted images representing diffuse white matter injury (see Figs. 15.20 and 15.21). This imaging characteristic is later associated with thinning of the corpus callosum and loss of white matter volume (see later). In several studies on preterm infants, brain diffuse excessive high signal intensity (DEHSI) in the cerebral white matter on T2-weighted imaging was reported to be present in up to 40% to 75% of low-birthweight-preterm infants imaged at term[100] (Fig. 15.21). MRI is further ideally equipped to assess delayed myelination. The absence of myelination in the posterior limb of the internal capsule (missing T1 high signal intensity, T2 low signal intensity) at term age is a good indicator of later neuromotor

impairment (Fig. 15.21)[1,14] but mild diffuse high signal intensity (DEHSI) is not associated with significant neurodevelopmental impairment.[101,102]

Conventional T1 and T2 weighted imaging can also show other signal abnormalities in the periventricular white matter. In the subacute phase of white matter injury, MRI detects punctate periventricular areas of T1 signal hyperintensities (see Fig. 15.22). The precise neuropathological correlate of these signal abnormalities is not completely known but may be due to some hemorrhagic components of the lesion but most likely represent the cellular reaction of glial cells and macrophages, which are known to contain lipid droplets (see neuropathology description) which explain perfectly the high signal intensity in T1-weighted MR images.[103] When MRI is performed within the DWI window, restricted diffusion can often be noted, suggestive of an ischemic lesion. By adding SWI to the imaging protocol, the absence of hemorrhage can be confirmed (Fig. 15.22). Risk factors for these punctate lesions differ if visible on SWI though involving hemosiderin associated with presence of IVH or SWI negative more frequently associated with intubation for respiratory distress syndrome.[104]

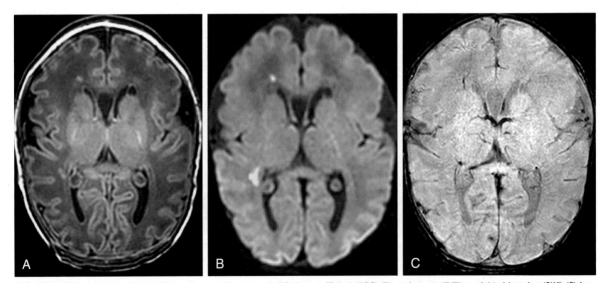

Fig. 15.22 MRI, axial planes, T2-weighted sequence (A), apparent diffusion coefficient (ADC) (B), and susceptibility-weighted imaging (SWI) (C) in a preterm infant with a gestational age of 34 weeks. The MRI was performed post surgery for an omphalocele. Several punctate lesions are present in the right hemisphere seen as increased signal intensity on T1 and DWI, but SWI does not show increased signal at the site of these lesions and hemorrhages can therefore be excluded. Also note a subependymal pseudocyst adjacent to the left frontal horn, which should not be confused with c-PVL.

The volume of the punctate white matter lesions (PWML) and their location on MRI was found to be related with motor and cognitive outcome.[105] In this study, punctate lesions were present in 24% of their preterm cohort and a dose-dependent relation was found to abnormalities in white matter microstructure, assessed with tract-based spatial statistics, and reduced thalamic volume ($p < 0.0001$), and predicted unfavorable motor outcome at a median (range) corrected age of 20.2 (18.4–26.3) months with sensitivity and specificity of 71 and 72, respectively.

In another study, templates were obtained of the PWMLs and larger frontal white matter injury (WMI) volumes predicted adverse cognitive outcomes and larger WMI volumes in frontal, parietal, and temporal lobes with adverse motor outcomes.[106] In their next study, they recommended a simple imaging rule, assessing whether the PWMLs were anterior or posterior only to the midventricle line on a reformatted axial plane.[107] Location of the PWMLs anterior to this line was predictive of cognitive and motor outcome at 4.5 years of age.

These localized T1 hyperintensities are less prominent at term[108] instead widened ventricles or periventricular cysts may appear, such as in Fig. 15.20.

Cortical differentiation can be qualitatively appreciated by conventional MRI and preterm infants with diffuse white matter abnormalities often show poor cortical gyrification at term with simple appearing gyri and sulci compared to complex tertiary sulci seen in the full-term infant (Fig. 15.21). Several semiquantitative scores have been developed to describe severity of abnormalities that relate to neurodevelopmental outcome[109,110] and classifications that include assessment of fetal compartments.[111] Absolute quantification of brain growth can be assessed by three-dimensional quantitative magnetic resonance imaging (3D-MRI) techniques described later.

DIFFUSION MAGNETIC RESONANCE IMAGING IN THE PRETERM INFANT

Early assessment of periventricular white matter in preterm infants with DWI can reveal bilateral periventricular diffusion restriction similar to the typical distribution of PVL when ultrasound and conventional MRI show no or nonspecific abnormalities[112] (see Fig. 15.23). A reduced ADC in an otherwise normal preterm brain is considered an early indicator of white matter damage (just as a reduced ADC is seen shortly after the onset of an acute cerebral ischemic lesion in the full-term newborn). The typical histologic changes in the acute phase of PVL outlined previously, like cellular and axonal swelling and astrocytic hyperplasia, are characterized by some of the same mechanisms leading to restriction of water diffusivity. They considerably change the microstructure of white matter and therefore change water diffusivity and may evolve into distinct cysts but also evolve into diffuse white matter loss ventricular dilatation and delay of myelination as illustrated in Fig. 15.23.

The diffuse T2 hyperintensities or DEHSI as indicators of the chronic phase of white matter injury are associated with higher ADC values which confirm the locally higher tissue water content and loss of microstructure impeding water diffusion in those areas[37,113,114] (see Fig. 15.21). These high ADC values are similar to those seen in the very immature healthy white matter; therefore, a potential explanation for the failure of ADC to decline from high levels in the extremely premature infant to lower levels in the term infant in the presence of DEHSI might be related to prior injury with destruction of normal cellular elements (e.g., axonal injury) or a delay in maturation.[115] Further quantitative measures of diffusion at term among premature infants with perinatal white matter lesions, when compared to preterm infants without white matter injury, showed lower anisotropy values in the area of the previous injury, i.e., central periventricular white matter, but also in the underlying posterior limb of internal capsule.[37] The lower anisotropy in the injured cerebral white matter suggests that white matter fiber tracts were destroyed or their subsequent development was impaired. The lower anisotropy in the internal capsule further suggests a disturbance in the development of the descending corticospinal tracts.[116] This finding might well be the basis for the reduction in myelination in the posterior limb of the internal capsule observed on conventional MR imaging which was shown to be highly correlated with development of motor deficits. DWI with diffusion tensor analysis (DTI) has provided new insights into the microstructural white matter development and seems to be an ideal tool to assess alteration of white matter pathways in neurologic

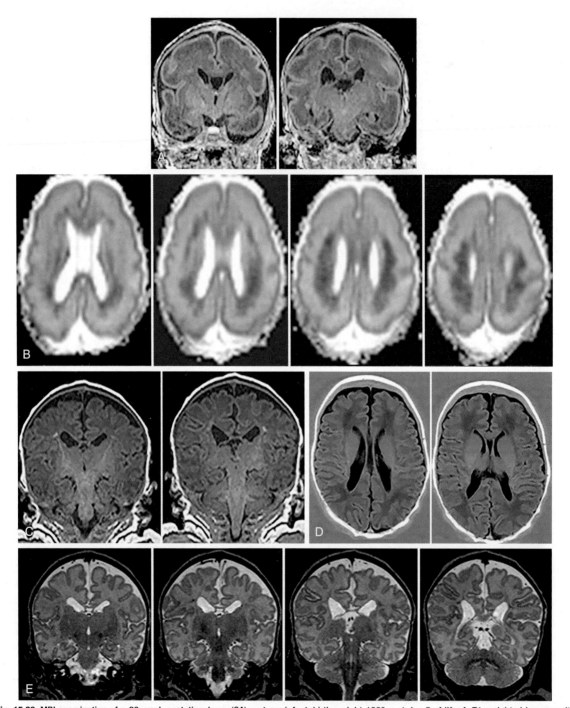

Fig. 15.23 MRI examination of a 28-week gestational age (GA) preterm infant, birth weight 1260 g at day 5 of life. A, T1-weighted images with periventricular T1 hyperintensities. B, Apparent diffusion coefficient (ADC) maps show bilateral extensive diffusion restriction in the periventricular white matter. C, T1-weighted MR images at term show some punctate lesions (T1 hyperintense) with loss of white matter and reduced T1 hypersignal in the capsula interna. D, Axial IR images showing squared off dilated ventricles (E) coronal T2-weighted images with dilated asymmetrical ventricles, loss of periventricular white matter. At 3 years of age, the child has cerebral palsy (CP) with distal predominant tetraspasticity and mild cognitive delay.

disease. DTI has further become a valuable tool to assess brain connectivity changes as a consequence of early brain injury summarized in recent reviews.[23]

MAGNETIC RESONANCE SPECTROSCOPY IN THE PRETERM INFANT

The biochemical characteristics of white matter damage in preterm infants have been studied in vivo using MRS.[117] Similar to the high diagnostic value of MRS in term asphyxia, MRS in acute phase immature white matter injury can detect indicators of anaerobic glycolysis with increased intracerebral lactate.[51] White matter damage in the preterm infant studied around term gestational age resulted in high Lac/Cr and high Myo-Inositol/Cr ratios[118] also seen in inflammatory models of brain injury.[89] The increased presence of lactate at the chronic stage was not associated with changes in pH while NAA, as marker of neuroaxonal integrity was reduced in the damaged periventricular white matter. Astrocytes further play a variety of complex nutritive and supportive roles in relation to neuronal metabolic homeostasis. For example, astrocytes take up glutamate and convert it to glutamine; this removal of glutamate from the extracellular space protects surrounding cells from excitotoxicity from glutamate. Glutamate uptake into astrocytes further stimulates glycolysis within the astrocyte with production of lactate that can be used by neurons as energy substrate.[119] Given that chronic phase white matter injury is characterized by widespread cerebral white matter astrocytosis, this change in metabolite composition might be an expression of altered cellular composition and substrate utilization. Recent reviews have concluded that in preterm-born infants, brain metabolism assessed using ^{1}H-MRS at term-equivalent age is associated with motor, cognitive, and language outcomes at 18 to 24 months with the ratio of NAA/Cho being the biomarker of interest.[120]

Advanced Quantitative MRI With Image Analysis Tools

In recent years, many 3D-MRI methods combined with image postprocessing techniques have been developed, which allow volumetric assessment of brain development and an absolute quantitation of myelination in the newborn.[121-125] These techniques allow

exact definition of brain volume and can therefore accurately monitor brain growth and measure CSF volume and volume changes in white matter and cortical gray matter, a recent metaanalysis providing reference values for these measures.[126] 3D-MRI volumetric techniques were used to evaluate the effect on subsequent brain development of early white matter injury in premature infants. In the premature infants with preceding white matter injury, the volume of myelinated white matter at term was significantly lower than in the premature infants without prior white matter injury and the infants born at term measuring the degree of delay of myelination. Furthermore, this study showed a marked decrease in cortical gray matter volume in the preterm infants with prior periventricular white matter injury indicating impaired cerebral cortical development after early white matter injury.[127] In a population study, similar volumetric changes of overall brain development in preterm infants were confirmed with significant reduction of myelinated white matter and cortical gray matter in preterm infants compared to full-term infants, with a reduction also of deep nuclear gray matter (basal ganglia) most pronounced in the lowest gestational ages.[128] Assessing moderately preterm infants without signs of white matter injury cortical development was similar to full-term infants.[129] Regional assessment of white matter myelination in preterm infants further revealed particular delay in myelination in the central and posterior part of the brain.[130] When assessing cerebellar volume at term, there was a significant reduction of cerebellar volume of preterm infants when compared to term infants[131] and were related to outcome.[132] Unilateral cerebral white matter lesions resulted in contralateral reduction of cerebellar volume indicating the trophic interplay due to loss of cerebro-cerebellar connectivity.[133]

Long-term follow-up studies of preterm infants have confirmed the permanent character of these disruptive/adaptive changes in brain development. Evaluation of 8-year-old preterm infants with volumetric brain assessment showed persistence of cortical gray matter reduction in preterm infants accompanied with a reduction in the volume of hippocampus, which correlated with cognitive scores indicating long-term functional consequences.[134] Both cortical volume and cortical thickness were shown to be reduced in

15-year adolescents born prematurely.[135] Voxel-based morphometry (VBM), an image analysis tool that compares brain tissue in groups after normalization to a template, has shown that adolescent and young adults born prematurely have smaller hippocampi with a correlation with performance IQ,[136] accompanied with a reduced gray matter volume in several regions of the brain, such as the orbitofrontal cortex when compared to infants born at term.[137-141] Cerebral white matter was shown in VBM studies to be equally affected by preterm birth. Overall white matter volume was reduced in former preterm infants with a significant impact in males born prematurely predominantly in the cingulum, the corpus callosum, and the corticospinal tracts.[142] What is less evident is the predictive value of these volumetric changes in the newborn period for neurodevelopmental outcome. Volumetric changes following brain imaging lesions show a good correlation with outcome[128] whereas volumetric changes in the absence of brain lesions have only limited predictive value.[122] Recent studies on growth from newborn period to 7 years observe correlations of basal ganglia and thalamic growth rates and cognitive outcome at 7 years.[143]

Effects of poor intrauterine growth and white matter lesions further result in considerable alteration of cortical surface, sulcation index, and cortical morphology.[144-148] A recent review summarizes a vast scientific literature looking at short-term and long-term effects of prematurity on brain tissue assessed by advanced MRI.[23]

In conclusion, the main advantages of MR techniques in the evaluation of the preterm infant are as follows:

1. Abnormal signal intensities in the white matter are more reliably detected by MRI than by ultrasound.
2. More widespread nonhemorrhagic white matter injury in the presence of IVH is more readily diagnosed with MR techniques than with ultrasound, both in the acute and chronic phases.
3. Diffuse white matter injury without frank cystic development can be detected by MRI both by conventional MRI (moderate to severe DEHSI) as well as DWI with measurement of ADC.
4. Myelination pattern at term defined by inversion recovery, T1- and T2-weighted MR sequences can predict neuromotor outcome.

5. Isolated punctate lesions identified as T1 hyperintensities can be further defined by adding SWI to assess hemorrhagic components.
6. More advanced MR image tools such as DTI, 3D-volumetric MRI, and fMRI can define plasticity and predict functional outcome of more complex brain functions.

Despite these advances in the field of neuroimaging in the newborn, there are several gaps that exist in our knowledge, including imaging characteristics of lesion progression during and after hypothermia, genetic background linked to imaging characteristics of perinatal HIE, the role of serial neuroimaging in the encephalopathy of prematurity, and the role of neuroimaging in the assessment of developmental plasticity.

REFERENCES

1. Volpe JJ. Perinatal brain injury: from pathogenesis to neuroprotection. *Ment Retard Dev Disabil Res Rev.* 2001;7:56.
2. van de Looij Y, Dean JM, Gunn AJ, Hüppi PS, Sizonenko SV. Advanced magnetic resonance spectroscopy and imaging techniques applied to brain development and animal models of perinatal injury. *Int J Dev Neurosci.* 2015;45:29-38.
3. Kiss JZ, Vasung L, Petrenko V. Process of cortical network formation and impact of early brain damage. *Curr Opin Neurol.* 2014;27(2):133-141.
4. Haacke EM, Liu S, Buch S, Zheng W, Wu D, Ye Y. Quantitative susceptibility mapping: current status and future directions. *Magn Reson Imaging.* 2015;33:1-25.
5. Neil J, Miller J, Mukherjee P, Hüppi PS. Diffusion tensor imaging of normal and injured developing human brain—a technical review. *NMR Biomed.* 2002;15:543.
6. Barkovich AJ, Miller SP, Bartha A, et al. MR imaging, MR spectroscopy, and diffusion tensor imaging of sequential studies in neonates with encephalopathy. *AJNR Am J Neuroradiol.* 2006;27:533.
7. Hüppi PS, Lazeyras F. Proton magnetic resonance spectroscopy (¹H-MRS) in neonatal brain injury. *Pediatr Res.* 2001;49:317-320.
8. Oz G, Alger JR, Barker PB, et al. Clinical proton MR spectroscopy in central nervous system disorders. *Radiology.* 2014;270:658-679.
9. Seghier ML, Hüppi PS. The role of functional magnetic resonance imaging in the study of brain development, injury, and recovery in the newborn. *Semin Perinatol.* 2010;34:79-86.
10. Perlman JM. Intrapartum asphyxia and cerebral palsy: is there a link? *Clin Perinatol.* 2006;33:335.
11. Volpe JJ. *Neurology of the Newborn.* 6th ed. Philadelphia: Elsevier; 2018.
12. Nelson KB, Ellenberg JH. Antecedents of cerebral palsy: multivariate analysis of risk. *N Engl J Med.* 1986;315:81.
13. de Vries LS, van Haastert IC, Benders MJ, Groenendaal F. Myth: cerebral palsy cannot be predicted by neonatal brain imaging. *Semin Fetal Neonatal Med.* 2011;16:279-287.
14. Sohma O, Mito T, Mizuguchi M, Takashima S. The prenatal age critical for the development of the pontosubicular necrosis. *Acta Neuropathol.* 1995;90:7-10.

15. Takizawa Y, Takashima S, Itoh M. A histopathological study of premature and mature infants with pontosubicular neuron necrosis: neuronal cell death in perinatal brain damage. *Brain Res.* 2006;1095:200-206.

16. Barkovich AJ, Sargent SK. Profound asphyxia in the premature infant: imaging findings. *AJNR Am J Neuroradiol.* 1995;16:1837.

17. Greisen G. Effect of cerebral blood flow and cerebrovascular autoregulation on the distribution, type and extent of cerebral injury. *Brain Pathol.* 1992;2:223-228.

18. Pasternak JF, Gorey MT. The syndrome of acute near-total intrauterine asphyxia in the term infant. *Pediatr Neurol.* 1998;18:391-398.

19. Shah P, Riphagen S, Beyene J, Perlman M. Multiorgan dysfunction in infants with post-asphyxial hypoxic-ischaemic encephalopathy. *Arch Dis Child Fetal Neonatal Ed.* 2004;89:F152.

20. Annink KV, de Vries LS, Groenendaal F, et al. The development and validation of a cerebral ultrasound scoring system for infants with hypoxic-ischaemic encephalopathy. *Pediatr Res.* 2020;87:59-66.

21. Cabanas F, Pellicer A, Perez-Higueras A, Garcia-Alix A, Roche C, Quero J. Ultrasonographic findings in thalamus and basal ganglia in term asphyxiated infants. *Pediatr Neurol.* 1991;7:211.

22. Kashman N, Kramer U, Stavorovsky Z, et al. Prognostic significance of hyperechogenic lesions in the basal ganglia and thalamus in neonates. *J Child Neurol.* 2001;16:591.

23. Dubois J, Alison M, Counsell SJ, Hertz-Pannier L, Hüppi PS, Benders M. MRI of the neonatal brain: a review of methodological challenges and neuroscientific advances. *J Magn Reson Imaging.* 2021;53:1318-1343.

24. Hüppi PS. Cortical development in the fetus and the newborn: advanced MR techniques. *Top Magn Reson Imaging.* 2011;22:33-38.

25. Annink KV, van der Aa NE, Dudink J, et al. Introduction of ultra-high-field MR imaging in infants: preparations and feasibility. *AJNR Am J Neuroradiol.* 2020;41:1532-1537.

26. Wisnowski JL, Wintermark P, Bonifacio SL, et al. Neuroimaging in the term newborn with neonatal encephalopathy. *Semin Fetal Neonatal Med.* 2021;26:101304.

27. Rutherford MA, Pennock JM, Counsell SJ, et al. Abnormal magnetic resonance signal in the internal capsule predicts poor neurodevelopmental outcome in infants with hypoxic-ischemic encephalopathy. *Pediatrics.* 1998;102:323.

28. Rutherford M, Ward P, Allsop J, Malamatentiou C, Counsell S. Magnetic resonance imaging in neonatal encephalopathy. *Early Hum Dev.* 2005;81:13.

29. Pasternak JF. Parasagittal infarction in neonatal asphyxia. *Ann Neurol.* 1987;21:202.

30. Volpe JJ, Pasternak JF. Parasagittal cerebral injury in neonatal hypoxic-ischemic encephalopathy: clinical and neuroradiologic features. *J Pediatr.* 1977;91:472.

31. Kwan S, Boudes E, Gilbert G, et al. Injury to the cerebellum in term asphyxiated newborns treated with hypothermia. *AJNR Am J Neuroradiol.* 2015;36:1542-1549.

32. Arca-Díaz G, Re TJ, Drottar M, et al. Can cerebellar and brainstem apparent diffusion coefficient (ADC) values predict neuromotor outcome in term neonates with hypoxic-ischemic encephalopathy (HIE) treated with hypothermia? *PLoS One.* 2017;12:e0178510.

33. Annink KV, Meerts L, van der Aa NE, et al. Cerebellar injury in term neonates with hypoxic-ischemic encephalopathy is underestimated. *Pediatr Res.* 2021;89:1171-1178.

34. Hayakawa K, Tanda K, Koshino S, Nishimura A, Kizaki Z, Ohno K. Pontine and cerebellar injury in neonatal hypoxic-ischemic encephalopathy: MRI features and clinical outcomes. *Acta Radiol.* 2020;61:1398-1405.

35. Lemmon ME, Wagner MW, Bosemani T, et al. Diffusion tensor imaging detects occult cerebellar injury in severe neonatal hypoxic-ischemic encephalopathy. *Dev Neurosci.* 2017;39:207-214.

36. Dubois J, Dehaene-Lambertz G, Mangin JF, Le Bihan D, Hüppi PS, Hertz-Pannier L. Brain development of infant and MRI by diffusion tensor imaging. *Neurophysiol Clin.* 2012;42:1-9.

37. Hüppi PS, Murphy B, Maier SE, et al. Microstructural brain development after perinatal cerebral white matter injury assessed by diffusion tensor magnetic resonance imaging. *Pediatrics.* 2001;107:455-460.

38. Kunz N, Zhang H, Vasung L, et al. Assessing white matter microstructure of the newborn with multi-shell diffusion MRI and biophysical compartment models. *Neuroimage.* 2014;96:288-299.

39. Moseley ME, Kucharczyk J, Minotorovitch J. Diffusion-weighted MR imaging of acute stroke: correlation with T2-weighted and magnetic susceptibility-enhanced MR-imaging in cats. *AJNR Am J Neuroradiol.* 1990;11:423.

40. Warach S, Chien D, Li W. Fast magnetic resonance diffusion-weighted imaging of acute human stroke. *Neurology.* 1992;42:1717.

41. Inder T, Hüppi PS, Zientara GP, et al. Early detection of periventricular leukomalacia by diffusion-weighted magnetic resonance imaging techniques. *J Pediatr.* 1999;134:631.

42. Li F, Han SS, Tatlisumak T, et al. Reversal of acute apparent diffusion coefficient abnormalities and delayed neuronal death following transient focal cerebral ischemia in rats. *Ann Neurol.* 1999;46:333.

43. Copen WA, Schwamm LH, Gonzalez RG, et al. Ischemic stroke: effects of etiology and patient age on the time course of the core apparent diffusion coefficient. *Radiology.* 2001;221:27.

44. McKinstry RC, Miller JH, Snyder AZ, et al. A prospective, longitudinal diffusion tensor imaging study of brain injury in newborns. *Neurology.* 2002;59:824.

45. Rutherford M, Counsell S, Allsop J, et al. Diffusion-weighted magnetic resonance imaging in term perinatal brain injury: a comparison with site of lesion and time from birth. *Pediatrics.* 2004;114:1004.

46. Imai K, de Vries LS, Alderliesten T, et al. MRI changes in the thalamus and basal ganglia of full-term neonates with perinatal asphyxia. *Neonatology.* 2018;114:253-260.

47. Robertson RL, Ben-Sira L, Barnes PD, et al. MR line-scan diffusion-weighted imaging of term neonates with perinatal brain ischemia. *AJNR Am J Neuroradiol.* 1999;20:1658.

48. Soul JS, Robertson RL, Tzika AA, du Plessis AJ, Volpe JJ. Time course of changes in diffusion-weighted magnetic resonance imaging in a case of neonatal encephalopathy with defined onset and duration of hypoxic-ischemic insult. *Pediatrics.* 2001;108:1211.

49. Oz G, Alger JR, Barker PB, et al. Clinical proton MR spectroscopy in central nervous system disorders. *Radiology.* 2014;270:658-679.

50. Groenendaal F, Veehoven RH, van der Grond J, Jansen GH, Witkamp TD, de Vries LS. Cerebral lactate and N-acetylaspartate/choline ratios in asphyxiated full-term neonates demonstrated in vivo using proton magnetic resonance spectroscopy. *Pediatr Res.* 1994;35(2):148.

51. Penrice J, Cady EB, Lorek A, et al. Proton magnetic resonance spectroscopy of the brain in normal preterm and term infants, and early changes after perinatal hypoxia-ischemia. *Pediatr Res.* 1996;40:6.

52. Hanrahan JD, Cox IJ, Edwards AD, et al. Persistent increases in cerebral lactate concentration after birth asphyxia. *Pediatr Res.* 1998;44:304.

53. Robertson NJ, Cowan FM, Cox IJ, Edwards AD. Brain alkaline intracellular pH after neonatal encephalopathy. *Ann Neurol.* 2002;52:732.

54. Zarifi MK, Astrakas LG, Poussaint TY, Plessis AA, Zurakowski D, Tzika AA. Prediction of adverse outcome with cerebral lactate level and apparent diffusion coefficient in infants with perinatal asphyxia. *Radiology.* 2002;225:859.

55. Kadri M, Shu S, Holshouser B, et al. Proton magnetic resonance spectroscopy improves outcome prediction in perinatal CNS insults. *J Perinatol.* 2003;23:181.

56. Ouwehand S, Smidt LCA, Dudink J, et al. Predictors of outcomes in hypoxic-ischemic encephalopathy following hypothermia: a meta-analysis. *Neonatology.* 2020;117:411-427.

57. Roelants-Van Rijn AM, van Der GJ, de Vries LS, Groenendaal F. wValue of ^{1}H-MRS using different echo times in neonates with cerebral hypoxia-ischemia. *Pediatr Res.* 2001;49:356.

58. Lally PJ, Montaldo P, Oliveira V, et al. Magnetic resonance spectroscopy assessment of brain injury after moderate hypothermia in neonatal encephalopathy: a prospective multicentre cohort study. *Lancet Neurol.* 2019;18:35-45. doi:10.1016/S1474-4422(18)30325-9.

59. Bach AM, Fang AY, Bonifacio S, et al. Early magnetic resonance imaging predicts 30-month outcomes after therapeutic hypothermia for neonatal encephalopathy. *J Pediatr.* 2021;238:94-101.e1.

60. Bednarek N, Mathur A, Inder T, Wilkinson J, Neil J, Shimony J. Impact of therapeutic hypothermia on MRI diffusion changes in neonatal encephalopathy. *Neurology.* 2012;78:1420-1427.

61. Rutherford M, Ramenghi LA, Edwards AD, et al. Assessment of brain tissue injury after moderate hypothermia in neonates with hypoxic-ischaemic encephalopathy: a nested substudy of a randomised controlled trial. *Lancet Neurol.* 2010;9:39.

62. Lodygensky GA, West T, Moravec MD, et al. Diffusion characteristics associated with neuronal injury and glial activation following hypoxia-ischemia in the immature brain. *Magn Reson Med.* 2011;66:839.

63. Wintermark P, Hansen A, Soul J, Labrecque M, Robertson RL, Warfield SK. Early versus late MRI in asphyxiated newborns treated with hypothermia. *Arch Dis Child Fetal Neonatal Ed.* 2011;96:F36.

64. Thoresen M, Penrice J, Lorek A, et al. Mild hypothermia after severe transient hypoxia-ischemia ameliorates delayed cerebral energy failure in the newborn piglet. *Pediatr Res.* 1995;37:667.

65. Corbett RJ, Purdy PD, Laptook AR, Chaney C, Garcia D. Noninvasive measurement of brain temperature after stroke. *AJNR Am J Neuroradiol.* 1999;20:1851.

66. Laptook AR, Corbett RJ, Sterett R, Burns DK, Garcia D, Tollefsbol G. Modest hypothermia provides partial neuroprotection when used for immediate resuscitation after brain ischemia. *Pediatr Res.* 1997;42:17.

67. Massaro AN, Kadom N, Chang T, Glass P, Nelson K, Baumgart S. Quantitative analysis of magnetic resonance images and neurological outcome in encephalopathic neonates treated with whole-body hypothermia. *J Perinatol.* 2010;30:596.

68. Martinez-Biarge M, Cheong JL, Diez-Sebastian J, Mercuri E, Dubowitz LM, Cowan FM. Risk factors for neonatal arterial ischemic stroke: the importance of the intrapartum period. *J Pediatr.* 2016;173:62-68.e1.

69. Nunez C, Arca G, Agut T, Stephan-Otto C, Garcia-Alix A. Precise neonatal arterial ischemic stroke classification with a three-dimensional map of the arterial territories of the neonatal brain. *Pediatr Res.* 2020;87:1231-1236.

70. Curtis C, Mineyko A, Massicotte P, et al. Thrombophilia risk is not increased in children after perinatal stroke. *Blood.* 2017;129:2793-2800.

71. Wagenaar N, Martinez-Biarge M, van der Aa NE, et al. Neurodevelopment after perinatal arterial ischemic stroke. *Pediatrics.* 2018;142:e20174164.

72. Boardman JP, Ganesan V, Rutherford MA, Saunders DE, Mercuri E, Cowan F. Magnetic resonance image correlates of hemiparesis after neonatal and childhood middle cerebral artery stroke. *Pediatrics.* 2005;115:321.

73. Kirton A, Shroff M, Visvanathan T, deVeber G. Quantified corticospinal tract diffusion restriction predicts neonatal stroke outcome. *Stroke.* 2007;38:974-980.

74. Wusthoff CJ, Kessler SK, Vossough A, et al. Risk of later seizure after perinatal arterial ischemic stroke: a prospective cohort study. *Pediatrics.* 2011;127:e1550-e1557.

75. Fox CK, Glass HC, Sidney S, Smith SE, Fullerton HJ. Neonatal seizures triple the risk of a remote seizure after perinatal ischemic stroke. *Neurology.* 2016;86:2179-2186.

76. Olivé G, Agut T, Echeverría-Palacio CM, Arca G, García-Alix A. Usefulness of cranial ultrasound for detecting neonatal middle cerebral artery stroke. *Ultrasound Med Biol.* 2019;45:885-890.

77. Seghier ML, Lazeyras F, Zimine S, Saudan-Frei S, Safran AB, Hüppi PS. Visual recovery after perinatal stroke evidenced by functional and diffusion MRI: case report. *BMC Neurol.* 2005;5:17.

78. Ramenghi LA, Cardiello V, Rossi A. Neonatal cerebral sinovenous thrombosis. *Handb Clin Neurol.* 2019;162:267-280.

79. Ballabh P. Intraventricular hemorrhage in premature infants: mechanism of disease. *Pediatr Res.* 2010;67:1-8.

80. Parodi A, Govaert P, Horsch S, Bravo MC, Ramenghi LA, eurUS.brain group. Cranial ultrasound findings in preterm germinal matrix haemorrhage, sequelae and outcome. *Pediatr Res.* 2020;87:13-24.

81. Cizmeci MN, de Vries LS, Ly LG, et al. Periventricular hemorrhagic infarction in very preterm infants: characteristic sonographic findings and association with neurodevelopmental outcome at age 2 years. *J Pediatr.* 2020;217:79-85.e1.

82. Deguchi K, Oguchi K, Takashima S. Characteristic neuropathology of leukomalacia in extremely low birth weight infants. *Pediatr Neurol.* 1997;16:296.

83. Deguchi K, Oguchi K, Matsuura N, Armstrong DD, Takashima S. Periventricular leukomalacia: relation to gestational age and axonal injury. *Pediatr Neurol.* 1999;20:370.

84. Hirayama A, Okoshi Y, Hachiya Y, et al. Early immunohistochemical detection of axonal damage and glial activation in extremely immature brains with periventricular leukomalacia. *Clin Neuropathol.* 2001;20:87.

85. Takashima S, Tanaka K. Development of cerebrovascular architecture and its relationship to periventricular leukomalacia. *Arch Neurol.* 1978;35:11.

86. Back SA, Han BH, Luo NL, et al. Selective vulnerability of late oligodendrocyte progenitors to hypoxia-ischemia. *J Neurosci.* 2002;22:455.

87. Haynes RL, Folkerth RD, Keefe RJ, et al. Nitrosative and oxidative injury to premyelinating oligodendrocytes in periventricular leukomalacia. *J Neuropathol Exp Neurol.* 2003;62:441.

88. McQuillen PS, Sheldon RA, Shatz CJ, Ferriero DM. Selective vulnerability of subplate neurons after early neonatal hypoxia-ischemia. *J Neurosci.* 2003;23:3308.

89. Lodygensky GA, Kunz N, Perroud E, et al. Definition and quantification of acute inflammatory white matter injury in the immature brain by MRI/MRS at high magnetic field. *Pediatr Res.* 2014;75:415-423.

90. Dammann O, Kuban KC, Leviton A. Perinatal infection, fetal inflammatory response, white matter damage, and cognitive limitations in children born preterm. *Ment Retard Dev Disabil Res Rev.* 2002;8:46.

91. Marin-Padilla M. Developmental neuropathology and impact of perinatal brain damage. II: white matter lesions of the neocortex. *J Neuropathol Exp Neurol.* 1997;56:219.

92. Volpe JJ. Brain injury in premature infants: a complex amalgam of destructive and developmental disturbances. *Lancet Neurol.* 2009;8:110.

93. El-Dib M, Limbrick Jr DD, Inder T, et al. Management of posthemorrhagic ventricular dilatation in the infant born preterm. *J Pediatr.* 2020;226:16-27.e3.

94. Leviton A, Gilles F. Acquired perinatal leucoencephalopathies. *Ann Neurol.* 1984;16:1.

95. Mohammad K, Scott JN, Leijser LM, et al. Consensus approach for standardizing the screening and classification of preterm brain injury diagnosed with cranial ultrasound: a Canadian perspective. *Front Pediatr.* 2021;9:618236.

96. DeVries LS, Eken P, Dubowitz LMS. The spectrum of leukomalacia using cranial ultrasound. *Behav Brain Res.* 1992;49:1.

97. Sarkar S, Shankaran S, Laptook AR, et al. Screening cranial imaging at multiple time points improves cystic periventricular leukomalacia detection. *Am J Perinatol.* 2015;32:973-979.

98. Kwon SH, Vasung L, Ment LR, Hüppi PS. The role of neuroimaging in predicting neurodevelopmental outcomes of preterm neonates. *Clin Perinatol.* 2014;41:257-283.

99. Leijser LM, Liauw L, Veen S, de Boer IP, Walther FJ, van Wezel-Meijler G. Comparing brain white matter on sequential cranial ultrasound and MRI in very preterm infants. *Neuroradiology.* 2008;50:799-811.

100. Maalouf EF, Duggan PJ, Rutherford MA, et al. Magnetic resonance imaging of the brain in a cohort of extremely preterm infants. *J Pediatr.* 1999;135:351.

101. Kidokoro H, Anderson PJ, Doyle LW, Neil JJ, Inder TE. High signal intensity on T2-weighted MR imaging at term-equivalent age in preterm infants does not predict 2-year neurodevelopmental outcomes. *AJNR Am J Neuroradiol.* 2011;32:2005-2010.

102. Leitner Y, Weinstein M, Myers V, et al. Diffuse excessive high signal intensity in low-risk preterm infants at term-equivalent age does not predict outcome at 1 year: a prospective study. *Neuroradiology.* 2014;56:669-678.

103. Schouman-Claeys E, Henry-Feugeas MC, Roset F, et al. Periventricular leukomalacia: correlation between MR imaging and autopsy findings during the first 2 months of life. *Radiology.* 1993;189:59.

104. Parodi A, Malova M, Cardiello V, et al. Punctate white matter lesions of preterm infants: risk factor analysis. *Eur J Paediatr Neurol.* 2019;23:733-739.

105. Tusor N, Benders MJ, Counsell SJ, et al. Punctate white matter lesions associated with altered brain development and adverse motor outcome in preterm infants. *Sci Rep.* 2017;7:13250.

106. Guo T, Duerden EG, Adams E, et al. Quantitative assessment of white matter injury in preterm neonates: association with outcomes. *Neurology.* 2017;88:614-622.

107. Cayam-Rand D, Guo T, Grunau RE, et al. Predicting developmental outcomes in preterm infants: a simple white matter injury imaging rule. *Neurology.* 2019;93:e1231-e1240.

108. Dyet LE, Kennea N, Counsell SJ, et al. Natural history of brain lesions in extremely preterm infants studied with serial magnetic resonance imaging from birth and neurodevelopmental assessment. *Pediatrics.* 2006;118:536.

109. Woodward LJ, Anderson PJ, Austin NC, Howard K, Inder TE. Neonatal MRI to predict neurodevelopmental outcomes in preterm infants. *N Engl J Med.* 2006;355:685.

110. Kidokoro H, Anderson PJ, Doyle LW, Woodward LJ, Neil JJ, Inder TE. Brain injury and altered brain growth in preterm infants: predictors and prognosis. *Pediatrics.* 2014;134:e444-e453. doi:10.1542/peds.2013-2336.

111. Pittet MP, Vasung L, Hüppi PS, Merlini L. Newborns and preterm infants at term equivalent age: a semi-quantitative assessment of cerebral maturity. *Neuroimage Clin.* 2019;24:102014.

112. Fu J, Xue X, Chen L, Fan G, Pan L, Mao J. Studies on the value of diffusion-weighted MR imaging in the early prediction of periventricular leukomalacia. *J Neuroimaging.* 2009;19:13-18.

113. Counsell SJ, Allsop JM, Harrison MC, et al. Diffusion-weighted imaging of the brain in preterm infants with focal and diffuse white matter abnormality. *Pediatrics.* 2003;112:1.

114. Miller SP, Vigneron DB, Henry RG, et al. Serial quantitative diffusion tensor MRI of the premature brain: development in newborns with and without injury. *J Magn Reson Imaging.* 2002;16:621.

115. Counsell SJ, Shen Y, Boardman JP, et al. Axial and radial diffusivity in preterm infants who have diffuse white matter changes on magnetic resonance imaging at term-equivalent age. *Pediatrics.* 2006;117:376.

116. Mazumdar A, Mukherjee P, Miller JH, Malde H, McKinstry RC. Diffusion-weighted imaging of acute corticospinal tract injury preceding Wallerian degeneration in the maturing human brain. *AJNR Am J Neuroradiol.* 2003;24:1057.

117. Groenendaal F, van de Grond J, Eken P, et al. Early cerebral proton MRS and neurodevelopmental outcome in infants with cystic leukomalacia. *Dev Med Child Neurol.* 1997;39:373.

118. Robertson NJ, Kuint J, Counsell TJ, et al. Characterization of cerebral white matter damage in the preterm infant using 1H and 31P magnetic resonance spectroscopy. *J Cereb Blood Flow Metab.* 2000;20:1446.

119. Pellerin L, Pellegri G, Bittar PG, et al. Evidence supporting the existence of an activity-dependent astrocyte-neuron lactate shuttle. *Dev Neurosci.* 1998;20:291.

120. Cebeci B, Alderliesten T, Wijnen JP, et al. Brain proton magnetic resonance spectroscopy and neurodevelopment after preterm birth: a systematic review. *Pediatr Res.* 2022;91(6):1322-1333. doi:10.1038/s41390-021-01539-x.

121. Hüppi PS, Warfield S, Kikinis R, et al. Quantitative magnetic resonance imaging of brain development in premature and mature newborns. *Ann Neurol.* 1998;43:224-235.

122. Gui L, Loukas S, Lazeyras F, Hüppi PS, Meskaldji DE, Borradori Tolsa C. Longitudinal study of neonatal brain tissue volumes in preterm infants and their ability to predict neurodevelopmental outcome. *Neuroimage.* 2019;185:728-741.

123. Inder TE, Warfield SK, Wang H, Hüppi PS, Volpe JJ. Abnormal cerebral structure is present at term in premature infants. *Pediatrics.* 2005;115:286.

124. Gui L, Lisowski R, Faundez T, Hüppi PS, Lazeyras F, Kocher M. Morphology-driven automatic segmentation of MR images of the neonatal brain. *Med Image Anal.* 2012;16:1565-1579.

125. Isgum I, Benders MJ, Avants B, et al. Evaluation of automatic neonatal brain segmentation algorithms: the NeoBrainS12 challenge. *Med Image Anal.* 2015;20:135-151.

126. Romberg J, Wilke M, Allgaier C, et al. MRI-based brain volumes of preterm infants at term: a systematic review and meta-analysis. *Arch Dis Child Fetal Neonatal Ed.* 2022;107(5): 520-526.

127. Inder TE, Hüppi PS, Warfield S, et al. Periventricular white matter injury in the premature infant is associated with a reduction in cerebral cortical gray matter volume at term. *Ann Neurol.* 1999;46:755.

128. Inder TE, Warfield SK, Wang H, Hüppi PS, Volpe JJ. Abnormal cerebral structure is present at term in premature infants. *Pediatrics.* 2005;115:286-294.

129. Zacharia A, Zimine S, Lovblad KO, et al. Early assessment of brain maturation by MR imaging segmentation in neonates and premature infants. *AJNR Am J Neuroradiol.* 2006;27:972.

130. Mewes AU, Hüppi PS, Als H, et al. Regional brain development in serial magnetic resonance imaging of low-risk preterm infants. *Pediatrics.* 2006;118:23.

131. Limperopoulos C, Soul JS, Gauvreau K, et al. Late gestation cerebellar growth is rapid and impeded by premature birth. *Pediatrics.* 2005;115:688.

132. Matthews LG, Inder TE, Pascoe L, et al. Longitudinal preterm cerebellar volume: perinatal and neurodevelopmental outcome associations. *Cerebellum.* 2018;17:610-627.

133. Limperopoulos C, Soul JS, Haidar H, et al. Impaired trophic interactions between the cerebellum and the cerebrum among preterm infants. *Pediatrics.* 2005;116:844.

134. Lodygensky GA, Rademaker K, Zimine S, et al. Structural and functional brain development after hydrocortisone treatment for neonatal chronic lung disease. *Pediatrics.* 2005;116:1-7.

135. Martinussen M, Fischl B, Larsson HB, et al. Cerebral cortex thickness in 15-year-old adolescents with low birth weight measured by an automated MRI-based method. *Brain.* 2005; 128:2588.

136. Isaacs EB, Edmonds CJ, Chong WK, Lucas A, Morley R, Gadian DG. Brain morphometry and IQ measurements in preterm children. *Brain.* 2004;127:2595.

137. Gimenez M, Junque C, Vendrell P, et al. Abnormal orbitofrontal development due to prematurity. *Neurology.* 2006;67:1818-1822.

138. Ganella EP, Burnett A, Cheong J, et al. Abnormalities in orbitofrontal cortex gyrification and mental health outcomes in adolescents born extremely preterm and/or at an extremely low birth weight. *Hum Brain Mapp.* 2015;36:1138-1150.

139. Liverani MC, Freitas LGA, Siffredi V, et al. Get real: orbitofrontal cortex mediates the ability to sense reality in early adolescents. *Brain Behav.* 2020;10:e01552.

140. Freitas LGA, Liverani MC, Siffredi V, et al. Altered orbitofrontal activation in preterm-born young adolescents during performance of a reality filtering task. *Neuroimage Clin.* 2021;30:102668.

141. Kesler SR, Ment LR, Vohr B, et al. Volumetric analysis of regional cerebral development in preterm children. *Pediatr Neurol.* 2004;31:318.

142. Ment LR, Hirtz D, Huppi PS. Imaging biomarkers of outcome in the developing preterm brain. *Lancet Neurol.* 2009;8:1042-1055.

143. Loh WY, Anderson PJ, Cheong JLY, et al. Longitudinal growth of the basal ganglia and thalamus in very preterm children. *Brain Imaging Behav.* 2020;14:998-1011.

144. Dubois J, Benders M, Borradori-Tolsa C, et al. Primary cortical folding in the human newborn: an early marker of later functional development. *Brain.* 2008;131:2028-2041.

145. Dubois J, Benders M, Cachia A, et al. Mapping the early cortical folding process in the preterm newborn brain. *Cereb Cortex.* 2008;18(6):1444–1454. doi:10.1093/cercor/bhm180.

146. Kapellou O, Counsell SJ, Kennea N, et al. Abnormal cortical development after premature birth shown by altered allometric scaling of brain growth. *PLoS Med.* 2006;3:e265.

147. Kersbergen KJ, Leroy F, Isgum I, et al. Relation between clinical risk factors, early cortical changes, and neurodevelopmental outcome in preterm infants. *Neuroimage.* 2016;142:301-310.

148. Dubois J, Lefevre J, Angleys H, et al. The dynamics of cortical folding waves and prematurity-related deviations revealed by spatial and spectral analysis of gyrification. *Neuroimage.* 2019;185:934-946.

Chapter 16

Congenital Heart Disease: An Important Cause of Brain Injury and Dysmaturation

Thiviya Selvanathan, Mike Seed and Vann Chau

Chapter Outline

Key Points

- Although there have been significant improvements in the survival of infants with congenital heart disease (CHD), they remain at high risk for neurodevelopmental impairments.
- Brain dysmaturation and brain injury are key brain changes contributing to adverse neurodevelopmental outcomes in CHD.
- Fetal neuroimaging studies have found that brain dysmaturation begins in utero and may be linked to altered cerebral blood flow and oxygenation in fetuses with CHD.
- With advances in genetic and genomic studies, there has been an expansion of our understanding of genetic risk factors for CHD. The associations between genetic abnormalities and neurodevelopmental outcomes in CHD require further study.
- Modifying environmental risk factors such as socioeconomic status and the home environment may be potential opportunities to optimize brain maturation and neurodevelopmental outcomes in CHD.

Introduction

Congenital heart disease (CHD) is the most common birth defect and occurs in approximately 1% of live births.[1–5] A recent systematic review and meta-analysis showed an increase in the birth prevalence of CHD globally from 1970 to 2017 with the highest prevalence seen in Asia (9.3 per 1000 live births) and lowest in Africa (2.3 per 1000 live births).[2] This increase was mainly driven by a change in the prevalence of mild CHD lesions (e.g., atrial septal defect, ventricular septal defect, patent ductus arteriosus) during the study period, likely reflecting improvements in the screening and detection of these lesions over time, although other studies have not observed a similar increase in prevalence.[1,6] This variation may be due to differences in definitions of CHD and study periods that were included across studies. Approximately one-third of infants with CHD have severe malformations requiring surgical interventions within the first year of life. This was previously associated with significant mortality, however, with advances in cardiac surgical and intensive care, there has been an increase in the survival of infants with CHD with now >85% surviving into adulthood.[1,7,8] This has led to an increase in the lifetime prevalence of CHD, and >65% of the entire CHD population are adults.[9] As a result, there has been an expanding body of research focused on understanding long-term outcomes in patients with CHD.

Neurodevelopmental impairments are common in severe CHD; they are present in over 50% of children.[10] The typical neurodevelopmental profile of children with CHD consists of mild but highly prevalent deficits across multiple domains: visual-spatial skills, executive function, memory, language, motor skills, social interactions, and behavior.[10–12] Although IQ scores in children with CHD on a group level are typically within the normal range, they are significantly lower when compared to population normative data or healthy control children.[13–18] Neurodevelopmental impairments emerge early in childhood with predominantly motor delays seen in infants with CHD.[19,20] However, as children with CHD become older, abnormalities in cognition, adaptive skills, and behavior become more apparent as cognitive and social expectations change with increasing age.[13,21–25] This highlights the importance of long-term neurodevelopmental follow-up in this population. These cognitive impairments persist throughout adolescence and adulthood.[16,18,26–30] Interestingly, a recent cohort study observed an increased risk of dementia, particularly early-onset dementia, in CHD adults compared to the general population, with the highest risk seen in severe CHD.[31] Adults with CHD are also more likely to be unemployed and achieve lower levels of education.[32–34] Further longitudinal studies following patients into late adulthood are needed to understand long-term neurological outcomes and psychosocial functioning in individuals with CHD.

Although mild, the highly prevalent neurodevelopmental and cognitive abnormalities in CHD have important functional consequences. Children and adolescents with CHD have an increased need for educational support, and lower employment rates are seen in adults with CHD.[10,15,35] Understanding the biologic basis of neurodevelopmental abnormalities in CHD and their key contributing factors are critical in developing effective interventions and management strategies that support optimal neurodevelopmental and cognitive outcomes. Neuroimaging studies have observed that brain *dysmaturation*, which begins antenatally, and brain injury are the key brain changes that underlie adverse neurodevelopmental outcomes in CHD. Several risk factors for neurodevelopmental impairments in CHD have been identified and include innate (genetic) as well as acquired and potentially modifiable (prenatal diagnosis, perioperative management, socioeconomic status [SES]) factors. This chapter reviews abnormalities in brain maturation and common types of brain injury observed in infants with CHD, as well as key contributors to these brain changes. Neuromonitoring and neuroprotective strategies that are currently in use or are under investigation to promote optimal brain health and neurodevelopment in CHD are also discussed. Finally, we highlight key knowledge gaps and areas in need of further study to improve neurodevelopmental outcomes in this population.

CHD Etiology and Malformation Grouping

The etiology of CHD is multifactorial with both environmental and genetic predisposing factors as shown in Fig. 16.1. Environmental contributors to CHD include antenatal exposures to infections (e.g., rubella),[36] teratogens (e.g., retinoic acid, phenytoin, lithium),[37] and maternal chronic conditions (e.g., obesity, diabetes mellitus, phenylketonuria).[38–41] The genetics of CHD is complex and heterogeneous; both inherited and de novo genetic alterations cause CHD.[42] Several genetic syndromes have been associated with CHD including aneuploidy syndromes (e.g., Down syndrome or trisomy 21), copy number variants (e.g., DiGeorge syndrome or 22q11.2 deletion), and single gene mutations (e.g., Noonan syndrome).[43,44] With advances in genetic and genomic technologies, recent studies have reported de novo single nucleotide variants across hundreds of genes involving multiple biological pathways that contribute to CHD, including in isolated (nonsyndromic) CHD.[45–47] Moreover, recent studies have shown gene-environment interactions

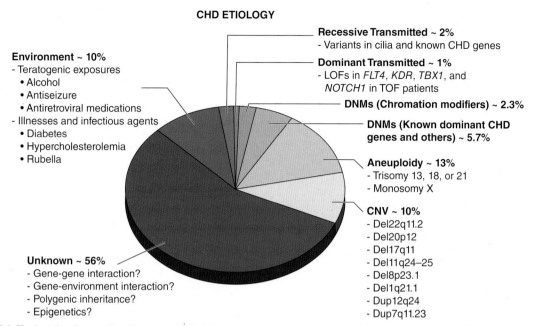

CHD ETIOLOGY

Fig. 16.1 Pie chart showing genetic and environmental etiologies of congenital heart disease. *CNM,* Copy number variation; *DNM,* de novo mutation. (Reproduced from Diab NS, Barish S, Dong W, et al. Molecular genetics and complex inheritance of congenital heart disease. *Genes* 2021;12(7):1020.)

between Notch signaling and maternal hyperglycemia and hypoxia resulting in an increased incidence of CHD in mice.[48,49] The complex interactions between environmental and genetic risk factors for CHD are an area that warrants further study.

Severe CHD is often categorized as single ventricle or biventricular lesions, and may be associated with aortic arch obstruction such as aortic coarctation and aortic valve atresia or stenosis. Severe CHD also frequently includes intracardiac (e.g., atrial septal defect or ventricular septal defect) or extracardiac (e.g., patent ductus arteriosus) shunts. The presence of shunts, along with abnormal cardiac connections, malformed valves, and obstructions to blood flow may result in reduced systemic oxygen delivery due to the mixing of venous and arterial blood. Two common forms of severe CHD accounting for a large proportion of surgeries performed in the neonatal period are transposition of the great arteries (TGA) and patients with single ventricle physiology, including those with hypoplastic left heart syndrome (HLHS), with much of the literature of neurodevelopment, brain maturation, and brain injury in infants with CHD focusing on these two high-risk populations.

TRANSPOSITION OF THE GREAT ARTERIES

TGA (Fig. 16.2) results from ventriculoarterial discordance when the aorta arises from the right ventricle and the pulmonary artery from the left ventricle.[50] This leads to the systemic circulation, being supplied with deoxygenated venous blood returning from the body, and the pulmonary circulation, being supplied with oxygenated blood returning from the lungs, to be in parallel rather than in series as they are in a normal heart. This results in the affected infant being cyanosed. TGA can be associated with other cardiac abnormalities, such as ventricular septal defects, left ventricular outflow tract obstruction, or coarctation of the aorta.[50] TGA can be difficult to diagnose antenatally with ultrasound, while affected infants can present with cyanosis and tachypnea. The severity of symptoms depends on the presence of other cardiac anomalies and the degree of mixing between the two parallel circulations.

The initial management of TGA is to stabilize the infant until the corrective surgery is performed. This includes maintaining the patency of the ductus arteriorus using prostaglandin E1 infusion to optimize circulatory mixing.[51] Balloon atrial septostomy may also

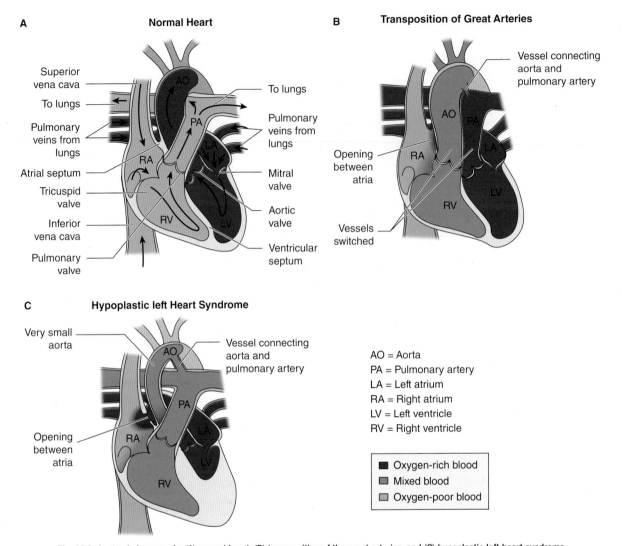

Fig. 16.2 Anatomic images of a (A) normal heart, (B) transposition of the great arteries, and (C) hypoplastic left heart syndrome.

be performed to improve oxygenation and survival in neonates with d-TGA.[52] In this intervention, a balloon is passed into the left atrium, inflated, and pulled vigorously across the atrial septum to create a larger atrial septal defect. The arterial switch operation is now the standard corrective procedure for TGA.[53]

HYPOPLASTIC LEFT HEART SYNDROME

HLHS (Fig. 16.2) describes a spectrum of cardiac malformations characterized by underdevelopment of the left heart with normally related great arteries, leaving

the right ventricle to perfuse both the pulmonary and systemic circulations. In HLHS, there is significant hypoplasia of the left ventricle which is associated with atresia, stenosis, or hypoplasia of the aortic and/or mitral valves, and hypoplasia of the ascending aorta and arch. The anatomic spectrum varies from almost complete absence of left ventricle combined with aortic and mitral atresia to milder hypoplasia of the left ventricle combined with aortic and mitral valve hypoplasia but without stenosis or atresia.[54] Survival is dependent on a patent ductus arteriosus and nonrestrictive atrial septal defect to ensure adequate systemic perfusion and mixing of oxygenated and deoxygenated blood. Affected infants become symptomatic when the ductus arteriosus closes and pulmonary vascular resistance decreases as expected after birth, progressing to cardiogenic shock and respiratory failure. Infants with a restrictive or intact atrial septal defect present with severe cyanosis and respiratory distress at birth because of pulmonary blood flow. Fortunately, a prenatal diagnosis is made in approximately 50% to 75% of cases with routine obstetrical ultrasound, typically between 18 and 24 weeks gestation, and is associated with improved survival and decreased morbidity.[55-58]

The initial management of infants with HLHS is focused on ensuring adequate systemic perfusion, which is achieved with intravenous prostaglandin E1 infusion to maintain patency of the ductus arteriosus. Balloon atrial septostomy may also be used in patients with a restrictive or intact atrial septum. The surgical palliation approach usually consists of a three-staged approach: (1) Norwood procedure (neonatal period), (2) bidirectional Glenn procedure (around 3–6 months of age), and (3) Fontan procedure (typically 2–5 years of age). In the Norwood procedure, a neoaorta is created by using the proximal pulmonary artery and homograft material, which is then connected to the native ascending aorta. A source of pulmonary blood flow is established either via a right ventricle to pulmonary artery conduit (Sano) or by connecting the innominate artery with the proximal right pulmonary artery via a Gore Tex tube (called modified Blalock-Taussig shunt). By 6 months of age, the arterial shunt can usually be substituted with a bidirectional cavo-pulmonary shunt (SVC to pulmonary artery anastomosis), which results in diminished volume loading for the ventricle. As the child grows further, the Fontan circulation can be completed. In this third stage, the inferior vena cava is connected to the pulmonary arteries, allowing the entire systemic venous return to pass through the lungs, driven by the suction force of the heart and finally achieving near normal arterial oxygen saturations.

Brain Dysmaturation and Brain Injury in CHD

Table 16.1 summarizes common neuroimaging and neuromonitoring studies performed in CHD infants and children, their utility, and expected findings.

BRAIN DYSMATURATION BEGINS IN UTERO IN CHD

Abnormalities in brain maturation and growth are common brain changes seen in CHD and are key

---

TABLE 16.1	Neuroimaging and Neuromonitoring Studies Performed in Infants With CHD and Typical Findings in CHD Infants
Investigation	**Indications and Typical Findings**
Cranial ultrasound	• Cranial ultrasound is a noninvasive and bedside procedure • Can provide an assessment of ventricular size, cystic WMI, large hemorrhages, and large infarcts, although up 1/3 of infarcts can be missed when compared to MRI[59] • Doppler measurements can also provide information about flow in the largest venous sinuses
CT	• Uses ionizing radiation • Can be performed rapidly • Can provide an assessment of ventricular size, hemorrhages, ischemic brain injury, although it is less likely to detect cortical and focal/multifocal brain injury when compared to MRI[60,61]
MRI	• Brain MRI is critical in identifying structural brain abnormalities and acquired brain injuries in infants with CHD • Advanced techniques allow for quantitative measures of brain development including brain volume, surface area, folding patterns which are abnormal in fetuses and infants with CHD[62,63]
MRS	• Measure regional concentrations of brain metabolites to assess metabolic maturation in neonates • NAA increases with advancing cerebral maturation and decreases with cerebral injury • CHD fetuses have lower NAA:choline ratio compared to healthy controls[62]

Continued

TABLE 16.1	**Neuroimaging and Neuromonitoring Studies Performed in Infants With CHD and Typical Findings in CHD Infants—cont'd**
Investigation	**Indications and Typical Findings**
DTI	• Anisotropy reflects the degree to which the movement of water molecules is restricted • Have increasing FA and decreasing MD as part of normal neonatal white matter development • CHD neonates have lower MD and FA preoperatively compared to healthy controls[64] • Can be combined with tractography to study at structural connectivity, which is altered in CHD neonates[65]
fMRI	• fMRI measures blood-oxygen-level-dependent (BOLD) signals which is an indirect measure of neural activity • Resting-state fMRI measures spontaneous neural activity to study brain functional network organization • Single study in CHD neonates reporting intact global network topology but altered regional network functional connectivity[66]
Aeeg	• aEEG is a continuous bedside monitoring tool of brain activity that can be helpful in assessing background activity and for seizures • Delayed/lack of return of aEEG background activity to normal associated with adverse neurodevelopmental outcomes in CHD[67,68,69] • Abnormal pre- and postoperative aEEG associated with brain injury in CHD[70,71]
Cerebral NIRS	• Noninvasive bedside monitoring tool to assess cerebral tissue oxygen saturation • Intraoperative NIRS can provide information about hypoxia and low cerebral perfusion • Associations between NIRS measures and neurodevelopmental outcomes unknown

aEEG, Amplitude-integrated electroencephalography; *CHD*, congenital heart disease; *CT*, computed tomography; *DTI*, diffusion tensor imaging; *FA*, fractional anisotropy; *fMRI*, functional MRI; *MD*, mean diffusivity; *MRI*, magnetic resonance imaging; *MRS*, magnetic resonance spectroscopy; *NAA*, N-acetylaspartate; *NIRS*, near-infrared spectroscopy; *WMI*, white matter injury.

contributors to adverse neurodevelopmental outcomes. Neonates with severe CHD have *preoperative* abnormalities in brain microstructural and metabolic maturation when compared to healthy controls.[64,72] Smaller head circumferences,[73] decreased total and regional brain volumes,[74–76] reduced cortical folding,[77,78] and alterations in structural and functional brain network connectivity[65,66,79] are also present at birth, even before neonates with CHD undergo surgery (Table 16.2). Some studies have observed a link between brain dysmaturation in the neonatal period and adverse neurodevelopmental outcomes later in childhood in CHD, although additional studies are required to further elucidate this relationship.[80–82] These alterations in brain maturation persist through childhood and adolescence and are also associated in long-term neurodevelopmental outcomes in CHD.[27,83–87] Recent studies have observed smaller brain volumes and altered white matter microstructure in adults with CHD, which are associated with cognitive function.[26,88] Table 16.3 summarizes a selected list of studies that have observed associations between brain abnormalities and neurodevelopment and cognition in CHD.

Brain dysmaturation in CHD begins during fetal brain development (Table 16.4). A fetal neuroimaging study of fetuses with CHD observed smaller total brain volumes and lower NAA:choline ratios (reflective of metabolic maturation) compared to controls. In this study, the differences in metabolic maturation and brain volumes between CHD and control fetuses widened over the third trimester during a period when brain growth and maturation is expected to accelerate, suggesting that the impairments in brain maturation observed in fetuses with CHD progress throughout gestation.[62] Fetuses with CHD also have smaller regional brain volumes,[108] slower head growth,[109,110] and delayed cortical development.[63,111] Interestingly, fetuses with CHD had less pronounced reductions in regional brain volumes when compared to fetuses with a family history of CHD rather than when compared to control fetuses with no family history of CHD, suggesting that genetic or shared environmental factors may contribute to brain dysmaturation in fetuses with CHD.[108]

TABLE 16.2 Selected Neuroimaging Studies in Neonates With CHD and Their Findings

Study: First Author (Year)	Study Design	Neuroimaging Modality	Risk Factors	Brain Abnormalities
Lynch et al. (2021)[89]	Prospective cohort CHD undergoing DHCA (n = 15)	MRI, diffuse optical spectroscopy, diffuse correlation spectroscopy	Cerebral oxygen extraction during DHCA	Larger decreases in cerebral oxygen saturation during DHCA associated with new postoperative WMI (p = 0.02).
Peyvandi et al. (2021)[90]	Prospective cohort TGA (n = 37) and HLHS (n = 26)	Fetal MRI, neonatal MRI	CHD lesion type	Lower brain volumes with more severe WMI in TGA (p = 0.04) but not HLHS.
Schlatterer et al. (2021)[91]	Prospective cohort Critical CHD (n = 34)	MRI	Autonomic dysfunction	Lower autonomic tone associated with preoperative brain injury (p < 0.01).
Feldmann et al. (2020)[65]		MRI, DTI, tractography	—	Reduced pre- and postoperative global network efficiency in CHD. Larger WMI volume associated with lower network strength and global efficiency.
Ng et al. (2020)[75]	Case-control CHD (64/256)	MRI (tensor-based morphometry)	—	Volume reduction in basal ganglia, thalami, corpus callosum, and cortical regions, and volume expansion in CSF in CHD.
Ni Bhroin et al. (2020)[79]	Case-control CHD (58/174)	MRI, DTI, tractography	—	Reduced structural connectivity in a cortico-striatal-thalamic subnetwork in CHD.
Claessens et al. (2019)[72]	Prospective cohort Surgical CHD (n = 74)	MRI, DTI	SVP	Increased preoperative fractional anisotropy in TGA and mean diffusivity highest in SVP.
Kelly et al. (2019)[92]	Case-control CHD (48/96)	MRI, NODDI	Impaired cerebral oxygen delivery	Increased cortical fractional anisotropy and reduced orientation dispersion index in CHD. Cortical orientation dispersion index associated with gyrification index and cerebral oxygen delivery.
Kelly et al. (2019)[93]	Prospective cohort Surgical CHD (n = 70)	MRI	BAS	Preoperative brain injury in 39%. Strokes (4%) were only seen in patients who had BAS.
De Asis-Cruz et al. (2018)[66]	Case-control Surgical CHD (30/112)	fMRI	—	Intact global network topology but reduced preoperative regional functional connectivity involving subcortical areas and brainstem.
Peyvandi et al. (2018)[94]	Prospective cohort TGA (n = 49) and HLHS (n = 30)	MRI	HLHS	More postoperative (p = 0.03) and severe (p = 0.01) brain injury in HLHS compared with TGA. Slower rate of brain growth in patients with severe brain injury (p < 0.01) and HLHS (p < 0.001).
Schmithorst et al. (2018)[95]	Case-control CHD (111/202)	MRI, DTI, tractography	—	Reduced global network efficiency and nodal efficiency in CHD pre- and postoperatively.
Fogel et al. (2017)[96]	Prospective cohort SVP (n = 168)	MRI	Surgical stage	More WMI post-BDG (OR 3.68) and post-Fontan (OR 2.0) compared to pre-BDG. Most focal tissue loss post-BDG (OR 8.75) and post-Fontan (OR 6.16) compared to pre-BDG.
Peyvandi et al. (2016)[97]	Prospective cohort TGA (n = 96) and SVP (n = 57)	MRI, DTI	Postnatal diagnosis of CHD	More brain injury with postnatal diagnosis (p = 0.003). Faster white matter (p = 0.04) and gray matter (p = 0.02) microstructural brain development with prenatal diagnosis.

Continued

TABLE 16.2   Selected Neuroimaging Studies in Neonates With CHD and Their Findings—cont'd

Study: First Author (Year)	Study Design	Neuroimaging Modality	Risk Factors	Brain Abnormalities
von Rhein et al. (2015)[74]	Case-control Surgical CHD (19/38)	MRI	—	Lower total brain and regional volumes in CHD ($p < 0.001$).
Andropoulos et al. (2010)[98]	Prospective cohort Surgical CHD (n = 67)	MRI, NIRS	SVP	Structural brain immaturity associated with pre- ($p < 0.01$) and postoperative brain injury ($p = 0.05$). SVP associated with postoperative WMI ($p < 0.01$).
Miller et al. (2007)[64]	Case-control TGA and SVP (41/57)	MRI, MRS, DTI	—	Lower preoperative NAA:choline ($p < 0.01$) and white matter fractional anisotropy ($p < 0.001$) in CHD.
McQuillen et al. (2006)[99]	Prospective cohort TGA (n = 29)	MRI	BAS	41% had focal preoperative brain injury, associated with BAS (number needed to harm 1.6).
Mahle et al. (2002)[100]	Prospective cohort Surgical CHD (n = 24)	MRI, MRS	—	WMI: preoperative 16%, postoperative 42% Stroke: preoperative 8%, postoperative 19% Elevated lactate in 53%, correlated with preoperative lesions ($p < 0.02$)

BAS, Balloon atrial septostomy; *BDG*, bidirectional Glenn; *CHD*, congenital heart disease; *DHCA*, deep hypothermic circulatory arrest; *DTI*, diffusion tensor imaging; *fMRI*, functional MRI; *HLHS*, hypoplastic left heart syndrome; *MRI*, magnetic resonance imaging; *MRS*, magnetic resonance spectroscopy; *NIRS*, near-infrared spectroscopy; *NODDI*, neurite orientation dispersion and density imaging; *SVP*, single ventricle physiology; *TGA*, transposition of the great arteries; *WMI*, white matter injury.

TABLE 16.3   Selected Neuroimaging Studies of Associations Between Brain Abnormalities and Neurodevelopment in CHD

Study: First Author (Year)	Study Design	Assessment Modality	Neuroimaging Modality	Key Findings
Bonthrone et al. (2021)[101]	Prospective cohort CHD (n = 56)	Bayley-III at 22 months	MRI	Cognitively stimulating parenting associated with cognitive outcomes at 2 years.
Ehrler et al. (2021)[88]	Case-control Adult CHD (45/99)	Extensive test battery	MRI, DTI	Lower fractional anisotropy in CHD adults. Lower executive function scores in CHD adults, associated with lower fractional anisotropy.
Kuhn et al. (2021)[102]	Prospective cohort TGA (n = 29), HLHS (n = 24)	PSOM, Glasgow Outcome Scale-Extended (Pediatric version) between 5 and 23 months of age	MRI	Mechanical ventilation >12 days (OR 17.9) and DHCA >40 minutes (OR 11.6) associated with moderate-severe deficits on PSOM. Longer stay in ICU associated with brain injury ($p < 0.001$).
Stegeman et al. (2021)[80]	Prospective cohort Surgical CHD (n = 51)	Bayley-III at 3, 6, 18 months.	MRI	WMI associated with worse gross motor outcomes ($p < 0.05$). Cortical gray matter and cerebellar volumes ($p < 0.05$) associated with fine motor outcomes. Repeated cardiac surgery associated with poorer motor outcomes.

TABLE 16.3   Selected Neuroimaging Studies of Associations Between Brain Abnormalities and Neurodevelopment in CHD—cont'd

Study: First Author (Year)	Study Design	Assessment Modality	Neuroimaging Modality	Key Findings
Verrall et al. (2021)[26]	Case-control Adolescent and adult Fontan (n = 107), controls (TGA, healthy controls)	Cogstate battery	MRI	Fontan group had lower cognitive scores, which were associated with more childhood inpatient days, younger age at Fontan surgery, longer duration since Fontan surgery. Fontan group had smaller brain volumes, which were associated with resting oxygen saturations.
Noorani et al. (2020)[83]	Case-control Adolescent SVP (23/60)	MoCA, Wide Range Assessment of Memory and Learning-2	MRI	Smaller caudate volumes in SVP. Caudate volumes correlated with cognitive scores.
Cabrera-Mino et al. (2020)[84]	Case-control Adolescent SVP (25/63)	MoCA, Wide Range Assessment of Memory and Learning-2	MRI	Smaller mammillary body volumes in SVP. Mammillary body volumes correlated with cognitive scores.
Ehrler et al. (2020)[27]	Case-control Adolescent CHD	Weschler Intelligence Scale for Children-IV	MRI, DTI	Lower fractional anisotropy in CHD. Lower working memory scores in CHD, which were associated with frontal lobe fractional anisotropy.
Hottinger et al. (2020)[103]	Case-control Neonate CHD (92/138)	Bayley-III at 1 year	MRI	Lower pre- ($p = 0.01$) and postoperative ($p = 0.03$) brain maturation scores in CHD. Brain maturation not associated with Bayley-III scores.
Morton et al. (2020)[85]	Case-control Adolescent SVP (115/160)	Weschler Intelligence Scale for Children-IV, Delis-Kaplan Executive Function System	MRI	Differences in sulcal patterns in CHD that are associated with cognitive outcomes.
Lim et al. (2019)[104]	Prospective cohort TGA neonates (n = 45)	Bayley-III at 18 months	MRI	Older age at repair and presence of VSD (both $p < 0.01$) associated with reduced perioperative neonatal brain growth. Older age at repair associated with lower language outcomes ($p < 0.01$).
Meuwly et al. (2019)[105]	Case-control CHD neonates (77/121)	Bayley-III at 12 months	MRI	Smaller brain volumes in CHD ($p < 0.01$). Lower cognitive and motor scores in CHD ($p < 0.001$). Postoperative brain volumes associated with cognitive and language scores ($p < 0.04$).
Claessens et al. (2018)[82]	Prospective cohort CHD neonates with aortic arch obstruction (n = 34)	Bayley-III at 2 years, WPPSI at 6 years	MRI	WMI associated with lower cognitive scores ($p < 0.05$). Injury to posterior limb of internal capsule associated with motor outcomes ($p = 0.03$). Smaller basal ganglia and brainstem volumes associated with lower IQ ($p = 0.03$).

Continued

TABLE 16.3   Selected Neuroimaging Studies of Associations Between Brain Abnormalities and Neurodevelopment in CHD—cont'd

Study: First Author (Year)	Study Design	Assessment Modality	Neuroimaging Modality	Key Findings
Peyvandi et al. (2018)[106]	Prospective cohort TGA (n = 84), SVP (n = 20)	Bayley-II at 12 and 30 months	MRI	WMI associated with motor outcomes at 30 months ($p \leq 0.05$).
Watson et al. (2018)[86]	Case-control Fontan children and adolescents (102/149)	Weschler Intelligence Scale for Children, Weschler Adult Intelligence Scale	MRI, DTI	Lower fractional anisotropy in multiple tracts in Fontan which were associated with more complications at first operation, more operations, and neurologic events. Fractional anisotropy correlated positively with processing speed and full-scale IQ.
Rollins et al. (2017)[107]	Case-control Biventricular CHD (48/61)	Bayley-II, MacArthur-Bates Communicative Development Inventories (CDI) at 1 year	MRI	Smaller total and regional brain volumes in CHD ($p < 0.01$). Brain volumes correlated with CDI language scores ($p < 0.05$).

CHD, Congenital heart disease; *DTI*, diffusion tensor imaging; *HLHS*, hypoplastic left heart syndrome; *MoCA*, Montreal Cognitive Assessment; *MRI*, magnetic resonance imaging; *PSOM*, Pediatric Stroke Outcome Measure; *SVP*, single ventricle physiology; *TGA*, transposition of the great arteries; *VSD*, ventral septal defect; *WPPSI*, Wechsler Preschool and Primary Scale of Intelligence; *WMI*, white matter injury.

TABLE 16.4   Selected Fetal Neuroimaging Studies in CHD and Key Brain Abnormalities Observed in Each

Study: First Author (Year)	Study Design	Neuroimaging Modality	Brain Abnormalities
Paladini et al. (2021)[112]	Case-control CHD (101/522)	Fetal ultrasound	Smaller frontal lobe anteroposterior diameter/occipitofrontal diameter ratio ($p < 0.001$) in CHD fetuses.
Peyvandi et al. (2021)[90]	Prospective cohort of TGA (n = 37) and HLHS (n = 26)	Fetal MRI, neonatal preoperative MRI	Lower total brain volume (fetal and neonatal scans) associated with increased risk of postnatal moderate-severe WMI in TGA, but not HLHS.
Ren et al. (2021)[113]	Case-control CHD (40/160)	Fetal MRI	Smaller gray matter, subcortical brain tissue, cerebellar and brainstem volumes and larger CSF and ventricular volumes in CHD fetuses.
Ren et al. (2021)[114]	Case-control CHD (50/150)	Fetal MRI, DWI	ADC values lower in frontal and periventricular white matter and pons and higher in thalamus in CHD fetuses.
Rollins et al. (2021)[108]	Case-control CHD: HLHS/TGA (24/179), other CHD (50/179)	Fetal MRI	Smaller brain volumes in HLHS/TGA fetuses ($p < 0.001$). Smaller subplate and intermediate zone volumes ($p < 0.01$) in HLHS/TGA fetuses.
Inversetti et al. (2020)[109]	Case-control CHD (79/229)	Fetal ultrasound	Lower head circumference in CHD fetuses after second trimester ($p < 0.01$). Fetuses with cyanotic CHD had slower head growth than acyanotic CHD ($p < 0.05$).

TABLE 16.4 Selected Fetal Neuroimaging Studies in CHD and Key Brain Abnormalities Observed in Each—cont'd

Study: First Author (Year)	Study Design	Neuroimaging Modality	Brain Abnormalities
Jaimes et al. (2020)[115]	Case-control CHD (48/69)	Fetal MRI	Lower fetal total (brain) maturation score ($p < 0.01$) in CHD fetuses.
Wu et al. (2020)[116]	Case-control CHD (48/140)	Fetal MRI	Maternal psychological distress associated with smaller hippocampal and cerebellar volumes ($p < 0.05$) in CHD fetuses.
Claessens et al. (2019)[117]	Prospective cohort CHD (n = 61)	Fetal MRI, neonatal pre- and postoperative MRI	Larger fetal brain volumes correlated with larger neonatal brain volumes. Smaller fetal brain volumes associated with neonatal ischemic brain injury.
Ortinau et al. (2019)[111]	Case-control CHD (17/36)	Fetal MRI	Altered global sulcation pattern of left hemisphere of CHD fetuses.
Olshaker et al. (2018)[118]	Retrospective CHD cohort (n = 46)	Fetal MRI	Smaller cerebellar volumes in CHD compared to population norm ($p < 0.05$)
Rajagopalan et al. (2018)[119]	Prospective cohort of biventricular (n = 7) and single ventricle (n = 10) CHD	Fetal MRI	Slower cerebral regional ($p < 0.05$) and cerebellar growth ($p < 0.01$) trajectories in single ventricle fetuses.
Ruiz et al. (2017)[110]	Prospective cohort CHD (n = 119)	Fetal ultrasound	Smaller biparietal diameter and head circumference throughout gestation compared to normative data.
Wong et al. (2017)[120]	Case-control CHD (11/62)	Fetal MRI, neonatal pre- and postoperative MRI	Delayed internal closure of bilateral opercula, enlargement of bilateral lateral ventricles, and smaller cerebellar vermis height in CHD fetuses and neonates (all $p < 0.05$).
Masoller et al. (2016)[121]	Case-control CHD (58/116)	Fetal MRI, MRS, fetoplacental Doppler ultrasound	Lower biparietal diameter, head circumference, and cerebral blood flow (all $p < 0.05$) in CHD fetuses. Lower NAA/choline values in basal ganglia and frontal lobe ($p < 0.05$) in CHD fetuses. Smaller brain volumes in CHD fetuses ($p < 0.05$).
Sun et al. (2015)[122]	Case-control CHD (30/60)	Fetal MRI	Smaller total brain volume correlated with reduced cerebral oxygen delivery and consumption in CHD ($p < 0.001$).
Clouchoux et al. (2013)[63]	Case-control HLHS (18/48)	Fetal MRI	Progressively lower subcortical gray ($p < 0.05$) and white matter ($p < 0.001$) volumes in third trimester. Smaller gyrification index and cortical surface area ($p < 0.001$).
Limperopoulos et al. (2010)[62]	Case-control CHD (55/105)	Fetal MRI, MRS	Lower total brain volumes ($p < 0.001$) and NAA/choline ($p < 0.001$) in CHD fetuses

CHD, Congenital heart disease; *DWI*, diffusion-weighted imaging; *HLHS*, hypoplastic left heart syndrome; *MRI*, magnetic resonance imaging; *MRS*, magnetic resonance spectroscopy; *NAA*, N-acetylaspartate; *TGA*, transposition of the great arteries; *WMI*, white matter injury.

Findings of animal studies suggest that hypoxia-ischemia plays a key role in fetal neuronal and white matter dysmaturation in CHD, possibly mediated by the hypoxia-inducible-factor signaling pathway and impaired angiogenesis.[123–128] This is of particular importance given alterations in cerebral blood flow and oxygenation that are observed in fetuses with CHD.[129] In particular, the immature white matter in the developing brain is especially vulnerable to hypoxia-ischemia. The primary myelinating cells in the brain are oligodendrocytes which undergo expected maturation from neural stem cells to oligodendrocyte precursor cells to immature pre-oligodendrocytes and finally into mature myelinating oligodendrocytes.[130] Hypoxia-ischemia causes pre-oligodendrocyte cell injury following which the injured pre-oligodendrocyte cells degenerate.[131,132] New pre-oligodendrocytes regenerate from the population of oligodendrocyte progenitor cells that are resistant to hypoxia-ischemia. However, these new pre-oligodendrocytes experience maturational arrest and do not differentiate into mature myelinating oligodendrocytes, resulting in impaired myelination and white matter microstructural abnormalities.[133–136]

Imaging studies of human fetuses with CHD in vivo have found an association between brain dysmaturation and altered fetal cerebral oxygenation and blood flow. Fetuses with CHD have decreased umbilical blood flow and streaming of oxygenated blood from the placenta to the ascending aorta, which is associated with lower oxygen saturations in the ascending aorta. These hemodynamic changes correlate with less cerebral oxygen delivery and smaller brain volumes in fetuses with CHD.[122] A recent study using a novel fetal imaging technique to quantify fetal cerebral oxygenation (measuring $T2^*$ decay) observed a similar association between reduced cerebral oxygenation in fetuses with CHD compared to control, which was associated with reduced brain volumes.[137] Reduced regional brain volumes in important structures containing maturing neurons and glial cells (subplate, intermediate zone, ventricular zone) in fetuses with CHD is also associated with less cerebral substrate delivery.[108] These studies support the hypothesis that altered fetal hemodynamics and cerebral oxygenation play a critical role in brain dysmaturation in fetuses with CHD. Thus, current studies are investigating the use of maternal hyperoxygenation as a potential neuroprotective strategy in CHD.[138]

BRAIN INJURY IN CHD

Neonates with CHD are at risk for acquired brain injuries, which may be present in up to 60% of cases and are mostly clinically silent.[93,100,102] White matter injury (WMI) and small arterial ischemic strokes are the most common types of ischemic brain injury seen in neonates with CHD; other acquired brain injuries in CHD include hypoxic-ischemic brain injury, cerebral venous sinus thrombosis, and intracranial hemorrhages. A study across two large pediatric cardiac centers reported arterial ischemic strokes in 18% of preoperative and 19% of postoperative MRI of neonates with severe CHD. New multifocal ischemic lesions (WMI or hypoxic-ischemic brain injury) were seen in 15% of preoperative and 30% of postoperative MRI.[139] As clinically asymptomatic acute ischemic strokes and WMI are common in CHD and have a low risk of progressing after surgery, most brain injury findings on MRI should not be an indication to delay clinically indicated surgical planning.[140,141]

Neonatal brain injury in infants with CHD, particularly WMI, has been linked to neurodevelopmental outcomes.[80,82,106] It is important to realize that the majority of injuries in neonates with CHD are clinically silent and are often present in well-appearing infants.[140,98] Thus, appropriate investigations are necessary to identify infants with CHD at greatest risk for developmental impairments and implement early interventions to promote optimal neurodevelopmental outcomes. MRI is an important tool for the investigation of neonates with CHD due to the high burden of radiation with CT and poor reliability of cranial ultrasound.[59] MRI with diffusion-weighted imaging (DWI), in combination with T1- and T2-weighted imaging, is useful in identifying tissue edema and is a sensitive test for acute brain ischemia and injury. In assessing for silent ischemic brain injury, MRI with DWI is best performed within the first week of life preoperatively, or within 1 week postoperatively, as there is postinjury pseudonormalization of the DWI signal beyond 5 to 7 days in the neonatal brain.

Neonatal Ischemic Brain Injury: White Matter Injury and Arterial Ischemic Stroke

WMI is the most common type of ischemic brain injury seen in term infants with CHD and is like the pattern of brain injury seen in preterm infants in response to hypoxia-ischemia. It contrasts with the typical pattern of hypoxic-ischemic brain injury seen in term infants, which usually involves neuronal structures: basal ganglia, thalamus, hippocampus, and cerebral cortex. WMI occurs secondary to the selective vulnerability of pre-oligodendrocytes cells, abundant cells in the immature white matter of CHD infants, to hypoxic-ischemic insults. Infants with CHD are also at

risk of impaired cerebral autoregulation and may not maintain adequate cerebral blood flow during periods of low cardiac output state or hemodynamic fluctuations, possibly further contributing to WMI.[142]

WMI in infants with CHD consists of punctate T1 hyperintense lesions in the periventricular white matter (Fig. 16.3E), which can be associated with hemorrhagic or cystic changes in a minority of infants. Compared to WMI in preterm infants, advanced brain lesion mapping studies have identified a predilection for the anterior and posterior instead of central periventricular white matter in infants with CHD. This correlates with the expected maturation of white

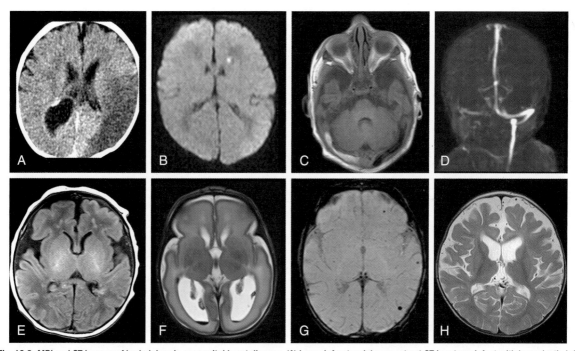

Fig. 16.3 MRI and CT images of brain injury in congenital heart disease. (A) Large infarct: axial noncontrast CT in a term infant with hypoplastic left heart syndrome status post-Norwood procedure showing a large hypodense area in the left middle cerebral artery territory. (B) Small acute infarct: axial diffusion-weighted MRI image of a term neonate with transposition of the great arteries (TGA) following balloon atrial septostomy showing a small diffusion restriction infarct in the left caudate. (C) Cerebral sinovenous thrombosis: axial T1-weighted MRI image of a neonate with TGA performed postoperatively showing a hyperintense right transverse sinus consist with thrombosis. Absent flow is seen through the right transverse and sigmoid sinuses in the MR venogram (D). (E) White matter injury: axial T1-weighted MRI image of a term neonate with TGA performed postoperatively showing multiple punctate hyperintense lesions in the periventricular white matter. (F) Intraventricular hemorrhage: axial T2-weighted MRI image of a preterm neonate with truncus arteriosus showing bilateral grade 3 intraventricular hemorrhages with posthemorrhagic ventricular dilatation. (G) Cerebral microhemorrhages: axial susceptibility-weighted MRI image in a term neonate with TGA performed postoperatively showing multiple areas of increased susceptibility consistent with microhemorrhages. (H) White matter volume loss: axial T2-weighted MRI image in a 9-month-old infant after heart transplant showing significant thinning of the white matter with increased extra-axial spaces anteriorly and enlarged lateral ventricles.

matter that begins in the central periventricular white matter, and then occurs anteriorly and posteriorly.[143] It is important to note that the punctate periventricular white matter lesions seen on clinical neuroimaging do not reflect the full spectrum of white matter abnormalities in infants with CHD; this also includes alterations in white matter microstructure, myelination, and structural network connectivity.

Arterial ischemic strokes are the second most common type of ischemic brain injury in infants with CHD (Fig. 16.3A and B). These are typically small, asymptomatic, and often missed on cranial ultrasound.[59] Arterial ischemic strokes may occur in up to 25% of neonates with severe CHD, and recent studies have demonstrated an increased risk for stroke in adult survivors of CHD compared to controls.[139,144–146] This increased risk in adulthood may be multifactorial with thromboembolism, need for repeat cardiac surgeries, and development of arrhythmias potentially playing a role, although further research is needed to identify risk factors associated with the greatest stroke risk.

Specific Risk Factors for Ischemic Brain Injury With CHD

Several risk factors for brain injury in infants with CHD have been identified.[147] Brain dysmaturation is an important *predisposing factor* for brain injury in infants with CHD, especially in the preoperative period (see above). In neonates with CHD, lower fractional anisotropy and NAA:choline ratios, reflecting less mature white matter microstructure and brain metabolism, were associated with more severe preoperative WMI.[148] A similar link between smaller fetal brain volumes and increased risk for more severe preoperative WMI has also been observed.[90] Interestingly, recent studies have observed that neonatal WMI may contribute to abnormalities in postnatal brain maturation, suggesting that there is a complex relationship between brain dysmaturation and brain injury in CHD that requires further study.[65,94] Finally, the transition from fetal to neonatal circulation may be a period of increased risk for preoperative brain injury in neonates with CHD. In the normal transition, air-breathing results in a dramatic reduction in pulmonary vascular resistance with associated increase in pulmonary blood flow which provides the increase in left ventricular preload that supports the severalfold

increase in left ventricular output that occurs in neonatal period. However, CHD neonates that depend on right ventricular output for cerebral perfusion, including those with TGA and HLHS, may be more susceptible to a transient episode of cerebral ischemia during umbilical cord clamping, which is associated with a reduction in right ventricular preload. In CHD neonates with right ventricle dependent systemic perfusion, the drop in pulmonary vascular resistance occurring at birth may exacerbate the impact of cord clamping through the development of a steal into the pulmonary circulation. This combined with abnormal cerebral autoregulation in neonates with CHD may lead to an increased risk for preoperative brain injury in CHD neonates.[149,150] Other important risk factors for preoperative ischemic brain injury include balloon atrial septostomy,[93,99] time to surgery,[151,152] and postnatal diagnosis of CHD.[97] Several intraoperative factors have been associated with increased risk for ischemic brain injury, including reduced cerebral oxygen saturation during deep hypothermic circulatory arrest (DHCA) and duration of DHCA.[141,89] A recent study of piglets exposed to cardiopulmonary bypass observed cortical dysmaturation with reduced neuronal migration, altered densities of inhibitory neurons, reduced gyrification index, and smaller cortical volumes.[153] However, there is significant variability seen across studies with some reporting associations while others have not, suggesting that operative factors may contribute less to brain injury than others. In the postoperative period, prolonged low cardiac output state and single ventricle physiology, a group of infants with persistent chronic hypoxemia after neonatal surgery, are key risk factors for new ischemic brain injury.[154,155] Collectively, these studies suggest that strategies to promote adequate cerebral oxygenation and hemodynamic monitoring are important for neuroprotection in CHD. These will be discussed in more detail in subsequent sections of this chapter.

Cerebral Sinovenous Thrombosis

Cerebral sinovenous thrombosis (CSVT) is a serious complication of hemostasis in the critically ill neonate and has been observed in up to 28% of infants with severe CHD (Fig. 16.3C and D).[156,157] In adults with CHD, hypoxemia has been associated with thrombosis and bleeding.[158–160] The etiology of these abnormalities remains incompletely understood, though chronic endothelial damage, increased blood volume and viscosity, low pulmonary artery velocity, biventricular dysfunction, and chronic right-to-left shunting have all been proposed to contribute.[160] In a study of neonates with CHD, CSVT was associated with prolonged use of a central venous catheter which may be associated with line-related thrombosis and local injury to the vessel wall endothelium with elevated coagulation factors.[157] Investigating suspected CSVT should include either a computerized tomography (CT) and/or MRI T1- and T2-weighted imaging, in addition to venography (CT venography or MRV) to investigate for clots within the venous sinuses as well as parenchymal injury with infarction or hemorrhage.[161]

Intracranial Hemorrhages

Intracranial hemorrhages in infants with CHD include: subdural hemorrhage (SDH), parenchymal hemorrhages (including cerebellar hemorrhage), intraventricular hemorrhage, and cerebral microhemorrhages/microbleeds. SDH is a common finding in neonates with CHD and occurs in up to 52% of infants with CHD.[156,162,163] This is higher than rates reported in healthy term infants; a recent MRI study reported a rate of SDH of 23% in healthy term neonates.[164] More SDH was observed in infants with CHD born by vaginal delivery than by cesarean section (46% vs. 27%, respectively).[162] Though SDH is a common finding in infants with CHD, SDHs are generally asymptomatic and resolve over time without treatment.[162] The impact of SDH on neurodevelopmental outcome in CHD is currently unknown. Infants with CHD are also at risk for intraventricular hemorrhage, with increasing incidence associated with lower gestational age (Fig. 16.3F).[156,165] Cerebral microhemorrhages are seen on postoperative MRI in infants with CHD and are a common finding after cardiac surgery with cardiopulmonary bypass in children and adults (Fig. 16.3G).[166,167] Some studies have reported a possible association of cerebral microhemorrhages with neurodevelopmental outcomes, although this link is not clear and requires further study.[107,168]

NEUROMONITORING STUDIES IN CHD

Amplitude-Integrated Electroencephalography

Amplitude-integrated electroencephalography (aEEG) is a continuous bedside monitoring tool that can be used to monitor brain activity during the perioperative period in infants with CHD. aEEG provides clinicians with valuable information about background electrical activity and identifies seizures. In a study of neonates with CHD, abnormal voltage patterns were identified on aEEG in 60% of neonates at some point in the first 72 hours, with severely abnormal patterns of burst-suppression, continuous low voltage or flat tracings in 15% of neonates.[169] Seizures were identified in 19% of neonates in this study, and 2/12 seizures were subclinical[169]; other studies have observed a similar prevalence of subclinical seizures.[67,68,70,170] This highlights the utility of aEEG in detecting seizures in infants with CHD who may experience "uncoupling" of clinical and electrographic seizures, a common phenomenon in neonates.[171] The sensitivity of aEEG for seizure detection ranges from 70% to 85%, but is lower for seizures that are brief, low amplitude, or distant from the electrodes.[172] Abnormal postoperative aEEG background pattern and delay or lack of return to normal background (continuous normal voltage, sleep-wake cycling) have been found to predict motor and cognitive neurodevelopmental outcomes in infants with CHD.[67,68,69] Abnormal pre- and postoperative aEEG patterns have also been associated with brain injury in infants with CHD suggesting that aEEG may be a useful bedside neuromonitoring tool for early identification of infants at greatest risk for developing brain injury.[70,71]

Continuous Electroencephalography

Neonates with CHD are at risk of seizures in both the pre- and postoperative periods.[70,170,173,174] In a study of continuous electroencephalography (cEEG) during the postoperative period at a single center, electrographic seizures were observed in 8% of all CHD infants with a median onset time at 20 hours (interquartile range 15–34 hours) after return to the cardiac ICU. Clinical seizures with electrographic correlate occurred in 15% of patients while 85% of seizures were electrographic only with no clinical correlate. Status epilepticus, defined as a single seizure lasting >30 minutes or recurrent seizures lasting for at least 30 minutes during a 60-minute period, occurred in 62% of infants with seizures or 5% of all CHD infants. All infants with seizures in this study had diffuse or multifocal lesions identified on head ultrasound or brain MRI. Longer DHCA duration was associated with an increased risk for seizures in this study, similar to previous findings.[173,175] Given the strong association between seizures and CHD, cEEG should be considered in all neonates with CHD, particularly in the postoperative period, in order to better identify seizures and assist in the identification of underlying brain injury. This is of particular importance given the large proportion of subclinical or electrographic-only seizures in infants with CHD. The American Clinical Neurophysiology Society guideline on neonatal EEG monitoring recommends consideration for cEEG monitoring in high-risk populations where neonatal seizures are common, including in infants with severe CHD.[176]

Near-Infrared Spectroscopy

Near-infrared spectroscopy (NIRS) is a noninvasive bedside monitor that utilizes tissue oximeters to monitor hemoglobin oxygen saturation in a localized tissue bed. When placed on the head, NIRS provides real-time information on oxygenation of the cerebral cortex. NIRS has been shown to correlate well with superior vena cava oxygen saturation highlighting its utility as a cerebral monitor and there has been an increase in the use of this technology in CHD infants.[177,178] As an intraoperative neuromonitoring

system, NIRS has been shown to be a valuable tool in the assessment of hypocarbia and hypoxia and can alarm the surgical team to low cerebral perfusion when there are deviations from the expected changes in cerebral tissue oxygen saturation during cardiac surgery with cardiopulmonary bypass. Whether intraoperative NIRS is associated with improvements in neurodevelopmental outcomes remains uncertain as adverse neurodevelopmental outcomes have not been consistently associated with lower cerebral tissue oxygen saturation.[179] Pre- and postoperative changes in cerebral oxygenation are also not well understood and require further study.[179] Regardless, NIRS as a marker of cerebral oxygenation during the perioperative period is well-supported by the literature, and its use in combination with other neuromonitoring strategies provides significant benefit to the infant with CHD as well as the surgical and clinical care teams.

Key Contributors to Neurodevelopmental Outcomes in CHD

There are many risk factors of adverse neurodevelopmental outcomes in CHD, and these can be divided as those in the pre-, intra-, and postoperative periods (Fig. 16.4).

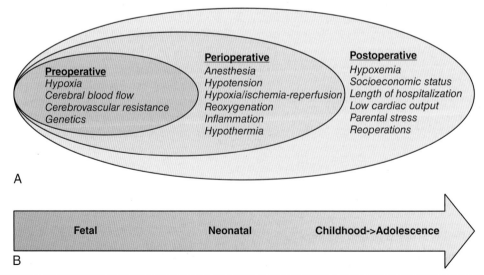

Fig. 16.4 Risk factors associated with neurodevelopment in congenital heart disease during progressive periods of brain development. (Reproduced with permission from Morton PD, Ishibashi N, Jonas RA, Gallo V. Congenital cardiac anomalies and white matter injury. *Trends Neurosci* 2015;38(6):353–363.)

PREOPERATIVE FACTORS

In the preoperative period, the presence of underlying genetic abnormalities is a significant risk factor for adverse neurodevelopmental outcomes in CHD.[10,11,19,180] Hypoxemia, beginning as early as the fetal period, contributes to brain dysmaturation in addition to brain injury, which has been linked to neurodevelopmental impairments in CHD.[122,181] Prenatal diagnosis has also been associated with improved brain maturation, reduced rates of brain injury, and improved neurodevelopmental outcomes in CHD. This is hypothesized to be due to improved hemodynamic stability in the preoperative period, although it requires further study.[97] Older age at neonatal surgical repair has also been associated with adverse neurodevelopmental outcomes in infants with TGA.[104]

INTRAOPERATIVE FACTORS

Several factors during the intraoperative period have been associated with neurodevelopmental outcomes in CHD including the use of cardiopulmonary bypass, lower hematocrit levels during cardiopulmonary bypass, and duration of DHCA. In two clinical trials investigating hematocrit levels during bypass, hematocrit levels lower than 24% were associated with poorer motor outcomes at 1 year of age; this has been observed in other studies and targeting higher hematocrits during cardiopulmonary bypass has been adopted widely.[182–184] The Boston Circulatory Arrest Trial, which compared neurodevelopmental outcomes in infants with TGA who underwent surgery with either DHCA or continuous low-flow cardiopulmonary bypass, observed poorer cognitive outcomes at 8 years of age in children who underwent DHCA for durations longer than 40 minutes.[185] However, there is significant variability of findings across studies suggesting that intraoperative management strategies likely contribute less to neurodevelopmental and cognitive abnormalities than previously believed.[19,186–188]

POSTOPERATIVE FACTORS

Postoperative complications such as prolonged mechanical ventilation, longer hospital stay, poor feeding, and growth have been associated with adverse neurodevelopmental outcomes in CHD.[10,189–191] Recent studies have also highlighted the importance of environmental influences on neurodevelopmental outcomes in CHD including SES, parental mental health, and the home environment.[101,116,192–194] Low SES and less maternal education have been associated with poorer neurodevelopmental outcomes in children with CHD.[193,194] Children and infants from low SES may also have alterations in brain structure and function.[195,196] Interestingly, higher maternal education, often used as a measure of SES, may mitigate the harmful effects of brain injury in preterm infants, a population with similar risk for brain injury and adverse neurodevelopmental outcomes as CHD infants.[197] Changes to public policies and providing additional support to families of children with CHD may potentially improve neurodevelopmental outcomes. Interdisciplinary cardiac neurodevelopmental follow-up programs are also critical for the early identification of high-risk children and implementation of neurodevelopmental supports.[10,198]

Neuroprotective Strategies Under Investigation

Through the 1990s and early 2000s, several large studies (e.g., Boston Circulatory Arrest Trial) focused on optimizing intraoperative factors such as cardiopulmonary bypass for the surgical management of CHD.[199] However, we have since learned that intraoperative surgical management strategies likely contribute less to neurodevelopmental and cognitive abnormalities in this population than previously believed.[18,24] Thus, there has been a shift in focus toward potential opportunities during the fetal, pre-, and postoperative periods to improve the brain health of neonates with CHD. Antenatally, brain dysmaturation has been associated with chronic hypoxia in fetuses with CHD. Given this link, recent studies have focused on maternal hyperoxygenation as a potential intervention to promote brain maturation and neurodevelopment in this population.[200] Maternal hyperoxygenation has been shown to increase cerebral blood oxygenation in fetuses with CHD,[137,201] however, further studies will need to determine whether this is associated with improved brain maturation. Several perioperative neuroprotection strategies are also currently under investigation. Most recently, erythropoietin was evaluated for neuroprotection in neonatal cardiac surgery; in a large pilot study, neurodevelopmental outcomes at 1 year of age were not improved by erythropoietin.[202] Studies of the role of corticosteroids, remote ischemic preconditioning, allopurinol, and mesenchymal stem cells in neuroprotection are currently underway.[203]

Knowledge Gaps and Future Directions

Although there have been significant advances in identifying and studying key contributors to neurodevelopmental outcomes in CHD, there are still several knowledge gaps that exist in understanding the ideal management of infants with CHD. With advances in genetic and genomic studies, there has been an increased understanding of the role of genetic alterations in etiology of CHD. Recent work has identified de novo mutations across hundreds of genes in individuals with isolated (nonsyndromic) CHD, with several genes involved in development of both the heart and the brain.[45–47] However, we still do not know the etiology of CHD in most patients or understand how these genetic alterations contribute to altered brain maturation and neurodevelopmental impairments in this population. Further, many de novo mutations have been found in histone-modifying genes; however, the contributions of epigenetic mechanisms to CHD are not well understood.[45,204] We have also gained significant insight into many potential mechanisms of brain dysmaturation in CHD; however, we do not yet have any treatments that may help to advance brain maturation during this period of rapid brain growth and maturation. Further, altered fetal circulation in fetuses with CHD coupled with impaired cerebral autoregulation in neonates with CHD may contribute to an increased risk for WMI during periods of hypoperfusion, including during transition after birth.[142,149] This link between alterations in cerebral blood flow and oxygenation during the perinatal transition period with preoperative brain injury in neonates with CHD requires further study. The survival of infants with CHD has improved significantly with advances in cardiac surgical and intensive care, and the current treatments with DHCA and cardiopulmonary bypass can be performed safely and without major injury to the infant's brain in the majority of cases. However, the ideal timing for surgery to optimize brain maturation and neurodevelopmental outcomes remains unknown. Finally, with an increasing proportion of patients with CHD being adults, longitudinal studies with neuroimaging and neuropsychological testing into adulthood are required to understand long-term neurocognitive and brain abnormalities in CHD.

Acknowledgments

We thank Dr. Steven P. Miller for his support and mentorship, as well as Ms. Vanna Kazazian for her contributions to a figure.

REFERENCES

1. Zimmerman MS, Smith AGC, Sable CA, et al. Global, regional, and national burden of congenital heart disease, 1990–2017: a systematic analysis for the Global Burden of Disease Study 2017. *Lancet Child Adolesc Health.* 2020;4(3):185-200. doi:10.1016/s 2352-4642(19)30402-x.
2. Liu Y, Chen S, Zühlke L, et al. Global birth prevalence of congenital heart defects 1970–2017: updated systematic review and meta-analysis of 260 studies. *Int J Epidemiol.* 2019;48(2): 455-463. doi:10.1093/ije/dyz009.
3. Reller MD, Strickland MJ, Riehle-Colarusso T, Mahle WT, Correa A. Prevalence of congenital heart defects in metropolitan Atlanta, 1998–2005. *J Pediatr.* 2008;153(6):807-813. doi:10.1016/j. jpeds.2008.05.059.
4. Hoffman JIE, Kaplan S. The incidence of congenital heart disease. *J Am Coll Cardiol.* 2002;39(12):1890-1900. doi:10.1016/ s0735-1097(02)01886-7.
5. Leirgul E, Fomina T, Brodwall K, et al. Birth prevalence of congenital heart defects in Norway 1994–2009—a nationwide study. *Am Heart J.* 2014;168(6):956-964. doi:10.1016/j.ahj.2014.07.030.
6. Wu W, He J, Shao X. Incidence and mortality trend of congenital heart disease at the global, regional, and national level, 1990–2017. *Medicine (Baltimore).* 2020;99(23):e20593. doi:10. 1097/MD.0000000000020593.
7. Oster ME, Lee KA, Honein MA, Riehle-Colarusso T, Shin M, Correa A. Temporal trends in survival among infants with critical congenital heart defects. *Pediatrics.* 2013;131(5):e1502-e1508. doi:10.1542/peds.2012-3435.
8. Warnes CA, Liberthson R, Danielson GK, et al. Task Force 1: the changing profile of congenital heart disease in adult life. *J Am Coll Cardiol.* 2001;37(5):1170-1175. doi:10.1016/ s0735-1097(01)01272-4.
9. Marelli AJ, Ionescu-Ittu R, Mackie AS, Guo L, Dendukuri N, Kaouache M. Lifetime prevalence of congenital heart disease in the general population from 2000 to 2010. *Circulation.* 2014;130(9):749-756. doi:10.1161/circulationaha.113.008396.
10. Marino BS, Lipkin PH, Newburger JW, et al. Neurodevelopmental outcomes in children with congenital heart disease: evaluation and management: a scientific statement from the American Heart Association. *Circulation.* 2012;126(9):1143-1172. doi:10. 1161/CIR.0b013e318265ee8a.
11. Wernovsky G. Current insights regarding neurological and developmental abnormalities in children and young adults with complex congenital cardiac disease. *Cardiol Young.* 2006; 16(S1):92-104. doi:10.1017/s1047951105002398.

12. Nattel SN, Adrianzen L, Kessler EC, et al. Congenital heart disease and neurodevelopment: clinical manifestations, genetics, mechanisms, and implications. *Can J Cardiol.* 2017; 33(12):1543-1555. doi:10.1016/j.cjca.2017.09.020.

13. Spillmann R, Polentarutti S, Ehrler M, Kretschmar O, Wehrle FM, Latal B. Congenital heart disease in school-aged children: cognition, education, and participation in leisure activities. *Pediatr Res.* 2021. doi:10.1038/s41390-021-01853-4.

14. Atallah J, Garcia Guerra G, Joffe AR, et al. Survival, neurocognitive, and functional outcomes after completion of staged surgical palliation in a cohort of patients with hypoplastic left heart syndrome. *J Am Heart Assoc.* 2020;9(4):e013632. doi:10.1161/jaha.119.013632.

15. Hiraiwa A, Ibuki K, Tanaka T, et al. Toddler neurodevelopmental outcomes are associated with school-age IQ in children with single ventricle physiology. *Semin Thorac Cardiovasc Surg.* 2020;32(2):302-310. doi:10.1053/j.semtcvs.2019.10.017.

16. Bellinger DC, Watson CG, Rivkin MJ, et al. Neuropsychological status and structural brain imaging in adolescents with single ventricle who underwent the Fontan procedure. *J Am Heart Assoc.* 2015;4(12):e002302. doi:10.1161/jaha.115.002302.

17. Gerstle M, Beebe DW, Drotar D, Cassedy A, Marino BS. Executive functioning and school performance among pediatric survivors of complex congenital heart disease. *J Pediatr.* 2016; 173:154-159. doi:10.1016/j.jpeds.2016.01.028.

18. Bellinger DC, Wypij D, Rivkin MJ, et al. Adolescents with d-transposition of the great arteries corrected with the arterial switch procedure. *Circulation.* 2011;124(12):1361-1369. doi:10.1161/circulationaha.111.026963.

19. Gaynor JW, Stopp C, Wypij D, et al. Neurodevelopmental outcomes after cardiac surgery in infancy. *Pediatrics.* 2015;135(5):816-825. doi:10.1542/peds.2014-3825.

20. Sananes R, Manlhiot C, Kelly E, et al. Neurodevelopmental outcomes after open heart operations before 3 months of age. *Ann Thorac Surg.* 2012;93(5):1577-1583. doi:10.1016/j.athoracsur.2012.02.011.

21. Gaudet I, Paquette N, Bernard C, et al. Neurodevelopmental outcome of children with congenital heart disease: a cohort study from infancy to preschool age. *J Pediatr.* 2021;239:126-135.e5. doi:10.1016/j.jpeds.2021.08.042.

22. Sananes R, Goldberg CS, Newburger JW, et al. Six-year neurodevelopmental outcomes for children with single-ventricle physiology. *Pediatrics.* 2021;147(2):e2020014589. doi:10.1542/peds.2020-014589.

23. Goldberg CS, Hu C, Brosig C, et al. Behavior and quality of life at 6 years for children with hypoplastic left heart syndrome. *Pediatrics.* 2019;144(5):e20191010. doi:10.1542/peds.2019-1010.

24. Bellinger DC, Newburger JW, Wypij D, Kuban KCK, Duplesssis AJ, Rappaport LA. Behaviour at eight years in children with surgically corrected transposition: The Boston Circulatory Arrest Trial. *Cardiol Young.* 2009;19(01):86-97. doi:10.1017/s1047951108003454.

25. Brosig CL, Mussatto KA, Kuhn EM, Tweddell JS. Psychosocial outcomes for preschool children and families after surgery for complex congenital heart disease. *Pediatr Cardiol.* 2007;28(4):255-262. doi:10.1007/s00246-006-0013-4.

26. Verrall CE, Yang JYM, Chen J, et al. Neurocognitive dysfunction and smaller brain volumes in adolescents and adults with a Fontan circulation. *Circulation.* 2021;143(9):878-891. doi:10.1161/CIRCULATIONAHA.120.048202.

27. Ehrler M, Latal B, Kretschmar O, Von Rhein M, O'Gorman Tuura R. Altered frontal white matter microstructure is associated with working memory impairments in adolescents with congenital heart disease: a diffusion tensor imaging study. *NeuroImage Clin.* 2020;25:102123. doi:10.1016/j.nicl.2019.102123.

28. Tyagi M, Fteropoulli T, Hurt CS, et al. Cognitive dysfunction in adult CHD with different structural complexity. *Cardiol Young.* 2017;27(5):851-859. doi:10.1017/S1047951116001396.

29. Ilardi D, Ono KE, Mccartney R, Book W, Stringer AY. Neurocognitive functioning in adults with congenital heart disease. *Congenit Heart Dis.* 2017;12(2):166-173. doi:10.1111/chd.12434.

30. Klouda L, Franklin WJ, Saraf A, Parekh DR, Schwartz DD. Neurocognitive and executive functioning in adult survivors of congenital heart disease. *Congenit Heart Dis.* 2017;12(1):91-98. doi:10.1111/chd.12409.

31. Bagge CN, Henderson VW, Laursen HB, Adelborg K, Olsen M, Madsen NL. Risk of dementia in adults with congenital heart disease: population-based cohort study. *Circulation.* 2018;137(18):1912-1920. doi:10.1161/CIRCULATIONAHA.117.029686.

32. Cocomello L, Dimagli A, Biglino G, Cornish R, Caputo M, Lawlor DA. Educational attainment in patients with congenital heart disease: a comprehensive systematic review and meta-analysis. *BMC Cardiovasc Disord.* 2021;21(1). doi:10.1186/s12872-021-02349-z.

33. Karsenty C, Maury P, Blot-Souletie N, et al. The medical history of adults with complex congenital heart disease affects their social development and professional activity. *Arch Cardiovasc Dis.* 2015;108(11):589-597. doi:10.1016/j.acvd.2015.06.004.

34. Zomer AC, Vaartjes I, Uiterwaal CS, et al. Social burden and lifestyle in adults with congenital heart disease. *Am J Cardiol.* 2012;109(11):1657-1663. doi:10.1016/j.amjcard.2012.01.397.

35. Mahle W, Clancy R, Moss E, Gerdes M, Jobes D, Wernovsky G. Neurodevelopmental outcome and lifestyle assessment in school-aged and adolescent children with hypoplastic left heart syndrome. *Pediatrics.* 2000;105(5):1082-1089. doi:10.1542/peds.105.5.1082.

36. Ye Z, Wang L, Yang T, et al. Maternal viral infection and risk of fetal congenital heart diseases: a meta-analysis of observational studies. *J Am Heart Assoc.* 2019;8(9):e011264. doi:10.1161/jaha.118.011264.

37. Lynch TA, Abel DE. Teratogens and congenital heart disease. *J Diagn Med Sonogr.* 2015;31(5):301-305. doi:10.1177/8756479315598524.

38. Helle E, Priest JR. Maternal obesity and diabetes mellitus as risk factors for congenital heart disease in the offspring. *J Am Heart Assoc.* 2020;9(8):e011541. doi:10.1161/jaha.119.011541.

39. Levy HL, Guldberg P, Güttler F, et al. Congenital heart disease in maternal phenylketonuria: report from the maternal PKU collaborative study. *Pediatr Res.* 2001;49(5):636-642. doi:10.1203/00006450-200105000-00005.

40. Dolk H, Mccullough N, Callaghan S, et al. Risk factors for congenital heart disease: The Baby Hearts Study, a population-based case-control study. *PLoS One.* 2020;15(2):e0227908. doi:10.1371/journal.pone.0227908.

41. Jenkins KJ, Correa A, Feinstein JA, et al. Noninherited risk factors and congenital cardiovascular defects: current knowledge. *Circulation.* 2007;115(23):2995-3014. doi:10.1161/circulationaha.106.183216.

42. Diab NS, Barish S, Dong W, et al. Molecular genetics and complex inheritance of congenital heart disease. *Genes.* 2021;12(7):1020. doi:10.3390/genes12071020.

43. Zaidi S, Brueckner M. Genetics and genomics of congenital heart disease. *Circ Res.* 2017;120(6):923-940. doi:10.1161/circresaha.116.309140.

44. Fahed AC, Gelb BD, Seidman JG, Seidman CE. Genetics of congenital heart disease. *Circ Res*. 2013;112(4):707-720. doi:10.1161/circresaha.112.300853.

45. Zaidi S, Choi M, Wakimoto H, et al. De novo mutations in histone-modifying genes in congenital heart disease. *Nature*. 2013;498(7453):220-223. doi:10.1038/nature12141.

46. Jin SC, Homsy J, Zaidi S, et al. Contribution of rare inherited and de novo variants in 2,871 congenital heart disease probands. *Nat Genet*. 2017;49(11):1593-1601. doi:10.1038/ng.3970.

47. Homsy J, Zaidi S, Shen Y, et al. De novo mutations in congenital heart disease with neurodevelopmental and other congenital anomalies. *Science*. 2015;350(6265):1262-1266. doi:10.1126/science.aac9396.

48. Basu M, Zhu JY, Lahaye S, et al. Epigenetic mechanisms underlying maternal diabetes-associated risk of congenital heart disease. *JCI Insight*. 2017;2(20):e95085. doi:10.1172/jci.insight.95085.

49. Chapman G, Moreau JLM, Eddie IP, et al. Functional genomics and gene-environment interaction highlight the complexity of congenital heart disease caused by Notch pathway variants. *Hum Mol Genet*. 2020;29(4):566-579. doi:10.1093/hmg/ddz270.

50. Warnes CA. Transposition of the great arteries. *Circulation*. 2006; 114(24):2699-2709. doi:10.1161/circulationaha.105.592352.

51. Freed MD, Heymann MA, Lewis AB, Roehl SL, Kensey RC. Prostaglandin E1 infants with ductus arteriosus-dependent congenital heart disease. *Circulation*. 1981;64(5):899-905. doi:10.1161/01.cir.64.5.899.

52. Rashkind WJ. Creation of an atrial septal defect without thoracotomy. *JAMA*. 1966;196(11):991. doi:10.1001/jama.1966.03100240125026.

53. Jatene AD, Fontes VF, Paulista PP, et al. Anatomic correction of transposition of the great vessels. *J Thorac Cardiovasc Surg*. 1976;72(3):364-370.

54. Tchervenkov CI, Jacobs JP, Weinberg PM, et al. The nomenclature, definition and classification of hypoplastic left heart syndrome. *Cardiol Young*. 2006;16(04):339-368. doi:10.1017/s1047951106000291.

55. Morris SA, Ethen MK, Penny DJ, et al. Prenatal diagnosis, birth location, surgical center, and neonatal mortality in infants with hypoplastic left heart syndrome. *Circulation*. 2014;129(3):285-292. doi:10.1161/circulationaha.113.003711.

56. Pinto NM, Morris SA, Moon-Grady AJ, Donofrio MT. Prenatal cardiac care: goals, priorities & gaps in knowledge in fetal cardiovascular disease: perspectives of the Fetal Heart Society. *Prog Pediatr Cardiol*. 2020;59:101312. doi:10.1016/j.ppedcard.2020.101312.

57. Brown DW, Cohen KE, O'Brien P, et al. Impact of prenatal diagnosis in survivors of initial palliation of single ventricle heart disease. *Pediatr Cardiol*. 2015;36(2):314-321. doi:10.1007/s00246-014-1005-4.

58. Mahle W, Clancy R, McGaurn S, Goin J, Clark B. Impact of prenatal diagnosis on survival and early neurologic morbidity in neonates with the hypoplastic left heart syndrome. *Pediatrics*. 2001;107(6):1277-1282. doi:10.1542/peds.107.6.1277.

59. Cowan F, Mercure E, Groenendaal F, et al. Does cranial ultrasound imaging identify arterial cerebral infarction in term neonates? *Arch Dis Child Fetal Neonatal Ed*. 2005;90(3):F252-F256. doi:10.1136/adc.2004.055558.

60. Sorokan ST, Jefferies AL, Miller SP. Imaging the term neonatal brain. *Paediatr Child Health*. 2018;23(5):322-328. doi:10.1093/pch/pxx161.

61. Chau V, Poskitt KJ, Sargent MA, et al. Comparison of computer tomography and magnetic resonance imaging scans on the third day of life in term newborns with neonatal encephalopathy. *Pediatrics*. 2009;123(1):319-326. doi:10.1542/peds.2008-0283.

62. Limperopoulos C, Tworetzky W, McElhinney DB, et al. Brain volume and metabolism in fetuses with congenital heart disease. *Circulation*. 2010;121(1):26-33. doi:10.1161/circulationaha.109.865568.

63. Clouchoux C, Du Plessis AJ, Bouyssi-Kobar M, et al. Delayed cortical development in fetuses with complex congenital heart disease. *Cereb Cortex*. 2013;23(12):2932-2943. doi:10.1093/cercor/bhs281.

64. Miller SP, Mcquillen PS, Hamrick S, et al. Abnormal brain development in newborns with congenital heart disease. *N Engl J Med*. 2007;357(19):1928-1938. doi:10.1056/nejmoa067393.

65. Feldmann M, Guo T, Miller SP, et al. Delayed maturation of the structural brain connectome in neonates with congenital heart disease. *Brain Commun*. 2020;2(2):fcaa209. doi:10.1093/braincomms/fcaa209.

66. De Asis-Cruz J, Donofrio MT, Vezina G, Limperopoulos C. Aberrant brain functional connectivity in newborns with congenital heart disease before cardiac surgery. *NeuroImage Clin*. 2018;17:31-42. doi:10.1016/j.nicl.2017.09.020.

67. Latal B, Wohlrab G, Brotschi B, Beck I, Knirsch W, Bernet V. Postoperative amplitude-integrated electroencephalography predicts four-year neurodevelopmental outcome in children with complex congenital heart disease. *J Pediatr*. 2016;178:55-60.e1. doi:10.1016/j.jpeds.2016.06.050.

68. Gunn JK, Beca J, Hunt RW, Olischar M, Shekerdemian LS. Perioperative amplitude-integrated EEG and neurodevelopment in infants with congenital heart disease. *Intensive Care Med*. 2012;38(9):1539-1547. doi:10.1007/s00134-012-2608-y.

69. Gunn JK, Beca J, Penny DJ, et al. Amplitude-integrated electroencephalography and brain injury in infants undergoing Norwood-type operations. *Ann Thorac Surg*. 2012;93(1):170-176. doi:10.1016/j.athoracsur.2011.08.014.

70. Claessens NHP, Noorlag L, Weeke LC, et al. Amplitude-integrated electroencephalography for early recognition of brain injury in neonates with critical congenital heart disease. *J Pediatr*. 2018;202:199-205.e1. doi:10.1016/j.jpeds.2018.06.048.

71. Mulkey SB, Yap VL, Bai S, et al. Amplitude-integrated EEG in newborns with critical congenital heart disease predicts preoperative brain magnetic resonance imaging findings. *Pediatr Neurol*. 2015;52(6):599-605. doi:10.1016/j.pediatrneurol.2015.02.026.

72. Claessens NHP, Breur J, Groenendaal F, et al. Brain microstructural development in neonates with critical congenital heart disease: an atlas-based diffusion tensor imaging study. *Neuroimage Clin*. 2019;21:101672. doi:10.1016/j.nicl.2019.101672.

73. Licht DJ, Shera DM, Clancy RR, et al. Brain maturation is delayed in infants with complex congenital heart defects. *J Thorac Cardiovasc Surg*. 2009;137(3):529-536; discussion 536-537. doi:10.1016/j.jtcvs.2008.10.025.

74. von Rhein M, Buchmann A, Hagmann C, et al. Severe congenital heart defects are associated with global reduction of neonatal brain volumes. *J Pediatr*. 2015;167(6):1259-1263.e1. doi:10.1016/j.jpeds.2015.07.006.

75. Ng IHX, Bonthrone AF, Kelly CJ, et al. Investigating altered brain development in infants with congenital heart disease using tensor-based morphometry. *Sci Rep*. 2020;10(1):14909. doi:10.1038/s41598-020-72009-3.

76. Claessens NHP, Moeskops P, Buchmann A, et al. Delayed cortical gray matter development in neonates with severe congenital heart disease. *Pediatr Res*. 2016;80(5):668-674. doi:10.1038/pr.2016.145.

77. Kelly CJ, Makropoulos A, Cordero-Grande L, et al. Impaired development of the cerebral cortex in infants with congenital heart disease is correlated to reduced cerebral oxygen

delivery. *Sci Rep*. 2017;7(1):15088. doi:10.1038/s41598-017-14939-z.

78. Ortinau C, Alexopoulos D, Dierker D, Van Essen D, Beca J, Inder T. Cortical folding is altered before surgery in infants with congenital heart disease. *J Pediatr*. 2013;163(5):1507-1510. doi:10.1016/j.jpeds.2013.06.045.

79. Ni Bhroin M, Abo Seada S, Bonthrone AF, et al. Reduced structural connectivity in cortico-striatal-thalamic network in neonates with congenital heart disease. *NeuroImage Clin*. 2020; 28:102423. doi:10.1016/j.nicl.2020.102423.

80. Stegeman R, Sprong MCA, Breur JMPJ, et al. Early motor outcomes in infants with critical congenital heart disease are related to neonatal brain development and brain injury. *Dev Med Child Neurol*. 2021;64(2):192-199. doi:10.1111/dmcn.15024.

81. Heye KN, Knirsch W, Latal B, et al. Reduction of brain volumes after neonatal cardiopulmonary bypass surgery in single-ventricle congenital heart disease before Fontan completion. *Pediatr Res*. 2018;83(1):63-70. doi:10.1038/pr.2017.203.

82. Claessens NHP, Algra SO, Ouwehand TL, et al. Perioperative neonatal brain injury is associated with worse school-age neurodevelopment in children with critical congenital heart disease. *Dev Med Child Neurol*. 2018;60(10):1052-1058. doi:10.1111/dmcn.13747.

83. Noorani S, Roy B, Sahib AK, et al. Caudate nuclei volume alterations and cognition and mood dysfunctions in adolescents with single ventricle heart disease. *J Neurosci Res*. 2020; 98(10):1877-1888. doi:10.1002/jnr.24667.

84. Cabrera-Mino C, Roy B, Woo MA, et al. Reduced brain mammillary body volumes and memory deficits in adolescents who have undergone the Fontan procedure. *Pediatr Res*. 2020; 87(1):169-175. doi:10.1038/s41390-019-0569-3.

85. Morton SU, Maleyeff L, Wypij D, et al. Abnormal left-hemispheric sulcal patterns correlate with neurodevelopmental outcomes in subjects with single ventricular congenital heart disease. *Cereb Cortex*. 2020;30(2):476-487. doi:10.1093/cercor/bhz101.

86. Watson CG, Stopp C, Wypij D, Bellinger DC, Newburger JW, Rivkin MJ. Altered white matter microstructure correlates with IQ and processing speed in children and adolescents post-Fontan. *J Pediatr*. 2018;200:140-149.e4. doi:10.1016/j.jpeds.2018.04.022.

87. Singh S, Kumar R, Roy B, et al. Regional brain gray matter changes in adolescents with single ventricle heart disease. *Neurosci Lett*. 2018;665:156-162. doi:10.1016/j.neulet.2017.12.011.

88. Ehrler M, Schlosser L, Brugger P, et al. Altered white matter microstructure is related to cognition in adults with congenital heart disease. *Brain Commun*. 2021;3(1):fcaa224. doi:10.1093/braincomms/fcaa224.

89. Lynch JM, Mavroudis CD, Ko TS, et al. Association of ongoing cerebral oxygen extraction during deep hypothermic circulatory arrest with postoperative brain injury. *Semin Thorac Cardiovasc Surg*. 2022;34(4):1275-1284. doi:10.1053/j.semtcvs.2021.08.026.

90. Peyvandi S, Lim JM, Marini D, et al. Fetal brain growth and risk of postnatal white matter injury in critical congenital heart disease. *J Thorac Cardiovasc Surg*. 2021;162(3):1007-1014.e1. doi:10.1016/j.jtcvs.2020.09.096.

91. Schlatterer SD, Govindan RB, Murnick J, et al. In infants with congenital heart disease autonomic dysfunction is associated with pre-operative brain injury. *Pediatr Res*. 2021. doi:10.1038/s41390-021-01931-7.

92. Kelly CJ, Christiaens D, Batalle D, et al. Abnormal microstructural development of the cerebral cortex in neonates with congenital heart disease is associated with impaired cerebral oxygen delivery. *J Am Heart Assoc*. 2019;8(5):e009893. doi:10.1161/jaha.118.009893.

93. Kelly CJ, Arulkumaran S, Tristão Pereira C, et al. Neuroimaging findings in newborns with congenital heart disease prior to surgery: an observational study. *Arch Dis Child*. 2019; 104(11):1042-1048. doi:10.1136/archdischild-2018-314822.

94. Peyvandi S, Kim H, Lau J, et al. The association between cardiac physiology, acquired brain injury, and postnatal brain growth in critical congenital heart disease. *J Thorac Cardiovasc Surg*. 2018;155(1):291-300.e3. doi:10.1016/j.jtcvs.2017.08.019.

95. Schmithorst VJ, Votava-Smith JK, Tran N, et al. Structural network topology correlates of microstructural brain dysmaturation in term infants with congenital heart disease. *Hum Brain Mapp*. 2018;39(11):4593-4610. doi:10.1002/hbm.24308.

96. Fogel MA, Li C, Elci OU, et al. Neurological injury and cerebral blood flow in single ventricles throughout staged surgical reconstruction. *Circulation*. 2017;135(7):671-682. doi:10.1161/circulationaha.116.021724.

97. Peyvandi S, De Santiago V, Chakkarapani E, et al. Association of prenatal diagnosis of critical congenital heart disease with postnatal brain development and the risk of brain injury. *JAMA Pediatr*. 2016;170(4):e154450. doi:10.1001/jamapediatrics.2015.4450.

98. Andropoulos DB, Hunter JV, Nelson DP, et al. Brain immaturity is associated with brain injury before and after neonatal cardiac surgery with high-flow bypass and cerebral oxygenation monitoring. *J Thorac Cardiovasc Surg*. 2010;139(3): 543-556. doi:10.1016/j.jtcvs.2009.08.022.

99. Mcquillen PS, Hamrick SEG, Perez MJ, et al. Balloon atrial septostomy is associated with preoperative stroke in neonates with transposition of the great arteries. *Circulation*. 2006;113(2): 280-285. doi:10.1161/circulationaha.105.566752.

100. Mahle WT, Tavani F, Zimmerman RA, et al. An MRI study of neurological injury before and after congenital heart surgery. *Circulation*. 2002;106(12 suppl 1):I109-I114. doi:10.1161/01.cir.0000032908.33237.b1.

101. Bonthrone AF, Chew A, Kelly CJ, et al. Cognitive function in toddlers with congenital heart disease: the impact of a stimulating home environment. *Infancy*. 2021;26(1):184-199. doi:10.1111/infa.12376.

102. Kuhn VA, Carpenter JL, Zurakowski D, et al. Determinants of neurological outcome in neonates with congenital heart disease following heart surgery. *Pediatr Res*. 2021;89(5):1283-1290. doi:10.1038/s41390-020-1085-1.

103. Hottinger SJ, Liamlahi R, Feldmann M, Knirsch W, Latal B, Hagmann CF. Postoperative improvement of brain maturation in infants with congenital heart disease. *Semin Thorac Cardiovasc Surg*. 2022 Spring;34(1):251-259. doi:10.1053/j.semtcvs.2020.11.029.

104. Lim JM, Porayette P, Marini D, et al. Associations between age at arterial switch operation, brain growth, and development in infants with transposition of the great arteries. *Circulation*. 2019;139(24):2728-2738. doi:10.1161/circulationaha.118.037495.

105. Meuwly E, Feldmann M, Knirsch W, et al. Postoperative brain volumes are associated with one-year neurodevelopmental outcome in children with severe congenital heart disease. *Sci Rep*. 2019;9(1):10885. doi:10.1038/s41598-019-47328-9.

106. Peyvandi S, Chau V, Guo T, et al. Neonatal brain injury and timing of neurodevelopmental assessment in patients with congenital heart disease. *J Am Coll Cardiol*. 2018;71(18):1986-1996. doi:10.1016/j.jacc.2018.02.068.

107. Rollins CK, Asaro LA, Akhondi-Asl A, et al. White matter volume predicts language development in congenital heart disease. *J Pediatr*. 2017;181:42-48.e2. doi:10.1016/j.jpeds.2016.09.070.

108. Rollins CK, Ortinau CM, Stopp C, et al. Regional brain growth trajectories in fetuses with congenital heart disease. *Ann Neurol.* 2021;89(1):143-157. doi:10.1002/ana.25940.

109. Inversetti A, Fesslova V, Deprest J, Candiani M, Giorgione V, Cavoretto P. Prenatal growth in fetuses with isolated cyanotic and non-cyanotic congenital heart defects. *Fetal Diagn Ther.* 2020;47(suppl 5):411-419. doi:10.1159/000493938.

110. Ruiz A, Cruz-Lemini M, Masoller N, et al. Longitudinal changes in fetal biometry and cerebroplacental hemodynamics in fetuses with congenital heart disease. *Ultrasound Obstet Gynecol.* 2017;49(3):379-386. doi:10.1002/uog.15970.

111. Ortinau CM, Rollins CK, Gholipour A, et al. Early-emerging sulcal patterns are atypical in fetuses with congenital heart disease. *Cereb Cortex.* 2019;29(8):3605-3616. doi:10.1093/cercor/bhy235.

112. Paladini D, Finarelli A, Donarini G, et al. Frontal lobe growth is impaired in fetuses with congenital heart disease. *Ultrasound Obstet Gynecol.* 2021;57(5):776-782. doi:10.1002/uog.22127.

113. Ren JY, Zhu M, Dong SZ. Three-dimensional volumetric magnetic resonance imaging detects early alterations of the brain growth in fetuses with congenital heart disease. *J Magn Reson Imaging.* 2021;54(1):263-272. doi:10.1002/jmri.27526.

114. Ren JY, Ji H, Zhu M, Dong SZ. DWI in brains of fetuses with congenital heart disease: a case-control MR imaging study. *Am J Neuroradiol.* 2021;42(11):2040-2045. doi:10.3174/ajnr.a7267.

115. Jaimes C, Rofeberg V, Stopp C, et al. Association of isolated congenital heart disease with fetal brain maturation. *Am J Neuroradiol.* 2020;41(8):1525-1531. doi:10.3174/ajnr.a6635.

116. Wu Y, Kapse K, Jacobs M, et al. Association of maternal psychological distress with in utero brain development in fetuses with congenital heart disease. *JAMA Pediatr.* 2020;174(3):e195316. doi:10.1001/jamapediatrics.2019.5316.

117. Claessens NHP, Khalili N, Isgum I, et al. Brain and CSF volumes in fetuses and neonates with antenatal diagnosis of critical congenital heart disease: a longitudinal MRI study. *Am J Neuroradiol.* 2019;40(5):885-891. doi:10.3174/ajnr.a6021.

118. Olshaker H, Ber R, Hoffman D, Derazne E, Achiron R, Katorza E. Volumetric brain MRI study in fetuses with congenital heart disease. *Am J Neuroradiol.* 2018;39(6):1164-1169. doi:10.3174/ajnr.a5628.

119. Rajagopalan V, Votava-Smith JK, Zhuang X, et al. Fetuses with single ventricle congenital heart disease manifest impairment of regional brain growth. *Prenat Diagn.* 2018;38(13):1042-1048. doi:10.1002/pd.5374.

120. Wong A, Chavez T, O'Neil S, et al. Synchronous aberrant cerebellar and opercular development in fetuses and neonates with congenital heart disease: correlation with early communicative neurodevelopmental outcomes, initial experience. *AJP Rep.* 2017;7(1):e17-e27. doi:10.1055/s-0036-1597934.

121. Masoller N, Sanz-Cortés M, Crispi F, et al. Mid-gestation brain Doppler and head biometry in fetuses with congenital heart disease predict abnormal brain development at birth. *Ultrasound Obstet Gynecol.* 2016;47(1):65-73. doi:10.1002/uog.14919.

122. Sun L, Macgowan CK, Sled JG, et al. Reduced fetal cerebral oxygen consumption is associated with smaller brain size in fetuses with congenital heart disease. *Circulation.* 2015;131(15):1313-1323. doi:10.1161/CIRCULATIONAHA.114.013051.

123. Chavali M, Ulloa-Navas M, Pérez-Borredá P, et al. Wnt-dependent oligodendroglial-endothelial interactions regulate white matter vascularization and attenuate injury. *Neuron.* 2020;108(6):1130-1145.e5. doi:10.1016/j.neuron.2020.09.033.

124. Kinnear C, Haranal M, Shannon P, Jaeggi E, Chitayat D, Mital S. Abnormal fetal cerebral and vascular development in hypoplastic left heart syndrome. *Prenat Diagn.* 2019;39(1):38-44. doi:10.1002/pd.5395.

125. Lange C, Turrero Garcia M, Decimo I, et al. Relief of hypoxia by angiogenesis promotes neural stem cell differentiation by targeting glycolysis. *EMBO J.* 2016;35(9):924-941. doi:10.15252/embj.201592372.

126. Morton PD, Korotcova L, Lewis BK, et al. Abnormal neurogenesis and cortical growth in congenital heart disease. *Sci Transl Med.* 2017;9(374):eaah7029. doi:10.1126/scitranslmed.aah7029.

127. Agematsu K, Korotcova L, Scafidi J, Gallo V, Jonas RA, Ishibashi N. Effects of preoperative hypoxia on white matter injury associated with cardiopulmonary bypass in a rodent hypoxic and brain slice model. *Pediatr Res.* 2014;75(5):618-625. doi:10.1038/pr.2014.9.

128. Yuen TJ, Silbereis JC, Griveau A, et al. Oligodendrocyte-encoded HIF function couples postnatal myelination and white matter angiogenesis. *Cell.* 2014;158(2):383-396. doi:10.1016/j.cell.2014.04.052.

129. Sun L, van Amerom JFP, Marini D, et al. MRI characterization of hemodynamic patterns of human fetuses with cyanotic congenital heart disease. *Ultrasound Obstet Gynecol.* 2021;58(6):824-836. doi:10.1002/uog.23707.

130. van Tilborg E, de Theije CGM, van Hal M, et al. Origin and dynamics of oligodendrocytes in the developing brain: implications for perinatal white matter injury. *Glia.* 2018;66(2):221-238. doi:10.1002/glia.23256.

131. Back SA, Han BH, Luo NL, et al. Selective vulnerability of late oligodendrocyte progenitors to hypoxia-ischemia. *J Neurosci.* 2002;22(2):455-463. doi:10.1523/jneurosci.22-02-00455.2002.

132. Back SA, Luo NL, Borenstein NS, Levine JM, Volpe JJ, Kinney HC. Late oligodendrocyte progenitors coincide with the developmental window of vulnerability for human perinatal white matter injury. *J Neurosci.* 2001;21(4):1302-1312. doi:10.1523/jneurosci.21-04-01302.2001.

133. Srivastava T, Diba P, Dean JM, et al. A TLR/AKT/FoxO3 immune tolerance-like pathway disrupts the repair capacity of oligodendrocyte progenitors. *J Clin Investig.* 2018;128(5):2025-2041. doi:10.1172/jci94158.

134. Segovia KN, Mcclure M, Moravec M, et al. Arrested oligodendrocyte lineage maturation in chronic perinatal white matter injury. *Ann Neurol.* 2008;63(4):520-530. doi:10.1002/ana.21359.

135. Buser JR, Maire J, Riddle A, et al. Arrested preoligodendrocyte maturation contributes to myelination failure in premature infants. *Ann Neurol.* 2012;71(1):93-109. doi:10.1002/ana.22627.

136. Back SA. White matter injury in the preterm infant: pathology and mechanisms. *Acta Neuropathol.* 2017;134(3):331-349. doi:10.1007/s00401-017-1718-6.

137. Peyvandi S, Xu D, Wang Y, et al. Fetal cerebral oxygenation is impaired in congenital heart disease and shows variable response to maternal hyperoxia. *J Am Heart Assoc.* 2021;10(1):e018777. doi:10.1161/jaha.120.018777.

138. Maternal Hyperoxygenation in Congenital Heart Disease (MATCH) ClinicalTrials.gov Identifier: NCT03136835. Updated April 13, 2021. Accessed January 31, 2022.

139. Claessens NHP, Chau V, De Vries LS, et al. Brain injury in infants with critical congenital heart disease: insights from two clinical cohorts with different practice approaches. *J Pediatr.* 2019;215:75-82.e2. doi:10.1016/j.jpeds.2019.07.017.

140. Block AJ, Mcquillen PS, Chau V, et al. Clinically silent preoperative brain injuries do not worsen with surgery in neonates

with congenital heart disease. *J Thorac Cardiovasc Surg.* 2010;140(3):550-557. doi:10.1016/j.jtcvs.2010.03.035.

141. Beca J, Gunn JK, Coleman L, et al. New white matter brain injury after infant heart surgery is associated with diagnostic group and the use of circulatory arrest. *Circulation.* 2013;127(9): 971-979. doi:10.1161/circulationaha.112.001089.

142. Votava-Smith JK, Statile CJ, Taylor MD, et al. Impaired cerebral autoregulation in preoperative newborn infants with congenital heart disease. *J Thorac Cardiovasc Surg.* 2017;154(3):1038-1044. doi:10.1016/j.jtcvs.2017.05.045.

143. Guo T, Chau V, Peyvandi S, et al. White matter injury in term neonates with congenital heart diseases: topology & comparison with preterm newborns. *NeuroImage.* 2019;185:742-749. doi:10.1016/j.neuroimage.2018.06.004.

144. Mandalenakis Z, Rosengren A, Lappas G, Eriksson P, Hansson PO, Dellborg M. Ischemic stroke in children and young adults with congenital heart disease. *J Am Heart Assoc.* 2016;5(2): e003071. doi:10.1161/jaha.115.003071.

145. Giang KW, Fedchenko M, Dellborg M, Eriksson P, Mandalenakis Z. Burden of ischemic stroke in patients with congenital heart disease: a nationwide, case-control study. *J Am Heart Assoc.* 2021;10(13):e020939. doi:10.1161/jaha.120.020939.

146. Rodan L, Mccrindle BW, Manlhiot C, et al. Stroke recurrence in children with congenital heart disease. *Ann Neurol.* 2012;72(1):103-111. doi:10.1002/ana.23574.

147. Morton PD, Ishibashi N, Jonas RA, Gallo V. Congenital cardiac anomalies and white matter injury. *Trends Neurosci.* 2015; 38(6):353-363. doi:10.1016/j.tins.2015.04.001.

148. Dimitropoulos A, Mcquillen PS, Sethi V, et al. Brain injury and development in newborns with critical congenital heart disease. *Neurology.* 2013;81(3):241-248. doi:10.1212/wnl. 0b013e31829bfdcf.

149. Peyvandi S, Donofrio MT. Circulatory changes and cerebral blood flow and oxygenation during transition in newborns with congenital heart disease. *Semin Pediatr Neurol.* 2018;28: 38-47. doi:10.1016/j.spen.2018.05.005.

150. Mcquillen PS, Goff DA, Licht DJ. Effects of congenital heart disease on brain development. *Prog Pediatr Cardiol.* 2010; 29(2):79-85. doi:10.1016/j.ppedcard.2010.06.011.

151. Petit CJ, Rome JJ, Wernovsky G, et al. Preoperative brain injury in transposition of the great arteries is associated with oxygenation and time to surgery, not balloon atrial septostomy. *Circulation.* 2009;119(5):709-716. doi:10.1161/ CIRCULATIONAHA.107.760819.

152. Lynch JM, Buckley EM, Schwab PJ, et al. Time to surgery and preoperative cerebral hemodynamics predict postoperative white matter injury in neonates with hypoplastic left heart syndrome. *J Thorac Cardiovasc Surg.* 2014;148(5):2181-2188. doi:10.1016/j.jtcvs.2014.05.081.

153. Dhari Z, Leonetti C, Lin S, et al. Impact of cardiopulmonary bypass on neurogenesis and cortical maturation. *Ann Neurol.* 2021;90(6):913-926. doi:10.1002/ana.26235.

154. Mcquillen PS, Barkovich AJ, Hamrick SEG, et al. Temporal and anatomic risk profile of brain injury with neonatal repair of congenital heart defects. *Stroke.* 2007;38(2):736-741. doi:10.1161/01.str.0000247941.41234.90.

155. Galli KK, Zimmerman RA, Jarvik GP, et al. Periventricular leukomalacia is common after neonatal cardiac surgery. *J Thorac Cardiovasc Surg.* 2004;127(3):692-704. doi:10.1016/j. jtcvs.2003.09.053.

156. Stegeman R, Feldmann M, Claessens NHP, et al. A uniform description of perioperative brain MRI findings in infants with severe congenital heart disease: results of a European collaboration. *Am J Neuroradiol.* 2021;42(11):2034-2039. doi:10.3174/ajnr.a7328.

157. Claessens NHP, Algra SO, Jansen NJG, et al. Clinical and neuroimaging characteristics of cerebral sinovenous thrombosis in neonates undergoing cardiac surgery. *J Thorac Cardiovasc Surg.* 2018;155(3):1150-1158. doi:10.1016/j.jtcvs.2017.10.083.

158. Egbe AC, Connolly HM, McLeod CJ, et al. Thrombotic and embolic complications associated with atrial arrhythmia after Fontan operation: role of prophylactic therapy. *J Am Coll Cardiol.* 2016;68(12):1312-1319. doi:10.1016/j.jacc.2016.06.056.

159. Egbe AC, Connolly HM, Niaz T, et al. Prevalence and outcome of thrombotic and embolic complications in adults after Fontan operation. *Am Heart J.* 2017;183:10-17. doi:10.1016/j. ahj.2016.09.014.

160. Martínez-Quintana E, Rodríguez-González F. Thrombocytopenia in congenital heart disease patients. *Platelets.* 2015; 26(5):432-436. doi:10.3109/09537104.2014.925104.

161. Ichord R. Cerebral sinovenous thrombosis. *Front Pediatr.* 2017;5:163. doi:10.3389/fped.2017.00163.

162. Kelly P, Hayman R, Shekerdemian LS, et al. Subdural hemorrhage and hypoxia in infants with congenital heart disease. *Pediatrics.* 2014;134(3):e773-e781. doi:10.1542/peds.2013-3903.

163. Tavani F, Zimmerman RA, Clancy RR, Licht DJ, Mahle WT. Incidental intracranial hemorrhage after uncomplicated birth: MRI before and after neonatal heart surgery. *Neuroradiology.* 2003;45(4):253-258. doi:10.1007/s00234-003-0946-8.

164. Carney O, Hughes E, Tusor N, et al. Incidental findings on brain MR imaging of asymptomatic term neonates in the Developing Human Connectome Project. *EClinicalMedicine.* 2021;38:100984. doi:10.1016/j.eclinm.2021.100984.

165. Ortinau CM, Anadkat JS, Smyser CD, Eghtesady P. Intraventricular hemorrhage in moderate to severe congenital heart disease. *Pediatr Crit Care Med.* 2018;19(1):56-63. doi:10.1097/ pcc.0000000000001374.

166. Patel N, Banahan C, Janus J, et al. Perioperative cerebral microbleeds after adult cardiac surgery. *Stroke.* 2019;50(2): 336-343. doi:10.1161/strokeaha.118.023355.

167. Kim PPC, Nasman BW, Kinne EL, Oyoyo UE, Kido DK, Jacobson JP. Cerebral microhemorrhage: a frequent magnetic resonance imaging finding in pediatric patients after cardiopulmonary bypass. *J Clin Imaging Sci.* 2017;7:27. doi:10. 4103/jcis.JCIS_29_17.

168. Soul JS, Robertson RL, Wypij D, et al. Subtle hemorrhagic brain injury is associated with neurodevelopmental impairment in infants with repaired congenital heart disease. *J Thorac Cardiovasc Surg.* 2009;138(2):374-381. doi:10.1016/ j.jtcvs.2009.02.027.

169. Ter Horst HJ, Mud M, Roofthooft MTR, Bos AF. Amplitude integrated electroencephalographic activity in infants with congenital heart disease before surgery. *Early Hum Dev.* 2010; 86(12):759-764. doi:10.1016/j.earlhumdev.2010.08.028.

170. Mebius MJ, Oostdijk NJE, Kuik SJ, et al. Amplitude-integrated electroencephalography during the first 72 h after birth in neonates diagnosed prenatally with congenital heart disease. *Pediatr Res.* 2018;83(4):798-803. doi:10.1038/pr.2017.311.

171. Scher MS, Alvin J, Gaus L, Minnigh B, Painter MJ. Uncoupling of EEG-clinical neonatal seizures after antiepileptic drug use. *Pediatr Neurol.* 2003;28(4):277-280. doi:10.1016/s0887-8994 (02)00621-5.

172. Rakshasbhuvankar A, Paul S, Nagarajan L, Ghosh S, Rao S. Amplitude-integrated EEG for detection of neonatal seizures: a systematic review. *Seizure.* 2015;33:90-98. doi:10.1016/j. seizure.2015.09.014.

173. Naim MY, Gaynor JW, Chen J, et al. Subclinical seizures identified by postoperative electroencephalographic monitoring are common after neonatal cardiac surgery. *J Thorac*

Cardiovasc Surg. 2015;150(1):169-180. doi:10.1016/j.jtcvs.2015.03.045.

174. Clancy RR, McGaurn SA, Wernovsky G, et al. Risk of seizures in survivors of newborn heart surgery using deep hypothermic circulatory arrest. *Pediatrics.* 2003;111:592-601.

175. Gaynor JW, Nicolson SC, Jarvik GP, et al. Increasing duration of deep hypothermic circulatory arrest is associated with an increased incidence of postoperative electroencephalographic seizures. *J Thorac Cardiovasc Surg.* 2005;130(5):1278-1286. doi:10.1016/j.jtcvs.2005.02.065.

176. Shellhaas RA, Chang T, Tsuchida T, et al. The American Clinical Neurophysiology Society's Guideline on continuous electroencephalography monitoring in neonates. *J Clin Neurophysiol.* 2011;28:611-617.

177. Reagor JA, Clingan S, Kulat BT, Matte GS, Voss J, Tweddell JS. The Norwood Stage 1 procedure—conduct of perfusion: 2017 Survey results from NPC-QIC member institutions. *Perfusion.* 2018;33(8):667-678. doi:10.1177/0267659118781173.

178. Harvey B, Shann KG, Fitzgerald D, et al. International pediatric perfusion practice: 2011 survey results. *J Extra Corpor Technol.* 2012;44:186-193.

179. Zaleski KL, Kussman BD. Near-infrared spectroscopy in pediatric congenital heart disease. *J Cardiothorac Vasc Anesth.* 2020;34(2):489-500. doi:10.1053/j.jvca.2019.08.048.

180. Homsy J, Zaidi S, Shen Y, et al. De novo mutations in congenital heart disease with neurodevelopmental and other congenital anomalies. *Science.* 2015;350(6265):1262-1266.

181. Khairy P, Poirier N, Mercier LAE. Univentricular heart. *Circulation.* 2007;115(6):800-812. doi:10.1161/circulationaha.105.592378.

182. Newburger JW, Jonas RA, Soul J, et al. Randomized trial of hematocrit 25% versus 35% during hypothermic cardiopulmonary bypass in infant heart surgery. *J Thorac Cardiovasc Surg.* 2008;135(2):347-354.e4. doi:10.1016/j.jtcvs.2007.01.051.

183. Wypij D, Jonas RA, Bellinger DC, et al. The effect of hematocrit during hypothermic cardiopulmonary bypass in infant heart surgery: results from the combined Boston hematocrit trials. *J Thorac Cardiovasc Surg.* 2008;135(2):355-360. doi:10.1016/j.jtcvs.2007.03.067.

184. Hirsch JC, Jacobs ML, Andropoulos D, et al. Protecting the infant brain during cardiac surgery: a systematic review. *Ann Thorac Surg.* 2012;94(4):1365-1373. doi:10.1016/j.athoracsur.2012.05.135.

185. Wypij D, Newburger JW, Rappaport LA, et al. The effect of duration of deep hypothermic circulatory arrest in infant heart surgery on late neurodevelopment: The Boston Circulatory Arrest Trial. *J Thorac Cardiovasc Surg.* 2003;126(5):1397-1403. doi:10.1016/s0022-5223(03)00940-1.

186. Wernovsky G, Licht DJ. Neurodevelopmental outcomes in children with congenital heart disease—what can we impact? *Pediatr Crit Care Med.* 2016;17:S232-S242. doi:10.1097/pcc.0000000000000800.

187. Gaynor JW, Stopp C, Wypij D, et al. Impact of operative and postoperative factors on neurodevelopmental outcomes after cardiac operations. *Ann Thorac Surg.* 2016;102(3):843-849. doi:10.1016/j.athoracsur.2016.05.081.

188. Newburger JW, Sleeper LA, Bellinger DC, et al. Early developmental outcome in children with hypoplastic left heart syndrome and related anomalies. *Circulation.* 2012;125(17):2081-2091. doi:10.1161/circulationaha.111.064113.

189. Khalid OM, Harrison TM. Early neurodevelopmental outcomes in children with hypoplastic left heart syndrome and related anomalies after hybrid procedure. *Pediatr Cardiol.* 2019;40(8):1591-1598. doi:10.1007/s00246-019-02191-3.

190. Reich B, Heye K, Tuura R, et al. Neurodevelopmental outcome and health-related quality of life in children with single-ventricle heart disease before Fontan procedure. *Semin Thorac Cardiovasc Surg.* 2017;S1043-0679(17)30288-5. doi:10.1053/j.semtcvs.2017.09.014.

191. Goldberg CS, Lu M, Sleeper LA, et al. Factors associated with neurodevelopment for children with single ventricle lesions. *J Pediatr.* 2014;165(3):490-496.e8. doi:10.1016/j.jpeds.2014.05.019.

192. Roberts SD, Kazazian V, Ford MK, et al. The association between parent stress, coping and mental health, and neurodevelopmental outcomes of infants with congenital heart disease. *Clin Neuropsychol.* 2021;35(5):948-972. doi:10.1080/13854046.2021.1896037.

193. Bucholz EM, Sleeper LA, Goldberg CS, et al. Socioeconomic status and long-term outcomes in single ventricle heart disease. *Pediatrics.* 2020;146(4):e20201240. doi:10.1542/peds.2020-1240.

194. Bucholz EM, Sleeper LA, Sananes R, et al. Trajectories in neurodevelopmental, health-related quality of life, and functional status outcomes by socioeconomic status and maternal education in children with single ventricle heart disease. *J Pediatr.* 2021;229:289-293.e3. doi:10.1016/j.jpeds.2020.09.066.

195. Brito NH, Troller-Renfree SV, Leon-Santos A, Isler JR, Fifer WP, Noble KG. Associations among the home language environment and neural activity during infancy. *Dev Cogn Neurosci.* 2020;43:100780. doi:10.1016/j.dcn.2020.100780.

196. Noble KG, Houston SM, Brito NH, et al. Family income, parental education and brain structure in children and adolescents. *Nat Neurosci.* 2015;18(5):773-778. doi:10.1038/nn.3983.

197. Benavente-Fernandez I, Synnes A, Grunau RE, et al. Association of socioeconomic status and brain injury with neurodevelopmental outcomes of very preterm children. *JAMA Netw Open.* 2019;2(5):e192914.doi:10.1001/jamanetworkopen.2019.2914.

198. Chorna O, Baldwin HS, Neumaier J, et al. Feasibility of a team approach to complex congenital heart defect neurodevelopmental follow-up. *Cir Cardiovasc Qual Outcomes.* 2016;9(4):432-440. doi:10.1161/circoutcomes.116.002614.

199. Newburger JW, Jonas RA, Wernovsky G, et al. A comparison of the perioperative neurologic effects of hypothermic circulatory arrest versus low-flow cardiopulmonary bypass in infant heart surgery. *N Engl J Med.* 1993;329(15):1057-1064. doi:10.1056/nejm199310073291501.

200. Lee FT, Marini D, Seed M, Sun L. Maternal hyperoxygenation in congenital heart disease. *Transl Pediatr.* 2021;10(8):2197-2209. doi:10.21037/tp-20-226.

201. You W, Andescavage NN, Kapse K, Donofrio MT, Jacobs M, Limperopoulos C. Hemodynamic responses of the placenta and brain to maternal hyperoxia in fetuses with congenital heart disease by using blood oxygen–level dependent MRI. *Radiology.* 2020;294(1):141-148. doi:10.1148/radiol.2019190751.

202. Andropoulos DB, Brady K, Easley RB, et al. Erythropoietin neuroprotection in neonatal cardiac surgery: a phase I/II safety and efficacy trial. *J Thorac Cardiovasc Surg.* 2013;146(1):124-131. doi:10.1016/j.jtcvs.2012.09.046.

203. Kobayashi K, Liu C, Jonas RA, Ishibashi N. The current status of neuroprotection in congenital heart disease. *Children.* 2021;8(12):1116. doi:10.3390/children8121116.

204. Wu Y, Jin X, Zhang Y, Zheng J, Yang R. Genetic and epigenetic mechanisms in the development of congenital heart diseases. *World J Pediatr Surg.* 2021;4(2):e000196. doi:10.1136/wjps-2020-000196.

Chapter 17

Neurodevelopmental Outcomes Following Very Preterm Birth: What Clinicians Need to Know

Peter Anderson (John) and Samudragupta Bora

Chapter Outline

Introduction

The vast majority of children born very preterm (<32 weeks' gestation) now survive, with survival rates increasing significantly over the past three decades due to advances in obstetric and neonatal care.[1] While important, survival is only one outcome, and it is possible that reductions in mortality are associated with increases in short- and long-term morbidity. Long-term outcome studies of children born very preterm are essential for determining the true benefits and consequences of new interventions and changes to management practices. Reliable outcome data is critical for clinical decision-making, counseling families, and structuring surveillance programs for individual children and their families. As such, it is recommended that perinatal health professionals have a strong understanding of the long-term outcomes following very preterm birth; however, this is not the case with health professionals tending to overestimate major disability in children born extremely preterm.[2,3]

While there is undeniable evidence that children born very preterm are at risk for a spectrum of developmental challenges, reviewing the literature can be daunting given the thousands of published papers on this topic. This chapter will begin with a brief summary of the long-term neurodevelopmental impairments associated with very preterm birth, followed by a discussion on how group-based data can often portray an overly negative perception of long-term outcomes. We propose that more emphasis should be given to interpreting the true rates of impairment, individual differences in severity and profile of impairments, whether or not impairments persist or diminish with increasing age, and consideration of the changes in long-term outcomes as a result of improved medical care.

Neurodevelopmental Outcomes Following Very Preterm Birth

General cognitive functioning is the most common domain assessed in long-term outcome studies of children born very preterm, and this is typically done by administering a measure of general intelligence, or IQ. A recent meta-analysis found that at a group level, the IQ of children born very preterm was 13 points lower than children born at term, representing a group difference of approximately 0.9 standard deviation (SD).[4] The authors also performed a meta-regression examining the standardized mean difference according to the birth year of the pooled cohorts (1990–2017), and found no evidence that the IQ discrepancy between children born very preterm and term is reducing in more recent cohorts. While IQ tests are generally sensitive at identifying cognitive problems, these measures are not particularly helpful for determining the nature of the cognitive deficits. Neuropsychological evaluations are required to establish the profile of cognitive strengths and weaknesses in children born very preterm, which is critical for determining appropriate remediate strategies.

Sensory and motor systems are impacted following very preterm birth. Meta-analyses report poorer performance in children born very preterm of 0.6 to 0.9 SD across tasks assessing visual perception and visual-motor integration when compared with term peers,[5] with the rate of impairment being 2 to 3 times higher for those born extremely preterm when compared with children born at term.[6] With regards to performance on standardized tests of motor functioning, the performance of children born very preterm is approximately 0.5 to 0.9SD below term peers.[7] In contrast to a rate of 0.1% to 0.2% in the general population, the prevalence of cerebral palsy (CP) is approximately 15% for infants born before 28 weeks' gestation and 6% for those born between 28 and 31 weeks' gestation.[8] Furthermore, it has been reported that approximately half of 5-year-olds born very preterm have functionally impaired motor coordination and balance which is not related to CP, and meeting criteria for developmental coordination disorder (DCD).[9]

Inattention is often noted to be an area of concern for children born very preterm by parents and teachers,[10] which is supported by numerous neuropsychological studies that have identified poorer performance by children born very preterm on formal tests of attention compared with term controls.[11-14] In a cohort of children born extremely preterm, it was

estimated that 75% had at least a mild attention impairment.[13] Deficits have been reported across all facets of attention functioning including selective, sustained, shifting, and divided attention,[13,14] and while there is inter-individual variability,[15] at a group level, the evidence suggests that very preterm birth is associated with a generalized attention impairment.

Executive function refers to those cognitive processes that are critical for goal-directed behavior and includes inhibitory control, working memory, cognitive flexibility, planning, and reasoning ability.[11-18] Meta-analyses have reported deficits across all elements of executive functioning, with the magnitude of the group differences with term controls ranging from 0.3 to 0.9 SD.[11,12,19] Executive dysfunction has been reported in preschoolers born very preterm,[20] but there is no evidence that these difficulties decline with age.[21,22]

Less research has studied memory following very preterm birth, but the evidence to date suggests that memory is also an area of concern.[23-25] The rate of verbal and visuospatial episodic deficits was approximately three-fold in a cohort of 7-year-olds born very preterm compared with term born controls.[25] Similar findings were reported in an older cohort (13-year-olds), although this study found the recall of visuospatial information to be particularly problematic for children born very preterm with a six-fold higher rate of impairment.[23] Prospective memory is also more likely to be impaired in children born very preterm, especially time-based tasks in which children are required to remember to perform a future action at a specific time.[23]

Language delay is common in infants and toddlers born very preterm, however, language challenges are ongoing with a meta-analysis revealing that school-aged children perform 0.6 SD below term controls for expressive language and 0.8 SD below for receptive language.[26] Children born extremely preterm seem particularly vulnerable, with reports of a 10-fold higher odds of a moderate to severe language impairment.[27]

Long-term outcome studies of children born very preterm often assess behavior and emotional status using parent-reported questionnaires. While differences are rarely found between children born very preterm and term on scales of externalizing behavior problems (i.e., aggression, conduct problems, defiance), there is a tendency for parents of children born very preterm to report more internalizing (i.e., anxiety, depression, social withdrawal)[12] and attention problems. Similarly, in adulthood, those born very preterm self-report more internalizing difficulties and fewer externalizing difficulties than term born peers.[28] Consistent with these findings, higher rates in specific psychiatric disorders have been reported in those born very preterm when structured clinical interviews have been conducted.[29,30] In a recent individual participant meta-analysis, those born very preterm were 10 times more likely to meet criteria for a diagnosis of autism spectrum disorder (ASD), 5 times more likely to meet criteria for attention-deficit hyperactivity disorder (ADHD), and twice as likely to meet criteria for anxiety.[31]

Given the increased risk for deficits across cognitive, motor, and behavioral domains, it is not surprising that children born very preterm are more likely to have academic difficulties. Multiple meta-analyses have reported poorer performance on standardized tests of reading and maths in children born preterm compared with term controls, especially those born very and extremely preterm, with group differences ranging from 0.5 SD to 0.8 SD.[12,32,33] Related to these findings, studies have reported a marked increase in the rate of children born very preterm who are receiving extra support and resources at school.[34,35]

This summary of the long-term outcomes following very preterm birth focuses on group-level findings and paints a pretty grim picture. However, it is important to note that the profile and severity of neurodevelopmental impairments for each child are unique. For example, a child may present with CP and intellectual impairment, another with ADHD and learning impairment, and a third with DCD and language impairment. There is also a significant proportion of children born very preterm who present with no developmental concerns. To demonstrate the considerable variability in outcomes at the individual level, the next two sections will highlight the importance of (1) analyzing the true rate of impairments and not just focusing on mean group differences and odds ratios and (2) utilizing person-centered analyses to examine profiles of functioning.

Rates of Impairments

Caution is needed when interpreting mean group differences as they can mask the breadth of outcomes at an individual level within a group. To illustrate this point, let's examine the findings from an 8-year follow-up of a cohort of children born extremely preterm or extremely low birth weight in the state of Victoria in 1997.[36] This cohort was assessed on measures of IQ, academic achievement and behavior problems, with their functioning compared with a group of children born term and normal birth weight, matched on birth hospital, due date, sex, mother's country of birth and health insurance status. The difference between the preterm and control groups for full-scale IQ was 12.5 points, or 0.83SD, which is widely considered a large effect.[37] Based on this finding alone, it is tempting to assume that a large proportion of this extremely preterm/extremely low birth weight cohort will have an intellectual impairment, which in turn could influence clinical decision-making and the way information is communicated to families. However, when using the control group distribution to classify intellectual impairment, nearly 50% of the preterm cohort had an IQ in the average range or above, and when using the test's norms to classify intellectual impairment as per normal clinical practice, over 75% of the preterm cohort had an IQ in the normal range or above.[36] Based on the control group distribution, only 15% of the preterm group had a major impairment (defined as <−2SD) and an additional 36% had a mild impairment (defined as between −1 and −2 SD); 13% of the control group had an intellectual impairment. This observation is not unique to IQ. In the same study, the extremely preterm/extremely low birth weight group performed 8 and 9 points lower on standardized tests of reading and spelling, respectively than the control group (0.5–0.6 SD).[36] Yet more than 70% of the preterm group performed in the average range or above for reading and maths, even when using a strict impairment classification. This data underlines the heterogeneity observed in long-term outcome, with the very preterm population having outcome distributions similar to that of the general population, albeit with a downward shift. We suggest that understanding the true rate of impairment, as described in this example, is equally, if not more, valuable than knowing that the preterm group had mean IQ deficit of 13 points.

Similarly, care is needed when evaluating odds ratios and relative risks, especially for low-prevalence disorders. A landmark study examined the association between preterm birth and psychiatric disorders using hospital psychiatric admissions for all individuals born in Sweden between 1973 and 1985 (n = 1,301,522).[38] In comparison to individuals born at term, individuals born very preterm had a 2.5-fold higher risk to be hospitalized for psychosis, 2.9-fold higher risk to be hospitalized for depressive disorder, and 7.4-fold higher risk to be hospitalized for bipolar disorder. On the surface, these findings are alarming, and in isolation can significantly distort their significance. This whole population data-linkage sample comprised 5125 individuals born very preterm, and the actual number hospitalized for psychosis, depressive disorder, and bipolar disorder was only 6 (0.12%), 22 (0.43%), and 4 (0.8%), respectively. Therefore while the relative risk of being hospitalized for these psychiatric disorders is higher for those born very preterm, the true rate is very low (<1%) and this context is crucial for reassuring families regarding the long-term prognosis for their children.

In summary, while the very preterm population perform significantly lower than term peers and are at increased risk for impairment across most neurodevelopmental domains, at an individual level, a significant proportion of the children are functioning within normal expectations and only a small minority experience severe impairment.

Neurodevelopmental Profiles

Clinicians monitoring the development of children born very preterm appreciate the heterogeneity in long-term neurodevelopmental outcomes in this population; however, this is difficult to illustrate when focusing on group-based data. Over the past 10 years, a number of groups have been applying person-centered multivariable approaches to investigate the existence of distinct subgroups of children born very preterm based on their neurodevelopmental profiles. While the studies vary in terms of the outcome domains of interest, the age of assessment, and sample size, all have reported marked heterogeneity with the identification of between 3 and 8 subgroups.[15,39-43]

The French EPIPAGE-2 study applied Latent Profile Analysis (LPA) to 1977 children born very preterm assessed at 5 years of age using a wide range of outcome domains including motor, cognitive, behavioral, and social functioning (15 outcome variables).[43] Four distinct profiles were identified for the very preterm cohort, the largest labeled as "favorable outcomes" (45%), with mean scores all above the test mean. The remaining three profiles included a subgroup that exhibited reasonable motor and cognitive functioning but specific behavioral difficulties (14%), a subgroup with mild cognitive and motor difficulties but good behavior and social functioning (31%), and the final profile reflected marked motor and cognitive difficulties. These findings highlight the considerable heterogeneity in the type and severity of impairments for children born very preterm.

Some studies have applied similar clustering approaches to neuropsychological data. For example, the ELGAN study is a large U.S. longitudinal observational study of children born before 28 weeks' gestational age.[39] Using LPA with nine measures of attention and executive function outcomes at 10 years of age, four different profiles or subgroups were identified. One-third of the preterm cohort had a "normal" cognitive profile, represented by group means in the average range for all outcomes. The largest subgroup (41%) was labeled "low-normal", with means falling between 0.5 and 1.0 SD below the test mean. The other two subgroups were children classified as having "moderately impaired" and "severely impaired" functioning, representing only 17% and 8% of the cohort, respectively. A study from Victoria, Australia, used LPA to examine distinct attention subgroups based on assessments performed at 7 and 13 years.[15] Three subgroups were identified at both timepoints, with the largest subgroup consisting of children exhibiting age-appropriate attentional skills, with the other two groups exhibiting suboptimal attention across different domains. Taking advantage of the longitudinal data, the very preterm children were categorized into four transition groups: (1) stable average attention (35%), (2) stable low attention (25%), (3) improving attention (23%), and (4) declining attention (17%).

At a group level, children born very preterm are reported to exhibit emotional and behavioral difficulties in the areas of anxiety, attention, and peer/social relations, leading to this pattern being labeled the "preterm behavioral phenotype."[44] Recently, a profile analysis was performed on a Victorian cohort of 8-year-old children born extremely preterm to determine whether the difficulties attributed to this phenotype co-occur at an individual level based on the four problem scales from the Strengths & Difficulties Questionnaire (SDQ).[41] The analysis revealed four profiles, including one profile that was similar to the "preterm behavioral phenotype", although this represented only 20% of the children born extremely preterm. The majority of the children (55%) were classified in a profile that reflected minimal emotional or behavioral problems. Therefore while there is strong evidence that children born very preterm are at increased risk for difficulties in attention, anxiety, and peer/social relations, this cluster of difficulties rarely co-occur within individual children.

In summary, there is considerable evidence from studies using techniques such as profile analysis that there is significant heterogeneity in the neurodevelopmental outcome for children born very preterm. These studies demonstrate that a significant proportion of this population perform within or above expected levels across neurodevelopmental domains, and for those who are exhibiting difficulties, the pattern varies both in terms of the severity and the type of deficits.

Developmental Stability

The neurodevelopment of children born very preterm is typically monitored by structured follow-up programs in early childhood but formal surveillance rarely extends beyond the preschool period. This is inadequate as many important cognitive and behavioral attributes do not emerge until the preschool period, followed by an extended developmental trajectory throughout childhood and into adolescence. As such, many skills and behaviors are difficult to reliably assess in early childhood. For example, the Bayley Scales for Infant and Toddler Development is only moderately predictive of school-aged outcomes.[45]

Understanding whether early neurodevelopmental issues reflect a delay or an ongoing deficit has important ramifications as to how to manage a child with developmental delay. There is considerable evidence that cognitive and behavioral difficulties are present in adults born very preterm,[46] suggesting that these children are unlikely to grow out of the neurodevelopmental problems that surface in early childhood. Furthermore, longitudinal studies have generally reported that the group differences observed between children born very preterm and term remain relatively stable at the group level, with little evidence of neurodevelopmental challenges resolving with age among survivors of very preterm birth.[47,48] However again, group-level data may mask significant changes occurring at the individual level.

A longitudinal study in Christchurch, New Zealand assessed the IQ for 110 children born very preterm and 113 children born at term at 4, 6, 9, and 12 years of age.[47] Despite some shift in IQ measures across these timepoints, the mean IQ for both groups remained very stable (mean IQ for very preterm group ranged from 94.7 to 96.6; mean IQ for term group ranged from 104.0 to 106.9), and as such the magnitude of the group difference also remained constant across these four timepoints (Cohen's d ranged from 0.6 to 0.9). Linear mixed-effects growth curve analysis was performed, which confirmed that the pooled trajectory for the groups was stable. However, the model also found evidence for marked individual variability, demonstrating that profiles at an individual level often do not mirror developmental profiles based on group-level data.

The inconsistency between group-level and individual-level developmental trajectories has been observed in outcome domains other than IQ. A Melbourne study examined language functioning in a cohort of children born very preterm and term at 2, 5, 7, and 13 years of age.[48] The linear effects model demonstrated (1) that the term group scored higher than the very preterm group at each timepoint, (2) the overall performance of both groups was remarkably similar at all timepoints resulting in very stable trajectories, and (3) there was no evidence that the language developmental trajectories differed between the very preterm and term groups. Further analysis of this dataset was undertaken to investigate the presence of distinct subgroups of children based on different developmental trajectories, with the latent growth mixture modeling revealing five profiles.[49] Approximately 30% of children born very preterm had consistently low to very poor language functioning between 2 and 13 years. The remaining children had better language functioning, although there was a subgroup who had very stable functioning, a subgroup who displayed strong early language skills that decreased across development, and another subgroup who displayed increasing language development between 2 and 7 years.

Instability across development at an individual level has also been observed in mental health disorders. The rate of any DSM-5 disorder was found to be 24% at age 7 years and 28% at age 13 years in a cohort of children born very preterm.[50] For specific disorders at 7 and 13 years, the rate of ADHD remained stable at 11%, while anxiety (11%–14%), mood (1%–3%), and autism (3%–6%) disorders increased marginally. Importantly, however, there was a considerable proportion of children who either moved into or out of a mental health diagnosis group. There are numerous explanations for this instability including a large group of subthreshold children who are on the borderline for a diagnosis. The instability may also be explained by normal maturational changes such as reductions in separation anxiety with age but an increase in generalized anxiety disorder and social anxiety during adolescence and early adulthood. Furthermore, the functional implications of subtle impairments, which are relevant when making a mental health diagnosis, may not become obvious until later in development with an increase in social and functional demands.

While the magnitude of group differences and rate of impairments may remain constant across childhood for the very preterm population, at an individual level, there is marked variability with some children displaying significant catch-up while others displaying decline. The nature of problems may also vary with age. For example, early expressive language delay may evolve into difficulties with higher-level pragmatics and discourse in adolescence. This highlights the care needed when counseling families regarding the long-term expectations for their child, as well as the importance of ongoing surveillance throughout childhood and into adolescence.

Changing Neurodevelopmental Outcomes With Medical Advances

Long-term outcomes studies of children born very preterm generally report on cohorts born 10 years or more earlier, and during that time, substantial improvements in perinatal and neonatal care may have occurred. While we have no choice other than to translate those findings of past cohorts to contemporary cohorts, an understanding of how medical advances have altered long-term neurodevelopmental outcomes is important. In particular, it is unwise to assume that long-term neurodevelopmental outcomes have improved alongside decreasing mortality because (1) it is possible that with more high-risk infants surviving, an increase in impairment will be observed, and (2) interventions that enhance survival may be associated with adverse long-term effects.[51,52]

There are only a few groups that have assessed long-term outcomes in geographic cohorts of children born early across multiple eras. The Victorian Infant Collaborative Study (VICS) group is unique in that they have adopted the same methodology to assess outcomes of children born extremely preterm/extremely low birth weight in four discrete eras, 1991–1992, 1997, 2005, and 2016–2017, alongside contemporaneous term/normal birth weight controls. A recent paper comparing the 2-year outcomes across these eras reported that the rate of CP has declined from 11%–12% in the 1990s to 6% in 2016–2017.[1] While there was no decline in developmental delay and neurodevelopmental disability over this 25-year period, there was a linear improvement in survival without major disability. Similarly, the EPICure group reported an 11% increase in survival without disability between 1995 and 2006 in infants born <26 weeks' gestation in England,[53] and the EPIPAGE group reported a 7% increase in survival without neuromotor or sensory disability and a 3% decrease in rate of CP between 1997 and 2011 in infants born very preterm in nine regions of France.[54] Thus when taking survival into account, there is considerable evidence to suggest that early neurodevelopmental outcomes have improved with advances in medical care.

However, as already noted, tools that assess neurodevelopment in early childhood cannot evaluate skills that are yet to emerge, and are not strongly predictive of long-term outcomes. While there are only a few reports of change across eras in terms of long-term outcomes, based on research to date, there is little evidence to suggest improved functioning in more recent cohorts. The VICS group examined IQ in the extremely preterm group at age 8 years relative to the matched control group in the 1991–1992, 1997, and 2005 cohorts and found that the IQ deficit remained relatively stable across eras after adjustment (1991–1992: –8.0; 1997: –10.5; 2005: –10.2).[55] There was also no improvement in academic functioning across eras, and in fact, there was some evidence that relative to term controls, the deficit in reading, spelling, and mathematics was greater in more contemporary cohorts.[55] The VICS group also reported an increase in executive function impairments at age 8 years for the 2005 cohort in comparison with the earlier cohorts, in particular in the working memory and the planning/organization domains.[56] Similarly, motor impairment increased from 23% in 1991–1992 to 37% in 2005[57] which was due to an increase in non-CP motor impairment and not an increase in CP. At 11 years of age, the EPICure group also found no significant improvement between the 1995 and 2006 cohorts in IQ and academic achievement for infants born <26 weeks' in England.[58]

While survival without early disability seems to be improving, there is currently no evidence that advances in care are associated with better long-term neurodevelopmental outcomes. More research is needed to investigate changing neurodevelopmental outcomes across eras, especially mental health and adaptive outcomes in adolescence and early adulthood.

Factors Contributing to Variable Outcomes

Moving forward, we need to understand the reasons for the marked variability in long-term outcomes in children born very preterm. Knowing the key factors associated with good and poor outcome across different domains will enhance the capacity to identify high-risk children early in life, enabling surveillance and interventions tailored to the needs of individual children to be initiated in early childhood and before the emergence of problems. At present, the capacity to predict developmental outcome following very preterm birth is poor. Gestational age, birth weight, small for gestational age, bronchopulmonary dysplasia, sepsis, necrotizing enterocolitis, and brain pathology are examples of neonatal clinical factors associated with neurodevelopmental outcomes, yet independently and collectively these clinical factors are unable to accurately predict long-term outcome.[59] This may be explained by the critical role of genetic predisposition, parenting, and the social environment in shaping child development, such that prediction models will always lack precision unless these additional factors are also included.

At a population level, social factors such as socioeconomic status, maternal education, and family structure are known to strongly influence child development.[60,61] This is also the case for children born very preterm such that these factors are likely to explain some of the heterogeneity in long-term outcome.[62-65] Determining the independent role of social factors on child neurodevelopment is challenging as they are interrelated and often co-occur.[66] Research to date suggests that social risk factors have both independent and additive effects on long-term developmental outcomes in children born very preterm. For example, a study with children born very low birth weight found higher maternal education, higher paternal education, and caregiver employment were all associated with an increase in cognitive functioning over time of 3 to 4 points, but the effect increased to 11 points for children in which all three social factors were present.[67]

The combined effect of clinical and social-environmental factors on cognitive and academic outcomes in children born very preterm has been examined across development.[68] Neonatal clinical factors associated with poorer neurodevelopment included lower gestational age, small for gestational age, male sex, Grade 3/4 IVH, postnatal corticosteroid treatment, and neonatal surgery, while important social factors included lower social class, maternal education, and language spoken at home. There is some evidence that the contribution of neonatal clinical factors on neurodevelopment diminishes with increasing age, while the impact of social factors is cumulative with the contribution increasing throughout development.[68] When examining language outcomes of children born very preterm, the contribution of social-environmental factors far outweighs the contribution of neonatal clinical factors, with parenting explaining the most variance.[69]

Very preterm birth affects the whole family, and there is strong evidence of the significant distress experienced by parents that can endure for many years.[70,71] The impact on the broader family needs to be considered when evaluating the long-term consequences of very preterm birth, especially given that parental mental health and parenting are likely to influence child outcome.[72] In fact, the family environment, including parenting practices and behaviors, is likely to be the strongest predictor of child development even in high-risk children such as those born very preterm. More research is needed investigating family outcomes and how environmental factors can play a protective role in supporting the child's development.

Key Points and Recommendations

1. Information on long-term neurodevelopmental outcomes can influence clinical decision-making, counseling families, and tailoring surveillance programs, and as such it is imperative that perinatal health professionals keep up-to-date with research in this area.

2. At a population level, children born very preterm perform more poorly and have higher rates of impairment across most neurodevelopmental domains than children born at term.

3. The long-term outcome literature focuses on group differences and increased risk; however, these data can be misleading due to the marked inter-individual variability.

4. The true rate of impairment is important information to relay to families, providing a context that is more relevant than group differences and relative risk.

5. Research now clearly demonstrates that children born very preterm are not a homogeneous group, with distinct subgroups exhibiting different profiles of strengths and weaknesses. This is also valuable information to be presented to families.

6. Neurodevelopment is a dynamic process, and early childhood assessments are not particularly predictive of longer-term functioning. Some children will demonstrate considerable catch-up to their peers with maturity, while others may start to struggle as specific skills emerge in later childhood and become more functionally relevant. Thus development is not stable and children display different developmental trajectories.

7. Surveillance programs should closely monitor developmental progress in early childhood in order to address developmental issues as they emerge and minimize persistent impairments. Ideally, surveillance programs for children born very preterm would continue throughout childhood and adolescence as some issues do not have functional consequences until they transition to independence and life demands become more complex.

8. There is no evidence that long-term neurodevelopmental outcomes have improved over the past 25 years. While this may be related to a greater number of the highest-risk infants surviving, it also highlights the importance of genetic and environmental factors.

9. Very preterm birth can have long-term consequences for the broader family. Managing parent and family issues will have a positive effect on the high-risk child.

REFERENCES

1. Cheong JLY, Olsen JE, Lee KJ, et al. Trends in neurodevelopment to two years after extremely preterm birth: prospective population-based studies spanning 25 years. *JAMA Pediatr.* 2021;175(10):1035-1042.
2. Boland RA, Davis PG, Dawson JA, Doyle LW. What are we telling the parents of extremely preterm babies? *Aust N Z J Obstet Gynaecol.* 2016;56:274-281.
3. Boland RA, Cheong JLY, Stewart MJ, Kane SC, Doyle LW. Disparities between perceived and true outcomes of infants born at 23–25 weeks' gestation. *Aust N Z J Obstet Gynaecol.* 2021. doi:10.1111/ajo.13443.
4. Twilhaar ES, Wade RM, De Kieviet J, Van Goudoever JB, Van Elburg RM, Oosterlaan J. Cognitive outcomes of children born extremely or very preterm since the 1990s and associated risk factors: a meta-analysis and meta-regression. *JAMA Pediatr.* 2018;172(4):361-367.
5. Geldof CJA, van Wassenaer AG, de Kieviet JF, Kok JH, Oosterlaan J. Visual perception and visual-motor integration in very preterm and/or very low birth weight children: a meta-analysis. *Res Dev Disabil.* 2012;33(2):726-736.
6. Molloy CS, Wilson-Ching M, Anderson VA, Roberts G, Anderson PJ, Doyle LW. Visual processing in adolescents born extremely low birth weight and/or extremely preterm. *Pediatrics.* 2013;132(3):e704-e712.
7. de Kieviet JF, Piek JP, Aarnoudse-Moens CS, Oosterlaan J. Motor development in very preterm and very low-birth-weight children from birth to adolescence: a meta-analysis. *JAMA.* 2009;302(20):2235-2242.

8. Himpens E, Van den Broeck C, Oostra A, Calders P, Vanhaese-brouck P. Prevalence, type, distribution, and severity of cerebral palsy in relation to gestational age: a meta-analytic review. *Dev Med Child Neurol.* 2008;50(5):334-340.

9. Spittle AJ, Dewey D, Nguyen TNN, et al. Rates of developmental co-ordination disorder throughout childhood in children born very preterm. *J Pediatr.* 2021;231:61-67.

10. de Kieviet JF, van Elburg RM, Lafeber HN, Oosterlaan J. Attention problems of very preterm children compared with age-matched term controls at school-age. *J Pediatr.* 2012;161(5):824-829.

11. Mulder H, Pitchford NJ, Hagger MS, Marlow N. Development of executive function and attention in preterm children: a systematic review. *Dev Neuropsychol.* 2009;34(4):393-421.

12. Aarnoudse-Moens CSH, Weisglas-Kuperus N, van Goudoever JB, Oosterlaan J. Meta-analysis of neurobehavioral outcomes in very preterm and/or very low birth weight children. *Pediatrics.* 2009;124(2):717-728.

13. Anderson PJ, De Luca CR, Hutchinson E, et al. Attention problems in a representative sample of extremely preterm/extremely low birth weight children. *Dev Neuropsychol.* 2011;36(1):57-73.

14. Wilson-Ching M, Molloy CS, Anderson VA, et al. Attention difficulties in a contemporary geographic cohort of adolescents born extremely preterm/extremely low birth weight. *J Int Neuropsychol Soc.* 2013;19(10):1097-1108.

15. Bogicevic L, Pascoe L, Nguyen TNN, et al. Individual attention patterns in children born very preterm and full term at 7 and 13 years of age. *J Int Neuropsychol Soc.* 2021;27:970-980.

16. Anderson P. Assessment and development of executive function (EF) during childhood. *Child Neuropsychol.* 2002;8(2):71-82.

17. Diamond A. Executive functions. *Annu Rev Psychol.* 2013;64(1):135-168.

18. Miyake A, Friedman NP, Emerson MJ, Witzki AH, Howerter A, Wager TD. The unity and diversity of executive functions and their contributions to complex "frontal lobe" tasks: a latent variable analysis. *Cogn Psychol.* 2000;41(1):49-100.

19. van Houdt CA, Oosterlaan J, van Wassenaer-Leemhuis AG, van Kaam AH, Aarnoudse-Moens CSH. Executive function deficits in children born preterm or at low birthweight: a meta-analysis. *Dev Med Child Neurol.* 2019;61(9):1015-1024.

20. Orchinik LJ, Taylor HG, Espy KA, et al. Cognitive outcomes for extremely preterm/extremely low birth weight children in kindergarten. *J Int Neuropsychol Soc.* 2011;17(6):1067-1079.

21. Taylor HG, Minich NM, Klein N, Hack M. Longitudinal outcomes of very low birth weight: neuropsychological findings. *J Int Neuropsychol Soc.* 2004;10(2):149-163.

22. Stålnacke J, Lundequist A, Böhm B, Forssberg H, Smedler AC. A longitudinal model of executive function development from birth through adolescence in children born very or extremely preterm. *Child Neuropsychol.* 2019;25(3):318-335.

23. Stedall PM, Spencer-Smith MM, Lah S, et al. Episodic and prospective memory difficulties in 13-year-old children born very preterm. *J Int Neuropsychol Soc.* 2022. doi:10.1017/S1355617722000170.

24. Taylor GH, Klein NM, Minich NM, Hack M. Verbal memory deficits in children with less than 750 g birth weight. *Child Neuropsychol.* 2000;6(1):49-63.

25. Omizzolo C, Scratch SE, Stargatt R, et al. Neonatal brain abnormalities and memory and learning outcomes at 7 years in children born very preterm. *Memory.* 2014;22(6):605-615.

26. Barre N, Morgan A, Doyle LW, Anderson PJ. Language abilities in children who were very preterm and/or very low birth weight: a meta-analysis. *J Pediatr.* 2011;158:766-774.

27. Wolke D, Samara M, Bracewell M, Marlow N. Specific language difficulties and school achievement in children born at 25 weeks of gestation or less. *J Pediatr.* 2008;152(2):256-262.

28. Pyhälä R, Wolford E, Kautiainen H, et al. Self-reported mental health problems among adults born preterm: a meta-analysis. *Pediatrics.* 2017;139(4):e20162690.

29. Treyvaud K, Ure A, Doyle LW, et al. Psychiatric outcomes at age seven for very preterm children: rates and predictors. *J Child Psychol Psychiatry.* 2013;54(7):772-779.

30. Johnson S, Hollis C, Kochhar P, Hennessy E, Wolke D, Marlow N. Psychiatric disorders in extremely preterm children: longitudinal finding at age 11 years in the EPICure study. *J Am Acad Child Adolesc Psychiatry.* 2010;49:453-463.

31. Anderson PJ, Marques de Miranda D, Albuquerque MR, et al. Psychiatric disorders in individuals born very preterm / very low birth weight: an individual participant data (IPD) meta-analysis. *EClinicalMedicine.* 2021;42:101216.

32. McBryde M, Fitzallen GC, Liley HG, Taylor HG, Bora S. Academic outcomes of school-aged children born preterm: a systematic review and meta-analysis. *JAMA Netw Open.* 2020;3(4):e202027.

33. Twilhaar ES, de Kieviet JF, Aarnoudse-Moens CS, van Elburg RM, Oosterlaan J. Academic performance of children born preterm: a meta-analysis and meta-regression. *Arch Dis Child Fetal Neonatal Ed.* 2018;103(4):F322-F330.

34. Johnson S, Fawke J, Hennessy E, et al. Neurodevelopmental disability through 11 years of age in children born before 26 weeks of gestation. *Pediatrics.* 2009;124(2):e249-e257.

35. Litt JS, Taylor HG, Margevicius S, Schluchter M, Andreias L, Hack M. Academic achievement of adolescents born with extremely low birth weight. *Acta Paediatr.* 2012;101(12):1240-1245.

36. Hutchinson EA, de Luca CR, Doyle LW, Roberts G, Anderson PJ. School-age outcomes of extremely preterm or extremely low birth weight children. *Pediatrics.* 2013;131:e1053-e1061.

37. Cohen J. A power primer. *Psychol Bull.* 1992;112(1):155-159.

38. Nosarti C, Reichenberg A, Murray RM, et al. Preterm birth and psychiatric disorders in young adult life. *Arch Gen Psychiatry.* 2012;69:1-8.

39. Heeren T, Joseph RM, Allred EN, O'Shea TM, Leviton A, Kuban KCK. Cognitive functioning at the age of 10 years among children born extremely preterm: a latent profile approach. *Pediatr Res.* 2017;82(4):614-619.

40. Stålnacke J, Lundequist A, Böhm B, Forssberg H, Smedler AC. Individual cognitive patterns and developmental trajectories after preterm birth. *Child Neuropsychol.* 2015;21(5):648-667.

41. Burnett AC, Youssef G, Anderson PJ, Duff J, Doyle LW, Cheong JLY. Exploring the "Preterm Behavioral Phenotype" in children born extremely preterm. *J Behav Dev Pediatr.* 2019;40(3):200-207.

42. Lean RE, Lessov-Shlaggar CN, Gerstein ED, et al. Maternal and family factors differentiate profiles of psychiatric impairments in very preterm children at age 5-years. *J Child Psychol Psychiatry.* 2020;61(2):157-166.

43. Twilhaar SE, Pierrat V, Marchand-Martin L, Benhammou V, Kaminski M, Ancel PY. Profiles of functioning in 5.5-year-old very preterm born children in France: The EPIPAGE-2 Study. *J Am Acad Child Adolesc Psychiatry.* 2021. doi:10.1016/j.jaac.2021.09.001.

44. Johnson S, Marlow N. Preterm birth and childhood psychiatric disorders. *Pediatr Res.* 2011;69:11-18.

45. Anderson PJ, Burnett A. Assessing developmental delay in early childhood—concerns with the Bayley-III scales. *Clin Neuropsychol.* 2016;31(2):371-381.

46. Cheong JLY, Haikerwal A, Anderson PJ, Doyle LW. Outcomes into adulthood of infants born extremely preterm. *Semin Perinatol.* 2021;45(8):151483.
47. Mangin KS, Horwood LJ, Woodward LJ. Cognitive development trajectories of very preterm and typically developing children. *Child Dev.* 2017;88:282-298.
48. Nguyen TNN, Spencer-Smith M, Zannino D, et al. Developmental trajectory of language from 2 to 13 years in children born very preterm. *Pediatrics.* 2018;141(5):e20172831.
49. Nguyen TNN, Spencer-Smith M, Haebich KM, et al. Language trajectories of children born very preterm and full-term from early to late childhood. *J Pediatr.* 2018;202:86-91.
50. Yates R, Treyvaud K, Doyle LW, et al. Rates and stability of mental health disorders in children born very preterm at 7 and 13 years. *Pediatrics.* 2020;145(5):e20192699.
51. Cheong JLY, Olsen JE, Huang L, et al. Changing consumption of resources for respiratory support and short-term outcomes in four consecutive geographical cohorts of infants born extremely preterm over 25 years since the early 1990s. *BMJ Open.* 2020;10:e037507.
52. Marlow N, Doyle LW, Anderson PJ, et al. Assessment of long-term neurodevelopmental outcome following trials of medicinal products in newborn infants. *Pediatr Res.* 2019;86:567-572.
53. Moore T, Hennessy EM, Myles J, et al. Neurological and developmental outcome in extremely preterm children born in England in 1995 and 2006: the EPICure studies. *BMJ.* 2012;345:e7961.
54. Pierrat V, Marchand-Martin L, Arnaud C, et al. Neurodevelopmental outcome at 2 years for preterm children born at 22 to 34 weeks' gestation in France in 2011: EPIPAGE-2 cohort study. *BMJ.* 2017;358:j3448.
55. Cheong JLY, Anderson PJ, Burnett AC, et al. Changing neurodevelopment at 8 years of children born extremely preterm since the 1990s. *Pediatrics.* 2017;139(6):e20164086.
56. Burnett AC, Anderson PJ, Lee KJ, Roberts G, Doyle LW, Cheong JLY. Trends in executive functioning in extremely preterm children across 3 birth eras. *Pediatrics.* 2018;141(1):e20171958.
57. Spittle AJ, Cameron K, Doyle LW, Cheong JL. Motor impairment trends in extremely preterm children: 1991–2005. *Pediatrics.* 2018;141:e20173410.
58. Marlow N, Ni Y, Lancaster R, et al. No change in neurodevelopment at 11 years after extremely preterm birth. *Arch Dis Child Fetal Neonatal Ed.* 2021;106:418-424.
59. Anderson PJ, Treyvaud K, Neil JJ, et al. Associations of newborn brain magnetic resonance imaging with long-term neurodevelopmental impairments in very preterm children. *J Pediatr.* 2017;187:58-65.
60. Brooks-Gunn J, Duncan GJ. The effects of poverty on children. *Future Child.* 1997;7:55-71.
61. Hackman DA, Farah MJ. Socioeconomic status and the developing brain. *Trends Cogn Sci.* 2009;13:65-73.
62. Linsell L, Malouf R, Morris J, Kurinczuk JJ, Marlow N. Prognostic factors for poor cognitive development in children born very preterm or with very low birth weight: a systematic review. *JAMA Pediatr.* 2015;169:1162-1172.
63. Asztalos EV, Church PT, Riley P, Fajardo C, Shah PS. Association between primary caregiver education and cognitive and language development or preterm neonates. *Am J Perinatol.* 2017;34:364-371.
64. Potharst ES, van Wassenaer AG, Houtzager BA, van Hus JWP, Last BF, Kok JH. High incidence of multi-domain disabilities in very preterm children at five years of age. *J Pediatr.* 2011;159:79-85.
65. Joseph RM, Hooper SR, Heeren T, et al. Maternal social risk, gestational age at delivery, and cognitive outcomes among adolescents born extremely preterm. *Paediatr Perinat Epidemiol.* 2021. doi:10.1111/ppe.12893.
66. McGowan EC, Vohr BR. Neurodevelopmental follow-up of preterm infants—what is new? *Pediatr Clin N Am.* 2019;66:509-523.
67. Manley BJ, Roberts RS, Doyle LW, et al. Social variables predict gains in cognitive scores across the preschool years in children with birth weights 500 to 1250 grams. *J Pediatr.* 2015;166:870-876.
68. Doyle LW, Cheong JLY, Burnett A, Roberts G, Lee KJ, Anderson PJ. Biological and social influences on outcomes of extreme-preterm/low-birth-weight adolescents. *Pediatrics.* 2015;136:1513-1520.
69. Nguyen N, Spencer-Smith M, Pascoe L, et al. Language skills in children born preterm (<30 wks' gestation) throughout childhood: associations with biological and socio-environmental factors. *J Dev Behav Pediatr.* 2019;40:735-742.
70. Yaari M, Treyvaud K, Lee KJ, Doyle LW, Anderson PJ. Preterm birth and maternal mental health—longitudinal trajectories and predictors. *J Pediatr Psychol.* 2019;44(6):736-747.
71. Treyvaud K, Lee KJ, Doyle LW, Anderson PJ. Very preterm birth influences parental mental health and family outcomes seven years after birth. *J Pediatr.* 2014;164(3):515-521.
72. Treyvaud K, Doyle LW, Lee KJ, et al. Parenting behavior at 2 years predicts school-age performance at 7 years in very preterm children. *J Child Psychol Psychiatry.* 2016;57(7):814-821.

Index

Note: Page numbers followed by "*f*" refer to illustrations; page numbers followed by "*t*" refer to tables; page numbers followed by "*b*" refer to boxes.

ESBLS. *see* Extended-spectrum β-lactamases
Ethamsylate, 61
Evans, N, 33–34
Excitatory amino acid antagonists, 140–141
Excitotoxic injury, 73
Executive dysfunction, in very preterm birth, 324
Executive function, 324
Extended-spectrum β–lactamases (ESBLs), 186
External ventricular drain, for post-hemorrhagic ventricular dilation, 110
Extracorporeal membrane oxygenation (ECMO), 201
Extremely-low-birth-weight (ELBW) neonate, blood pressure threshold for, 30, 30f

F

Facioscapulohumeral dystrophy (FSHD), 226
infantile, 226
Fatal infantile myopathy, 231
Fatty acid oxidation defects, 231–232
Fetal Neurobehavior Coding System (FENS), 16
Fetal neuroimaging, in CHD, 304, 308–309t
Fiber type disproportion, congenital, 230
Fick's principle, 37–38
Flat tracing (FT) pattern, aEEG, 24, 240f
"Floppy infant syndrome," 213–214
Focal and multifocal ischemic brain necrosis
etiologies of, 277t
MRI, 278
without asphyxia, 277–278, 278b, 280f
Focal clonic seizures, 147–148
Fontan procedure, 303
Free radical-mediated injury, posthemorrhagic ventricular dilation and, 107–108
French EPIPAGE-2 study, 326
Fukuyama muscular dystrophy (FMD), 223–224
Full-term neonate, cerebrospinal fluid indices in, 183t
Functional blood pressure threshold, 30, 31f
Functional MRI (fMRI), 261
in CHD infants, 303–304t

G

Ganciclovir, for congenital CMV infection, 204–205
General Movement Assessment (GMA), 14
Genetic disorders, aEEG and, 250, 256f
Genetic epilepsies, 153
Genital HSV infection, in neonatal herpes, 197
Gentamicin, for late-onset sepsis, 185
Germinal matrix (GM), 281–283
Girolami, G, 16–17
Glenn procedure, bidirectional, 303
Glucose, 165–176
blood concentration, 136–137
blood-glucose measurement, 170
blood glucose variability, 174
perinatal brain injury and, 165–176
perinatal glucose regulation and, 165–167
Glucose-6-phosphatase, 166
Glutamate-mediated excitotoxicity, 73
Glycogen storage disease II, 230
GMA. *see* General Movement Assessment
Gore Tex tube, 303
Graham-Rosenblith Scale, 3
Gray matter, loss of, posthemorrhagic ventricular dilation and, 108
Group B streptococcal (GBS) infection, intrapartum antimicrobial chemoprophylaxis in, 182

H

Habituation, 6
Hagmann, CF, 248

Hammersmith Neonatal Neurological Examination (HNNE), 14–15
Hemodynamics, impact of intensive care on, 44–45, 45f
Hemorrhage
cerebellar, 86–98
adult cerebellar infarct, 91
case history, 86–87, 87f, 88f
cerebellar development and vasculogenesis, 88–90, 89f
cerebellar organization, 90, 90f
consequences on developing cerebellum, 96
epidemiology and diagnosis with imaging, 91–92, 92f, 93f
experimental models, 95
functional topography, 90–91
key points, 86
outcomes, 96–98
pathogenesis and risk factors, 92–94, 94b
pathology, 94–95, 95f
preterm, 91–96
punctate *vs.* larger, 92t
returning to case, 98
intraventricular, 55–62
background on, 55
case history on, 55–56
clinical features of, 58
complications of, 58
cranial ultrasound of, 57f
factors associated with, 60, 60b
gaps in knowledge, 62
neuropathology of, 56, 57f
nursing care interventions, 61
outcome, 61–62
pathogenesis of, 56–57
perinatal strategies for, 58–59
postnatal medication administration for, 61
postnatal strategies for, 60
prevention of, 58–60
route of delivery for, 59
white matter injury associated with, 58
Hemorrhagic stroke, 151–152
Hereditary motor and sensory neuropathies (HMSN), 218–219
Herpes simplex virus infection, neonatal, 195–208
clinical manifestations of, 199
CNS, 201–204, 203f
diagnosis of, 206–207
diagnostic approach to, 206–207
disseminated, 201–204, 203f
management of, 208
mortality and morbidity outcomes of, 202–203, 202t
natural history of, 208
occurrence of, 196
risk factors for, 197, 198f
treatments and outcomes of, 201–204
monitoring, 207
HIE. *see* Hypoxic-ischemic encephalopathy
High angular resolution diffusion imaging (HARDI), 274
High Dose Erythropoietin for Asphyxia and Encephalopathy (HEAL) updates, 128
Hip and knee flexion, 5
HLHS. *see* Hypoplastic left heart syndrome
Horizontal suspension, 215
Hydrocephalus, posthemorrhagic, 101–113, 281–283
cerebral blood flow velocity spectra, 105f
cranial ultrasound in, 103f
excessive head enlargement defined for, 104–105
infant A and, 102
intracranial pressure and, 105–106
PHVD and, 102–104, 104f

Hyperalert infant, 3–4
Hyperbilirubinemia, severe, aEEG and, 250, 253–254f
Hypercapnia, 44–45
Hypercarbia, 56–57
Hyperekplexia, 150
Hypertension, pregnancy-induced, 59
Hypocapnia, 44–45
Hypoglycemia, 165
controversies in, 175–176
definitions of, 170–171, 171f
and developmental outcomes, 171–174
-induced brain injury mechanism, 167–169, 167f, 167t
and neurologic markers, 169–170
prevention and treatment of, 174–175
severity of, 171–174, 172–173t
symptomatic, 171
Hypoplastic left heart syndrome (HLHS), 302–303, 302f
Hypotension
amplitude-integrated EEG for, 39–40
approach to, 40–42
associated with PDA, treatment of, 42
definition of, 26–32, 28f, 29f
diagnosis of, 45–46
dopamine and, 42, 43
Doppler ultrasound and, 36–37
impedance electrical cardiometry and, 37
near-infrared spectroscopy and, 37–39
postmenstrual age-dependent approach to, 47, 48f
in premature infant, 24–47
summary and recommendations for, 45–47
systemic, 40–42
treated, 26
treatment of, 46–47
strategies for, 40–45
true, 28
uncertainties surrounding, 40–42
Hypothermia
MRI after, 276–277
MRI during, 276
Hypothermia, for hypoxic-ischemic encephalopathy, 117–129
components of, 118
knowledge gap of, 122, 125
therapeutic, 117–118
animal work and, 122
components of, 118
cooling on transport and, 126–127, 127f
death or disability outcomes of, 124
High Dose Erythropoietin for Asphyxia and Encephalopathy (HEAL) updates, 128
investigations of, 118–119
optimal temperature and duration for, 118f, 119–120, 120f
used in low- and middle-income countries, 128
time of initiation of, 121, 123f
Hypotonia, neonatal, 22
approach to, 232–234, 233f
cerebral (central), 215, 216t, 217b
combined cerebral and motor unit, 215–216, 216b
congenital muscular dystrophies of, 221–222
congenital myopathies of, 226–230, 227t
congenital myotonic dystrophy of, 225
congenital neuropathies of, 218–219
definition of, 214
differential anatomic diagnosis of, 215–216, 215b
lower motor unit, 215, 216t
metabolic myopathies of, 230–232
neuromuscular disorders and, 217–232, 217t